NEUROIMAGING – METHODS

Edited by **Peter Bright**

Neuroimaging – Methods
Edited by Peter Bright

Published by InTech
Janeza Trdine 9, 51000 Rijeka, Croatia

Publishing Process Manager Sandra Bakic

Technical Editor Teodora Smiljanic

Cover Designer InTech Design Team

Additional hard copies can be obtained from orders@intechopen.com

Neuroimaging – Methods, Edited by Peter Bright
p. cm.
ISBN 978-953-51-0097-3

For EU product safety concerns:
IN TECH d.o.o., Prolaz Marije Krucifikse Kozulić 3, 51000 Rijeka, Croatia,
info@intechopen.com or visit our website at intechopen.com.

Meet the editor

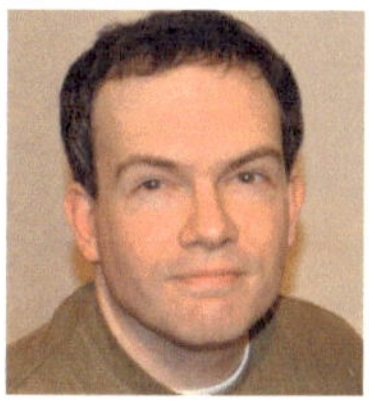

Dr Peter Bright was educated at the Universities of Surrey (BSc, 1991), Reading (MSc, 1993) and Cambridge (PhD, 1999). His research in the fields of memory and conceptual knowledge are well known. He has held research positions at the MRC Cognition and Brain Sciences Unit in Cambridge (1994-1995), King's College London (1998-2001), and the University of Cambridge (2001-2005). He currently holds the position of Reader at Anglia Ruskin University in Cambridge (since 2005).

Contents

Preface

Neuroimaging methodologies continue to develop at a remarkable rate, providing ever more sophisticated techniques for investigating brain structure and function. The scope of this book is not to provide a comprehensive overview of methods and applications but to provide a "snapshot" of current approaches using well established and newly emerging techniques. Taken together, these chapters provide a broad sense of how the limits of what is achievable with neuroimaging methods are being stretched. In cognitive neuroscience research, however, it is increasingly recognised that key theoretical debates about brain function are only likely to be resolved with reference to converging evidence from a range of methods. All neuroimaging techniques have important limitations which should always be acknowledged. For example, functional magnetic resonance imaging (fMRI) is a correlational, indirect method of measuring brain activation and interpretation of signal should always reflect this fact. Spatial resolution and sensitivity is improving with the commercial availability of ultra-high field human scanners, but a single voxel (the smallest unit of measurement) still corresponds to many thousands of individual neurons. Haemodynamic response to input is slow (in the order of seconds) and the relationship between this function and neural activity remains incompletely understood. Furthermore, choice of image preprocessing parameters can appear somewhat arbitrary and an obvious rationale for selection of statistical thresholds, correction for multiple corrections, etc. at the analysis stage can likewise be lacking. Therefore, to advance our knowledge about the neural bases of cognition, rigorous methodological control, well developed theory with testable predictions, and inferences drawn on the basis of a range of methods is likely to be required.

The first chapter (Zago, Lorusso and Priori) provides an informative (and sometimes surprising) historical overview of functional neuroimaging techniques, drawing a direct line of influence from cerebral thermometry and brain "pulsation" recordings through Roy and Sherrington's late eighteenth century studies linking neural activity with energy consumption and blood flow to the development of photon emission tomography (PET), computed tomography (CT), and measurement of the blood-oxygen-level dependent effect with magnetic resonance imaging (MRI). Chapter 2 (Nierhaus, Margulies, Long and Villringer) provides a brief but excellent introduction to the BOLD effect and a more comprehensive consideration of functional connectivity with specific reference to measurement of baseline or so called "resting state" networks. Principles and applications of functional near-infrared spectroscopy (fNIRS) are presented by León-Carrión and León-Domínguez (Chapter 3). These authors provide a strong case for more widespread application of fNIRS in a range of clinical populations and conditions. The size and portability of fNIRS devices provides opportunities for enhancing ecological validity of research investigations (in comparison to the restrictive conditions of fMRI), an argument also proposed by Tsunashima, Yanagisawa and Iwadate (Chapter 4). Tsunashima et al. provide a detailed consideration of NIRS signal analysis and offer a direct comparison of NIRS and fMRI data associated with systematic variations in cognitive demand.

Neuroinformatics is concerned with advancing neuroscience through a process of sharing and integrating data and techniques across all levels and scales of investigation. Schwabe (Chapter 5) argues convincingly for the importance of neuroinformatics tools, able to accommodate a range of spatial and temporal scales, for the development of detailed computational models of complex cognitive functions. Karanasiou (Chapter 6) discusses strengths and limitations associated with multimodal data acquisition (including simultaneous fMRI and electroencephalography (EEG), fNIRS with EEG, magnetoencephalography (MEG) with fNIRS, and fMRI with fNIRS) and also considers the viability and potential for integrating optogenetics with fMRI (ofMRI).

Diffusion tensor imaging is an MRI technique used to characterise white matter, specifically the directionality of pathways (or "tracts"). Visualisation of these tracts therefore provides the opportunity for examining structural connectivity in vivo. Lanyon (Chapter 7) presents an excellent overview of this technique, including consideration of its application for clinical diagnostic purposes. Transcranial magnetic stimulation (TMS) offers a number of important potential advantages over the classical neuropsychological (lesion-behaviour) approach to understanding neural basis of cognition. Through the creation of a "virtual lesion" in normal participants, the potential issues of cortical reorganisation, additional pathological substrates, distal pressure effects, psychiatric factors etc. in patient populations are avoided. Additionally, there is a great advantage in being able to study the same participants in control (i.e., pre-"lesion") and experimental (post-"lesion") conditions. Clinically, repetitive transcranial magnetic stimulation (rTMS) has proved successful (although not in all cases) in the treatment of a range of neurological or psychiatric conditions through the excitation or inhibition of target areas. However, among a number of methodological and interpretative challenges, perhaps the most critical is placement precision of the TMS coil. Andoh and Martinot (Chapter 8) present a validated and freely available triangulation-based MRI-guided manual method for ensuring accurate coil placement.

Mishra et al. (Chapter 9) describe in vivo neuronal tract tracing in the rat brain using biocytin-based tracers which clearly indicated their suitability for visualising cortical connectivity under MRI. Their research provides compelling evidence for the suitability of newly synthesized imaging probes for detecting and quantifying distributed tracer uptake across the cortex. Puri and Treasaden (Chapter 10) describe limitations of using conventional 31-phosphorus neurospectroscopy for quantifying membrane phospholipid metabolism (estimated indirectly by the ratio of phosphomonoesters to phosphodiesters). Rather than focusing on signals associated with narrow resonances, the authors argue that the broad component in the 31-phosphorous neurospectroscopy signal offers a more direct measure of brain cell membrane motion-restricted phospholipids.

Modern cranial ultrasound provides a number of advantages over neuroimaging methods such as MRI and CT, particularly with respect to costs and clinical practicalities of assessing intracranial pathology in gravely ill infants. Fickenscher, Bailey, Saettele, Dahl, and Lowe (Chapter 11) present a highly detailed overview of the approach which benefits greatly from the beautifully presented figures outlining normal and abnormal structure.

Level of recovery in survivors of ischemic stroke is highly variable and contingent upon success and speed with which blood flow can be restored to the affected area. Recovery can be gradual (months or even years), consistent with cerebral plasticity, i.e., the capacity for the structure and function of unaffected brain regions (e.g., the homologous contralesional site) to adapt to the behavioural or motor consequences of the stroke. Lindenberg and Seitz (Chapter 12) describe methodological issues associated with using DTI to assess post-stroke white matter integrity, and discuss evidence for structural changes possibly occurring in response to rehabilitative therapy. Their review indicates the clinical importance of DTI as a tool for predicting whether (and the extent to which) recovery is possible and the potential for understanding behavioural response to therapy in the context of underlying structural changes in the brain.

Identification of the extent of penumbral tissue (and differentiation from irreversibly infarcted tissue) following stroke is critical for predicting optimal intervention (if any) and tissue outcome. However, while best practice guidelines are typically available, there is considerable debate in the literature concerning important factors (including time-window for successful outcome, statistical thresholds for differentiating viable from unrecoverable areas, etc.). Scalzo, Hu and Liebeskind (Chapter 13) evaluate different flow parameters from perfusion weighted images during the acute stroke phase in terms of their predictive power for estimating tissue fate four days post onset. Using nonlinear regression models, their results indicate that tissue outcome is best predicted by a regional rather than single-voxel based approach. Recovery from stroke is also considered in a targeted review by Fabien et al. (Chapter 14). Specifically, these authors address possible explanations for why clinical trials of anti-inflammatory treatments have failed despite overwhelming evidence for an inflammatory response after stroke. They argue for the use of MRI to enable selection of patients most likely to benefit from anti-inflammatory treatment, to identify the therapeutic time-window, and to promote the development of interventions targeting specific pathophysiological processes. Arboix and Grive (Chapter 15) consider seven sites of intracerebral haemorrhage from the perspective of typical clinical spectrum and early outcome.

With the exception of the familial early onset form, the genetic risk factors of Alzheimer's disease remain poorly understood. Reitz (Chapter 16) discusses the potential of imaging genetics for exploring specific candidate genes on brain imaging phenotypes. Dementia with Lewy bodies (DLB), like some other forms of progressive dementing illness (e.g., semantic dementia), tends to be under-diagnosed. Baglio, Preti and Farina (Chapter 17) provide a valuable overview of DLB, with particular focus on neuroimaging findings. They convincingly argue for the employment of a range of MRI-based methods to improve differential diagnosis of DLB from other forms of dementia. In the final chapter, Jimenez-Vazquez provides an overview of endoscopic intracranial imaging for diagnosis and treatment of lesions within or adjacent to fluid-filled cavities.

I hope that, cumulatively, these chapters convey a broad sense of what can be achieved with neuroimaging methods. Rate of technological progress is encouraging increasingly sophisticated lines of enquiry in cognitive and clinical neuroscience and shows no sign of slowing down in the foreseeable future.

Dr. Peter Bright
Anglia Ruskin University,
Cambridge Campus,
East Road, Cambridge
United Kingdom

1

Functional Neuroimaging: A Historical Perspective

Stefano Zago[1], Lorenzo Lorusso[2],
Roberta Ferrucci[3] and Alberto Priori[3]
[1]*Dipartimento di Neuroscienze ed Organi di Senso, Università degli Studi di Milano,*
U.O.C. di Neurologia, Fondazione IRCCS Ca' Granda Ospedale Maggiore Policlinico,
[2]*Unità Operativa di Neurologia, Azienda Ospedaliera*
'M. Mellini' Chiari, Brescia,
[3]*Centro Clinico per la Neurostimolazione, le Neurotecnologie e i Disordini del Movimento,*
Dipartimento di Neuroscienze ed organi di Senso,
Università degli Studi di Milano,
Italy

1. Introduction

Modern in *vivo* functional neuroimaging techniques produce colorful computer images of the pattern of metabolic neuronal activity in living humans while engaged in performing cognitive and/or emotional tasks, and provide an unprecedented opportunity to examine how brain function supports activities in normal and abnormal conditions. The idea of the relation between blood flow and brain activity dates back to the second half of the 19th century, a time when some scientists made important contributions to this subject. In this period, functional brain activity began to be studied in the intact human brain by thermal recording from the scalp or by using techniques providing indirect graphical measurements of changes in cerebral flow when different mental tasks were performed. This relationship began to be quantified by measuring whole brain blood in animals and humans. The development of technologies that could measure these changes safely in normal human subjects would take another 60 years. Detailed mapping of regional flow changes during various mental and motor activities was achieved in 1970s and 1980s using new techniques (CT, PET and MRI) with further new valuable information about brain function in normal and in pathological conditions. This chapter will focus on a review of the historical background of functional brain imaging techniques.

2. The first evidence: Changes in scalp and cortex temperatures

Today, we know that brain temperature is a physiological parameter determined primarily by neural metabolism, regulated by cerebral blood flow, and affected by various environmental factors and drugs (Kiyatin, 2007). This aspect was already conjectured by some scientist in the mid-19th century. For example, the French physiologist Claude Bernard (1813-1878) in 1872 observed: '*If we now try to understand the relationship that one can obtain between the intensification of the circulatory function and the functional state of the organs, it is easy to see that the increase in blood supply is related to the increased intensity of the chemical metamorphoses that take place in tissues, and to the increment in thermogenetic phenomena which are the immediate and necessary consequence of those. . . . Each time the spinal or a nerve exhibit sensitivity or movement, each time the brain performs intellectual work, a corresponding amount of heat is produced'* (Bernard, 1872; Conti, 2002). The famous psychologist William James (1842-1910), in 1892, concluded that : '*. . . brain-activity seems accompanied by a local disengagement of heat'* and speculated that cerebral thermometry may be valuable for experimental psychology to correlate cognitive and emotional states focally to brain regions (James, 1892).

Starting from this interesting hypothesis, researchers placed thermometers or more sensitive thermoelectric piles on the scalp to measure regional changes in temperature. Several measurements of brain temperature, in normal and abnormal subjects, engaged in performing cognitive, motorial or emotional tasks or after administration of drugs were conducted from the second half of the 19th century (see Albers, 1861; Lombard, 1867, 1879; Gray, 1878; Maragliano and Seppili, 1879; Bert, 1879; Amidon, 1880; Maragliano, 1880; François-Franck, 1880; Sciamanna and Mingazzini, 1882; Bianchi, Montefusco e Bifulco, 1884; Tanzi, 1888; Mosso, 1894; Berger, 1901). In at least two studies, thermometers were placed also in direct contact with the cerebral cortex via skull cracks in patients responding to sensory stimuli, doing mental tasks, and undergoing emotional experiences (Mosso, 1894; Berger, 1901).

Among the most famous researchers using the cerebral thermometry approach were Josiah Stickney Lombard in the United States (Lombard, 1867, 1879; Marshall and Fink, 2003), Pierre Paul Broca in France (Broca, 1879), Angelo Mosso in Italy (Mosso, 1894) and Hans Berger in Germany (Berger, 1901).

In 1866, Lombard, first commenced a series of experiments, with thermoelectric apparatus, to determine the amount of blood circulating in the brain and the exterior temperature of the human head, in the quiescent mental condition, and in states of intellectual and emotional activity. He demonstrated that the exercise of the higher intellectual faculties, as well as the different emotions, caused a rise of temperature in the head perceptible through the medium of delicate apparatus. Lombard reviewed the results on cerebral temperature in his 1879 monograph on *Experimental Researches on the Regional Temperature of the Head under Conditions of Rest, Intellectual Activity and Emotion'*. He observed: '*. . . there is good reason to suppose that a slight change of temperature at the surface of the brain can show itself in a degree readily perceptible by means of delicate apparatus, at the exterior surface of the head; and we shall see, in the experiments now to be given, that the changes of temperature observed in the integument during increased mental activity are usually of a degree which may be fairly accounted for by the direct propagation outward, through the intervening tissues, of slight thermal changes at the cerebral surface'* (Lombard, 1879).

Mosso, in his book *La temperatura del cervello. Studi termometrici* [The temperature of the brain. Thermometric studies] set out a very large number of sophisticated experiments on cerebral thermometry. The temperature was ascertained by means of a delicate thermometer which gave to the naked eye a reading of 0.01 degrees. Mosso made observations directly on the cerebral human cortex. For example, he examined Delfina Parodi, a girl of twelve years who had a wound on the right side of the skull (see Fig. 1).

A

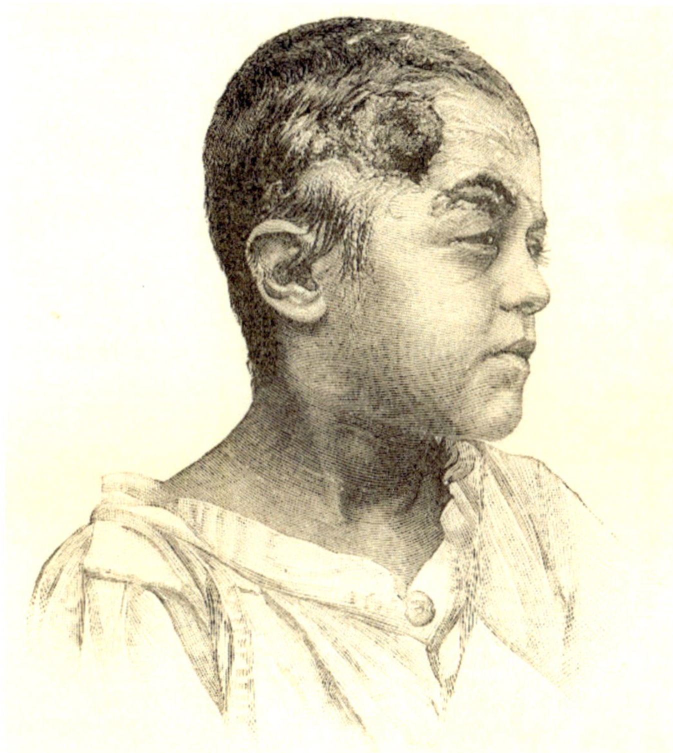

B

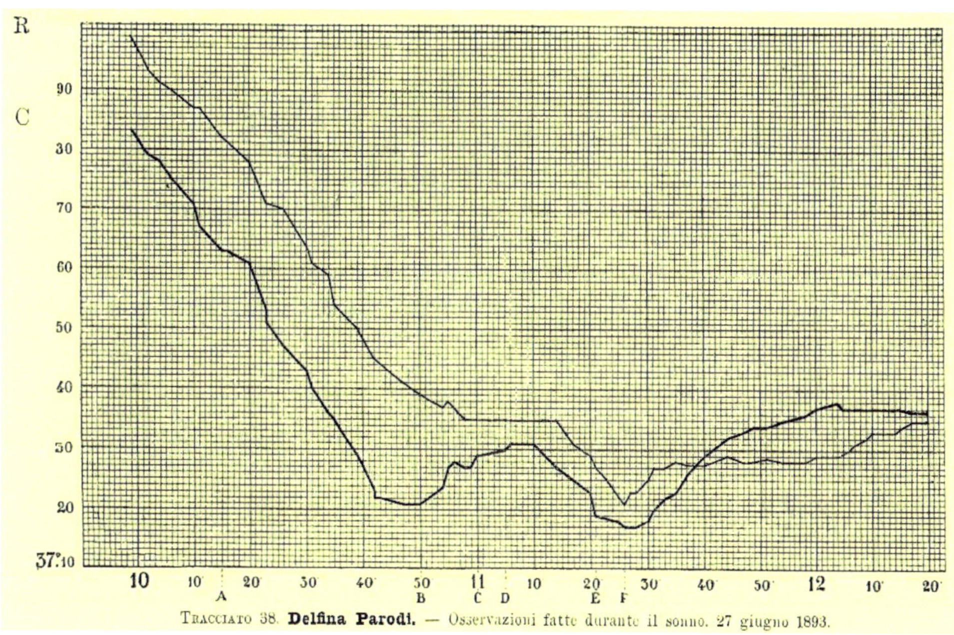

Fig. 1. (A) Delfina Parodi (B) Tracing obtained during sleep showed an increase in brain temperature when a dog began to bark in the next garden (A and D) and when the girl was called by name, Delfina (F), R=rectum, C=brain. Source: Mosso (1894).

Neither mental nor motor exertions had any influence upon the brain temperature, but emotions such as fear of the administration of chloroform caused a rise of temperature of 0.01 degrees. Berger (1901) stated that his principal aim was to find: '. . . *and equivalence between the chemical and thermic energy of the brain and psychic 'energy'*. Broca tried to demonstrate the effect of different mental tasks, especially language, on the localized temperature of the scalp of normal subjects, and also studied the diagnostic value of the thermogenic exploration of the scalp to discover focal lesion of the brain (Broca, 1877). Studies of brain localisation were also carried out by other researchers (Gray, 1878; Maragliano, 1880; Putnamm Iacobi, 1880; Bianchi, Montefusco and Bifulco, 1884).

3. Brain volume produced through mental activity: The Mosso methods

Though cerebral thermometry was abandoned owing to methodological difficulties and contradictory results, it provided the basic rationale for later studies on the relationship between function and blood circulation in overlying brain tissue.

A researcher who championed the idea of studying changes in brain blood flow was the Italian physiologist Angelo Mosso (1848-1910) who, at about the same time when he conducted his research on regional temperatures in the head and brain, began to investigate brain blood flow during certain emotional and cognitive tasks (Zago, Ferrucci, Marceglia and Priori, 2009). In his textbook on blood circulation in the human brain, printed in Germany in 1881, Mosso observed: '*Of all the body's organs, the brain is that in which the most frequent and most radical changes in the state of the blood vessels occur. Physiology has not yet determined which of these changes are produced reflexively by the action of a central motion vessel and which arise from purely local actions as an effect of the chemical transformations which occur in a given brain region. That there are, however, local changes due to local chemical action is undeniable*' (Mosso, 1881). The concepts expressed by Mosso engender the idea that when brain areas are active, changes in the amount of blood flowing in circumscribed brain regions, and specific biochemical processes, in the same areas, increase to ensure adequate energetic support to the active neurons. This mechanism, is actually termed *functional hyperaemia* (Iadecola, 2004).

In his investigations on human cerebral circulation Mosso proposed some new and valuable non-invasive procedures for detecting the functional correlates of various physiological and psychological states. The first method involves the development of a bed scales in which the body was placed in perfect balance and where it was possible to measure small tilts of a few millimeters of its longitudinal axis determined by the passage of blood from the legs to the head and vice versa (see Fig. 2).

With this apparatus Mosso verifies that the breath and sleep rhythms, the effect of pharmacological substance, and the response to particular mental states, determined minimal oscillations of the balance corresponding to changes in the distribution of blood (Mosso, 1882,1883). He observed that: '. . . *the spontaneous movements of the blood vessels and the undulations corresponding to psychic acts are equally visible by means of the balance*' (Mosso, 1882). Further research on bodily changes during mental activity appears to have been attempted with the Mosso apparatus, although with conflicting results (e.g. Weber, 1910; Lowe, 1935).

The second method used by Mosso consisted of recording the pulsations of the human cortex in individuals through the open skull, during mental tasks, by means of a system of pistons. For some time, the study of cerebral circulation within the cranial cavity presented

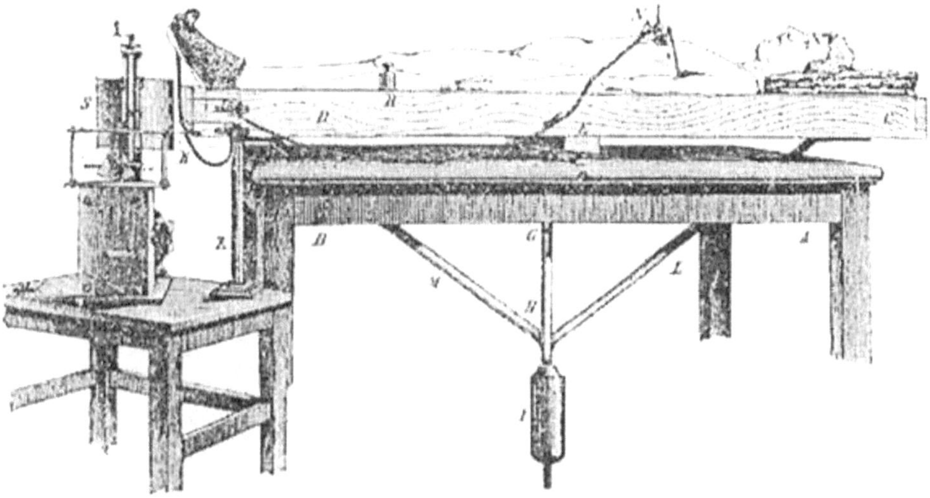

Fig. 2. Mosso's balance apparatus. Source: Mosso (1882).

difficulties due to relative inaccessibility of the brain *in vivo*. Mosso was inspired in his studies by some animals works carried out during the late 18th and early 19th centuries, which were designed to record pulsations of the brain during respiratory changes and modifications in cerebral blood circulation. In particular, he mentioned the work of the Italian physiologist Antonio Ravina, who invented a direct observation through a glass window for recording the change in volume of the cranial content of animal resulting from variations in the amount of blood present within the intracranial vessel (Ravina, 1811). Another researcher to deal with this type of investigation was the Dutch physiologist, Franciscus Cornelius Donders (1818-1889) who conceived the cranial window to observe in animals the ability of *pia mater* vessels to change their caliber in response to various kinds of stimulation (Donders, 1850).

The *Mosso method* consisting of recording simultaneous intracranial pressure changes in humans through a traumatic bone injury in the skull, compared to the pressure to the forearm or foot, to graphically demonstrate, the peculiar cerebral hemodynamic patterns during emotional and cognitive experiences. Hence, his work brought a modern perspective to the study of the central nervous system. Fig. 3 reports Mosso's instruments to analyse pressure changes in man.

The most famous case studied by Mosso was published in 1880. The report, titled, *Sulla circolazione del sangue nel cervello dell'uomo* [On the blood circulation in the human brain] presented the case of Michele Bertino, a 37-year-old farmer who had a large fracture to the skull (Mosso, 1880). The fractured bone pieces were removed and the cerebral mass was exposed through a bone breach measuring about 2 centimeters in diameter in the right frontal region. Intelligence, memory, language, motility and sensitivity all remained almost unchanged. Changes in brain volume related to cerebral blood flow were recorded through a button fixed to the wooden cupola with a sheet of gutta-percha resting on Bertino's exposed dura mater and connected to a screw on the recording drum (see Figure 4).

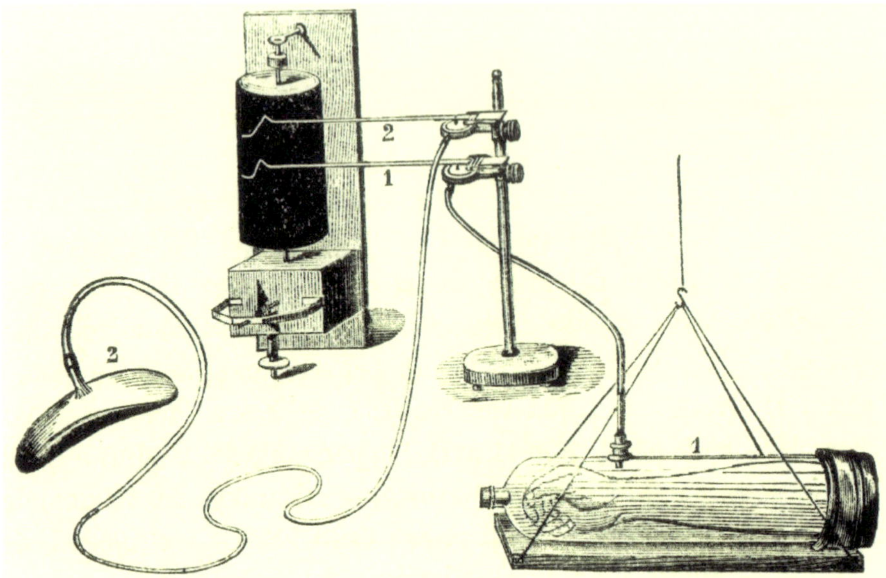

Fig. 3. Mosso's devices for recording the blood volumes in arm and brain.
Source: Patrizi (1896).

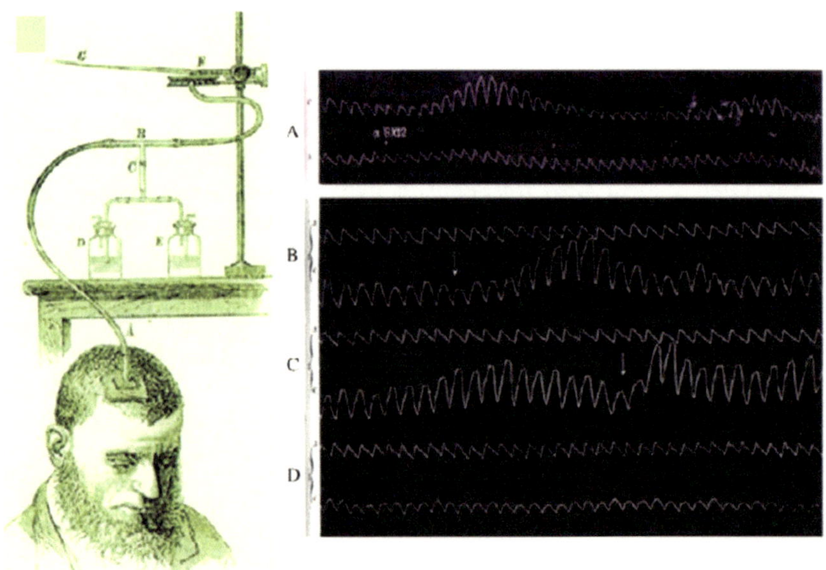

Fig. 4. Brain pulsation recordings when (A) Bertino was requested to multiply 8×12. Top trace is brain pulsation and bottom trace is the forearm pulsation. α: when the question was made, (B) a room clock strikes 12 (arrows). Top trace is forearm pulsation and bottom trace the brain pulsation; (C) Mosso asked (arrows) Bertino if Ave Maria should have been said. Top trace is forearm pulsation and bottom trace the brain pulsation (D) resting state condition. Top trace is the forearm pulsation and bottom trace the brain pulsation. Source: Mosso (1880).

When the brain volume changed, the pulsation of the brain increased, the pressure on the button also increased as did pressure on the screw, thus compressing the air inside the drum. Changes in air compression were trasmitted to a second recording drum, and then written on a rotating cylinder. When Mosso asked Bertino to multiply 8×12, the pulsations increased within a few seconds after the request. Similarly, when Mosso asked him if the chiming of the local church bell reminded him that he had forgotten his midday prayers, Bertino said yes, and his brain pulsated again. Mosso also demonstrated in this patient that the fluctuations in the blood supply to the brain were independent of respiratory changes. In another passage he also tackled the modern issue of the 'resting state' (Gusnard and Raichle, 2001; Morcom and Fletcher, 2007). He wrote: '*Because the brain is an organ that escapes our will why can we not arbitrarily bring it to absolute rest? The variations that the movement of blood in the brain can undergo during wakefulness refer far more often to variations in the energy needed for intellectual work, rather than to a real change in this organ's functions from a state of absolute rest to one of full activity*' (Mosso, 1880).

The work of De Sarlo and Bernardini (1891), who studied the variations of cerebral circulation during mental activity in a 50-year-old farmer, admitted for traumatic epilepsy, is also illustrative of the application of the Mosso's method (De Sarlo and Bernardini, 1891). At the age by 24, F. Carlo, while working in a petrol well was hit by falling rocks causing cranial fracture in the left parietal region. The injury resulted in a more or less triangular shaped opening, measuring between 1.5 cm and 2.5 cm approx. on each side. The posterior side was aligned with the Rolandic fissure. The inner side, parallel to the sagittal line, measured 1.5 cm. The opening was about one centimeter deep. After positioning a specially designed copper helmet of 5 cm in diameter over the cranial breach, using glazier's putty, a funnel-shaped part of the helmet was connected above to a Marey's drum. The cerebral pulse was not evident when the head was held straight, and the patient was asked to rest the bowed head on a special support (see Fig. 5A). Figure 5B shows the outline in different emotional situations.

Mosso's cerebral pulse method was used by numerous experimenters to study changes in the brain blood flow during mental effort, as well as after the administration of drugs (e.g. Fleming, 1877; François-Franck, 1877; Burckhardt, 1881; Mays, 1882; Sciamanna, 1882; Sciamanna and Mingazzini, 1882; Bergesio and Musso, 1884; Morselli and Bordoni-Uffreduzzi, 1884; Musso and Bergesio, 1885; Petrazzani, 1888; Binet and Sollier, 1895; Patrizi, 1896, 1897; Berger, 1901).

Mosso's method was hindered by the technical limitations of his time that precluded him from correlating specific regional changes in brain activity to cognitive and emotional processes. Although present imaging techniques do not use the same principle as Mosso's, his idea of monitoring the cerebral blood flow nonetheless anticipated the main concepts of modern brain imaging tools such as SPECT, PET and fMRI, and could in this sense be considered a precursor to modern functional neuroimaging (Raichle, 2008; Zago, Ferrucci, Marceglia and Priori, 2009).

After only 50 years, a new work on a human being was performed by the American neurosurgeon John Farquhar Fulton (1899-1960), a resident of Cushing in Boston and attendant at the Oxford University with Sherrington, who reported the clinical study of the patient Walter K.. The patient had a gradually decreasing visual disorder caused by a vascular malformation of the occipital lobe. Surgery removal was unsuccessful leaving a bony defect above the primary visual cortex. Walter K. complained that he perceived a noise (i.e. bruit) at the back of his head during visual activity. See Fig. 6.

A

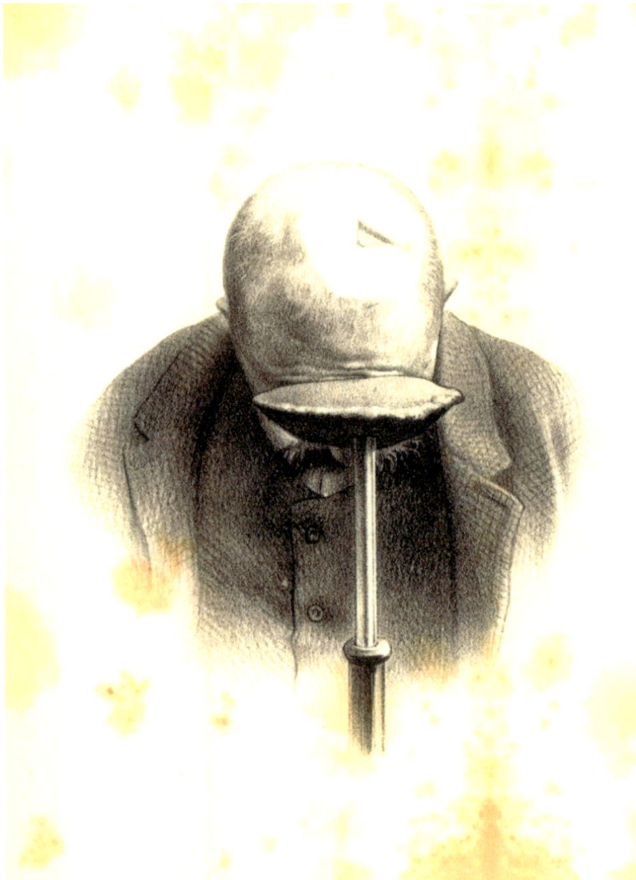

B

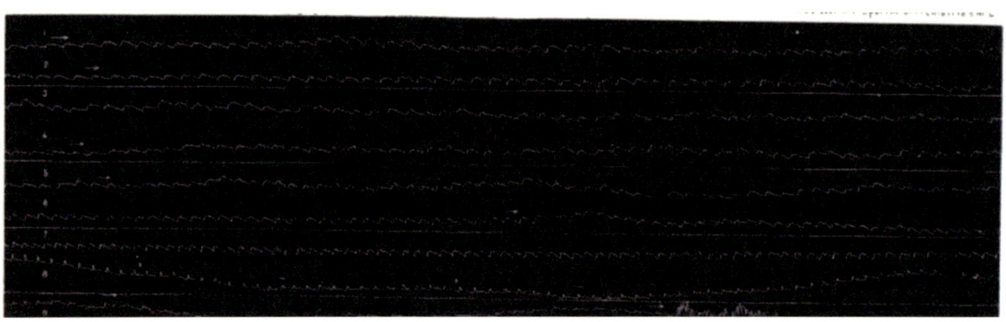

Fig. 5. (A) F. Carlo, the patient studied by De Sarlo and Bernardini (1891). The cranial fracture in the left parietal region is visible. (B). Brain pulsation recordings when: (1) F. Carlo was threatened with a penalty (2) He was promised a prize (3) At the beginning of the trace the subject looked for a focal point on the floor. At half way he found it (attention effort) (4) He was given different images of the Holy Virgin and kissed one of them (5) A nurse entered the room talking excitedly about something terrible that had happened (6) At the beginning of the trace he finds himself in pleasant spirits (he spoke about his return home) (7) He was shown images of scantily dressed women. He became irritate (8) Continued from trace six. Source: De Sarlo and Bernardini (1891).

A

B

1

2

3

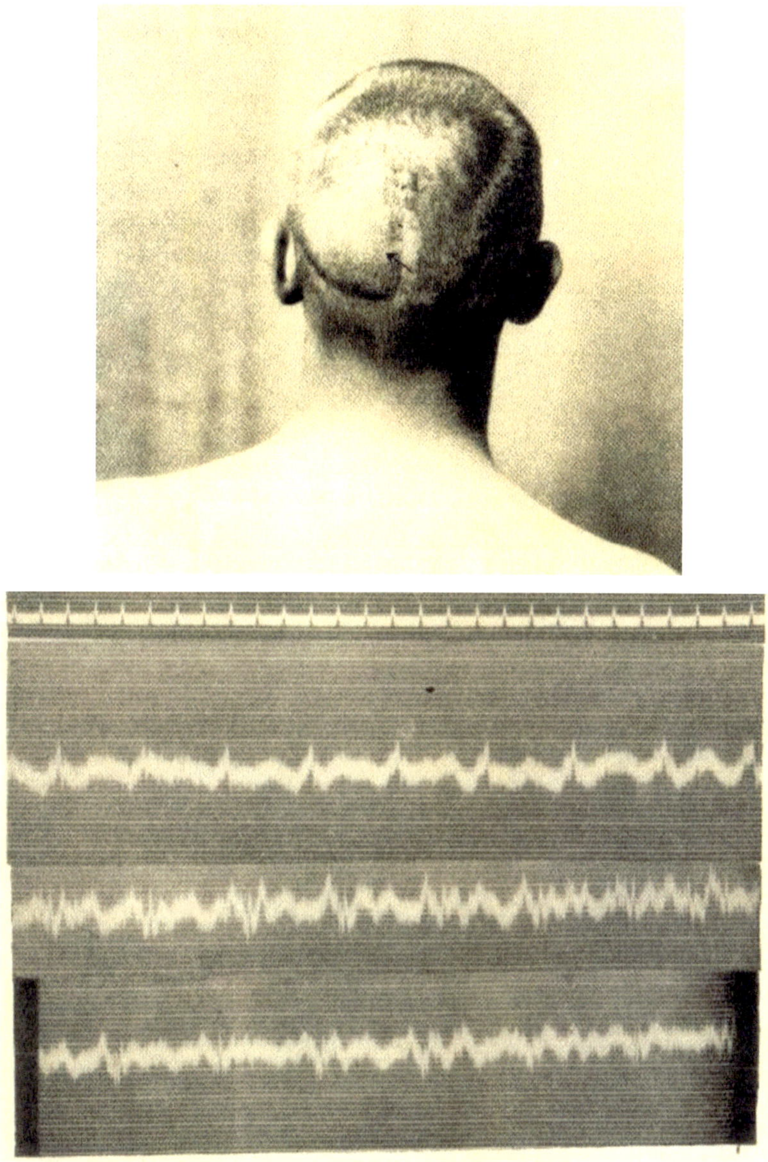

Fig. 6. (A) Walter K, the patient studied by Fulton in 1928. The arrow indicates the point of maximum intensity of the bruit. This overlies the region of greatest vascularity of the angioma. (B) Typical electrophonograms. (1) after ten minutes rest in a darkened room; (2) after two minutes reading small print illuminated by a single 40-watt tungsten bulb at 5 feet; (3) three minutes later, after two and half minutes rest in darkened room. It is evident an increased size of main deflections in b and the greater number of secondary deflections. Source: Fulton (1928).

This disturbance persisted for several years but he had: '. . . *never thought much of it*'. Fulton underlined: '*It was not difficult to convince ourselves that when the patient suddenly began to use his eyes after a prolonged period of rest in a dark room, there was a prompt and noticeable increase in the intensity of his bruit. Activity of his other sense organs, moreover, had no effect upon his bruit'.* This single case showed that blood flow to the occipital lobe was sensitive to the attention paid to objects in the environment. Fulton elicited a history of a cranial bruit audible to the patient whenever he engaged in a visual task. Remarkably consistent changes in the character of the bruit could be appreciated depending upon the visual activities of the patient (Fulton, 1928).

4. Functional activity, metabolism and blow flow in animal brain

In their seminal animal experimental observation on the cerebral circulation, Charles Smart Roy (1854-1897) and Charles Scott Sherrington (1857-1952), both working in the Cambridge Pathological Laboratory in England, mentioned the 'Mosso method' as one of the main techniques for investigating brain blood flow, however nothing the limitations (Roy and Sherrington, 1890).They remarked that studies with the Mosso apparatus had not '. . . *sufficiently recognized the necessity of taking, simultaneously with the curve from the cranial cavity, graphic records both of the arterial and venous pressures. The influence of changes in these latter where this method is employed, is so great that results obtained without due control of them must, we think, be looked upon as likely to mislead'* (Roy and Sherrington, 1890).

In their work, Roy and Sherrington suggested two distinct mechanisms for the control of the cerebral circulation, one of them acting through the vasomotor nervous system, and another intrinsic one by which the blood supply of various parts of the brain can be varied locally in accordance with regional requirements.

Roy and Sherrington's experiments were applied chiefly on exposed dogs' brains but controlled by repeating them on cats and rabbits using a trepanation near the middle line of the vertex of the cranium. They then registered pressure and blood variation after stimulations by inducing currents through parts of the body. Their experimental conclusion was that: '. . . *the chemical products of cerebral metabolism contained in the lymph which bathes the walls of the arterioles of the brain can cause variations of the caliber of the cerebral vessels: that in this re-action the brain possesses an intrinsic mechanism by which its vascular supply can be varied locally in correspondence with local variations of functional activity'.* This statement, implying that cerebral functional activity, energy metabolism, and blood flow are closely related, and presumably most responsible for the concept of '*tight coupling*' that has played an important role in recent years.

It was observed that experimental data obtained by Roy and Sherrington were inadequate to support the interrelation between functional activity, metabolism and blood flow, because they hadn't examined any of the relevant processes, energy metabolism and functional activity, but only an indicator of cerebral cortical blood volume rather than cerebral blood flow (Sokoloff, 2001). They believed that cerebral blood flow was regulated mainly by arterial blood pressure and fine-tuned chemical substances in that they affirmed that '*the blood supply of the brain varies directly with blood pressure in the systemic arteries*' (Roy and Sherrington, 1890).

Later in 1914, Joseph Barcroft (1872-1947), at the University of Cambridge, contended that an enhanced functional level in a tissue can be sustained only by increasing the rate at which oxygen is consumed. Blood flow was measured without use of extensive surgery or profound anaesthetic procedures, and its mechanism was based on the autoregulation of the cerebral circulation and the influence of chemical factors. Barcroft supported the association between functional activity and energy metabolism and he wrote: '*There is not instance in which it can be proved that an organ increase its activity, under physiological condition without also increasing its demand for oxygen'* (Barcroft, 1914).

In the case of the brain interrelation between functional activity, metabolism and blood flow experimental studies on animals by the physiologist Edward Horne Craigie was also of note. He demonstrated that the vascular demand in different parts of the brain parts related to functional activity, and that increases found in localized areas parts due to a major metabolic demand of these regions associated with functional activity (Craigie, 1924).

5. Subsequent investigations: The diffusible indicators for the determination of brain circulation and metabolism in animals and humans

As pointed out by Raichle (2008), despite this promising study interest in brain circulation and metabolism decreased during the first quarter of the 20th century for two main reasons: (1) a lack of sufficiently sophisticated tools to pursue this line of research, and (2) criticism by some influential researchers who concluded that no relationship existed between brain function and brain circulation.

In particular, the work of Leonard Erskine Hill (1866-1952), physiologist and professor of the *Royal College of Surgeons in England*, was very influential on the research that followed. His eminence as physiologist covered the inadequacy of his results and led him to affirm that there was no relationship between brain function and cerebral circulation and resolutely denied the existence of local metabolic regulation. He proclaimed that: *'We have been entirely unable to confirm the result of Roy and Sherrington obtained with acids and have not found the slightest evidence of active dilation of the cerebral vessels . . . In every experimental condition the cerebral circulation passively follows the changes in the general arterial and venous pressures . . . The brain has no vasomotor mechanism . . .'* (Hill, 1896).

Progress in the field of cerebral circulation and metabolism was correlated with technological development. In the early 20th century, measurement methods were confined to indices of brain tissue volume or blood volume and the diameter of retinal or superficial cerebral vessels. Following, thermoelectric instruments such as thermostromuhrs, heated or cooled thermocouples with other devices were inserted into cerebral vessels or tissue.

Subsequent investigators determined that cerebral metabolism and blood flow increased during the normal activation of the specific region when engaged in brain activity. In 1937, Carl Frederik Schmidt (1893-1988) and James P. Hendrix of the *University of Pennsylvania School of Medicine* recorded a localized increase in the blood flow through the visual cortex of a cat when a small spot on the animal's retina was illuminated (Schmidt and Hendrix, 1937). It is now clear that there is local change in nerve-cell activity and metabolic rate that gives a rise in the increasing blood flow in the active region. This discovery gave a suggestion to study brain regional variation in blood flow related to its function. Dumke and Schimdt in 1943 studied, for the first time, the circulation of blood to the brain of an anesthetized rhesus monkey, by means of a flow meter inserted directly into the cerebral arteries (Dumke and Schmidt, 1943).

On this basis, studies followed to apply quantitative in measuring cerebral blood flow associated with cerebral metabolic rates. The turning point was the mid 1940s, in which the American Seymour Kety (1915-2000) and colleagues at the *University of Pennsylvania and National Institutes of Health*, introduced the first technique for measuring whole brain blood flow in unanesthetized humans (Raichle, 2010). In 1944, Kety took part in a meeting of the *Federation of American Societies for Experimental Biology* (FASEB), where there was a symposium on the cerebral circulation. The main theme of the symposium was measurement methods for cerebral blood flow in unanesthetized men. At that time, there were two non quantitative methods of detection of cerebral blood flow in humans: the thermoelectric probe placed into the internal jugular to detect changes in flow within the vein, and the measurement of cerebral arteriovenous oxygen differences, which varies inversely with changes in cerebral blood flow and consumption of oxygen if it remains constant. Both techniques were unable to distinguish between blood flow and the constant oxygen consumption. The only practicable method for detecting the two parameters: the *bubble-flow technique of Dumke and Schmidt*, required anesthesia in addition to extensive surgery and only ever been tried on monkeys (Dumke and Schmidt, 1943). Kety attended this symposium and explained his idea on the observation rate at which the brain was satured or desatured using an inert gas. The method was based on the venerable *'Fick Principle'* on the conservation of matter (Fick, 1870). According to the principle, cerebral blood flow (volume per unit of mass per unit of time) is related to the time course of the arterovenous difference and to the final tissue concentration of a diffusible trace. Following this, Kety with Schmidt applied the central idea that the amount of an inhaled, highly diffusible, inert gas (*nitrous oxide*) taken up by the brain per unit of time is equal to the amount of that gas brought to the brain by the arterial blood minus the amount carried away in the cerebral venous blood. The subject inhaled 15 percent *nitrous oxide* for ten minutes, during which time the concentration of the gas was followed by drawing samples of arterial and venous blood from the brain. The area between the arterial and the venous saturation curves yielded a measure of the average blood flow, which is normally about 50 milliliters of blood per 100 grams of brain tissue per minute. As pointed out by Kety: *'A method is described applicable to unanesthetized man for the quantitative determination of cerebral blood flow by means of arterial and internal jugular blood concentration of an inert gas . . . human subjects by this method have thus far been made and suggest the feasibility of applying this method to clinical investigations'* .

The first measurements were obtained in a group of young male volunteers, yelding a mean value for blood flow of 54 ml/100 g/min or 750 ml/100 g/min for the whole brain (Kety and Schmidt, 1945, 1948). This indirect, minimally invasive technique, applicable to normally conscious animals and humans, made a great contribution to estimate the overall brain blood flow and metabolic activity of the brain.

With numerous collaborators, Kety's methods was applied in neurology, psychiatry, and medicine leading to greater knowledge of normal physiology, pathophysiology, and pharmacology of the circulation and metabolism of the human brain in healthy and diseased conditions, especially regarding the role of glucose in brain metabolism (Kety, 1950).

In the cat, Kety's team used a soluble gaseous radioactive tracer, fluorinated methane labelled with ^{131}I, and a quantitative application to obtain values for perfusion connected with functional activity in 28 cerebral structures (Landau, Freygang, Rowland, Sokoloff and Kety, 1955). This method used a unique quantitative autoradiographic technique in which the optical densities in autoradiographs of brain sections were quantitatively related to the local tissue concentrations of the radioactive tracer. These concentrations were in turn determined by the rate of blood flow to the tissue. In summary, the method provided pictorial maps of the local rates of blood flow throughout the brain exactly within each of its anatomic structures. This technique was called autoradiography because images were acquired by laying radioactive brain sections directly onto X-ray film (Kety, 1960; Taber, Black and Hurley, 2005). The study included CBF images showing clear changes between a baseline (sedated) and stimulated (awake, restrained) state (see Figure 7).

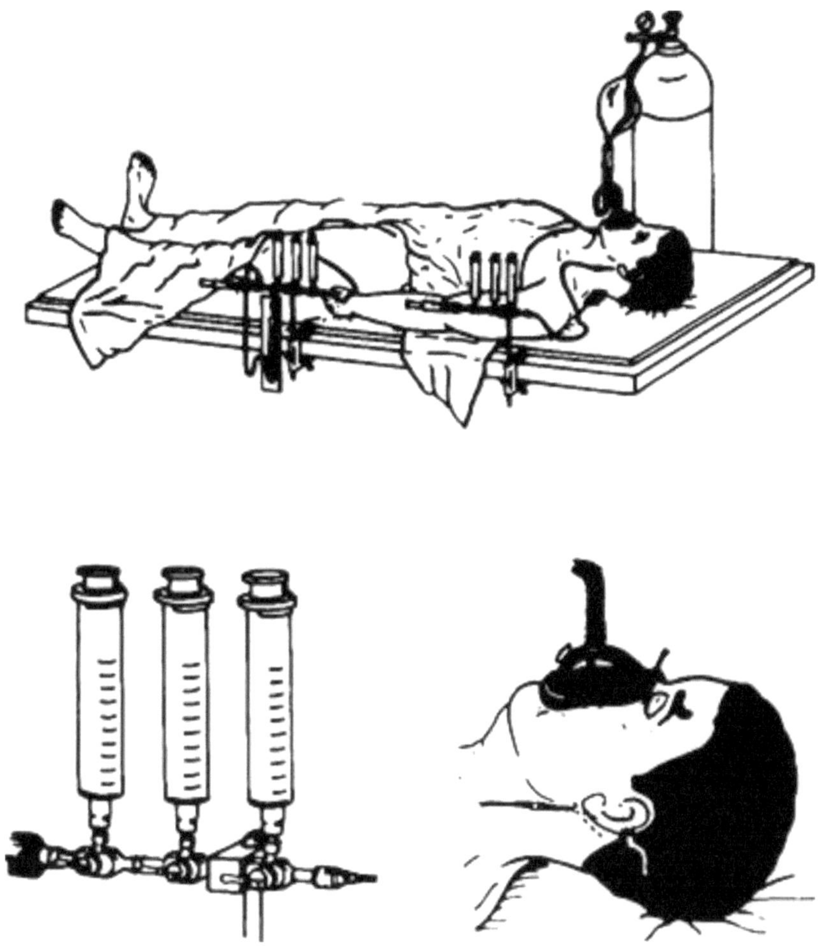

Fig. 7. Whole-brain, inert-gas (nitrous oxide) technique for the measurement of blood flow and metabolism in humans. Source: Kety and Schmidt (1948).

Kety and Sokoloff emphasized that the metabolic homeostasis hypothesis of Roy and Sherrington does not fully explain the increase in cerebral blood flow accompanying increased metabolic activity. Moreover, the association of two events (metabolism and flow) does not prove one (metabolism) to be determinant of the other (flow). Other factors on the coupling between cerebral metabolism and perfusion can describe the concept of perfusion governed by the effects of change in the metabolic rate. Metabolic demands of the cerebral tissue is accompanied by focal neural activation and modification of vessels, which may be mediated by neurotransmitters or the action of drugs on the cerebral circulation (Freygang 1958; Sokoloff, 1959, 1961; Lou, 1987).

These studies were a catalyst for the development of new cerebral blood flow modifications to the original Kety-Schmidt nitrous oxide method. Kety's group continued to refine the measurement of CBF introducing new radiotracers; in particular ^{131}I-antipyrine, ^{14}C-antipyrine, and C-antipyrine, an inert and freely diffusible tracer that had many advantages over previous diffusible indicators (Kety, 1965; Reivich, Jehle, Sokoloff et al., 1969).

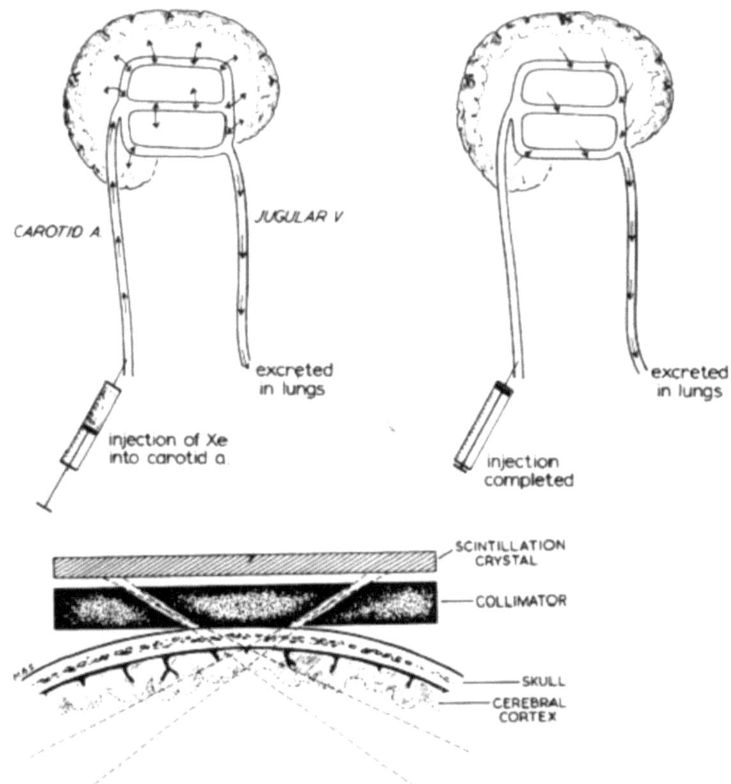

Fig. 8. The rationale of inert gas clearance method with a diagram of simple collimator. Following its injection into the carotid artery, xenon diffuses in a known ratio between the blood and brain tissue. After a sufficiently long injection period the brain tissue and venous blood will be in equilibrium. On cessation of the injection the carotid arterial blood, now containing virtually no radioactive xenon, will wash out the xenon in the brain tissue and the rate at which this takes place will depend on the quantity of blood perfusing the brain. Source: Harper, Glass, Steven and Granat (1964).

Lassen and Munck (1955) modified the classical Kety-Schmidt technique by substituting the inhalation of a radioactive inert gas, the ^{85}Kr, in place of nitrous oxide (see also Lassen, Munck and Tottey, 1957). In the early 1960s, thanks to the studies with radioactive tracers by Niels Alexander Lassen (1926-1997), David Henschen Ingvar (1924-2000) and their Scandinavian colleagues, it was becoming possible to measure local blood flow in the cerebral cortex. Lassen and Ingvar, injected a radioactive isotopes into the internal carotid artery (^{85}Kr), measuring the rate of clearance from the underlying cortex of the beta emissions of the isotope (Lassen and Ingvar, 1961; Ingvar and Lassen, 1961, 1962).
(Lassen and Edt-Rasmussen, 1966). Another report described the measurement of regional blood flow evoked by brain activity in the cerebral cortex of man through intact skull monitoring the low incidence gamma emissions of ^{85}Kr using scintillation detectors arrayed

like a helmet over the head (Lassen, Høedt-Rasmussen, Sørensen, Skinhøj, Cronquist, Bodforss and Ingvar, 1963). The use of collimated scintillation detectors allowed blood flow measurement in small neural populations of the cortex. Sveinsdottir and Lassen (1973) calculated that a regional blood flow was simultaneously measured in about 256 regions of a hemisphere. This application signalled the dawn of the modern era in human brain imaging. The rationale of inert gas clearance methods with a diagram of simple collimator is illustrated in Figure 8 as reported by Harper, Glass, Steven and Granat (1964).

The method devised by Lassen and Ingvar was suitable for clinical use, following the injection of ^{133}Xe, a radioactive tracers originally introduced by the group of *University of Glasgow* headed by Glass and Harper (Glass and Harper, 1963; Harper, Glass, Steven and Granat, 1964).

Some years after, Lassen, Ingvar and Skinhøj, wrote about their application: '*The radioactive gas was dissolved in a sterile saline solution, and a small volume (two to three milliliters, containing from three to five millicuries of radioactivity) is injected as a bolus into one of the main arteries to the brain. The arrival and subsequent washout of the radioactivity from many brain regions is followed for one minute with a gamma-ray camera consisting of a battery of 254 externally placed scintillation detectors, each of which is collimated to scan approximately one square centimetre of brain surface. Information from the detectors is processed by a small digital computer and is displayed in graphical form on a colour-television monitor, with each flow level being assigned a different colour or hue. Owing to the attenuation of radiation from structure deeper in the brain, the gamma radiation detected comes from the superficial cortex. Thus the radioactive-xenon technique provides a fairly specific picture of the activity of the cerebral cortex directly below the detector array*' (Lassen, Ingvar and Skinhǿj, 1978).

The ^{133}Xe tecnique has been extensively and very effectively used as a clinical and research tool for several decades (Glass and Harper, 1963; Lassen and Ingvar, 1963; Ingvar, Cronqvuist, Ekber, Risberg and Hǿedt-Rasmussen, 1965; Hǿedt-Rasmussen, Sveindottir and Ingvar, 1966; Ingvar and Risberg, 1967; Olesen, Paulson and Lassen, 1971; Ingvar and Lassen, 1973; Ingvar and Schwartz, 1974; Ingvar and Franzen, 1974; Soh, Larsen, Skinhøj and Lassen, 1978; Lassen, 1985). The Figure 10 adapted by Lassen and Ingvar (1972) illustrates their apparatus to detect rCBF changes and the results in a normal male adult using ^{133}Xe at rest and during a mental task.

Early techniques such as ^{133}Xe inhalation provided the first blood flow maps of the brain as they able to demonstrate directly in normal human change of blood flow within discrete parts of the cerebral cortex during mental activation. The first study on induced variation of brain blood circulation using this method was reported by Ingvar and Risberg in 1965 at the first *International Meeting on the Brain Blood Metabolism*, held in Lund. This research was received with caution because of its potential importance regarding human studies of regional change in blood flow using these techniques in normal humans and in conditions with neurological disorders.

6. The origin of new functional imaging techniques: PET, SPECT and fMRI

The introduction of an *in vivo* tissue autoradiographic measurement of blood flow in laboratory animals by Kety's group many years later became important for the measurement of blood flow in humans when positron emission tomography (PET) provided a means of quantifying the spatial distribution of radiotracers in tissue without the need for invasive autoradiography (Kety, 1999).

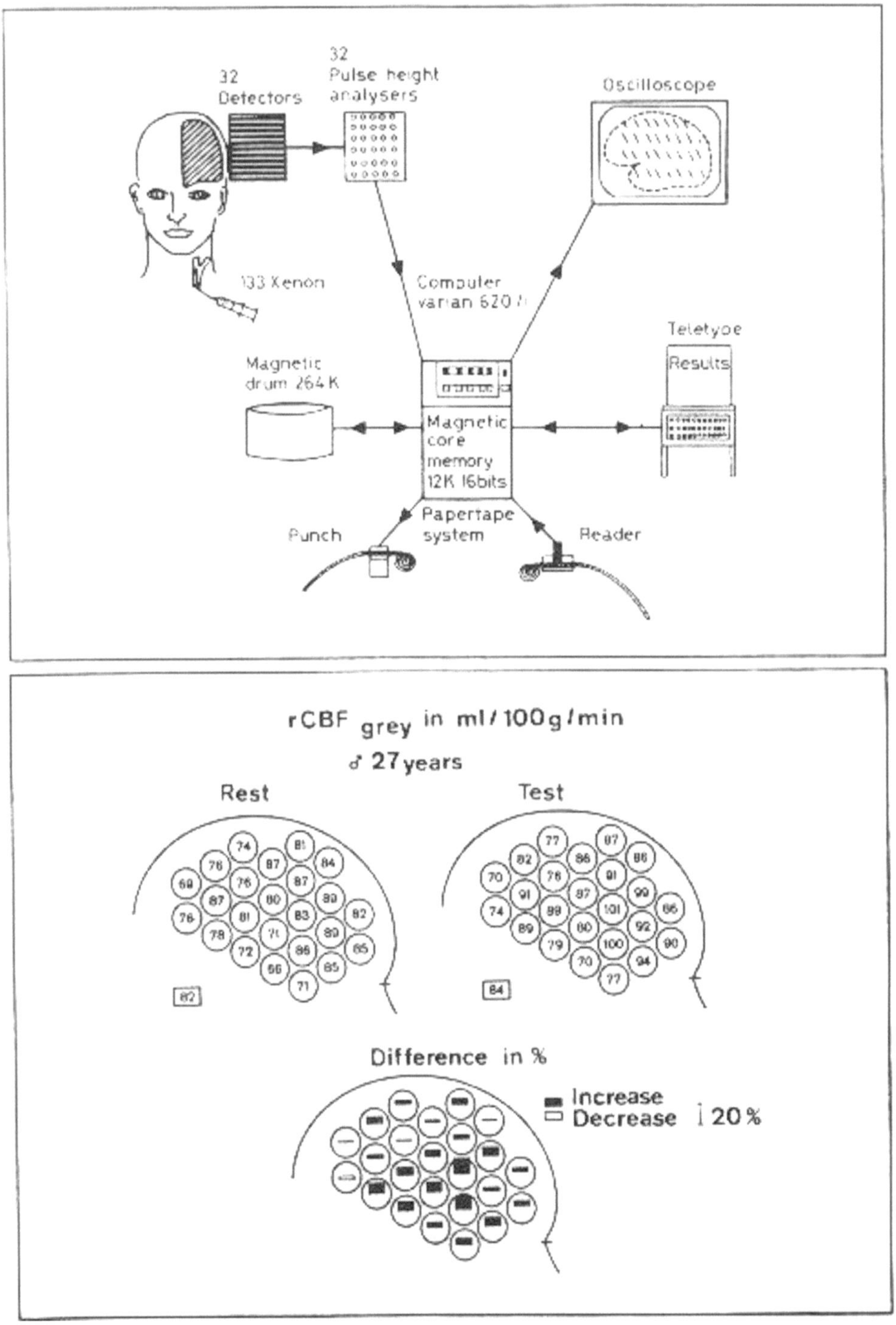

Fig. 9. Regional cerebral blood flow estimated from counts of arterially xenon-133 in a normal male adult at rest and during a mental task. Areas of large blood flow increase were found in temporal and precentral regions of gray matter. Source: Lassen and Ingvar, (1972).

PET, based on the decay of radioactive atoms that release positrons, derives its name and its fundamental properties from a group of radionuclides (^{15}O, ^{11}C, ^{18}F and ^{13}N). The properties of these radionuclides include short half-lives, a unique decay scheme involving the emission of positrons and chemical properties whose relevance to studies in biology and medicine arises from the fact that these chemical elements are building blocks of most biological molecules (Raichle, 2010).

The concept of emission and transmission tomography was introduced in the late 1950s by the American physic David Edmund Kuhl, who has been called the father of emission tomography. In the early 1960s, with the collaboration of Roy Edwards, Kuhl designed and made a detector which scanned in a series of tangential traverses, rotating about the patient on a circular path between scan passes. Their work later led to the design and construction of several tomographic instruments (Kuhl and Edwards, 1963). At the *University of Pennsylvania in Philadelphia,* Kuhl headed a group that developed a series of SPECT (single photon emission computed tomography) devices, the Mark II in 1964, the Mark III in 1970 and the Mark IV in 1976. The group also advanced the medical use of tomographic image reconstruction based on numerical computation, and made the transaxial section tomography of a living body possible. In the mid-1960s, Kuhl and collaborators, who improved tomographic image quality, proved their clinical efficacy for image separation pathological conditions of the brain and succeeded in the axial transverse tomographic imaging of humans. One such important milestone was the introduction of a new instrument: X-ray computed tomography (CT), that had enormous impact on the development and evolution of various methods of computed tomography, including PET (Kuhl, Hale and Eaton, 1966).

The CT method was invented by a British electronic engineer Godfrey Newbold Hounsfield (1919-2004), at the *Atkinson Morley Hospital* in London, who in 1971 built an instrument that combined an X-ray machine and a computer and used certain principles of algebraic reconstruction to scan the body (Hounsfield, 1973). Unknown to Hounsfield, the American nuclear physicist Allan MacLeod Cormack (1924-1998) had published essentially the same idea in 1963 (Cormack, 1963), using a reconstruction technique called the *Radon transform.* Although Cormack's work was not widely circulated, in 1979 he and Hounsfield shared the Nobel prize in Medicine and Physiology for the development of CT (www-Nobelprize.org). In creating CT, Hounsfield had arrived at a practical solution to the problem of the three-dimensional transaxial tomographic images of an intact object using data obtained from by passing highly focused X-ray beams through the object and recording their attenuation. Hounsfield's invention was fundamental in changing the approach for observing the human brain.

During the mid-1970s, at the *Washington University School of Medicine in St. Louis,* the Armenian-American physic Michel Ter-Pogossian (1925-1996) lead a research team of physicists scientist, chemists, and physicians to build the first PET scanner for medical application. Previously, Ter-Pogossian performed a quantitative measurement of regional brain blood flow and oxygen consumption in humans using a radiotracer technique developed by him (Ter-Pogossian et al. 1969, 1970). A fundamental role was played by Ed Hoffman and Michael E Phelps which led to the production of the first PET camera, PET III (Ter-Pogossian, Phelps and Hoffman, 1975; Phelps, Hoffman, Mullani and Ter-Pogossian, 1975; Phelps, Hoffman, Mullani, Higgins, Ter-Pogossian, 1976; Hoffman, Phelps, Mullani,

Higgins and Ter-Pogossian, 1976). As pointed by Raichle (2010): '*With PET, we had a tool that brought quantitative tissue autoradiography from the laboratory into the clinic. Such things as brain blood flow, blood volume, oxygen consumption, and glucose utilization, not to mention tissue pH and receptors pharmacology, could now be measured safely in humans*'.

At approximately the same time of the Kulh's and Ter-Pogossian's studies, at the *Laboratory of Cerebral Metabolism at the National Institutes of Health in Bethesda*, Sokoloff and colleagues, directly disclosed, in the brain of experimental animals (rats and monkeys), cerebral utilization of an energy-rich substrate, 2-deoxyglucose tagged with carbon-14 (Sokoloff, Reivich, Kennedy, Des Rosiers, Patlak, Pettigrew, Sakurada and Shinohara, 1977). Sokoloff and colleagues studied cerebral metabolism on a microscopic scale by injecting a radioactive analogue of glucose into the brain demonstrating that the rate at which the substance is taken up by nerve cells reflects their functional activity. The brain's oxygen consumption is almost entirely determined by the oxidative metabolism of glucose which in normal physiological conditions is the exclusive substrate for the brain's energy metabolism (Clarke and Sokoloff, 1999).

Aiming to employ the [^{14} C] deoxyglucose technique clinically, Kuhl's team conducted joint research with Alfred P Wolf of the *Brookhaven National Laboratory* and with Sokoloff's group, ultimately reaching the conclusion that ^{18}F-2-fluoro-2-deoxy-D-glucose or 'FDG' was the most appropriate positron emitting tracer for human use (Ido, Wan, Casella, Fowler, Wolf, Reivich and Kuhl, 1978; Reivich, Kuhl, Wolf, Greenberg, Phelps, Ido, Casella Fowler, Hoffman, Alavi and Sokoloff, 1979; Phelps, Huang, Hoffman, Selin, Sokoloff and Kuhl, 1979).

The development of the [^{14}C] deoxyglucose method made it possible to measure the local rate of glucose utilization throughout the brain. The method employed a quantitative autoradiographic technique like that of the [^{131}I] trifluoroiodomethane method but, subsequently, added computerized processing techniques which scanned the autoradiographs and redisplayed them in colour with the actual rate of glucose utilization encoded in a calibrated colour scale. This was the first use of the deoxyglucose technique for the regional measurement of glucose metabolism in laboratory animals and the basis for an application for clinical purpose (Sokoloff, Reivich, Kennedy, Des Rosiers, Patlak, Pettigrew, Sakurada and Shinohara, 1977). These [^{131}I] trifluoroiodomethane and [^{14} C] deoxyglucose methods were used to measure local cerebral blood flow and glucose utilization in studies in animals. Both methods were subsequently were adapted for use in humans by substituting positron-emitting tracers and PET in place of autoradiography: [^{18}F] fluorodeoxyglucose in place of [^{14} C] deoxyglucose to measure glucose utilization (Raichle, Phelps, Larson, Grubb, Welch and Ter-Pogossian, 1973; Reivich, Kuhl, Wolf, Greenberg, Phelps, Ido, Casella Fowler, Hoffman, Alavi and Sokoloff, 1979; Phelps, Huang, Hoffman, Selin, Sokoloff and Kuhl, 1979) and $^{15}H_20$ instead [^{131}I] trifluoroiodomethane to measure blood flow (Herscovitch, Markham and Raichle, 1983).

PET method has had some advantage, such as: the blood flow was measured quickly (<1 min) by using an easily produced radiopharmaceutical ($^{15}H_20$) with a short half life (123 sec) that allowed many repeat measurements in the same subject. However, PET present some disadvantages: few spatial resolution than the autoradiography methods, in the mm instead of μm range; they contributed very little to define mechanisms that relate blood flow and energy metabolism to functional activity in the brain, their application did initiate and establish the field of functional brain imaging in humans (Sokoloff, 2008).

Raichle and his colleagues, at the *Mallinckrodt Institute of Radiology of the Washington University of St Louis,* used PET technology to measure cerebral blood volume (CBV) in normal right-handed human volunteers following inhalation of trace quantities of cyclotron-produced, ^{11}C-labeled carbon monoxide. The CBV was significantlylarger in the temporal left cerebral hemisphere in the tomographic scans during speech, a region which is thought to be larger in individuals with left cerebral dominance for speech. As pointed out the authors: *'This observation is the first in vivo demonstration of a structural correlate of a known functional difference in the cerebral hemispheres of man'* (Grubb, Raichle, Higgins, Eichling, 1978).

In the 1980s, Raichle and colleagues systematically applied PET technique to the normal human brain, using oxygen-15 labelled water and to demonstrate regional metabolic activation induced by cognitive tasks. The labelled water, which emits positrons as it decays with a half-life of approximately two minutes, accumulates in the brain in less than a minute, forming an accurate image of blood flow. In a series of original works Raichle and colleagues firstly studied the manner in which the normal human brain processes single words, from perception to speech (Raichle, 1996) (see. Fig. 10).

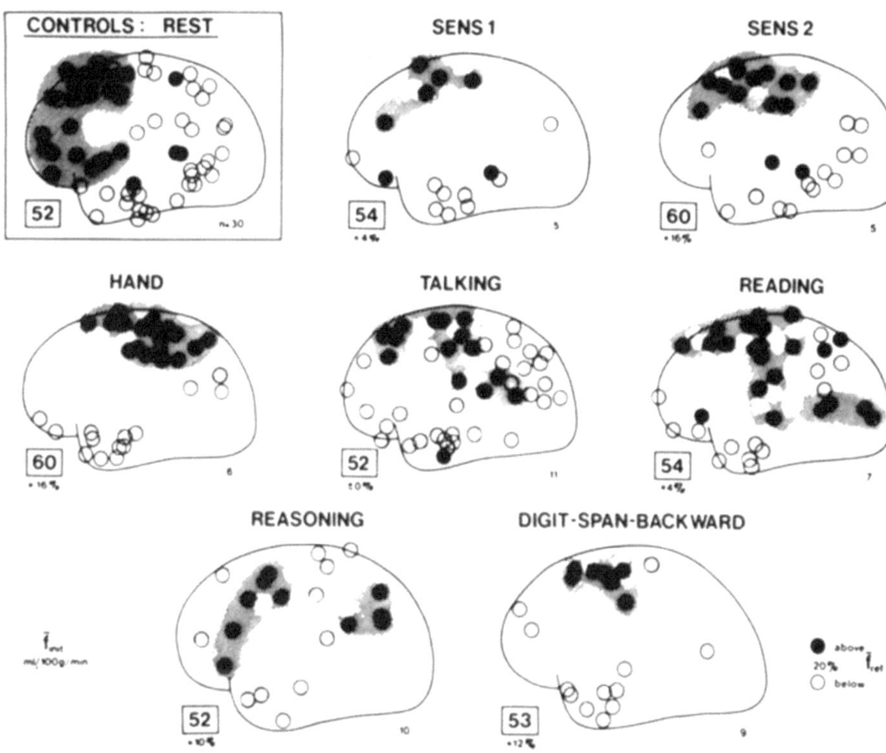

Fig. 10. Four different hierarchically organized conditions are represented in these mean blood flow difference images obtained with PET. All of the changes shown in these images represent increases over the control state for each task. Source: Raichle (1996).

This approach was not embraced by most neuroscientists or cognitive scientists until the 1980s after increase of technological, procedural and conceptual sophistication at the beginning of the 20th century (Raichle, 1987; 1998; 2008).

The advent of the nuclear magnetic resonance imaging (MRI) introduced a new and now the most convenient and widely used technique for functional brain imaging (fMRI) in both animals and humans. It is based on the physical property of atomic nuclei that, when first oriented in an magnetic field and then reoriented by radiofrequency pulses, emit during their return to their chemical species, concentrations, and environments. The strongest signals are those obtained from hydrogen nuclei because they are in water and thus prevalent.
The physical principles associated with MRI were discovered independently by the Swiss-American Felix Bloch (1905-1983), at *Stanford University*, and the American Edward Mills Purcell (1912-1997), at *Harvard University*. In December 1945, at the American Physical Society, they met and discussed their research. Both recognized that the theoretical basis of their respective projects was the same, although they had been using slightly different techniques to achieve experimental results. So they decided to split up the field: Bloch would use the effect in the study of liquids; Purcell would examine crystals. The Stanford group gathered its first positive results in January 1946 (Bloch, Hansen and Packard, 1946; Purcell, Torrey and Pound, 1946). In 1952, Bloch and Purcell were awarded the Nobel Prize for Physics for the 'development of new methods for nuclear magnetic precision measurements and discoveries in connection therewith' (Nobelprize.org). Many years of research followed, in which the technique was used for basic research in chemistry. During this time it was known as nuclear magnetic resonance (NMR).
In 1973, the American-chemist Paul C Lauterbur (1929-2007) came up with a strategy in which the NMR signals could be used to create cross-sectional images in much the same manner as a CT (Lauterbur, 1973). In 2003, he was awarded with the Nobel Prize in Medicine along with the British physicist Peter Mansfield for their research on NMR. Mansfield is credited with showing how the radio signals from MRI can be mathematically analyzed, making interpretation of the signals into a useful image a possibility. He is also credited with discovering how fast imaging was possible by developing the MRI protocol called echo-planar imaging. Echo-planar imaging allows T2* weighted images to be collected many times faster than previously possible. It has also made functional magnetic resonance imaging (fMRI) feasible (Mansfield and Baines 1976). This method had an immediate use because the technique was free of ionizing radiation, but also for the quality of images of the human body with detailed information, when compared to CT it proved more sensitive to soft tissue. An opening for MRI in the area of functional brain imaging emerged when it was discovered that during changes in neuronal activity there are local changes in the amount of oxygen in the tissue (Fox and Raichle, 1986). By combining the above observation with another much earlier one by Linus Pauling (1901-1994) and Charles D Coryell (1912-1971) it was shown that change in the amount of oxygen carried by the hemoglobin alters the degree to which hemoglobin disturbs a magnetic field (Pauling and Coryell 1936).
It was Michael Faraday (1791-1867) who first studied the magnetic properties of hemoglobin. In 1845, he noted (to his surprise that hemoglobin contains iron) that dried blood was not magnetic, noting '*Must try fluid blood*' (Faraday, 1933). Many years later Pauling and Coryell found that the magnetic susceptibility of oxygenated and deoxygenated hemoglobin differed significantly. In 1982, Keith Thulborn and collaborators found the difference in magnetic susceptibility of oxy and deoxyhemoglobin for the measurement of brain oxygen consumption with MRI (Thulborn, Waterton, Matthews and Radda, 1982).

They demonstrated clearly the feasibility of measuring the state of oxygenation of blood *in vivo* with MRI. This step was important for the further study of Sieji Ogawa and colleagues for the so-called Blood-Oxygen-Level Dependent (BOLD) effect. The physical effect is based on the difference between reduced hemoglobin in venous blood, paramagnetic, and oxyhemoglobin prevalent in the arterial blood is diamagnetic and has no such effect. During the oxygen consumption from the blood by the tissue, the venous system draining the tissue within the field of view, contains more oxyhemoglobin and less in deoxthemoglobin. This leads to a small increase in the MRI signal, i.e.: the BOLD effect. Owaga labeled his finding 'BOLD contrast' and noted that BOLD contrast adds an additional feature to MRI and complements other techniques that are attempt to provide PET-like measurements related to regional neural activity (Ogawa, Lee, Kay and Tank, 1990). The potential for BOLD fMRI was seen in three groups in 1992 (Ogawa, Tank, Menon et al 1992, Kwong, Belliveau, Chesler et al., 1992, Bandettini, Wong, Hinks et al, 1992), in especially from the group at the *Massachuttes General Hospital* led by Ken Kwong. Although MRI also offers additional approaches to the measurement of brain function, it is BOLD imaging that has dominated the research agenda to date.

fMRI is the new non-invasive imaging tool for its remarkable high quality and it is considered by Raichle a tool for the 'masses' (Raichle, 2010). fMRI could be viewed as a logical extension of PET although fMRI can acquire images every few seconds and secondly is the neuronal responses occurring in the brain are 'filtered' by a hemodynamic response, which is responsible for the fMRI signals that can give the most powerful strategies for neurocognitive studies. According to Raichle, the future in functional brain imaging research has two developmental routes. The first is the research on individual differences improving the functional imaging in the clinical area. The combination of anatomical and functional imaging with genetic information opens new areas of research on the human brain in healthy and pathological conditions (Raichle, 2010). The second is an attempt to integrate work from functional brain imaging with neurophysiology in relation to various kinds of intrinsic rhythmic activity of the brain (Buzsaki, 2006).

However, the success of human brain imaging was not only the involvement of physiologists, who provided information on basic mechanism of neuronal activity, but also of different figures such as neurologists, neuropsychologists, psychiatrists who had the strategies and influence to provide an important tool in the understanding of '*how the mind works*' in normal and pathological conditions.

The scope of brain function imaging in future is to study the brain without requiring the subject to remain in a scanner approaching the organization of intrinsic activity of the neuronal cells in normal functional activity not only to addresses a specific feature of its activity. Another important step is to achieve rapidly changing electrical events instead of changes in slow activity of the brain's intrinsic work after an '*environmental stimuli* '. A possible anticipatory signal that could prevent negative behavior neural activity of latent brain diseases.

7. References

Albers JFH (1861) Die temperatur der äusseren oberfläche, namentlich des kopfes bei irren. Allgemeine Zeitschrift für Psychiatrie, 18, 450-473

Amidon RW (1880) The effect of willed muscular movements on the temperature of the head: new study of cerebral localisation. Archives of Medecine. Cited in: Bianchi L, Montefusco A and Bifulco F (1884). Contributo alla dottrina della temperature cefalica. Ricerche cliniche e sperimentali. La Psichiatria, 2, 193-242

Bandettini PA, Wong EC, Hinks RS et al (1992) Time course EPI of human brain function during task activation. Magnetic Resonance Medicine 25: 390-397

Barcroft J (1914) The respiratory function of the blood. Macmillan, New York

Berger H (1901) Zur Lehre von der Blutzirkulation in der Shändelhöle des Menschen namentlich unter dem Einfluss von Medikamenten. Verlag von Gustav Fischer, Jena

Bergesio B, and Musso G (1884) Contribuzione allo studio della circolazione cerebrale. Giornale della R. Accademia Medica di Torino, 24, 136-161

Bernard C (1872) Des fonctions du cerveau. Revue Deux Mondes, 98, 373-385

Bert P (1879) De la termometrie cérebrale. Societè de Biologie, January 1879. Cited in: Bianchi L, Montefusco A and Bifulco F (1884). Contributo alla dottrina della temperature cefalica. Ricerche cliniche e sperimentali. La Psichiatria, 2, 193-242

Bianchi L, Montefusco A and Bifulco F (1884). Contributo alla dottrina della temperature cefalica. Ricerche cliniche e sperimentali. La Psichiatria, 2, 193-242

Binet, A and Sollier P (1895) Recherches sur le pouls cerebral dans ses rapports avec les attitudes du corps, la respiration et le actes psychiques. Archives de Physiologie, 27, 718-734

Bloch F, Hansen WW, Packard M (1946) Nuclear induction. Physical Review, 70, 474-485

Broca PP (1879) Sur les températures morbides locale. Bulletin de l'Academie de Mèdecine 8, 1331-1347

Burckhardt G (1881) Ueber Gehirnbewegungen. Eine Experimental Studien, Bern

Buzsaki G (2006) Rhythms of the brain. New York, Oxford University Press.

Clarke DD and Sokoloff L (1999) Circulation and energy metabolism of the brain. In: Siegel G, Agranoff RW, Fisher S (Eds) Basic neurochemistry: molecular, cellular, and medical aspects. 6th Edition. Lippincott-Raven, Philadelphia

Conti, F. (2002). Claude Bernard's Des Fonctions du Cerveau: an ante litteram manifesto of the neurosciences? Nature Review Neuroscience 3, 979-985

Cormack A M (1963) Representation of a function by its line integrals, with some radiological applications. Journal of Applied Physiology 34, 2722-2727

Craigie EH (1924) Changes in vascularity in the brain stem and cerebellum of the albino rat between birth and maturity. Journal of Comparative Neurology 38, 27-48

De Sarlo F and Bernardini C (1891) Ricerche sulla circolazione cerebrale durante l'attività psichica. Rivista Sperimentale di Freniatria e di Medicina Legale 17, 503-528

Donders FC (1850) De bewegingen der hersenen en de veranderingen der vaatvulling van de pia mater, ook bij gesloten onuitzetbaren schedel regtstreeks onderzocht. Nederland Lancet 5: 521-553

Dumke, PR and Schmidt CF (1943) Quantitative measurements of cerebral blood flow in the macacque mondkey. American Journal of Physiology 138, 421-431

Faraday M (1933) Faraday's diary. Being the various philosophical notes of experiment investigation during the year 1820-1862. G. Bell and Sons

Fick A (1870) Ueber die Messung des Blutquantum in den Herzventrikeln. Versammlung der physikalisch-medizinischen Gesellschaft zu Würzburg 2, 16-28

Fleming W (1877). The motions of the brain. The Glasgow Medical Journal. Abstract in Psychological Retrospect 187, 424-425.

Fox PT, Raichle ME (1986) Focal physiological uncoupling of cerebral blood flow and oxidative metabolism during somatosensory stimulation in human subjects. Proceeding of the National Academy of Sciences USA 83, 1140-1144

François-Franck CE (1877) Recherches critiques et expérimentales sur les mouvements alternatifs d'expansion et de resserements du cerveau. Journal de l'Anatomie et de la Physiologie de Ch. Robin 13, 267-307

François-Franck CE (1880) Température du cerveau at differentes hauteurs. Societè de Biologie, May 1880. Cited in: Bianchi L, Montefusco A and Bifulco F. (1884). Contributo alla dottrina della temperature cefalica. Ricerche cliniche e sperimentali. La Psichiatria 2, 193-242

Freygang WH and Sokoloff L (1958) Quantitative measurement of regional circulation in the central nervous system by the use of radioactive inert gas. Advances in Biological and Medical Physics 6, 263-279

Fulton JF (1928) Observations upon the vascularity of the human occipital lobe during visual activity. Brain 51, 310-328

Glass HI and Harper AM (1963) Measurement of regional blood flow in cerebral cortex of man through intact skull. British Medical Journal 1, 593

Gray LC (1878) Cerebral thermometry. New York Medical Journal. August 1878. Cited in: Bianchi L, Montefusco A and Bifulco F. (1884). Contributo alla dottrina della temperature cefalica. Ricerche cliniche e sperimentali. La Psichiatria 2, 193-242

Grubb RL Jr, Raichle ME, Higgins CS and Eichling JO (1978) Measurement of regional cerebral blood volume by emission tomography. Annals of Neurology 4, 322-328

Gusnard DA, and Raichle ME (2001) Searching for a baseline: functional imaging and the resting human brain. Nature Review Neuroscience 2, 685-694

Harper AM, Glass H, Steven JL and Granat AH (1964) The measurement of local blood flow in the cerebral cortex from the clearance of xenon133. Journal of Neurology, Neurosurgery and Psychiatry, 27, 255-258

Herscovitch P, Markham J, Raichle M (1983) Brain blood flow measured with intravenous $^{15}H_20$. I. Theory and error analysis. Journal of Nuclear Medicine 24: 782-789

Hill L (1896) The physiology and pathology of the cerebral circulation: an experimental research. Churchill, London

Høedt-Rasmussen K, Sveinsdottir E and Lassen NA (1966) Regional Cerebral low in Man Determined by Intral-artrial Injection of Radioactive Inert Gas. Circulation Research, 18, 237-247

Hoffmann EJ, Phelps ME, Mullani NA, Higgins CS, Ter-Pogossian MM. (1976) Design and performance characteristics of a whole-body positron transaxial tomography. Journal of Nuclear Medicine, 17, 493-502

Hounsfield GN (1973) Computerised transverse axial scanning (tomography): Part I. Description of system. British Journal of Radiology 46, 1016-1022

Iadecola C (2004) Neurovascular regulation in the normal brain and in Alzheimer's disease. Nature Reviews 5, 347-360

Ido T, Wan CN, Casella V, Fowler JS, Wolf AP, Reivich M, and Kuhl D (1978) Labeled 2-deoxy-D-glucose analogs. 18F-labeled 2-deoxy-2-fluoro-D-glucose, 2-deoxy-2-

fluoro-D-mannose and 14C-2-deoxy-2-fluoro-D-glucose. Journal of Labelled Compounds and Radiopharmaceuticals 14, 175-183
Ingvar DH and Lassen NA (1961) Quantitative determination of regional cerebral flood flow in man. Lancet 278, 806-807
Ingvar, D.H., Lassen, N.A. (1962): Regional blood flow of the cerebral cortex determined by Krypton-85. Acta Physiologica Scandinavica 54, 325-338
Ingvar DH and Risberg J (1965). Influence of mental activity upon regional cerebral blood flow in man. Acta Neurologica Scandinavica, Supplement 14, 183-186
Ingvar DH, Cronqvist S, Ekbehg R, Risberg, J and Høedt-Rasmussen K (1965) Normal values of regional cerebral blood flow in man, including flow and weight estimates of gray and white matter. Acta Neurologica Scandinavica, Supplement 14, 72-78
Ingvar DH Risberg J (1967) Increase of regional cerebral blood flow during mental effort in normal and in patients with focal brain disorders. Experimental Brain Research 3: 195-211
Ingvar DH and Lassen NA (1973) Cerebral Complications Following Measurements of Regional Cerebral Blood Flow (rCBF) With the lntra-arterial 133 Xenon Injection Method. Stroke 4, 658-665
Ingvar DH and Schwartz M (1974) Blood flow patterns induced in the dominant hemisphere by speech and reading. Brain 97, 273-288
Ingvar DH and Franzen G (1974) Abnormalities of cerebral blood flow distribution in patients with chronic schizophrenia. Acta Psychiatrica Scandinavica 50, 425-462.
James W (1892) Psychology. Briefer course. New York, Henry Holt
Kety SS (1950) Circulation and metabolism of the human brain in health and disease. American Journal of Medicine 8: 205-217
Kety SS (1960) Measurement of local blood flow by the exchange of an inert, diffusible substance. Methods in Medical Research 8, 228-236
Kety SS (1965) Measurement of local contribution within the brain by means of inert, diffusible tracers: examination of the theory, assumptions and possible sources of error. Acta Neurologica Scandinavica, 14, 20-23
Kety SS (1999) Circulation and metabolism of the human brain. Brain Research Bulletin 50: 415-416
Kety SS and Schmidt CF (1945) Determination of cerebral blood flow in man by the use of nitrous oxide in low concentration. American Journal of Physiology 143, 53-66
Kety SS and Schmidt CF (1948) The nitrous oxide method for the quantitative determination of cerebral blood flow in man: theory, procedure and normal values. Journal of Clinical Investigation 27, 476-483
Kiyatkin EA (2007) Brain temperature fluctuations during physiological and pathological conditions. European Journal of Physiology 101, 3-17
Kuhl DE and Edwards RQ (1963) Image Separation Radioisotope Scanning. Radiology 80, 653-662
Kuhl DE, Hale J, and Eaton WL (1966) Transmission scanning: A useful adjunct to conventional emission scanning for accurately keying isotope deposition to radiographic anatomy. Radiology 87, 278-284
Kwong KK, Belliveau JW, Chesler DA et al (1992) Dynamic magnetic resonance imaging of human brain activity during primary sensory stimulation. Proceeding of the National Academy of Sciences USA 89, 5675-5679

Landau WM, Freygang WH, Rowland LP, Sokoloff L and Kety SS (1955) The local circulation of the living brain: values in the unanesthetized and anesthetized cat. Transactions of the American Neurological Association 80, 125-129

Lassen NA and Munck O (1955) The cerebral blood flow in man determined by the use of radioactive Krypton. Acta Physiologica Scandinavica 33, 30-49

Lassen NA, Munck O and Tottey ER (1957) Mental function and cerebral oxygen consumtion in organic dementia. Archives of Neurology and Psychiatry 77, 126-133

Lassen NA and Ingvar DH (1961) The blood flow of the cerebral cortex determined by radioactive krypton^{85} Experimentia 17, 42-43

Lassen NA and Ingvar DH (1963) Regional cerebral blood flow measurement in man. Archives of Neurology and Psychiatry 9, 615-622

Lassen NA, Høedt-Rassmussen K, Sørensen SC, Skinhøj E, Cronquist S, Bodforss B and Ingvar DH (1963) Regional cerebral blood flow in man determined by Krypton^{85} Neurology 13, 719-727

Lassen NA and Edt-Rasmussen KH (1966) Comparison of the Kety-Schmidt Method and the Intra-Arterial Injection Method Human Cerebral Blood Flow Measured by Two Inert Gas Techniques. Circulation Research 19, 681-688

Lassen NA and Ingvar DN (1972) Radioisotopic assessment of regional blood flow. Progress in Nuclear Medicine, 1, 376-409

Lassen NA, Ingvar DH and Skinhøj E (1978) Brain function and blood flow. Scientific American 239, 62-71

Lassen NA (1985) Cerebral blood flow tomography with xenon-133. Seminars in Nuclear Medicine 15, 347-356

Lauterbur P (1973) Image formation by induced local interactions: examples employing nuclear magnetic resonance. Nature 242: 190-191

Lombard JS (1867) Experiments on the relation of heat to mental works. New York Medical Journal 5, 198-205

Lombard JS (1879) Experimental researches on the regional temperature of the head under conditions of rest, intellectual activity, and emotion. Lane Medical Library, San Francisco

Lou HC, Edvinsson L, MacKenzie ET (1987) The concept of coupling blood flow to brain function: revision required? Annals of Neurology 22, 289-297

Lowe MF (1935) The application of the balance to the study of the bodily changes occurring during periods of volitional activity. British Journal of Psychology 26, 245-262

Mansfield P, Maudsley AA, Baines T (1976) Fast scan proton density imaging by NMR. Journal of Physics E: Scientific Instruments 9, 271-278

Maragliano D, Seppili G (1879) Studi di termometria cerebrale negli alienati. Rivista Sperimentale di Freniatria 5, 94-115

Maragliano D (1880) La temperatura cerebrale, ricerche cliniche e sperimentali, Bologna

Marshall JC and Fink GR (2003) Cerebral localization, then and now. Neuroimage 20 (Supplement 1), S2–7.

Mays K (1882) Ueber die Bewegungen des menschlichen Gehirn. Virchow's Archiv 88. Cited in: Bergesio B, and Musso G (1884) Contribuzione allo studio della circolazione cerebrale. Giornale della R. Accademia Medica di Torino, 24, 136-161

Morcom, A.M., Fletcher, P.C., 2007. Does the brain have a baseline? Why we should be resisting a rest. Neuroimage 37, 1073–1082

Morselli E, Bordoni-Uffreduzzi C (1884) Sui cangiamenti della circolazione cerebrale prodotti dalle diverse percezioni semplici. Archivio di Psichiatria, Scienze Penali e di Antropologia Criminale 4, 111-112

Mosso A (1880) Sulla circolazione del sangue nel cervello dell'uomo. Memorie della Reale Accademia dei Lincei della Classe di Scienze Fisiche, Matematiche e Naturali 5, 237-358

Mosso A (1881) Ueber den Kreislauf des Blutes im Menschlichen Gehirn. Leipzig, Viet.

Mosso A (1882) Application de la balance. A L'étude de la circulation du sang chez l'homme. Archives Italiennes de Biologie, 5, 130-143

Mosso A (1883) Applicazione della bilancia allo studio della circolazione del sangue nell'uomo. Reale Accademia delle Scienze di Torino 17, 534-535

Mosso A. La temperatura del cervello. Studi termometrici. Milano, Fratelli Trevers, 1894

Musso G and Bergesio B (1885) Influenza di alcune applicazioni idroterapiche sulla circolazione cerebrale nell'uomo. Rivista Sperimentale di Freniatria e di Medicina Legale 11, 124-138

Ogawa S, Lee TM, Kay AR, Tank TW (1990) Brain magnetic resonance imaging with contrast dependent on blood oxygenation. Proceedings of the National Academy of Sciences USA 87, 9868-9872

Ogawa S, Tank DW, Menon R et al. (1992) Intrinsic signal changes accompanying sensory stimulation: functional brain mapping with magnetic resonance imaging. Proceeding of the National Academy of Sciences USA 89, 5951-5955

Olesen J, Paulson OB and Lassen NA (1971) Regional cerebral blood flow in man determined by the initial slope of the clearance of intra-arterially injected ^{133}Xe. Stroke 2, 519-540

Patrizi ML (1896) Primi esperimenti intorno all'influenza della musica sulla circolazione del sangue nel cervello dell'uomo. Rivista Musicale Italiana 3, 275-294

Patrizi ML (1897) Il tempo di reazione semplice studiato in rapporto colla curva pletismografia cerebrale. Rivista Sperimentale di Freniatria, Medicina Legale e delle Alienazioni Mentali 34, 257-269

Pauling L and Coryell CD (1936) The magnetic properties and structure of hemoglobin, oxyhemoglobin and carbonmonoxyhemoglobin. Proceedings of the National Academy of Sciences USA 22, 210-216

Petrazzani P (1888) Intorno all'azione di talune sostanze sul polso cerebrale. Ricerche grafiche. Rivista Sperimentale di Freniatria e di Medicina Legale 14: 270-314

Phelps ME, Hoffman EJ, Mullani NA and Ter-Pogossian MM (1975) Application of annihilation coincidence detection to transaxial reconstruction tomography. Journal of Nuclear Medicine 16, 210-240

Phelps M.E., Hoffman E., Mullani N., Higgins C., Ter-Pogossian M (1976) Design considerations for a positron emission transaxial tomograph (PET III). IEEE Transactions on Biomedical Engineering 23, 516-522

Phelps ME, Huang SC, Hoffman EJ, Selin C, Sokoloff L and Kuhl DE (1979) Tomographic measurement of local cerebral glucose metabolic rate in humans with (^{18}F)2-fluoro-2-deoxy-D-glucose: validation of method. Annals of Neurology 6, 371-388

Purcell EM, Torrey HC, Pound RV (1946) Resonance absorption by nuclear magnetic moments in a solid. Physical Review 69, 37-38

Putnamm Jacobi MC (1880) Case of tubercular meningitis with measurements of cranial temperatures. Chicago, Cited in: Bianchi L, Montefusco A and Bifulco F (1884). Contributo alla dottrina della temperatura cefalica. Ricerche cliniche e sperimentali. La Psichiatria 2, 193-242

Raichle ME, Phelps ME, Larson KB, Grubb Jr. RL, Welch MJ, Ter-Pogossian MM. (1973) In vivo measurement of cerebral glucose metabolism employing 11C-labeled glucose. Transactions of the American Neurological Association 98,11-13

Raichle ME (1987) Circulatory and metabolic correlates of brain function in normal humans. In: The handbook of physiology. Second 1: The nervous system, Vol V. Higher function of the brain. Part 1 (eds F. Plum and V. Mountcastle). Bethesda, American Phisiology Society.

Raichle ME (1996) What words are telling us about the brain. Cold Spring Harbor Symposia on Quantitative Biology 61, 9-14

Raichle EM (1998) Behind the scenes of functional brain imaging: a historical and physiological perspective. Proceedings of the National Academy of Sciences USA 95, 765-772

Raichle ME (2008) A brief history of human brain mapping. Trends of Neurosciences 32, 118-126

Raichle ME (2010) The origins of functional brain imaging in humans. In: History of Neurology. S Finger, F Boller, KL Tyler (eds). In: Handbook of Clinical Neurology, vol 95 (3rd series). Elservier, Amsterdam

Ravina A (1811) Specimen de motu cerebri. Mémoires dell'Académie des Sciences de Turin.

Reivich M, Jehle J, Sokoloff L, et al (1969) Measurement of regional cerebral blood flow with antipyrine 14C in awake cats. Journal of Applied Physiology 27, 296-300

Reivich M, Kuhl D, Wolf A Greenberg J, Phelps M, Ido T, Casella V, Fowler J, Hoffman E, Alavi, A, Som P and Sokoloff L (1979) The [18F]fluorodeoxyglucose method for the measurement of local cerebral glucose utilization in man. Circulation Research 44, 127-137

Roy CS and Sherrington CS (1890) On the regulation of the blood supply of the brain. Journal of Physiology 11, 85-108

Schmidt CF and Hendrix JP (1937). The action of chemical substances on cerebral blood vessels. Research Publications - Association for Research in Nervous and Mental Disease 18, 229-276

Sciamanna E (1882) Fenomeni prodotti dall'applicazione della corrente elettrica sulla dura madre e modificazione del polso cerebrale. Ricerche sperimentali sull'uomo. Memorie della Classe di scienze fisiche, matematiche e naturali 13, 25-42

Sciamanna E and Mingazzini G (1882) Ricerche sul polso cerebrale. Archivio di Psichiatria, Scienze Penali ed Antropologia Criminale 2, 310-311

Soh K, Larsen, B, Skinhøj E, and Lassen NA (1978) Regional cerebral blood flow in aphasia. Archives of Neurology 35, 625-632

Sokoloff L (1959) The action of drugs on the cerebral circulation. Pharmacological Reviews 11, 1–85

Sokoloff L (1961) Local cerebral circulation at rest and during altered cerebral activity induced by anesthesia or visual stimulation. In: Kety SS, Elkes J, (eds). The regional chemistry, physiology and pharmacology of the nervous system. Oxford, Pergamon Press

Sokoloff L, Reivich M, Kennedy C et al (1977) The [^{14}C] deoxyglucose method for the measurement of local cerebral glucose utilization: theory, procedure, and normal values in the conscious and anesthetized albino rat. Journal of Neurochemistry 28: 897-916

Sokoloff L (2001) Historical review of developments in the field of cerebral blood flow and metabolism. In: Fukuuchi Y, Tomita M, Koto A (eds) Ischemic blood flow in the brain. Keio University Symposia for Life Science and Medicine, Vol. 6. Tokio, Springer-Verlag.

Sokoloff L (2008) The physiological and biochemical bases of functional brain imaging. Cognitive Neurodynamics 2, 1-5

Sveinsdottir E and Lassen NA (1973) Detector system for measuring regional cerebral blood flow (abstr.). Stroke 4, 365, 1973

Taber KH, Black KJ, and Hurley, RA (2005) Blood flow imaging of the brain: 50 years experience. The Journal of Neuropsychiatry and Clinical Neurosciences 17, 441-446

Tanzi E (1888) Ricerche termo-elettriche sulla corteccia cerebrale in relazione con gli stati emotivi. Rivista Sperimentale di Freniatria e di Medicina Legale 14, 234-269

Ter-Pogossian MM, Eichling JO, Davis DO, Welch MJ and Metzger JM (1969) The determination of regional cerebral blood flow by means of water labeled with radioactive oxygen 15. Radiology 93, 31-40

Ter-Pogossian MM, Eichling JO, Davis DO and Welch MJ (1970) The measure of regional cerebral oxigen utilization by means of oxyhemoglobin labeled with radioactive oxygen-15. The Journal of Clinical Investigation 49, 381-391

Ter-Pogossian MM, Phelps ME, Hoffman EJ, and Mullani NA (1975) A positron-emission transaxial tomograph for nuclear imaging (PETT). Radiology 114, 89–98

Thulborn KR, Waterton JC, Matthews PM, Radda GK (1982) Oxygenation dependence of the transverse relaxation time of water protons in whole blood at high field. Biochimica et Biophysica Acta 714, 265-270

Zago S, Ferrucci, R, Marceglia S and Priori A (2009) The Mosso method for recording brain pulsation: the forerunner of functional neuroimaging. Neuroimage 48, 652-656

Weber E (1910) Der einfluss psychischer vorgänge auf den körper. Cited in: Lowe MF (1935) The application of the balance to the study of the bodily changes occurring during periods of volitional activity. British Journal of Psychology 26, 245-262

www-Nobelprize.org

2

fMRI for the Assessment of Functional Connectivity

Till Nierhaus, Daniel Margulies, Xiangyu Long and Arno Villringer
Max-Planck-Institute for Human Cognitive and Brain Sciences, Leipzig
Germany

1. Introduction

The advantage of modern brain imaging techniques is the ability to non-invasively investigate human brain function during mental work. Therefore, most functional neuroimaging studies have investigated brain activity evoked by certain types of stimulation or tasks. Related brain function is then localized by contrasting task-states, or often, with a baseline-state acquired during rest. However, in wakeful human subjects this resting condition cannot be associated with neutral brain activity, in part, because there is always a relatively high level of neuronal background activity. Thus, the question arises whether spontaneous fluctuations of resting brain activity can be dismissed as stochastic noise, or whether they contain functionally relevant information.

In the past decade, numerous studies have investigated brain activity during the resting state. Background activity has been shown to fluctuate spontaneously, i.e. unrelated to any obvious task, and that these fluctuations are not random. Rather, this spontaneous activity is characterized by several distinct pattern of correlated brain activity, so called: "resting state networks". Network activity, usually derived from temporal correlation of neuronal activity measured in different brain regions ("functional connectivity"), describes the functional relationship between brain regions. Functional connectivity networks have been identified by different methods, such as positron emission tomography (PET), optical imaging, magneto- and electroencephalography (M/EEG), whereas by far most studies made use of functional magnetic resonance imaging (fMRI) data. Traditionally, functional connectivity measures rely on correlation analyses, however in recent years the analytic tools for describing the functional organization of the brain has increased dramatically.

This chapter will provide insight into different ways to assess functional connectivity from resting-state fMRI data and describe applications of functional connectivity analyses to specific scientific questions. We will start with a description of the BOLD-effect, the underlying neurophysiological parameter in resting-state fMRI, followed by a résumé of the use of BOLD in functional neuroimaging, stating its history from simple "baseline-task-contrasts" to the nowadays widely-used concept of functional connectivity. In the following sub-chapters, we will briefly describe analytic categories as applied to resting-state fMRI data, including "seed-based functional connectivity", "independent component analysis (ICA)", "clustering", "multivariate pattern analysis (MVPA)", "graph theory" and "centrality". Finally, we will discuss two specific applications of functional connectivity analyses: (1) investigation of anatomy, and (2) investigation of dynamics using simultaneous EEG-fMRI measurements.

2. History of BOLD in functional neuroimaging, and the beginnings of functional connectivity in both task-states and rest

fMRI is the most widely used imaging technique in modern cognitive neuroscience. It allows for non-invasive (albeit indirect) studying of neuronal processes in the brain with excellent spatial resolution. While the first functional MRI experiment was performed with an exogenous contrast agent (Belliveau et al., 1991), fortunately another method was developed using magnetic properties of blood itself, so that such a contrast agent was no longer required for functional imaging (Bandettini et al., 1992; Frahm et al., 1992; Kwong et al., 1992; Ogawa et al., 1992). The fMRI signal depends on the vascular response to functional brain activation and is typically implemented by imaging of the blood oxygenation-level dependent (BOLD) contrast.

2.1 The BOLD-effect

The use of the BOLD effect for imaging brain activation relies on the fact that changes in neuronal activity are associated with changes in energy consumption and cerebral blood flow (Roy & Sherrington, 1890; Villringer & Dirnagl, 1995)[1]. Since changes in oxygen consumption and blood flow are associated with changes in haemoglobin oxygenation, the latter can also be used as an indirect measure of neuronal activity, assuming that activated neuronal circuits have an increased metabolic demand.

The magnetic susceptibility of blood depends on the magnetic properties of haemoglobin, the molecule carrying the oxygen necessary for aerobic cellular metabolism. During brain activation, blood focally changes its oxygenation level, which depends on the proportion of oxygenated haemoglobin ([oxy-Hb]) and deoxygenated haemoglobin ([deoxy-Hb]). [oxy-Hb] is a diamagnetic molecule, whereas [deoxy-Hb] is paramagnetic. The presence of [deoxy-Hb] causes local field inhomogeneities, which are responsible for a dephasing of the local transversal magnetization[2], leading to a reduction in the transverse relaxation time T_2.

---

[1] Although fMRI is widely used in scientific and clinical approaches, the complex mechanism describing the coupling of neuronal activity and metabolic demand ("neurovascular coupling") is not yet fully understood. Not only the role of the different mediators dealing with neurovascular coupling is under debate, also the formation of the vascular response obtained with fMRI is unclear (Buxton et al. 1998; Steinbrink et al. 2006; Villringer & Dirnagl 1995).

[2] In medicine, the MR signal is usually based on the magnetic dipole moment of hydrogen nuclei (protons) in water, by far the most abundant nuclei in the human body. In a static magnetic field B_0, these magnetic dipole moments generate a magnetisation vector M_L longitudinal oriented to B_0. Applying an adequate radio frequency pulse induces an additional magnetic field B_1, that flips M into the plane perpendicular to B_0. According to classical mechanics, this transversal magnetisation vector M_T starts rotating about the direction of B_0, inducing a voltage in a receiver coil proportional to the proton density. In the absence of B1, however, the excited magnetic spins will return to equilibrium. This relaxation is characterised by (1) a re-growth of M_L with the time constant T_1, and (2) by a decay of M_T with the time constant T_2. The values of T1 and T2 depend on tissue composition, structure and surroundings. The setting of a long echo time TE, that is the time between excitation and read-out, produces T_2-weighted images, because only tissue with a long T_2 decay constant will contribute to the signal intensity.

As a diamagnetic molecule, [oxy-Hb] does not produce the same dephasing. Thus, changes in [deoxy-Hb] can be observed as the BOLD contrast in T_2-weighted MR-images, serving as an indirect measure of neuronal activity. Since neuronal activation is accompanied by a focal increase in oxygenated blood, overshooting the actual metabolic demand, activated brain areas are characterised by positive BOLD responses in fMRI measurements.

2.2 From 'baseline' to 'resting' to 'intrinsic' dynamics

For functional investigations of the human brain, typically, a task or a stimulus is administered to a subject in a block or event-related experimental design and the resulting changes in neuronal activity are detected by contrasting a "task-state" and a "control- or baseline-state". The term "baseline-state" thereby cannot be associated with "zero brain activity", since even during so called "rest conditions", there is always some neuronal activity (spikes, synaptic activity) associated with a relatively high level of (baseline) cerebral blood flow and oxygen consumption (Clarke & Sokoloff, 1999; Sokoloff et al., 1955 for a review Raichle, 2010). Such task-state contrasts are by far the most used data analysis approach in fMRI assuming more or less constant baseline activity to be independent from task- or stimulation-evoked activity.

Given that baseline activity is not zero, the question arises whether spontaneous fluctuations of resting brain activity are stochastic ("noise") and thus can be simply attenuated by averaging procedures. Furthermore, it is of relevance whether fluctuations of the baseline influence the shape and amplitude of task-evoked activity during the stimulation period. In recent years, the issue of "physiological noise" and brain activity during resting states has become accessible for investigation. Numerous studies have been published examining spontaneous fluctuations of baseline activity (i.e. unrelated to any obvious task) in the low-frequency range <0.1 Hz (Biswal et al., 1995; Fox et al., 2005). These fluctuations contain important function-related information and it has been shown that "resting states" are characterized by several distinct patterns of correlated intrinsic brain activity, so called "resting state networks", describing intrinsic functional connectivity (Gusnard & Raichle, 2001). Resting state activity has been identified by different methods, such as fMRI, PET, Optical Imaging, EEG, and MEG, and in several instances simultaneous combinations of methods such as EEG/fMRI have been particularly useful. In addition, numerous studies have addressed the influence of ongoing activity on behavioural responses and the relationship between ongoing activity and evoked activity (Becker et al., 2011; Scheeringa et al., 2011; for a review Nierhaus et al., 2009; Sadaghiani et al., 2010).

2.2.1 Task-state contrasts (evoked brain activity)

Despite the fact that vascular responses are only indirectly related to changes in brain activity and that they develop with time constants of several seconds to the underlying neuronal activity, vascular methods, in particular fMRI, have become the most widely used method for the assessment of evoked brain activity. Stimuli or tasks are organized either in an event-related design, a block design, or a mixture of those two. Data analysis typically employs a general linear model of evoked brain activity (Friston et al., 1995). By contrasting the "activated state" with the "control state", changes in brain activity due to task or stimulation are visualized. Figure 1 shows a typical fMRI response for a somatosensory stimulation paradigm, where subjects received 4-Hz electrical stimulation of the left middle finger at amplitude twice of the sensory perception threshold.

Alternating stimulation blocks with resting periods allowed for contrasting two activation states, revealing a positive BOLD signal change in the contralateral primary somatosensory cortex, whereas the secondary somatosensory cortices are bilaterally activated (Fig.1A). The time course of the activated region shows a high correlation with the stimulation, and the peak of the hemodynamic response occurs with a delay of several seconds. This approach of contrasting rest- and task-state assumes fluctuations of baseline activity to appear merely stochastic and independent from evoked activity, thus vanishing in the averaging process.

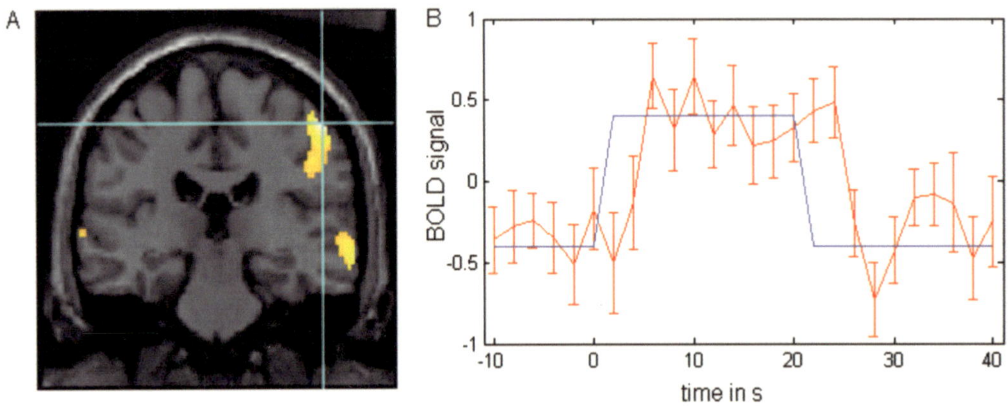

Fig. 1. Evoked brain activity. BOLD fMRI response on 4 Hz electrical stimulation of the left middle finger (adapted from Taskin et al., 2006). Stimulation was applied in blocks of 20 s alternating with periods of rest of the same duration. (A) The activation map generated by contrasting stimulation- with resting-periods (statistical T-maps, n=6, $p<0.05$ corrected for multiple comparisons). (B) BOLD dynamics as average time course over 30 blocks (red, mean+ S.E.M.) of the labelled region in A and stimulation paradigm (blue).

2.2.2 Resting state (ongoing brain activity)

The apparent "noise" in the BOLD signal was quite early assessed to have neuronal components, however, only in recent years has its investigation become a wide-spread research endeavour. Bharat Biswal and colleagues at the Medical College of Wisconsin demonstrated in 1995 that low frequency fluctuations of baseline (resting state) fMRI contain information about background neuronal activity (Biswal et al., 1995), which was subsequently elaborated by other groups (Fox et al., 2005; Greicius et al., 2003). Such correlations in the patterns of spontaneous activity specifically within the low-frequency band (<0.1 Hz) have given rise to the study of "resting state networks", an example of which is depicted in Figure 2.

The approach of measuring BOLD signal independent of any task makes the method independent of any differences of performance between sessions and/or subjects. Therefore, resting-state fMRI can be easily employed in patients with potentially limited ability for participation in task paradigms. Indeed it has been successfully applied in many clinical populations e.g., with Alzheimer disease (Greicius et al., 2004; Sorg et al., 2007), schizophrenia (Calhoun et al., 2009), stroke (van Meer et al., 2010), and different age-groups (Madden et al., 2010).

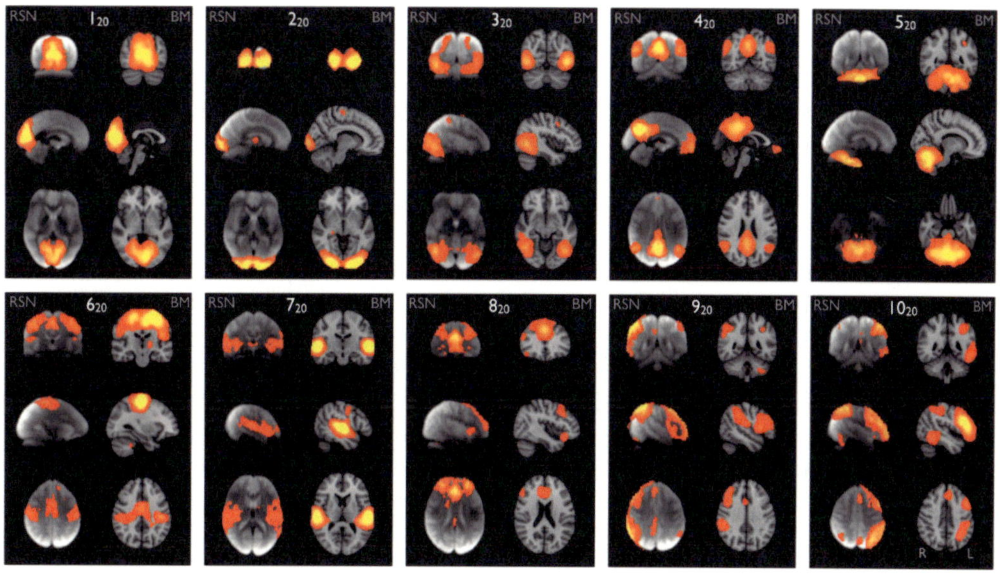

Fig. 2. Figure from Smith et al. (2009) depicting similarity between 'resting-state network' (left) and task-coactivation derived networks (right).

Many questions remain open regarding the mechanisms underlying the coherence of these spatially-distributed, low-frequency fluctuations. However, the rapid employment of these techniques by the imaging community over the past decade is due, in part, to both the ease of data acquisition and the similarity of results to previous finding using task-induced approaches. Since the methods for analysing resting-state activity are not limited to data acquired during 'rest', the term 'functional connectivity' has gained popularity, describing functional interplay of spatially distinct brain regions.

3. A brief overview of analytic methods to assess functional connectivity

Different post-processing techniques can be used for identifying spatial patterns of coherent BOLD activity in fMRI data, allowing for interpretation regarding functional connectivity[3] between spatially distributed brain areas. Since the following subchapters will explain only very briefly the idea and theoretical presuppositions of each analytic tool, for a more detailed description, we refer to a recent review by our group (Margulies et al., 2010).

3.1 Seed-based functional connectivity

This technique makes use of correlation from an *a priori* region-of-interest (ROI) or "seed region". In its simplest form, an averaged ROI time series is correlated with the time series of

[3] Functional Connectivity is often described in contrast to Effective Connectivity. While the former describes different brain regions which are functionally connected, the latter addresses the direction of these neuronal interactions. Causality models, such as Dynamic Causal Modelling, Structural Equation Modelling or Granger Causality are used to estimate effective connectivity from neuroimaging data. Assuming that better prediction is an indication of influence, the common idea is to determine whether activity in one brain region can be predicted by the dynamics in other brain regions.

all the other voxels in the brain, or with the average time series of several distributed ROIs. The resulting matrix of correlation coefficients then can be interpreted as the functional connectivity of the selected seed region, where a high correlation coefficient indicates strong functional connectivity to the respective area. From such correlation maps, a number of different functional networks have been derived, e.g. a motor network, a visual network, the default-mode network and others. Seed-based functional connectivity analysis was initially applied to resting-state data by Biswal et al. (1995), showing motor cortex functional connectivity being similar to motor task activity patterns. Mapping the default-mode network - which is implicitly linked to the brains resting state - was much later achieved (Greicius et al., 2003).

Correlation of time series implies quantifying the relation of two signals in the time-domain (such as 'covariance' or 'cross-correlation'). Of course, different mathematical methods can be used to quantify the relationship between the seed region time series and the time series of other voxels or ROIs. While 'coherence' operates equivalently in the frequency-domain (Sun et al., 2004), another approach would be to explore the 'phase-spectrum delay' between regions (Sun et al., 2005). Thus, the choice of the proper mathematical method, and the selection, size and shape of the *a priori* defined seed region are critical variables for assessing functional connectivity with the seed-based method (Van Dijk et al., 2010).

3.2 Independent Component Analysis (ICA)

One of the features of resting-state analysis is that there is no stimulation paradigm for researchers to be dependent on. Therefore, many data-driven solutions have been employed for identification of low-frequency resting state patterns (Beckmann et al., 2005; Fox & Raichle, 2007). The most widely used approach is Independent Component Analysis (ICA). By using blind source separation techniques[4], ICA methods decompose the entire BOLD data set into statistically independent components (Hyvärinen & Oja, 2000) without any hypothesis paradigms, i.e. prior seed definition is not required any more. Researchers found that several separated spatial components could accurately represent specific functional networks during resting state. Many neuroimaging studies have demonstrated that ICA is a productive tool for investigating resting-state fMRI data. Some widely studied functional networks e.g., the default mode network and motor network, show consistency across subjects (Damoiseaux et al., 2006; Zuo et al., 2010). ICA has also been successfully applied to demonstrate significant differences in connectivity patterns between patients and healthy controls (Calhoun et al., 2009; Greicius et al., 2004; Sorg et al., 2007). In addition to identifying functionally relevant networks, ICA also enables automatic separation of artificial and physiological noise sources from fMRI data (De Martino et al., 2007; Tohka et al., 2008).

Still, two controversial issues should be considered: specifying the number of components and selecting those that are functionally meaningful. The number of independent

---

[4] Blind source separation techniques underlie the assumption that the measured signal is a linear mixture of independent signals from a number of spatially distributed sources. Decomposition algorithms separate multi-channel data into a set of such independent spatial or temporal components. Temporal decomposition is widely used in EEG research, generating sources, each given by a time course of its activity and a weighting-vector, describing its contribution to the signal recorded in each sensor. As fMRI data usually consists of more spatial than temporal data points, spatial decomposition is more widely applied.

components appropriate to resting-state data is an issue of ongoing debate, and several data driven approaches for optimising the selection of this number have been developed (Beckmann & Smith, 2004; Li et al., 2007). However, it is worthwhile to consider that due to the multiple scales of functional organisation in the brain, determining the number of functionally relevant components is also a product of the spatial scale of interest. Thus, even with data driven approaches like ICA, certain assumptions about brain organization are still required. Selecting components that are of functional relevance is another challenging issue with ICA. While automatic rejection of artefact components can be implemented rather easily (through assessing the frequency spectrum or high spatial scattering), the most commonly used method for identifying functionally relevant components, such as the default-mode network, remains visual inspection by an expert—though several automated network selection approaches have also been proposed (Greicius et al., 2004; De Martino et al., 2007).

3.3 Multivariate Pattern Analysis (MVPA)

In recent years the use of pattern-classification algorithms has gained increasing importance in fMRI data analysis (for reviews Haynes & Rees, 2006; Norman et al., 2006). In general, these algorithms use specific features of objects to identify classes to which they belong. In fMRI data, spatially distributed brain activation or connectivity patterns are used as features to classify different brain or cognitive states. Applying this technique requires in the beginning a training of the classification algorithm with the features and the prespecified classes. Thereby a subset of the data (training-set) must be used to attune the classifier on the relationship between features and classes, before the rest of the data (testing-set) can be used to verify the classifiers capability for new/unknown data.

Feature selection and the choice of a proper classifier are critical issues to achieve good results. While mathematical methods allow for a data driven, automated selection of discriminative features, a manual selection method can be beneficial for designing application specific features. For pattern classification, usually supervised[5] machine learning algorithms, such as support vector machines (SVM), neural networks, or linear discriminant analysis (LDA), are used. Knowledge about the relationship between features and classes (i.e. a linear or non-linear relation is assumed) should be taken into account for classifier selection.

Revealing disease-related differences in resting-state functional connectivity, MVPA has been successfully used for disease-state prediction, discriminating patients and healthy controls (Craddock et al., 2009; Shen et al., 2010; Zhu et al., 2008).

3.4 Clustering

Similar to MVPA, clustering is a family of mathematical techniques that can be applied to fMRI data to search for characteristic patterns. However, clustering algorithms tend to find patterns without specific knowledge about classes. This means that data is partitioned (classified) into subsets (clusters) in an unsupervised manner, such that observations assigned to the same cluster are similar. Different clustering algorithms[6] have been applied

---

[5] Unsupervised algorithms, such as clustering, tend to find pattern without prior knowledge about the desired classes, inevitably increasing uncertainty of the whole procedure.

[6] Different clustering approaches are e.g. 'hierarchical clustering', 'partitional clustering', 'spectral clustering' or 'non-metric clustering', and the development and improvement of clustering methods is an intense research field (Margulies et al., 2010).

to fMRI data in several studies deriving clusters of voxels or regions that represent known functional or anatomical subdivisions in the brain (Bellec et al., 2010; van den Heuvel et al., 2008; Salvador et al., 2005). Another approach is division of the data into functional units by clustering voxels that have similar pattern of functional connectivity (Cohen et al., 2008). Although a model-free approach (in this sense similar to ICA) which finds specific pattern without prior assumptions (as e.g. seed selection in model based approaches), clustering still involves human judgement. Usually, the user has to define a number of clusters in which the data should be partitioned, and the clustering results need comparison with known functional networks.

3.5 Graph theory

Characterising aspects of network structure is a common mathematical problem in which graphs represent mathematical structures describing pairwise relations between objects in a certain network. A graph consists of a collection of *vertices* or *nodes*, and a collection of *edges* connecting pairs of vertices. A *path* in a graph is a sequence of vertices which are connected by edges, and the *distance* between two vertices is the shortest path connecting them. The *degree* of a vertex is the number of terminating edges. Vertices with very high degrees are termed *hubs*. Translated to fMRI data, a voxel or ROI constitute a vertex and their connections are represented by edges. Thus, the theoretical framework of graph theory can be used to analyse brain networks obtained from imaging data (for a review see Bullmore & Sporns, 2009). Given a functional connectivity map, a graph representation can be derived either by assigning an edge if the correlation between two vertices exceeds a certain threshold, or the correlation coefficients themselves can be used to weight each edge.

Numerous tools can be used for characterising such network organisation, which can be conceptually divided into 'local' measures (characterising vertices individually) and 'global' measures (characterising the whole graph). The latter is e.g. realised by the degree distribution $P(k)$, that represents the probability that a randomly chosen vertex has the degree k (Achard et al., 2006; Eguíluz et al., 2005; Nakamura et al., 2009). It also offers information about the number of *hubs* in a graph - obviously regions of special interest for connectivity analyses (Buckner et al., 2009). The ability to separate a network into clusters with high internal connectivity is described by *modularity*, whereas the degree of integration of a graph can be described by the *average path length*. Combining these measures brings up the fundamental approach of the brain being characterised as a *small-world network*, supporting both modular processing of information by high clustering and distributed information processing via short wiring distances (Bassett & Bullmore, 2006).

3.6 Centrality

One of the graph-based approaches is the centrality measure. The centrality of a node within a network is an estimation of the relative importance of that node within a network.

Eigenvector centrality mapping (ECM) was recently implemented to estimate the centrality of human brain regions with fMRI data (Lohmann et al., 2010). In their study, the linear correlation was proposed to generate a network of every voxel within the entire brain. Then centrality of each voxel was estimated within its own brain network. They found that some brain regions, e.g. precuneus, cerebellum, showed higher centrality than other brain regions during resting state scan. In addition, by comparing centrality between a hungry and sated condition, the results showed that the precuneus has higher centrality in a hungry state than in a sated state.

The ECM analysis is a data-driven method and therefore it is an appropriate tool for data analysis of "resting-state" studies. There are only few studies on centrality of brain regions but if validity is confirmed, centrality measures will probably be of wide interest for many studies on the human brain in experimental and clinical settings.

4. Applications of functional connectivity analyses to specific scientific questions

As we have just described, functional connectivity provides a means of investigating underlying organization of functional systems in the brain. While each of these methodologies allows for the description of specific aspects of network structure, interaction, and organization, the research question we are now stuck with is how to meaningfully apply such techniques. We will here describe two main avenues of research, broadly categorized by anatomical and dynamical lines of investigation. More specifically, anatomical questions will relate to spatial aspects of brain organization, how regions connect to one another, and how those patterns differ between mental states, or between patients and healthy control populations. Dynamical aspects address the interactions in time between brain regions, and can likewise be evaluated for the aforementioned categorical differences. We consider the anatomical/dynamical distinction valuable because each set of research questions brackets a different set of analytic tools. For instance, in evaluating neuroanatomy, the relation between two regions can be quantified using a variety of correlation-based metrics, however, the aim of such analyses lies predominantly in the resulting spatial maps.

4.1.1 Investigation of anatomy

Brain mapping is mostly based on anatomical structures, e.g., Brodmann areas. Numerous schemas have been proposed over the past century for describing subdivisions in various areas of the cortex and subcortical regions. Among them, cytoarchitectonics, the mapping of the cellular structure within the cortical layers, has maintained popularity as a method for describing cortical areas within the functional neuroimaging literature. However, cytoarchitectonic mapping has the disadvantage of only being discernable using histological techniques, making it difficult to subsequently conduct functional imaging studies on the same research subjects. Function-based brain mapping is strongly demanded because of the value of precisely localizing functional areas in the brain. Intrinsic functional connectivity approaches, a synonym of resting-state functional connectivity, however, take advantage of a primary characteristic of the brain: namely, its connectivity. Connectivity has previously been applied extensively in the macaque monkey using axonal labelling tract-tracing techniques. The success of this approach in the macaque suggests that a non-invasive approach in humans also holds great promise.

In humans, resting-state functional connectivity has been successfully used to map divisions with complex structures such as the anterior cingulate (Margulies et al., 2007), precuneus (Margulies et al., 2009), striatum (Di Martino et al., 2008), lateral parietal lobule (Cohen et al., 2008; Mars et al., 2011; Nelson et al., 2010), motor cortex (Cauda et al., 2010; van den Heuvel & Hulshoff Pol, 2010), to name a few examples. In addition, functional connectivity has been demonstrated to map closely to anatomical connectivity methods, such as diffusion tensor imaging (DTI) tractography (Greicius et al., 2009; Skudlarski et al., 2008) and tract tracing studies in the macaque monkey (Margulies et al., 2009; Mars et al., 2011; Vincent et al., 2007). Therefore, several studies have begun to use functional networks to find functional areas within some anatomical brain regions. For instance, precuneus has been found to show similar sub-regions distribution in human and monkey (Margulies et al., 2009). In addition, supplementary motor area has been demonstrated to be organized into two functional anterior-posterior structures based on their respective functional networks (Kim et al., 2010), and a lateral-medial structure has been found in anterior bank of central gyrus (Long et al., 2010). These findings strongly suggest that functional network is a useful approach to delineating functionally unique brain regions. Underlying the strength of this approach is the hypothesis that differential functional connectivity is associated with differentiable functional roles.

4.1.2 Methods for investigating neuroanatomy

As previously described, the seed-based correlation approach creates a spatial map for an individual seed. These spatial maps can then be used as features to distinguish seed regions from one another. This can be done through both visual inspection, direct contrasts of the respective functional connectivity maps, and also through computationally based clustering techniques (e.g., Cohen et al., 2008; Kelly et al., 2010)

As the seed-based functional connectivity approach aims to describe the connectivity of a single region-of-interest, regions can also be delineated as whole networks (or 'functional systems'). The ICA approach previously described aims to pull out whole networks simultaneously using a multivariate approach. The primary advantage of this approach is that it can describe independent systems without a priori hypotheses about the spatial location of such systems. Notable early examples of this approach aimed to characterize the number of unique "resting-state networks" throughout the brain (Beckmann et al., 2005; Damoiseaux et al., 2006; De Luca et al., 2006; Smith et al., 2009). Discriminating the appropriate number of networks is still a challenge to the community, as the number of networks derived using ICA requires a priori assumptions. However, this data-driven approach also offers the advantage of not requiring prior assumptions about the location of networks.

4.2.1 Investigation of dynamics: simultaneous EEG-fMRI

Although fMRI is widely used in clinical and scientific approaches, many fundamental questions are still unknown; most notably, the precise relationship to the underlying neuronal activity. Despite significant progress in understanding this relationship (Lauritzen & Gold, 2003; Logothetis et al., 2001; Shibasaki, 2008), based on BOLD signal alone, the underlying neuronal activity cannot be recovered unambiguously ("Inverse Problem of fMRI"). This is not only due to the poor temporal resolution of the vascular response but also due to the fact that different types of neuronal (and non-neuronal) events such as excitatory/inhibitory postsynaptic potentials (EPSP/IPSP), action potentials, glia-activity, etc., are being translated into only a one-dimensional variable of "more or less" BOLD signal. Additional sources of information are frequently needed for further clarification of the underlying processes in the respective brain areas. Particularly, the combination of fMRI with electrophysiological methods such as EEG may be useful for this purpose. Simultaneous EEG-fMRI approaches allow for investigation of the link between changes in

EEG patterns and changes in the vascular signal. For functional connectivity studies, investigating intrinsic brain activity at rest, the EEG signal then can be used as independent variable, classifying brain states in the absence of any stimulation or task paradigm.

Of special interest for the investigation of intrinsic brain activity is spectral analysis of the ongoing EEG. Many perceptual and cognitive processes emerge from recurrent network interactions, which are induced by, but not necessarily phased-locked to external events. Analysis of event-related potentials (ERP)[7] excludes these non-phase-locked signal components from investigation. Different background rhythms in a large range of frequency bands have been described, not only recorded during 'rest', but also with relation to various cognitive states, mental activity, and showing specific temporal pattern following external events (for a review see Nierhaus et al., 2009). Since different sensory networks were found to exhibit distinct background rhythms[8], resting rhythmic activity denotes a network specific attribute, describing network activity from a different angle. Thus, investigating the relationship of spectral EEG phenomena and functional connectivity maps derived from fMRI data is an obvious and promising challenge.

4.2.2 Associating EEG rhythms and resting-state networks

Simultaneous EEG-fMRI measurements have been applied to investigate the relationship of electrophysiological background rhythms and BOLD signal fluctuations (for reviews see Laufs 2008; Ritter & Villringer 2006). Most of these studies show an inverse correlation of the background rhythm strength with the spontaneous BOLD signal fluctuations in the cortical sensory area generating the respective rhythm. However, positive correlations between subcortical, i.e., thalamic BOLD signals and occipital EEG alpha power have also been reported. Investigation of stimulus driven responses revealed a close coupling between gamma-band (40-100 Hz) activity and BOLD signal of sensory cortical regions, demonstrated using intracranial recordings in human (Lachaux et al., 2007; Mukamel et al., 2005) and in animals (Logothetis et al., 2001; Niessing et al., 2005). Since gamma-band activity is associated with sensory information processing, further investigation with simultaneous EEG-fMRI should allow for a better understanding of resting-state network behaviour during mental work. First attempts of such investigations were recently performed using direct intracerebral recordings in the default-mode network (Jerbi et al., 2010). Execution of attention-demanding tasks were shown to suppress gamma power accompanied by BOLD deactivation.

The default-mode network (DMN) has also been investigated in several EEG-fMRI studies. Using the power of spontaneous EEG oscillations, a positive correlation of the *beta* frequency band with the DMN was shown (Laufs et al., 2003). The DMN activity has also been found to be negatively correlated to frontal theta power derived using ICA on the EEG data in a

---

[7] Repeated measures of external events with subsequent averaging enables investigation of the isolated neural response phase-locked to the event.

[8] Most prominent is the occipital *alpha* rhythm with a frequency between 8-12 Hz. Since occipital alpha is strongest in the absence of visual input, it is referred to as the "idle rhythm" of the visual system. Such inverse relationship of rhythm strength and sensory input is also found for pericentral rhythms, with peak frequencies around 12 Hz (*mu*) and 20 Hz (*beta*), which are known to desynchronise following motor activation or somatosensory stimulation. Oscillations with a frequency of 3-8 Hz are termed *theta,* which are most prominent in hippocampus and frontal cortex and are associated with the neural basis of learning and memory. *Delta* oscillations (1-3 Hz) are a characteristic feature of deeper sleep stages.

resting state experiment (Scheeringa et al., 2008) and, in a second study, even at the single trial level increases of frontal theta power induced by a working memory task were correlated to decreased DMN activity (Scheeringa et al., 2009).
Mantini et al. used ICA to identify resting-state networks in fMRI data and then correlated the time courses of these networks with the power of five specific EEG frequency bands (*delta, theta, alpha, beta, gamma*), averaged across the entire scalp (Mantini et al., 2007). Four of six networks, including a dorsal attention network and a somatomotor network, showed exclusively negative correlations with EEG frequency band power. Again, the DMN showed a positive correlation with *beta* activity, and here additionally with *alpha* power. Also gamma power was found to be positively correlated with one network, well in line with the previous described invasive findings. Improved results could be expected from EEG source separation with direct correlation of source and network activity.
A common way to integrate EEG data into fMRI analyses is to take EEG frequency band power as a regressor in a general linear model, thus, investigating how well fMRI data is explained by certain features of the EEG. Vice versa it would be interesting if the EEG data can be explained by fMRI activity pattern. To address this question, MVPA might be a helpful technique: brain activation or connectivity pattern could be used as features to train a classifier, which capability then would be verified using EEG data.
Also "centrality mapping" could be a promising approach for analysing simultaneous acquired EEG-fMRI data. Therefor, the average time course of regions indicated by high centrality must be correlated with the time course of frequency band power of EEG source activity. The results would show whether regions of high "hubness" are also involved in EEG rhythm generation.

5. Conclusion

In the past decades the view on background fluctuations in brain activity, which were previously assumed to reflect (stochastic) "physiological noise", has changed dramatically: Spontaneous fluctuations have been identified to contain important information reflecting brain function. Specifically, it has been shown that the brain 'at rest' is characterised by several distinct pattern of correlated brain activity - resting state networks - and that changes in network activity can be associated with cognitive states, mental activity and pathophysiological conditions.
Numerous techniques can be applied to fMRI data for investigating functional connectivity, each with different weaknesses and strengths, depending on the experimental design and the kind of research question/hypothesis. Although described very briefly, we endeavoured to provide insight into each of the various options for investigating functional brain organisation with fMRI data. Further, two main research fields were broadly categorized by anatomical and dynamical lines of investigation, covering meaningful applications of the aforementioned analysis techniques.
The use of functional connectivity to investigate spatial aspects of brain organization is based on the assumption that brain areas with different functional roles exhibit differential functional connectivity pattern. Parcellating brain regions by their functional network patterns allows for a more precise localisation of brain function and there is no doubt that a well-investigated function-based human mapping will be created in future studies.
Investigating dynamical changes using EEG and fMRI indicate that EEG background rhythms and fMRI-based resting state measures are closely related, revealing network

specific attributes from different angles. Furthermore, simultaneous EEG/fMRI provides insights into the spatio-temporal organization of intrinsic signal fluctuations, whether measured at rest or during stimulation or task. Thereby, the interplay of these rhythmic fluctuations measured with different modalities at rest can be analysed in a straightforward manner. However, tasks involving perception and cognition are accompanied by fast changes in EEG signals, and it is still a major challenge for cognitive neuroscience to link these transient EEG features to measures of functional connectivity. A proper combination of the aforementioned analytic tools will help to further understand this link with task-based approaches, and will enable future investigation of the interaction between ongoing dynamical changes and transient activations evoked by task or stimulation.

6. Acknowledgment

The authors would like to thank The Neuro Bureau (www.neurobureau.org) and its affiliated team of researchers for continued creative support.

7. References

Achard, S., Salvador, R., Whitcher, B., Suckling, J., & Bullmore, E. (2006). A resilient, low-frequency, small-world human brain functional network with highly connected association cortical hubs. *The Journal of Neuroscience*, *26*(1), 63-72.

Bandettini, P. A., Wong, E. C., Hinks, R. S., Tikofsky, R. S., & Hyde, J. S. (1992). Time course EPI of human brain function during task activation. *Magnetic resonance in Medicine*, *25*(2), 390-7.

Bassett, D. S., & Bullmore, E. (2006). Small-world brain networks. *The Neuroscientist*, *12*(6), 512-23.

Becker, R, Reinacher, M., Freyer, F., Villringer, A., & Ritter, P. (2011). How ongoing neuronal oscillations account for variability of evoked fMRI responses. *The Journal of Neuroscience, in press.*

Beckmann, C. F., & Smith, Stephen M. (2004). Probabilistic independent component analysis for functional magnetic resonance imaging. *IEEE transactions on medical imaging*, *23*(2), 137-52.

Beckmann, C. F., DeLuca, M., Devlin, J. T., & Smith, Stephen M. (2005). Investigations into resting-state connectivity using independent component analysis. *Philosophical transactions of the Royal Society of London. Series B, Biological sciences*, *360*(1457), 1001-13.

Bellec, P., Rosa-Neto, P., Lyttelton, O. C., Benali, H., & Evans, A. C. (2010). Multi-level bootstrap analysis of stable clusters in resting-state fMRI. *NeuroImage*, *51*(3), 1126-39.

Belliveau, J. W., Kennedy, D. N., McKinstry, R. C., Buchbinder, B. R., Weisskoff, R. M., Cohen, M. S., Vevea, J. M., et al. (1991). Functional mapping of the human visual cortex by magnetic resonance imaging. *Science*, *254*(5032), 716-9.

Biswal, B. B., Yetkin, F. Z., Haughton, V. M., & Hyde, J. S. (1995). Functional connectivity in the motor cortex of resting human brain using echo-planar MRI. *Magnetic resonance in Medicine*, *34*(4), 537-41.

Buckner, R. L., Sepulcre, J., Talukdar, T., Krienen, F. M., Liu, H., Hedden, T., Andrews-Hanna, J. R., et al. (2009). Cortical hubs revealed by intrinsic functional connectivity: mapping, assessment of stability, and relation to Alzheimer's disease. *The Journal of Neuroscience, 29*(6), 1860-73.

Bullmore, E., & Sporns, O. (2009). Complex brain networks: graph theoretical analysis of structural and functional systems. *Nature reviews. Neuroscience, 10*(3), 186-98.

Buxton, R. B., Wong, E. C., & Frank, L. R. (1998). Dynamics of blood flow and oxygenation changes during brain activation: the balloon model. *Magnetic resonance in Medicine, 39*(6), 855-64.

Calhoun, V. D., Eichele, T., & Pearlson, G. (2009). Functional brain networks in schizophrenia: a review. *Frontiers in human neuroscience, 3*, 17.

Cauda, F., Giuliano, G., Federico, D., Sergio, D., & Katiuscia, S. (2010). Discovering the somatotopic organization of the motor areas of the medial wall using low-frequency bold fluctuations. *Human brain mapping*.

Clarke, D. D., & Sokoloff, L. (1999). Circulation and energy metabolism of the brain. In B. W. Agranoff & G. J. Siegel (Eds.), *Basic Neurochemistry. Molecular, Cellular and Medical Aspects* (6th ed., pp. 637-670). Philadelphia: Lippincott-Raven, ISBN-10: 0-397-51820-X.

Cohen, A. L., Fair, D. A., Dosenbach, N. U. F., Miezin, F. M., Dierker, D., Van Essen, David C, Schlaggar, B. L., et al. (2008). Defining functional areas in individual human brains using resting functional connectivity MRI. *NeuroImage, 41*(1), 45-57.

Craddock, R. C., Holtzheimer, P. E., Hu, X. P., & Mayberg, H. S. (2009). Disease state prediction from resting state functional connectivity. *Magnetic resonance in Medicine, 62*(6), 1619-28.

Damoiseaux, J. S., Rombouts, S. A. R. B., Barkhof, F., Scheltens, P., Stam, C. J., Smith, Stephen M, & Beckmann, C. F. (2006). Consistent resting-state networks across healthy subjects. *Proceedings of the National Academy of Sciences USA, 103*(37), 13848-53.

Van Dijk, K. R. A., Hedden, T., Venkataraman, A., Evans, K. C., Lazar, S. W., & Buckner, R. L. (2010). Intrinsic functional connectivity as a tool for human connectomics: theory, properties, and optimization. *Journal of neurophysiology, 103*(1), 297-321.

Eguíluz, V. M., Chialvo, D. R., Cecchi, G. A., Baliki, M., & Apkarian, A. V. (2005). Scale-free brain functional networks. *Physical review letters, 94*(1), 018102.

Fox, Michael D, & Raichle, Marcus E. (2007). Spontaneous fluctuations in brain activity observed with functional magnetic resonance imaging. *Nature reviews. Neuroscience, 8*(9), 700-11.

Fox, Michael D, Snyder, Abraham Z, Vincent, Justin L, Corbetta, Maurizio, Van Essen, David C, & Raichle, Marcus E. (2005). The human brain is intrinsically organized into dynamic, anticorrelated functional networks. *Proceedings of the National Academy of Sciences USA, 102*(27), 9673-8.

Frahm, J., Bruhn, H., Merboldt, K. D., & Hänicke, W. (1992). Dynamic MR imaging of human brain oxygenation during rest and photic stimulation. *Journal of magnetic resonance imaging : JMRI, 2*(5), 501-5.

Friston, K. J., Holmes, A. P., Poline, J. B., Grasby, P. J., Williams, S. C., Frackowiak, R. S. J., & Turner, R. (1995). Analysis of fMRI time-series revisited. *NeuroImage, 2*(1), 45-53.

Greicius, M. D., Krasnow, B., Reiss, A. L., & Menon, V. (2003). Functional connectivity in the resting brain: a network analysis of the default mode hypothesis. *Proceedings of the National Academy of Sciences USA, 100*(1), 253-8.

Greicius, M. D., Srivastava, G., Reiss, A. L., & Menon, V. (2004). Default-mode network activity distinguishes Alzheimer's disease from healthy aging: evidence from functional MRI. *Proceedings of the National Academy of Sciences USA, 101*(13), 4637-42.

Greicius, M. D., Supekar, K., Menon, V., & Dougherty, R. F. (2009). Resting-state functional connectivity reflects structural connectivity in the default mode network. *Cerebral cortex (New York, N.Y. : 1991), 19*(1), 72-8.

Gusnard, D. A., & Raichle, Marcus E. (2001). Searching for a baseline: functional imaging and the resting human brain. *Nature reviews. Neuroscience, 2*(10), 685-94.

Haynes, J.-D., & Rees, G. (2006). Decoding mental states from brain activity in humans. *Nature reviews. Neuroscience, 7*(7), 523-34.

van den Heuvel, M. P., & Hulshoff Pol, H. E. (2010). Specific somatotopic organization of functional connections of the primary motor network during resting state. *Human brain mapping, 31*(4), 631-44.

van den Heuvel, M., Mandl, R., & Hulshoff Pol, H. (2008). Normalized cut group clustering of resting-state FMRI data. *PloS one, 3*(4), e2001.

Hyvärinen, A., & Oja, E. (2000). Independent component analysis: algorithms and applications. *Neural networks, 13*(4-5), 411-30.

Jerbi, K., Vidal, J. R., Ossandon, T., Dalal, S. S., Jung, J., Hoffmann, D., Minotti, L., et al. (2010). Exploring the electrophysiological correlates of the default-mode network with intracerebral EEG. *Frontiers in systems neuroscience, 4*, 27.

Kelly, C., Uddin, Lucina Q., Shehzad, Zarrar, Margulies, Daniel S., Castellanos, F. Xavier, Milham, Michael P., & Petrides, M. (2010). Broca's region: linking human brain functional connectivity data and non-human primate tracing anatomy studies. *European Journal of Neuroscience, 32*(3), no-no.

Kim, J.-H., Lee, J.-M., Jo, H. J., Kim, S. H., Lee, J. H., Kim, S. T., Seo, S. W., et al. (2010). Defining functional SMA and pre-SMA subregions in human MFC using resting state fMRI: functional connectivity-based parcellation method. *NeuroImage, 49*(3), 2375-86.

Kwong, K. K., Belliveau, J. W., Chesler, D. A., Goldberg, I. E., Weisskoff, R. M., Poncelet, B. P., Kennedy, D. N., et al. (1992). Dynamic magnetic resonance imaging of human brain activity during primary sensory stimulation. *Proceedings of the National Academy of Sciences USA, 89*(12), 5675-9.

Lachaux, J.-P., Fonlupt, P., Kahane, P., Minotti, L., Hoffmann, D., Bertrand, O., & Baciu, M. (2007). Relationship between task-related gamma oscillations and BOLD signal: new insights from combined fMRI and intracranial EEG. *Human brain mapping, 28*(12), 1368-75.

Laufs, H, Krakow, K., Sterzer, P., Eger, E., Beyerle, A., Salek-Haddadi, A., & Kleinschmidt, A. (2003). Electroencephalographic signatures of attentional and cognitive default modes in spontaneous brain activity fluctuations at rest. *Proceedings of the National Academy of Sciences USA, 100*(19), 11053-8.

Laufs, Helmut. (2008). Endogenous brain oscillations and related networks detected by surface EEG-combined fMRI. *Human brain mapping, 29*(7), 762-9.

Lauritzen, M., & Gold, L. (2003). Brain function and neurophysiological correlates of signals used in functional neuroimaging. *The Journal of Neuroscience, 23*(10), 3972-80.

Li, Y.-O., Adali, T., & Calhoun, V. D. (2007). Estimating the number of independent components for functional magnetic resonance imaging data. *Human brain mapping, 28*(11), 1251-66.

Logothetis, N. K., Pauls, J., Augath, M., Trinath, T., & Oeltermann, A. (2001). Neurophysiological investigation of the basis of the fMRI signal. *Nature, 412*(6843), 150-7.

Lohmann, G., Margulies, Daniel S., Horstmann, A., Pleger, B., Lepsien, J., Goldhahn, D., Schloegl, H., et al. (2010). Eigenvector Centrality Mapping for Analyzing Connectivity Patterns in fMRI Data of the Human Brain. (O. Sporns, Ed.)*PLoS ONE, 5*(4), e10232.

Long, X., Margulies, Daniel S., & Villringer, A. (2010). Functional subregions within postcentral gyrus revealed by resting-state fMRI. *OHBM 2010, poster, Barcelona, Spain.*

De Luca, M., Beckmann, C. F., De Stefano, N., Matthews, P. M., & Smith, Stephen M. (2006). fMRI resting state networks define distinct modes of long-distance interactions in the human brain. *NeuroImage, 29*(4), 1359-67.

Madden, D. J., Costello, M. C., Dennis, N. A., Davis, S. W., Shepler, A. M., Spaniol, J., Bucur, B., et al. (2010). Adult age differences in functional connectivity during executive control. *NeuroImage, 52*(2), 643-57.

Mantini, D., Perrucci, M. G., Del Gratta, C., Romani, G. L., & Corbetta, Maurizio. (2007). Electrophysiological signatures of resting state networks in the human brain. *Proceedings of the National Academy of Sciences USA, 104*(32), 13170-5.

Margulies, Daniel S, Böttger, J., Long, X., Lv, Y., Kelly, C., Schäfer, A., Goldhahn, D., et al. (2010). Resting developments: a review of fMRI post-processing methodologies for spontaneous brain activity. *Magma (New York, N.Y.).*

Margulies, Daniel S, Kelly, A M Clare, Uddin, Lucina Q, Biswal, B. B., Castellanos, F Xavier, & Milham, Michael P. (2007). Mapping the functional connectivity of anterior cingulate cortex. *NeuroImage, 37*(2), 579-88.

Margulies, Daniel S, Vincent, Justin L, Kelly, C., Lohmann, G., Uddin, Lucina Q, Biswal, B. B., Villringer, A., et al. (2009). Precuneus shares intrinsic functional architecture in humans and monkeys. *Proceedings of the National Academy of Sciences USA, 106*(47), 20069-74.

Mars, R. B., Jbabdi, S., Sallet, J., O'Reilly, J. X., Croxson, P. L., Olivier, E., Noonan, M. P., et al. (2011). Diffusion-Weighted Imaging Tractography-Based Parcellation of the Human Parietal Cortex and Comparison with Human and Macaque Resting-State Functional Connectivity. *The Journal of Neuroscience, 31*(11), 4087-4100.

Di Martino, A, Scheres, A., Margulies, D S, Kelly, A M C, Uddin, L Q, Shehzad, Z, Biswal, B., et al. (2008). Functional connectivity of human striatum: a resting state FMRI study. *Cerebral cortex (New York, N.Y.: 1991), 18*(12), 2735-47.

De Martino, F., Gentile, F., Esposito, F., Balsi, M., Di Salle, F., Goebel, R., & Formisano, E. (2007). Classification of fMRI independent components using IC-fingerprints and support vector machine classifiers. *NeuroImage, 34*(1), 177-94.

van Meer, M. P. A., van der Marel, K., Wang, K., Otte, W. M., El Bouazati, S., Roeling, T. A. P., Viergever, M. A., et al. (2010). Recovery of sensorimotor function after experimental stroke correlates with restoration of resting-state interhemispheric functional connectivity. *The Journal of Neuroscience, 30*(11), 3964-72.

Mukamel, R., Gelbard, H., Arieli, A., Hasson, U., Fried, I., & Malach, R. (2005). Coupling between neuronal firing, field potentials, and FMRI in human auditory cortex. *Science, 309*(5736), 951-4.

Nakamura, T., Hillary, F. G., & Biswal, B. B. (2009). Resting network plasticity following brain injury. *PloS one, 4*(12), e8220.

Nelson, S. M., Cohen, A. L., Power, J. D., Wig, G. S., Miezin, F. M., Wheeler, M. E., Velanova, K., et al. (2010). A Parcellation Scheme for Human Left Lateral Parietal Cortex. *Neuron, 67*(1), 156-170.

Nierhaus, T., Schön, T., Becker, Robert, Ritter, P., & Villringer, A. (2009). Background and evoked activity and their interaction in the human brain. *Magnetic resonance imaging, 27*(8), 1140-50. Elsevier Inc.

Niessing, J., Ebisch, B., Schmidt, K. E., Niessing, M., Singer, W., & Galuske, R. A. W. (2005). Hemodynamic signals correlate tightly with synchronized gamma oscillations. *Science, 309*(5736), 948-51.

Norman, K. A., Polyn, S. M., Detre, G. J., & Haxby, J. V. (2006). Beyond mind-reading: multi-voxel pattern analysis of fMRI data. *Trends in cognitive sciences, 10*(9), 424-30.

Ogawa, S., Tank, D. W., Menon, R., Ellermann, J. M., Kim, S. G., Merkle, H., & Ugurbil, K. (1992). Intrinsic signal changes accompanying sensory stimulation: functional brain mapping with magnetic resonance imaging. *Proceedings of the National Academy of Sciences USA, 89*(13), 5951-5.

Raichle, Marcus E. (2010). Two views of brain function. *Trends in cognitive sciences, 14*(4), 180-90.

Ritter, P., & Villringer, A. (2006). Simultaneous EEG-fMRI. *Neuroscience and biobehavioral reviews, 30*(6), 823-38.

Roy, C. S., & Sherrington, C. S. (1890). On the Regulation of the Blood-supply of the Brain. *The Journal of Physiology, 11*(1-2), 85-158.17.

Sadaghiani, S., Hesselmann, G., Friston, K. J., & Kleinschmidt, Andreas. (2010). The relation of ongoing brain activity, evoked neural responses, and cognition. *Frontiers in Systems Neuroscience, 4*(June), 20.

Salvador, R., Suckling, J., Coleman, M. R., Pickard, J. D., Menon, D., & Bullmore, E. (2005). Neurophysiological architecture of functional magnetic resonance images of human brain. *Cerebral cortex, 15*(9), 1332-42.

Scheeringa, R., Bastiaansen, M. C. M., Petersson, K.-M., Oostenveld, R., Norris, D. G., & Hagoort, P. (2008). Frontal theta EEG activity correlates negatively with the default mode network in resting state. *International Journal of Psychophysiology, 67*(3), 242-51.

Scheeringa, R., Mazaheri, A., Bojak, I., Norris, D. G., & Kleinschmidt, Andreas. (2011). Modulation of visually evoked cortical FMRI responses by phase of ongoing occipital alpha oscillations. *The Journal of Neuroscience, 31*(10), 3813-20.

Scheeringa, R., Petersson, K.-M., Oostenveld, R., Norris, D. G., Hagoort, P., & Bastiaansen, M. C. M. (2009). Trial-by-trial coupling between EEG and BOLD identifies networks related to alpha and theta EEG power increases during working memory maintenance. *NeuroImage, 44*(3), 1224-38. Elsevier Inc.

Shen, H., Wang, L., Liu, Y., & Hu, D. (2010). Discriminative analysis of resting-state functional connectivity patterns of schizophrenia using low dimensional embedding of fMRI. *NeuroImage, 49*(4), 3110-21.

Shibasaki, H. (2008). Human brain mapping: hemodynamic response and electrophysiology. *Clinical Neurophysiology, 119*(4), 731-43.

Skudlarski, P., Jagannathan, K., Calhoun, V. D., Hampson, M., Skudlarska, B. A., & Pearlson, G. (2008). Measuring brain connectivity: diffusion tensor imaging validates resting state temporal correlations. *NeuroImage, 43*(3), 554-61.

Smith, S. M., Fox, P. T., Miller, K. L., Glahn, D. C., Fox, P. M., Mackay, C. E., Filippini, N., et al. (2009). Correspondence of the brain's functional architecture during activation and rest. *Proceedings of the National Academy of Sciences USA, 106*(31), 13040-13045.

Sokoloff, L., Mangold, R., Wechsler, R. L., Kenney, C., & Kety, S. S. (1955). The effect of mental arithmetic on cerebral circulation and metabolism. *The Journal of clinical investigation, 34*(7, Part 1), 1101-8.

Sorg, C., Riedl, V., Mühlau, M., Calhoun, V. D., Eichele, T., Läer, L., Drzezga, A., et al. (2007). Selective changes of resting-state networks in individuals at risk for Alzheimer's disease. *Proceedings of the National Academy of Sciences USA, 104*(47), 18760-5.

Steinbrink, J., Villringer, A., Kempf, F., Haux, D., Boden, S., & Obrig, H. (2006). Illuminating the BOLD signal: combined fMRI-fNIRS studies. *Magnetic resonance imaging, 24*(4), 495-505.

Sun, F. T., Miller, L. M., & D'Esposito, M. (2004). Measuring interregional functional connectivity using coherence and partial coherence analyses of fMRI data. *NeuroImage, 21*(2), 647-58.

Sun, F. T., Miller, L. M., & D'Esposito, M. (2005). Measuring temporal dynamics of functional networks using phase spectrum of fMRI data. *NeuroImage, 28*(1), 227-37.

Tohka, J., Foerde, K., Aron, A. R., Tom, S. M., Toga, A. W., & Poldrack, R. A. (2008). Automatic independent component labeling for artifact removal in fMRI. *NeuroImage, 39*(3), 1227-45.

Villringer, A., & Dirnagl, U. (1995). Coupling of brain activity and cerebral blood flow: basis of functional neuroimaging. *Cerebrovascular and brain metabolism reviews, 7*(3), 240-76.

Vincent, J L, Patel, G. H., Fox, M D, Snyder, A Z, Baker, J. T., Van Essen, D C, Zempel, J. M., et al. (2007). Intrinsic functional architecture in the anaesthetized monkey brain. *Nature, 447*(7140), 83-6.

Zhu, C.-Z., Zang, Y.-F., Cao, Q.-J., Yan, C.-G., He, Y., Jiang, T.-Z., Sui, M.-Q., et al. (2008). Fisher discriminative analysis of resting-state brain function for attention-deficit/hyperactivity disorder. *NeuroImage, 40*(1), 110-20.

Zuo, X.-N., Kelly, C., Di Martino, Adriana, Mennes, M., Margulies, Daniel S, Bangaru, S., Grzadzinski, R., et al. (2010). Growing together and growing apart: regional and sex differences in the lifespan developmental trajectories of functional homotopy. *The Journal of neuroscience: the official journal of the Society for Neuroscience, 30*(45), 15034-43.

3

Functional Near-Infrared Spectroscopy (fNIRS): Principles and Neuroscientific Applications

José León-Carrión[1] and Umberto León-Domínguez[2]
[1]*Human Neuropsychology Laboratory, Department of Experimental Psychology, University of Seville*
[2]*Center for Brain Injury Rehabilitation (C.RE.CER.) Seville, Spain*

1. Introduction

fNIRS is a device designed to detect changes in the concentration of oxygenated (oxyHb) and deoxygenated (deoxyHb) haemoglobin molecules in the blood, a method commonly used to assess cerebral activity. Over the last decade, functional near-infrared spectroscopy (fNIRS) has widely extended its applications due to its capacity to quantify oxygenation in blood and organic tissue in a continuous and non invasive manner (Chance & Leigh, 1977; Villringer & Chance, 1997). This technique is an effective, albeit 'indirect', optical neuroimaging method that monitors hemodynamic response to brain activation, on the basis that neural activation and vascular response are tightly coupled, so termed 'neurovascular coupling'. Different studies show that neural activity and hemodynamic response maintain a lineal relationship (Arthurs & Boniface, 2003; Logothetis et al., 2001), suggesting that these changes in hemodynamic response could provide a good marker for assessing neural activity. In neuroscience, functional near-infrared spectroscopy (fNIRS) is used to measure cerebral functions through different chromophore mobilization (oxygenated haemoglobin, deoxygenated haemoglobin and cytochrome c-oxidase) and their timing with concrete events. Due to methodological and theoretical problems associated with cytochrome c-oxidase functioning (Cyt-Ox) (see section 3.2.), current neuroscience studies on cerebral functions only assesses and analyzes oxyHb and deoxyHb mobilizations. These chromophore mobilizations are directly related to the cerebral blood flow (CBF) associated with an event and the physiological reactions provoked by the brain's functional state (fNIRS measures these reaction in the cerebral cortex). The assessment of these task-related mobilizations performed in light of a base line established by the researcher him/herself. The difference in oxyHb and deoxyHb concentrations at baseline and at task performance determines the location in the cortex of an increase or decrease in CBF. An increase in CBF is associated with cerebral activity, making the temporal and spatial correlation between CBF and task a determinant of cerebral function. This capacity to study cerebral functions, both spatial and temporal, is what gives name to the technique described in this chapter: functional near-infrared spectroscopy (fNIRS).

fNIRS has become a valuable neuroimaging technique, novel in its easy application and characterized by its small size, portability, and reliability. Although relatively new to the field of health care, fNIRS use is growing rapidly in clinical settings and research, particularly in work involving higher level cognitive control. fNIRS measures of hemodynamic response have been used in numerous studies to assess cerebral functioning during resting state (Lu et al., 2010) and tasks on motor skills (Leff et al., 2011; Obrig et al., 1996_a), vision (Gratton et al., 1995; Herrmann et al., 2008), hearing (Zaramella et al., 2001), speech (Cannestra et al., 2003) social skills (Ruocco et al., 2010), learning (León-Carrión et al., 2010), emotion (León-Carrión, 2006, 2007_a, 2007_b), and executive functions (Chance et al., 1993; León-Carrion et al., 2008; Nakahachi et al., 2010). fNIRS is a proven medical device for monitoring hemodynamic activity through the intact brain cortex in normal adult subjects, a powerful and original functional neuroimaging technique which charts cerebral functioning in a non-invasive and relatively low-cost manner. The application of fNIRS in cerebral functioning studies has been validated by other neuroimaging techniques, showing that the NIR signal maintains a strong correlation with PET measures of changes in regional cerebral blood flow (rCBF), and the fMRI Blood Oxygen Level Dependent (BOLD) signal (Hock et al., 1997; Huppert et al., 2006; Kleinschmidt et al., 1996; MacIntosh et al., 2003; Toronov, 2001, 2003; Villringer and Chance, 1997). Yet compared to traditional neuroimaging technology, fNIRS is non-invasive, safe, portable and inexpensive (Gratton, et al. 1995; Strangman, 2002; Totaro et al., 1998; Villringer & Chance, 1997; Wolf, et al., 2002; Zabel & Chute, 2002). Given these characteristics, fNIRS makes it possible for research to be done more ecologically, in clinical and social settings, without the restrictions of more traditional scanners. Furthermore, fNIRS technology is ideal for studies in which subjects may have a more difficult time with traditional neuroimaging techniques, namely children, patients with dementia, etc. The flexibility of fNIRS also makes it ideal for studies involving patients who are in movement (Milla et al., 2001), patients who are bed-ridden (von Pannwitz et al, 1998), and new-borns (Goff et al., 2010).

In this paper, we review the literature to determine the principles of fNIRS, which could help create experimental designs and data analysis techniques objectively and effectively. We also provide a description of articles carried out by our research team on the use of fNIRS as a paradigm in the study of cognitive functions and in clinical applications. Specifically, we consider fNIRS use in studies on learning processes and affective dimensions in dorsolateral prefrontal cortex (DLPFC), and their influence on evoked hemodynamic changes.

2. The principles of fNIRS

Spectroscopy is based on the study of light signals. Many fields of science use this technique to study the composition of objects, both organic and inorganic. In 1949, Hill and Keynes (1949) reported that nervous system cell activity was associated with changes in the optical properties of light. NIRS has thus far the unique feature of being able to measure intravascular (oxyHb and deoxyHb) (Jöbsis, 1977) and intracellular (cytochrome c-oxidase) (Heekeren et al., 1999) events simultaneously.

In the study of cerebral functioning, a ray of light is used near the visible spectrum of light (NIR). More specifically, a light source known as a light-emitting diode (LED), emits a ray of quasi-infrared light at the scalp, half the wave absorbed by the chromophores (oxyHb, deoxyHb and cytochrome c-oxidase) found in the nervous tissue. A photo detector captures the light wave resulting from the interaction with the chromophores, following a banana-shaped path back to the surface of the skin (see Fig 1.) (Gratton et al, 1994). The characteristics of this light wave have changed in respect to the original emitted by the LED due to the absorption and dispersion capacity of the nervous tissue and chromophores.

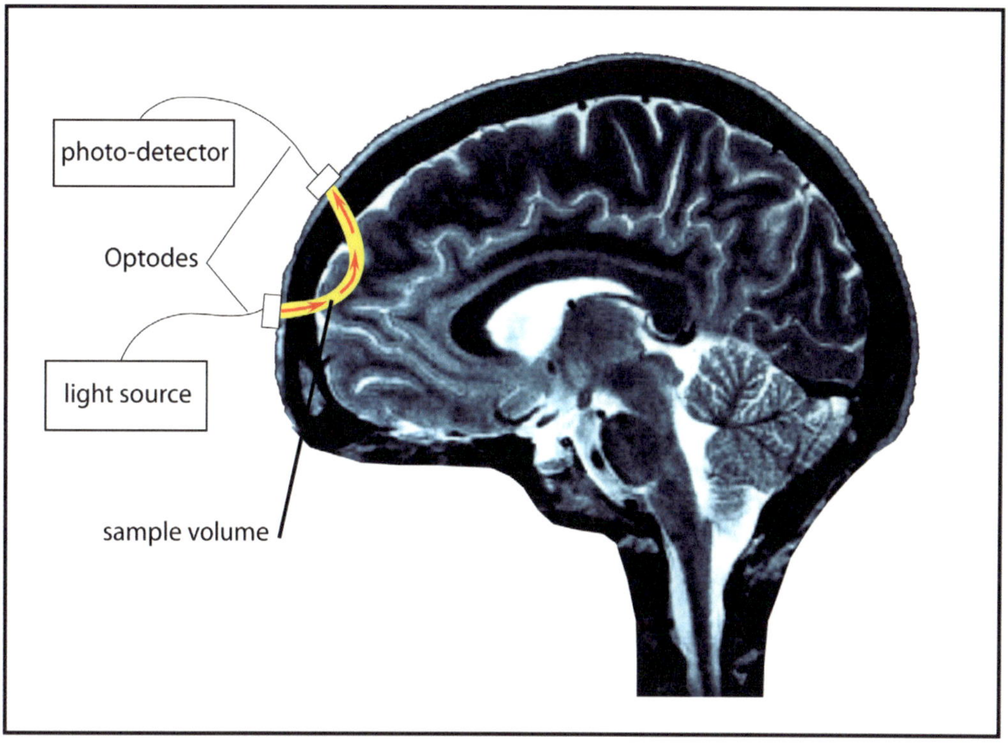

Fig. 1. Light from the light source is guided to the head by an optode. A photo-detector will collect the light which leaves the head at a distance of some centimetres. The photons follow a banana-shaped path from light source to detector.

The absorption spectra of light absorbing molecules (chromophores) are used to interpret the attenuated light levels as changes in chromophore concentration. The low absorption capacity of biological tissue (composed mostly of water) is one reason why light waves pierce different extracerebral tissue with hardly any absorption of NIR rays. In contrast, chromophores have characteristic optical properties which absorb rays close to the light. The transparency of the biological tissue, along with the absorption capacity of the diverse chromophores, makes it possible for optic methods to be used to measure hemodynamic responses (Chance, et al. 1998; Villringer and Chance, 1997). The optimal light spectrum for studying cognitive functions ranges between 700-900nm, which could be considered the biological "optical window", framed by chromophore mobilization (Jöbsis, 1977) (see Fig 2). This optical window lends itself to non-invasive, low-risk methods for studying cerebral processes.

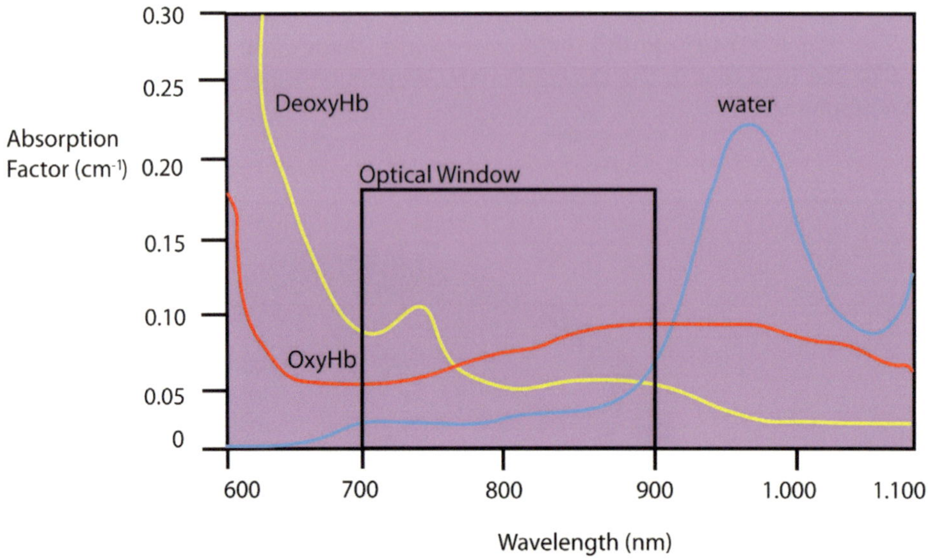

Fig. 2. Absorption spectrum in NIR window: different absorption spectra of oxyHb and deoxyHb at 700-900 (optical window) allow spectroscopy methods to assess their respective concentrations. Beyond 900 nm, the majority of the photons are absorbed by the water, making measurements difficult.

One of the limitations of the fNIRS is its scarce depth measurement capacity. This depth is determined mostly by two factors: wavelength and interopmode distance (IOD). Wavelength is one of the variables which determine a light's penetration capacity. In confocal microscopy at 488/514 nm, a penetration into cerebral tissue of approximately 0.25mm can be achieved (Dirnagl et al., 1991). When using dual photon technology with an excitation of 830 nm (Kleinfeld et al., 1998), penetration depth can surpass 0.6 mm below the brain surface. Nevertheless, penetration depth is limited by the optic window, given that a wavelength greater than 900nm penetrates tissue poorly due to the spectrum's high water absorption capacity at those depths (See Fig 2). The other parameter determining light penetration into nervous tissue is the distance between light source and detector. In general terms, the greater the source-detector distance, the deeper the penetration. However, a greater distance can also lead to a lower intensity of light captured by the detector. The ideal distance between source and detector depends on the capillary depth and demographic variables of the subjects being studied. Dark skin and very dark hair can absorb most wavelengths, hence a shorter distance between light source and detector would be recommended, which increases the intensity of the wavelength.

The main interaction between light and tissue is absorption, although the latter coexists with another phenomenon capable of modifying the optic characteristics of a light wave. This phenomenon, known as dispersion, illustrates photon loss which is not due to chromophore absorption (the loss depending on the size of the photo detector and the system's geometry). A photon's trajectory could vary when crossing nervous tissue with chromophores. A few photons will reach the photo detector without undergoing any dispersion or absorption effects (ballistic photon), some will be absorbed by chromophores (absorption), others--scattered out of the sampling volume--will not reach the photo detector (scatter), and the remainder will make it, but by travelling a path longer than the geometrical distance between light source and detector (scatter) (See Fig 3). Dispersion alters the attenuated light wave captured by the photo detector and hence the reflected chromophore absorption capacity. If we interpret this light wave solely on the basis of chromophores absorption, we would lose analytic access to the biological processes which underlie cerebral functions.

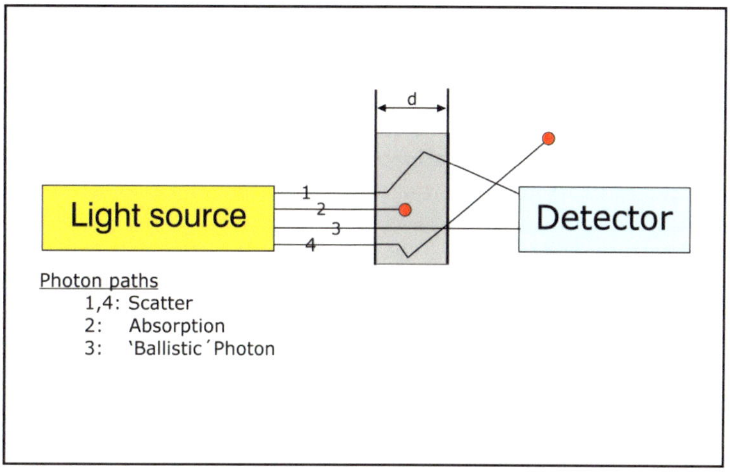

Fig. 3. Possible trajectory of a photon passing through biological tissue.

To offset dispersion and obtain a wider analytical scope of a light wave's optical characteristics, we applied the modified Beer-Lambert Law (Table 1). This version differs from the original in its conception of the effect of dispersion. In a typical trans-cranial study of the human brain, the mean path length of light is six times as long as the distance between sender and receiver (Duncan et al., 1995). In the modified Beer-Lambert Law, a new term (B) is added to represent the longest path length of light. A second modification to this equation is also necessary, given that not all photons reach the photo detector due to the dispersion effect. A second term is added (G) which measures photon loss due to dispersion. The process of modification of this law is as follows:

Original/Modified Beer-Lambert Law	Equation
Original Beer-Lambert Law	$A = \varepsilon \times c \times d$
Modified Beer-Lambert Law	$A = \varepsilon \times c \times d \times B + G$
Assuming constant B and C gives	$\Delta A = \varepsilon \times \Delta c \times d \times B$

Table 1. Variations of the original Beer-Lambert Law due to the dispersion effect.
A: absorbance, light attenuation (no units, since $A = \log10\ P0 / P$); **ε** is the molar absorption with units of L mol^{-1} cm^{-1};**c**: concentration of the compound in solution, expressed in mol^{-1}; **d**: path length of the sample; **G**: photon loss due to dispersion; **B**: longer path length due to dispersion effect.

3. Technical approaches for functional near-infrared spectroscopy and neuroimaging

Neuroscience interprets the optical characteristics of wavelengths reflected by different endogenous chromophores in nervous tissue, to discern the locations of cerebral functions at a specific moment. The functional state of the chromophores will determine how much spectrum light is absorbed, thereby revealing the functional state of the cortex. For example, the absorption spectrum for haemoglobin depends on whether or not it is oxygenated (venous vs. Arterial blood) (see Fig 2). Another important chromophore is cytochrome c-oxidase (Cyt-Ox), the terminal enzyme of oxidative phosphorylation whose absorption spectrum depends on its redox-state. Many other agents with absorption capacity are found in cerebral tissue, including melanin or water, although the spectral light of near-infrared rays practically nullifies their absorption capacity.

Apart from the changes in concentration of molecules with absorption capacity, dispersion causes changes in light's optical characteristics. The changes provoked by dispersion have been described as a result of changes in neural basal state. It is believed that rapid dispersion changes are temporally linked to changes in membrane potential (Stepnoski et al., 1991), whereas slow changes in dispersion probably reflect changes in cellular volume. The following section provides a description of the different parameters and elements used to analyze wavelengths and interpret study results.

3.1 OxyHb and DeoxyHb

To create cerebral activity, neurons require nutrients in order to generate energy and produce action potentials. Glucose, like oxygen and other substances, are sent to metabolically active neurons by means of blood perfusion via capillaries, which produces an increase in rCBF and in regional cerebral blood oxygenation (rCBO). Hence, changes in rCBF or rCBO can be used to map brain activity with high spatial resolution ("functional neuroimaging").

During functional activation, oxygen metabolism (cerebral metabolic rate of oxygen, $CMRO_2$) increases substantially (Ances et al., 2001_a; Dunn et al., 2005; Gjeddeet al., 2002) This increased oxygen consumption during neuronal activity results in a decrease in tissue oxygenation which is counteracted by the increase in O_2 supply when CBF and cerebral blood volume (CVB) increase (Ances et al., 2001_b; Enager et al., 2009; Offenhauser et al., 2005; Thompson et al., 2003), thanks to a mechanism known as neurovascular coupling. If the stimulus is lasting, glucose and oxygen consumption must be kept constant by increasing capillary density, which in turn increases total cerebral blood volume (Clarke & Sokoloff, 1994; Gross et al., 1987; Klein et al., 1986). However, when the stimulus is short-lived, the aforementioned hemodynamic and metabolic changes are not produced in the same manner.

CBF and oxygen metabolism is produced not only to counteract the effects of tissue oxygenation, but also to oxygenate haemoglobin. When haemoglobin transports oxygen, it is called oxyhaemoglobin (oxyHb). When it releases oxygen via an increase in oxygen metabolism, it transforms into deoxyhaemoglobin (deoxyHb). A cerebral region, therefore, could be considered active when its rCBF increases, producing a decrease in deoxyHb and an increase in oxyHb (Lindauer et al., 2001; Obrig et al., 1996_b), which in experimentation is generally associated with a specific event.

The increased oxygen transported to the brain area typically exceeds the local $CMRO_2$ utilization, causing an overabundance of cerebral blood oxygenation in active areas (Fox et al., 1988; Frostig et al., 1990; Lin et al., 2008; Lindauer et al., 2001; Mayhew et al., 2001). When there is an increase in CBF, tissue hyperoxygenation takes place (See Fig 4). Different optic studies using fNIRS and fMRI have reported that when neural activity commences, hyperoxygenation (due to an increase in CBF--increased oxyHb) is preceded by low oxygenation (increase in deoxyHb). This vascular response is difficult to measure and very controversial (Buxton, 2001; Frostig et al., 1990; Malonek & Grinvald, 1996; Obrig & Villringer, 2003).

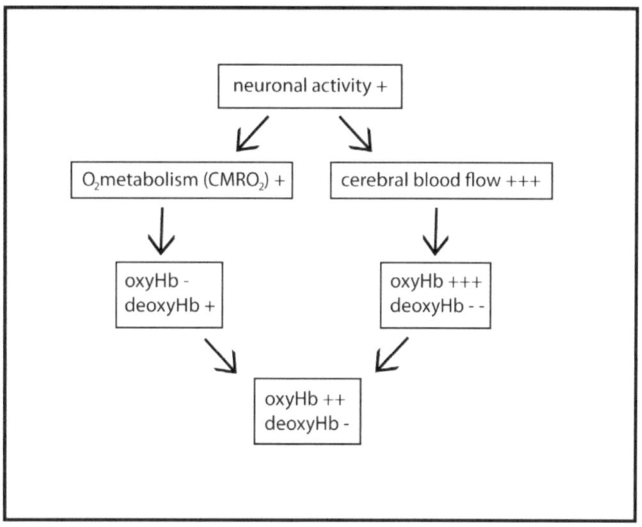

Fig. 4. Diagram of metabolic and hemodynamic changes during brain activity.

Scientific debate ensues as to which molecule possesses the highest discriminatory capacity for measuring neural activity. Currently, this is attributed to the deoxyHb molecule, the gold standard neuroscience neuroimaging technique. The deoxyHb molecule for cortical activity analysis has a high correlation with the BOLD response in fMRI (R=0.98; P<10-20), compared to that of the oxyHb molecule (R=0.71) or the Hb_{TOTAL} (R=0.53) (Huppert et al., 2006). These same results were obtained by other researchers (MacIntosh et al., 2003; Toronov 2001, 2003). In addition, concentrations of deoxyHb are reported to have more discriminatory power in humans than oxyHb (Herrmann et al., 2008).

In current research, our team is studying deoxyHb mobilization in different levels of consciousness during general anaesthesia. This mobilization has been correlated using Bispectral Index System (BIS) technology, the gold standard for controlling depth of anaesthesia. Preliminary results show a strong correlation between an increase in deoxyHb and a decrease in BIS as the patient reaches the lowest levels of consciousness. These results highlight the discriminatory power of the deoxyHb molecule in measuring deactivation in different brain areas.

As we mentioned earlier, oxyHb and deoxyHb possess characteristic optical properties in the near-infrared light range as well as wide-ranging sensibility to different wavelengths (See Figure 2), making it possible to use optics methods to quantify changes in chromophore concentration during neurovascular coupling (Chance et al., 1993; Chance et al., 1998;

Gratton et al., 1995; Hoshi et al., 1993; Villringer et al., 1993; Villringer & Chance 1997). To calculate the different levels of oxyHb, deoxyHb, and Hb_{TOTAL} concentration, the modified Beer-Lambert Law is used. The attenuation of light intensity after absorption and scattering by biological tissue is expressed as:

$$I = GI_0 e^{-(\alpha_{HB} C_{HB} + \alpha_{HBO2} C_{HBO2})L}$$

where G is a factor that accounts for the measurement geometry and is assumed constant when concentration changes. I_o is input light intensity; a_{HB} and a_{HBO2} represent molar extinction coefficients; C_{HB} and C_{HBO2} indicate concentrations of deoxyHb and oxyHb chromophores, respectively; and L represents the photon path, a function of absorption and scattering coefficients μ_a and μ_b (Izzetoglu et al., 2007).

By measuring optical density (OD) changes at two wavelengths, the relative change of oxy- and deoxy-haemoglobin versus time can be obtained. If the intensity measurement at the initial time (baseline) is I_b, and at another time is I, the OD change due to variation in C_{HB} and C_{HBO2} during that period is:

$$\Delta OD = \log (I_b/I) = \alpha_{HB}\Delta C_{HB} + \alpha_{HBO2}\Delta C_{HBO2}.$$

Measurements performed at two different wavelengths allow the calculation of ΔC_{HB} and ΔC_{HBO2}. Oxygenation and blood volume (Hb_{TOTAL}) can then be deduced (Izzetoglu et al., 2007):

1. Oxygenation = $\Delta C_{HBO2} - \Delta C_{HB}$
2. Blood Volume (Hb_{TOTAL}) = $\Delta C_{HBO2} + \Delta C_{HB}$

When baseline is taken, it is important to take into account that the subject is medicated or anxious, variables which could have a quantitative effect on CBF. Since NIRS measures changes in oxyHb and deoxyHb concentrations in the arterial and venous intracerebral compartments, comparisons of different measurements depend on the assumption that the proportion of arterial and venous compartments remains constant. For this reason, factors that alter venous volume should be considered. Changes in head position, likely to occur in the clinical use of NIRS, might influence venous pressure and alter the proportion of arterial and venous compartments in the cerebral vasculature. In addition, body position might modify the tone of the resistive vessels to maintain a constant cerebral blood flow. According to Toraro et al (1998), cerebrovascular reactivity measurements may be performed without taking into account changes of head position.

Other variables to take into account when interpreting oxyHb and deoxyHb results are those which affect CBF:

1. In hypercapnia, when baseline perfusion was increased by up to 100% (stronger hypercapnia), the deoxyHb response almost disappeared (Jones et al., 2005).
2. During hyperoxia, the deoxyHb outwash was significantly reduced under normobaric conditions (Lindauer et al., 2003) or even abolished under hyperbaric conditions of 3 or 4 ATA (Lindauer et al., 2010), while neuronal activity and CBF responses remained unaltered.
3. OxyHb and deoxyHb effects remained lineal when the stimulus lasted between 6-24 seconds. However, during shorter stimulation periods, strong nonlinear effects came into play (Wobst et al., 2001).
4. Although hypothermia reduced baseline CBF by almost 50%, neurovascular coupling was preserved. Reduction of functional changes in CBF, deoxyHb and $CMRO_2$ followed reductions in neuronal activity during hypothermia (Royl et al., 2008)

5. A recent study reported that the amplitude of the functional deoxyHb decrease in rat somatosensory cortex was reduced when ICP was elevated to 7 mmHg. At an ICP of 14 mmHg, the deoxyHb response was close to 0 and even reversed at an ICP of 28 mmHg (Füchtemeier et al., 2010).
6. Changes in oxyHb, deoxyHb and Hb_{TOTA} correlated significantly with changes in blood velocity (Totaro et al., 1998).
7. NIRS parameters, induced by CO, reflect variations in resistive vessels, and could thus be considered an index of cerebrovascular reactivity (Totaro et al., 1998).

3.2 Cytochrome-c oxidase

Cytochrome-c oxidase (Cyt-Ox), an enzyme found in the mitochondria, is responsible for more than 90% of cellular oxygen consumption. In isolated mitochondria, Cyt-Ox redox states showed transient oxidation during increased cellular activity (Chance & Williams, 1956), indicating that Cyt-Ox redox state could provide a good approximation for assessing transitory changes in cellular metabolism during neuronal activity (Wong Riley, 1989). Cyt-Ox has a characteristic light absorption pattern in the visible (Keilin, 1925) and near-infrared parts of the electromagnetic spectrum (band centred around 830 nm) (Wharton and Tzagoloff, 1964), and it is in principle feasible to measure changes in the Cyt-Ox redox state in vivo (Cooper et al., 1994; Ferrari et al., 1990; Jöbsis, 1977).

Cytochrome-c oxidase theoretically could be a biological marker for cellular metabolic demand, with the potential to provide more direct information on neuronal activity than haemoglobin (Heekeren et al., 1999; Jöbsis, 1977). The theoretical advantage of using this enzyme as a marker for neuronal activity is that it is much more exact than oxyHb and deoxy-Hb, given that the demand by neurons for oxygen exceeds the need for their activation (Fox et al., 1988). Nevertheless, while Cyt-Ox may be a more precise marker for measuring neuronal activity, its use in neuroscience as a parameter has been limited by two fundamental issues:

1. The use of non-invasive NIRS to detect redox changes in Cyt-Ox in response to cerebral activation is hampered by methodological spectroscopic issues related to the modification of the Beer-Lambert law. However, the separation of the haemoglobin signal from the Cyt-Ox signal has been regarded as questionable and mere cross talk (Cooper 1994, 1998; Matcher et al., 1995). Methodologically, the calculation of the enzyme's redox change may be erroneous due to the simplified assumptions inherent in the modified Beer - Lambert approach.
2. From a physiological standpoint, there is ongoing debate on as to whether or not the redox state of Cyt-Ox changes in response to the functional activation of cerebral cortex.

Recent studies have attempted to resolve these two questions. New algorithms are being developed that can help discern the role of Cyt-Ox and its functions during cerebral activity. A recent study reported that the differential stimulation of areas rich and poor in cytochrome-c-oxidase content results in optical changes which cannot be solely explained by the presently available models of cross talk (Uludağ et al., 2004). One of the most renowned studies tackling the physiological question reported that the spectra obtained in a state of increased brain activity cannot be explained solely by the well-known changes in oxyHb and deoxyHb, but must include Cyt-Ox in the analysis. The inclusion of Cyt-Ox to explain spectra changes is also applied to explain how Cyt-Ox transient oxidation increases significantly during visual stimulation in 9 out of 10 subjects (Heekeren, 1999).

For these reasons, Cyt-Ox is not widely used in research on normal cerebral functions, whereas other fields are finding use for its capacity as a direct maker for tissue oxygenation to study pathologies related to metabolic dysfunction of the mitochondria (Atamna et al., 2010; Levy et al., 2007; Pickrell et al., 2009). The mechanisms and control of this enzyme have been discussed in various reviews (Cooper, 1990; Brown, 1992).

3.3 Fast and slow light scattering signals

Another method used for measuring neuronal activation is known as the event-related optical signal, or EROS, which capitalizes on the changes in the optical properties of the cell membranes themselves that occur as a function of the ionic fluxes during firing (Gratton et al., 1995). It is well established that the optical properties of cell membranes change in the depolarized state relative to the resting state (Obrig & Villringer, 2003; Rector et al., 1997; Stepnoski et al., 1991). Optical technology can be used to study these changes.

The ability to measure neuronal membrane depolarization provides us with the opportunity to study neuronal activity more directly. There are two approaches to studying neuronal depolarization via light wave dispersion, one with fast and the other with slow scattering signals. These signals differ both in terms of duration (milliseconds vs. seconds) and magnitude and their subsequent physiological processes. Fast light scattering signals occur in milliseconds (Hill & Keynes, 1949). In isolated nerves cells, Stepnoski et al. (1991) showed that changes in light scattering were associated with membrane potentials. Slow light scattering signals, reported in bloodless brain slices, occurred in seconds after the onset of stimulation (MacVicar & Hochman, 1991). The origin of slow light scattering is still unclear, although the primary candidates are changes in intracellular volume and/or in extracellular volume (MacVicar & Hochman, 1991; Holthoff & Witte 1996).

The study of cerebral functions in humans using EROS signals is hampered by numerous limitations. The principal shortcoming is that the fast scattering signal represents the low signal-to-noise ratio (SNR) resulting from optical properties in the skin, skull and cerebral-spinal fluid, which are traversed by the quasi infra-red light wave. Furthermore, basic sensory and motor movements such as tactile stimulation and finger tapping require between 500–1,000 trials to establish a reliable signal (Franceschini et al., 2004).

Other difficulties have been encountered in attempts to replicate experiments both on fast and slow scattering signals, limiting data collection, for example, on the optic characteristics of the fast scattering signal in response to a visual stimulus among normal adult humans (Obrig & Villringer, 2003). A final constraint is that these methods, apart from requiring a more expensive and cumbersome laser-based light source, have an increased risk of inadvertent damage to the eyes in comparison to other systems measuring hemodynamic response. In spite of these current limitations, the fast optical signal continues to be an important area of investigation because it offers glimpses of the "holy grail" of neuroimaging: the direct measurement of neuronal activity with millisecond time resolution and superior spatial resolution (Izzetoglu et al., 2004).

4. Instrumentation

Functional near-infrared (fNIR) instrumentation is composed of various light-emitting diodes (LEDs) and photo detectors which pick up light waves after they have interacted with brain tissue. The fNIRS normally used for neuroimaging has numerous channels. Each channel represents a cerebral region covered by the light wave and which coincides with the separation between the LED and its corresponding photo detector. Due to the dispersion effect, a photo detector, which can detect light coming from cerebral tissue, is placed 2-7 cm from the LED. The relative contribution of extracranial tissue decreased as the interoptode distance increased, for an interoptode distance greater than 4.5 cm, the extracranial contribution was negligible (Smielewski 1995, 1997). The contribution of the scalp might be minimized by applying moderate pressure on the optodes (Owen et al., 1996). The ideal separation between source and photo detector is 4 cm, given that the fNIR signal becomes sensitive to hemodynamic changes within the top 2–3 mm of the cortex and extends laterally 1 cm to either side, perpendicular to the axis of source-detector spacing. Studies have shown that at interoptode distances as short as 2–2.5 cm, gray matter is part of the sample volume (Chance et al., 1998).

Three distinct types of fNIR implementation systems have been developed: time-resolved, frequency-domain, and continuous wave spectroscopy, each with its own strengths and limitations. (For review, see Minagawa-Kawai et al., 2008; Wolf et al., 2007). Our research team used the fNIRS system developed by Drexel University's Optical Engineering Team. This low-cost functional neuroimaging system provides a variety of clinical, research, and educational applications. Our NIRS system (NIM, Inc., Philadelphia, PA) applies light to tissue at constant amplitude and can provide measurements of oxy- and deoxy-Hb relative to baseline concentrations (see Bunce et al., 2006). The fNIRS probe is 17.5 cm long and 6.5 cm wide. It contains four light sources surrounded by ten detectors, for a total of 16 channels of data acquisition, covering an area of 14 X 3.5 cm on the forehead (see Figure 1). A source-detector distance of 2.5 cm provides a penetration depth of 1.25 cm. The probe positioning is such that the line of sources is set at the line of fronto-polar electrodes [FP1–FP2] (in the International 10–20 system). This is designed to image cortical areas that correspond to DLPFC (Izzetoglu, 2005). The DLPFC generally occupies the upper and side regions of the frontal lobes. It is comprised of BA 9 and 46. Area 9 occupies the dorsal region of lateral PFC and extends medially to the paracingulate of humans. Area 46 is generally located at the anterior end of the middle frontal sulcus. The fronto-polar PFC, BA 10, is a region positioned above the Orbito Frontal Cortex (OFC), inferior to Area 9, and anterior to Area 46, serving as a junction point between the OFC and DLPFC (Krawczyk, 2002). A complete data acquisition cycle lasts approximately 330ms, making the temporal resolution approximately 3 Hz.

5. fNIRS research

5.1 Prefrontal activity and learning processes

Understanding the processes which underlie learning has become a central theme in current society, whether it is in the scope of education or in the field of neurorehabilitation. The proper functioning of learning processes can determine the efficacy of an individual's adaptation in society. By identifying these processes, we can identify learning problems early on in childhood and intervene. This is also true in the rehabilitation of patients with brain injury, or with memory-related neuropathology, where learning processes can determine the path of neurorehabilitation within a therapeutic program.

During learning, different brain structures begin to function, regardless of content, channel or mode of information. PFC participates in memory control (Luria 1973; Blumenfeld & Ranganath, 2006), particularly dorsolateral PFC (DLPFC), which plays a relevant role in temporal integration by means of functions that are complimentary and temporally reciprocal. The capacity to learn and remember highlights the plastic, adaptive ability of the neural system to change in response to experience. This capacity to integrate information is

widely considered to be a product of working memory (WM) (D'Esposito et al., 1998; Owen, 1997, 2000). The following two articles provide evidences on how prefrontal cortex is related to learning capacity and working memory.
The first study (León-Carrión et al., 2010) was designed to measure the physiological effects of repetition on learning and working memory using an adaptation of Luria's Memory Word-Task (LMWT). The study focused on the physiological effects of repetition on learning and working memory. We have used an adaptation of Luria's Memory Word-Task (LMWT) to study functional hemodynamic changes related to learning by verbal repetition. Functional near infrared spectroscopy (fNIRS) is used to test the hypotheses that repeated verbal presentation of information will produce an increase in DLPFC activation only during learning, followed by a decrease in activation once the information has been learned. This study assessed the hemodynamic response of DLPFC in 13 healthy subjects while performing a Luria task. All subjects successfully completed the task. A significant result from our data was that during the learning process, an increase in activation takes place in right and left DLPFC, which then decreases or ceases when the learning is complete. Our findings show neural repetition suppression (NRS) (see Grill-Spector et al., 2006 for a review) in DLPFC after effective verbal learning, an adaptation of hemodynamic activity in DLPFC during multiple repetitions. The correlations between memory recall and fNIRS activation evidences the neurophysiological substrates related to LWMT (see Tables 1 and 2). In psychobiological terms, this indicates that NRS must be present in successful verbal learning to maximize the effectiveness and accuracy of learning, and also to free up space in working memory. This optimization of neural responses stems from a verbal learning process that to be effective, requires time and repetition of the material being learned. Thus effective learning by repetition produces a reduced demand on WM through decreased DLPFC oxygenation as a consequence of a shift from controlled to automatic processing. Our results also point out that NRS is necessary not only to complete or close learning, but to keep DLPFC free and available for engagement in other tasks upon demand.
The second study used fNIRS and the N-Back paradigm to assess prefrontal activation. The N-Back paradigm and its variations have been used in numerous neuroimaging studies investigating the neural bases of working memory processes (Owen et al., 2005). In the current study, a modified version of the N-back task is applied (see Fig 5), which includes working memory manipulation to explore PFC activation during tasks requiring working memory (Baddeley, 1986).

The N-back task is designed to increase the manipulative character of information, producing more activation in regions associated with working memory. We hypothesized that as task difficulty increased, so would the differentiation in activation among different areas of DLPFC. The study included 20 healthy volunteers (14 female, 6 male), all right-handed and between 22 - 39 years of age (mean age = 26.6; SD = 4.15). fNIRS and oxyHb molecule mobilization were also used to measure DLPFC activation. The preliminary results showed that like classic verbal N-back tasks, the modified version activated the same regions of PFC but with greater intensity. The main result showed that while both N-back tasks (modified and classic) activated the same left DLPFC regions, the modified version registered greater differential activation. One possible explanation for the differential activation could be that the modified N-back had a deeper processing of information, with its manipulation involving semantic category and chronological order (days of the week). This higher information processing implies greater executive control, and an increase in regional cerebral blow flow in areas related to verbal working memory. In our study, areas

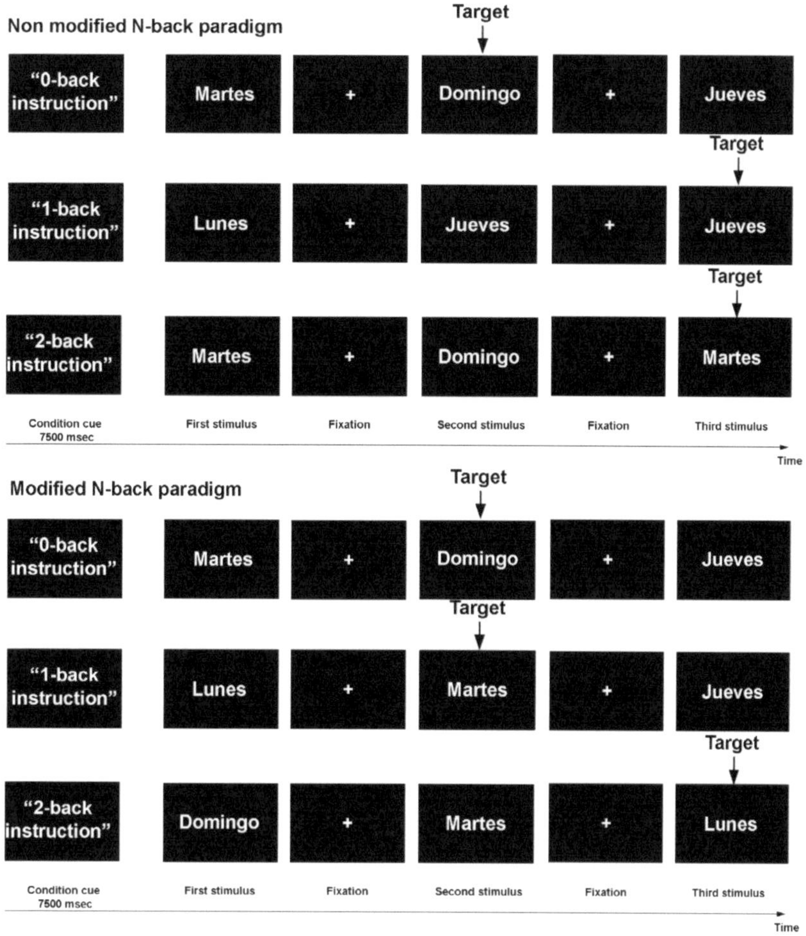

Fig. 5. Paradigms for unmodified N-back tasks (above) *and modified N-back tasks* (below). The *0-back condition for both sets of tasks* required a response when the word "Domingo" appeared. A fixation point (+) was located between stimuli. In the *unmodified 1-back condition,* the subject had to respond when a stimulus was repeated. In the *unmodified 2-back condition,* the subject had to respond when the present stimulus coincided with the prior stimulus. The *modified 1-back condition* required the subject to respond if the stimulus coincided with day after the prior stimulus. The *modified 2-back condition* requested a response if the present stimulus coincided with the day after the stimulus presented two positions back.

with significant differential activation, associated with verbal manipulation and maintenance, corresponded with DLPFC and left frontal operculum (Brodmann Areas 9, 10, 45 y 46) (See Fig 6).

Overall, these two studies carried out with fNIRS indicate the importance of DLPFC in learning processes. The learning of verbal information, both auditory and verbally, is determined by the capacity of working memory to load information temporarily and manipulate it. The increased load and manipulation of verbal information result in increased physiological activation in related zones. This increased activation translates to an increase in CBF in areas related to verbal tasks, mostly in the left hemisphere.

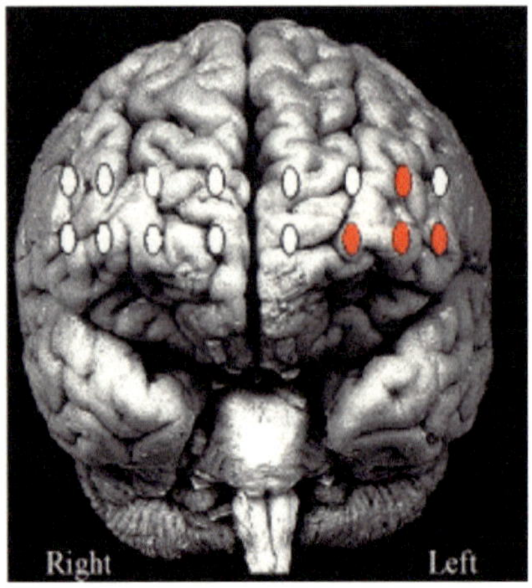

Fig. 6. Channels significantly activated during *modified* N-back task

5.2 Prefrontal activity and the affective dimension

The fNIRS is an excellent tool for studying the temporal dimension of hemodynamic activity, in terms of both reaction time (measured in ms) and residual activation after stimulus cessation. This residual activation could shed light on the characteristics of human behaviour. It is generally accepted that brain activation is elicited by direct cognitive/affective stimulation and that this activation decreases with stimulus cessation (Huettel & McCarthy, 2001). The DLPFC (Brodmann areas 9 and 46) has been selected as region of interest (ROI) based on a review of the literature which guarantees that emotional stimuli will produce some kind of activation in our ROI. These findings include DLPFC's sensitivity to emotional and motivationally significant aspects of stimuli (Hikosaka & Watanabe, 2000; Williams et al., 2001). The following articles display DLPFC activation during the viewing of scenes with different emotional content.

This first paper introduces a new paradigm in the study of emotional processes, emphasizing the role of affective dimensions in DLPFC and their influence on the neuroimaging of evoked hemodynamic changes (Leon-Carrion et al., $2007_{a)}$. Two affective dimensions have been studied extensively in neuroimaging research on emotional stimuli: arousal (exciting or calming) and valence (positive or negative) (Bradley et al., 1992). Another question that needs to be studied is whether the value (valence) and intensity (arousal) of an emotional stimulus evokes the same type of neural activation.

By using fNIRS, our intent was to image PFC oxyHb (oxygenated haemoglobin) changes and the duration of activation in relation to how subjects rated emotional stimuli (valence and arousal). We studied evoked-cerebral blood oxygenation (CBO) changes in DLPFC during direct exposure to emotion-eliciting stimuli ('on' period) and during the period directly following stimulus cessation ('off' period). Our hypothesis was that the evoked-CBO, rather than return to baseline after emotional stimulus cessation, would show either a significant increase (overshoot) or a significant decrease (undershoot) in oxyHb.

This study used visual emotional stimuli (film clips) of moderate length (approx. 20 s) and different emotional content to study the duration of DLPFC activation and provoke strong, lasting responses that could be easily registered. The content of the scenes ranged from mutilation, repulsive acts, and violence to walking along the street, cartoons, and scenes with explicit sex. The results showed that by using subjective ratings in analyzing PFC activation to account for individual differences in emotional response to salient stimuli, and by incorporating subjective data on emotional arousal, more robust activation occurred within DLPFC during the 'off' period than the 'on' period. In other words, when the subjective degree of arousal is high, the representation of the stimulus remains in the prefrontal cortex, even when the stimulus is no longer present. The persistence of sources of DLPFC activation during the 'off' period is closely related to the degree of arousal that the subject assigns to the stimulus (Fig 7).

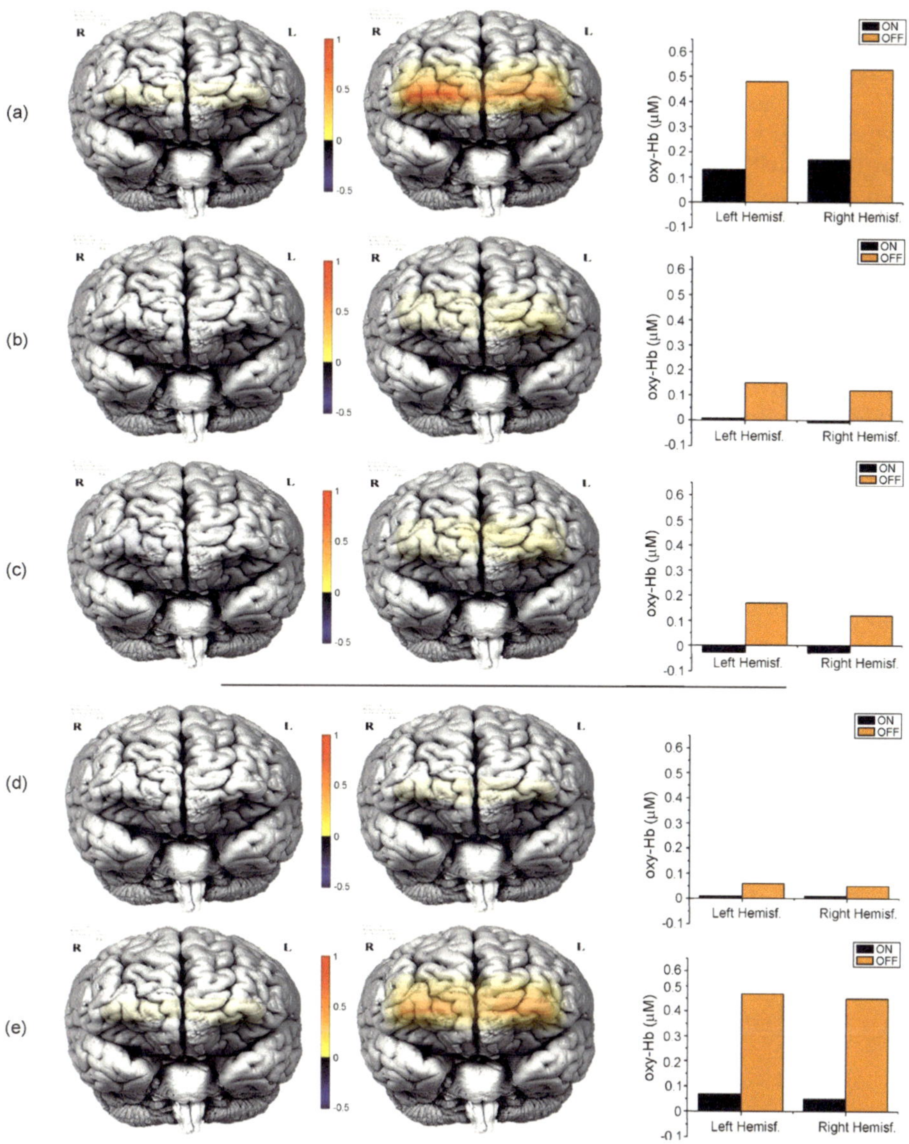

Fig. 7. Figure displays relative oxyHb concentrations, interpolated from the DLPFC channels of data acquisition in both on and off period for each emotional condition. The brain templates on the left and right represent the mean oxygenation during 'on' and 'off' periods, respectively. Valence category: (a) for unpleasant clips; (b) for neutral; and (c) for pleasant. Arousal category: (d) for non-arousing; and (e) for arousing. (Leon-Carrion et al., 2007_a)

The principle finding of this study was that an overshoot related to level of arousal in the DLPFC persists even when the arousing stimulus has disappeared. Our data also confirmed that valence and arousal have different effects on the course of evoked-CBO response in DLPFC. We also found significant post-stimulus overshoot related to arousal ratings. Significant differences between 'on' and 'off' periods of DLPFC activation based on valence ratings were not observed. In conclusion, our findings provide the first fNIRS evidence directly showing that an increment in subjective arousal leads to activation within DLPFC. This paper introduces a new paradigm in the study of emotional processes using functional neuroimaging techniques. Since arousing stimuli produce longer periods of brain activation than do non-arousing stimuli, neuroimaging studies must consider the duration and affective dimensions of the stimulus as well as the duration of the scanning. It will be necessary to specify how long a subject is exposed to a stimulus and how much of the recorded response is analyzed.

The second study (Leon-Carrion et al., 2007_b) explored DLPFC structures involved in the processing of erotic and non-sexual films. DLPFC plays a specific role in working memory in order to guide the inhibition or elicitation of sexual action. Different neurosurgery studies have demonstrated that frontal cortex is involved in the inhibitory control of human sexual behaviour (Freeman, 1973; Terzian & Ore, 1955). Here, we measured stimulus response both during direct viewing of the stimulus and for a short time after stimulus cessation, and recorded the temporal course of activation in DLPFC. Our hypothesis was that the sexual stimulus would produce a DLPFC overshoot during the period of direct perception ("on" period) that would continue after stimulus cessation ("off" period), whereas the non-sexual stimulus would not produce overshoot during either period.

Changes in pre-frontal concentrations of oxygenated haemoglobin (oxyHb) were measured during the two experimental conditions ("on" and "off" periods). Figure 8 shows a diagram of stimuli presentation and the sequence of fNIRS data acquisition. At the end of the presentation, participants were asked to rate each scene from 1 to 9 on a 2-dimensional scale. The first dimension, valence, corresponded to the subject's personal evaluation of the degree of pleasantness/unpleasantness of each scene, and the second, arousal, referred to how exciting or relaxing the subject perceived the scene to be.

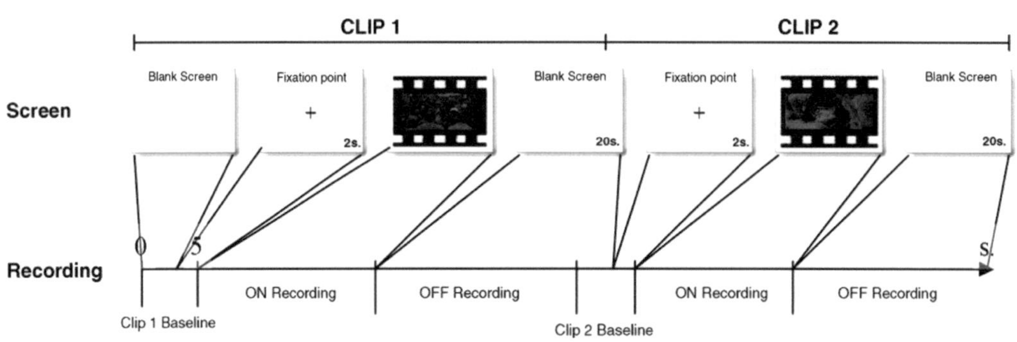

Fig. 8. Diagram of stimuli presentation and sequence of fNIRS recording. Note that to avoid accumulative effect, independent local baselines were recorded. (Leon-Carrion et al., 2007_b)

This is the first study to show that exposure to a sexually explicit scene produces strong overshoot in DLPFC, while exposure to a non-sexual scene does not. A significantly rapid and ascendant course in DLPFC overshoot was observed during direct viewing ("on" period) of the sexual scene, which became even more pronounced directly after viewing ("off" period), whereas a strong undershoot was observed for the non-sexual condition during the "off" period. We also found that the hemodynamic response to visual sexual stimuli differed between genders, with men registering higher oxyHb levels in DLPFC than women. Men seemed to be more interested in arousing visual stimuli as soon as these were perceived, and they experienced greater conflict in controlling their response. Men and women could differ in the urgency of response to a sexual stimulus, with men experiencing a greater degree of urgency than women. Compared to baselines, both genders showed significant overshoot in response to the sexual stimulus, but men showed a higher activation in absolute values. In men, activation was rapid and quickly increased, right from the onset of the stimulus, whereas women generally had a more delayed initial activation, which remained more stable than in men. This indicates that women, in general, would be more capable than men of controlling their response once aroused, and that this control, in both men and women, is a function of DLPFC. We therefore conclude that DLPFC plays a critical role in the self-regulation of sexual arousal. This study also demonstrates the feasibility of examining brain activation/sexual response relationships in an fNIRS environment.

Summarizing, the fNIRS is proven to be a useful tool for research on cognitive as well as emotional processes. Its high temporal resolution facilitates research of cerebral processes in their most dynamic and lasting form.

5.3 Near-Infrared Spectroscopy and its clinical use

In recent years, the use of near-infrared spectroscopy (NIRS) has steadily increased. It is now being applied in clinical settings, primarily in the field of medical monitoring and diagnosis (Frangioni, 2008; Kurth et al., 1995; Ward et al., 2006). One significant development has been the Infrascanner©, a tool which uses NIRS technology for the early diagnosis of cerebral haematomas (Leon-Carrion et al., 2010).

Traumatic brain injury (TBI) is a leading cause of death and disability and a major public health problem in the US, Canada (Leon-Carrion et al., 2005; Zygun et al., 2005) and Europe (Bruns & Hauser, 2003; Tagliaferri et al., 2006). Delayed medical attention is the strongest independent predictor of mortality in TBI patients. Early detection and surgical evacuation of mass-occupying lesions have decreased mortality and improved outcome in these patients. This reduction in mortality and morbidity requires rapid identification of the patient's cerebral and cranial status. Any further delay in haematoma evaluation severely increases mortality and worsens functional outcome in patients who survive (Seeling et al., 1985). NIRS technology could improve existing methods of identification of intracranial haematomas in these patients in situ. The Infrascanner test lasts 3 minutes and is easy to use in assessment applications as well as data organization and transmission. The purpose of this pilot investigation was to evaluate the Infrascanner as a handheld medical screening tool for the in situ detection of brain haematomas in patients who sustained a head injury.

The Infrascanner includes two main components: a NIRS-based sensor and a wireless personal digital assistant (PDA). The sensor includes a safe Class I NIRS diode laser, optically coupled to the patient's head by means of two disposable light guides in a 'hairbrush' like configuration. This configuration allows the sensor to contact the skin of the scalp. The 4.0cm separation between light source and detector allows NIRS absorbance measurement (~2cm wide and 2-3cm deep) in tissue volume. The light source uses an

808nm wavelength. The detector is covered by a band pass filter to minimize interference from background light. Electric circuitry is also included to control laser power and detector signal amplifier gain. Signals acquired from the detector are digitized and transmitted by a wireless link to the PDA. This link is also used to receive and set the sensor's hardware parameters. The PDA receives the data from the sensor and automatically adjusts its settings to ensure good data quality. The data is further processed and the results are displayed on the PDA screen (Fig 9).

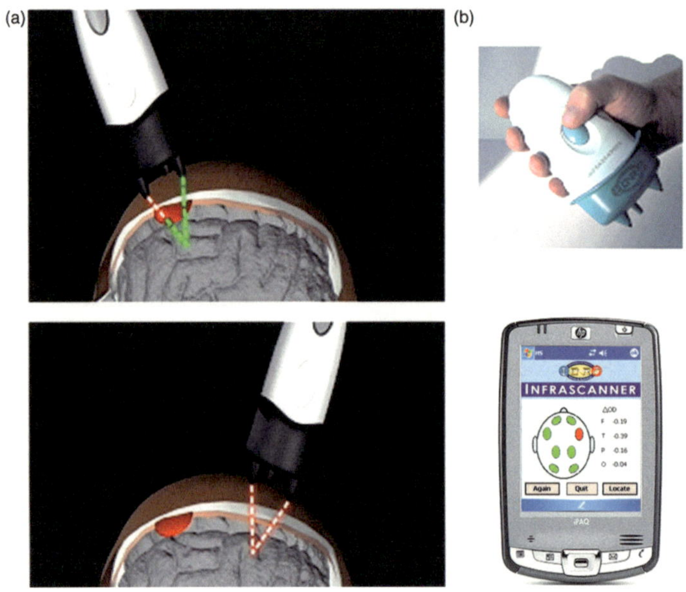

Fig. 9. Scanning sequence for brain haematoma. (a) The NIRS Sensor has two components: a 808nm diode laser and a silicon detector. The NIRS light source emits a light that penetrates the brain and is registered by the NIRS detector connected to the scalp through two optical fibres. The light intensity determines approximately how much blood volume is present. The Infrascanner performs symmetrical readings in the four main brain lobes: frontal, temporal, parietal and occipital. Haematoma detection derives from the difference in optical density between left and right readings for each brain lobe. (b) The detected signal is digitized and transmitted to a Bluetooth wireless personal digital assistant (PDA) that displays the results on the screen. (Leon-Carrion et al., 2010).

The results of this pilot study showed that handheld near-infrared Infrascanner demonstrates high sensitivity and specificity in detecting intra- and extra-axial hemorrhagic haematomas and, even more importantly, it could detect small haematomas (<25 mL) within the first 24 hours following injury. Data showed that the Infrascanner achieves 89.5% sensitivity when used on patients with TBI. Its on-site capacity to identify patients that have suffered an intracranial haematoma may be considered very high. The Infrascanner also

showed excellent specificity (81.2%) or the capacity to detect true negatives, identifying patients with TBI that have not suffered an intracranial haematoma. When compared to gold standard CT scans, its probability of positive predictive value was 85% and 86.7% for negative predictive value. This means that the Infrascanner is very accurate when confirming the presence or the absence of a haematoma.
This study demonstrated that the Infrascanner is a useful tool in the initial examination and screening of patients with head injury. It has proven utility as an adjunct to CT scans or as a preliminary exam given within 24 hours post-injury, when a CT scan is not available. In conclusion, the data shows that the Infrascanner is a sound portable device for detecting pre-operative intracranial subdural, epidural and subarachnoid haematomas in intensive care fields and emergency care units. It could aid paramedics, emergency room physicians and hospital staff, permitting earlier treatment and reducing secondary injury caused by present and delayed haematomas.

6. Conclusion

fNIRS has been approved by the FDA for clinical purposes and can be used simultaneously with other neuroimaging technologies. Studies show that fNIRS is a valid and reliable assessment tool for task-associated oxygenated blood, and while it may be early to define all the applications of this new technology, we believe it promises to find utility far beyond this in clinical practice. There are several types of clinical applications that could benefit from the unique attributes of fNIRS neuroimaging technology (Izzetoglu et al., 2004):

- Populations that may not be able to readily tolerate the confines of an fMRI magnet or be able to remain sufficiently still, e.g., schizophrenics, autistic children, neonates.
- Populations that require the long-term monitoring of cerebral oxygenation, e.g., premature and other high-risk infants.
- Studies that require repeated, low-cost neuroimaging, e.g., treatment studies that image the cortex for efficacy.
- Applications where an fMRI system would be too expensive or cumbersome, e.g., for use in a clinical office.
- Applications that require ecological validity, e.g., working at a computer or in an educational setting.

Furthermore, its current use is widely accepted by the neuroscientific community for studying cerebral functions due to its high level of consistency with findings based on traditional neuroimaging techniques. Like these, it measures neuronal activity indirectly via hemodynamic response. However, fNIRS is the only technique which can measure both extracellular and intracellular activation, with the latter still under development. fNIRS holds great potential for growth and application in clinical and research settings, offering new possibilities in neuroimaging techniques and expanding our knowledge about the functional organisation of the brain.

7. Acknowledgements

We would like to thank Drexel University, Philadelphia, PA, with special thanks to Banu Onaral, Kurtulus Izzetoglu, Kambiz Pourrezaei, Meltem Izzetoglu and Baruch Ben Dor. We would also like to extend our gratitude to the Center for Brain Injury Rehabilitation CRECER, especially to Dr. María del Rosario Domínguez Morales, Neurobirds and the department of experimental psychology (University of Seville, Spain) and its dedication to neuroscientific research.

8. References

Ances, B.M., Wilson, D.F., Greenberg, J.H. & Detre, J.A. (2001_a). Dynamic changes in cerebral blood flow, O2 tension, and calculated cerebral metabolic rate of O_2 during functional activation using oxygen phosphorescence quenching. *Journal of cerebral blood flow & metabolism*, Vol. 21, No. 5, (May 2001), pp. 511-6, ISSN 1559-7016

Ances, B.M., Buerk, D.G., Greenberg, J.H. & Detre, J.A. (2001_b). Temporal dynamics of the partial pressure of brain tissue oxygen during functional forepaw stimulation in rats. *Neuroscience letters*, Vol. 306, No. 1-2, (June 2001), pp. 106-10, ISSN 1872-7972

Arthurs, O.J. & Boniface, S., (2003). What aspect of the fMRI BOLD signal best reflects the underlying electrophysiology in human somatosensory cortex? *Clinical Neurophysiology*, Vol. 114, No. 7, (July 2003), pp. 1203-9, ISSN 1872-8952

Atamna, H. & Kumar, R. (2010). Protective role of methylene blue in Alzheimer's disease via mitochondria and cytochrome c oxidase. Journal of *Alzheimer's disease: JAD*, Vol. 20, No. Suppl 2, pp. S439-52, ISSN 1875-8908

Baddeley, A.D. (1986). *Working memory*. Oxford University Press, ISBN 0-19-852133-2, New York.

Blumenfeld, R.S. & Ranganath, C. (2006). Dorsolateral prefrontal cortex promotes long-term memory formation through its role in working memory organization. *Journal of Neuroscience*, Vol. 26, No. 3, (January 2006), pp. 916-25, ISSN 1529-2401

Bradley, M.M., Greenwald, M.K., Petry, M.C. & Lang, P.J. (1992). Remembering pictures: pleasure and arousal in memory. Journal of experimental psychology. *Learning, memory, and cognition*, Vol. 18, No. 2, (March 1992), pp. 379-90, ISSN 1939-1285

Brown, G.C. (1992). Control of respiration and ATP synthesis in mammalian mitochondria and cells. *The Biochemical journal*, Vol. 284, No. 1, (May 1992), pp. 1-13, ISSN 1470-8728

Bruns, Jr.J. & Hauser, W.A. (2003). The epidemiology of traumatic brain injury: A review. *Epilepsia*, Vol. 44, No. Suppl 10, pp. 2-10, ISSN 1528-1167.

Bunce, S.C., Izzetoglu, M., Izzetoglu, K., Onaral, B. & Pourrezaei K. (2006) Functional near-infrared spectroscopy. *Engineering in medicine and biology magazine*, Vol. 25 No. 4, (July-August 2006), pp. 54-62, ISSN 1937-4186

Buxton, R.B. (2001). "Commentary: The elusive initial dip," *NeuroImage*, Vol. 13, No. 6 Pt 1, (June 2001), pp. 953-8. ISSN 1095-9572

Cannestra, A.F., Wartenburger, I., Obrig, H., Villringer, A. & Toga, A.W. (2003). Functional assessment of Broca's area using near infrared spectroscopy in humans. *NeuroReport*, Vol. 14, No. 15, (October 2003), pp. 1961-5, ISSN 1473-558X

Chance, B. & Williams, G.R. (1956). The respiratory chain and oxidative phosphorylation. *Advances in enzymology and related subjects of biochemistry*, No. 17, pp. 65-134, ISSN 0096-5316

Chance, B. & Leigh Jr. J.S. (1977). Oxygen intermediates and mixed valence. states of cytochrome oxidase: infrared absorption difference spectra of compounds A, B, and C of cytochrome oxidase and oxygen. *Proceedings of the National Academy of Sciences of the United States of America* , Vol. 74, No.11, (November 1977), pp. 4777-80, ISSN 1091-6490

Chance, B., Leigh, J.S., Miyake, H., Smith, D.S., Nioka, S., Greenfeld, R., Finander, M., Kaufmann, K., Levy, W., Young, M., Choen, P., Yoshioka, H. & Boretsky, R. (1988). Comparison of time-resolved and -unresolved measurements of deoxyhemoglobin in brain. *Proceedings of the National Academy of Sciences of the United States of America*, Vol. 85, No. 14, (July 1988), pp. 4971-5, ISSN 1091-6490

Chance, B., Zhuang, Z., UnAh, C., Alter, C. & Lipton, L. (1993). Cognition-activated low-frequency modulation of light absorption in human brain. *Proceedings of the National Academy of Sciences of the United States of America*, Vol. 90, No. 8, (April 1993), pp. 3770-4, ISSN 1091-6490

Chance, B., Anday, E., Nioka, S., Zhou, S., Hong, L., Worden, K., Li, C., Murray, T., Ovetsky, Y., Pidikiti, D. & Thomas, R. (1998). A novel method for fast imaging of brain function, non-invasively, with light. *Optics express*, Vol. 2, No. 10, (May 1998), pp. 411-23, ISSN 1094-4087

Clarke, D.D. & Sokoloff, L. (1994). Circulation and energy metabolism of the brain, In: *Basic Neurochemestry*, Siegel, G.J. & Agranoff, B.W. (Ed.), pp. 645-80, Raven, ISBN 0-397-51820-X, New York.

Cooper, C.E. (1990). The steady-state kinetics of cytochrome c oxidation by cytochrome oxidase. *Biochimica et biophysica acta*, Vol. 1017, No. 3, (June 1990), pp. 187-203, ISSN 0006-3002

Cooper, C.E., Matcher, S.J., Wyatt, J.S., Cope, M., Brown, G.C., Nemoto, E.M. & Delpy, D.T. (1994). Near-infrared spectroscopy of the brain: relevance to cytochrome oxidase bioenergetics. *Biochemical Society transactions*, Vol. 22, No. 4, (November 1994), pp. 974-80, ISSN 1470-8752

Cooper, C.E., Delpy, D.T. & Nemoto, E.M. (1998). The relationship of oxygen delivery to absolute haemoglobin oxygenation and mitochondrial cytochrome oxidase redox state in the adult brain: a near-infrared spectroscopy study. The *Biochemical journal*, Vol. 332, No. Pt 3, (June 1998), pp. 627-32, ISSN 1470-8728

D'Esposito, M., Aguirre, G.K., Zarahn, E., Ballard, D., Shin, R.K. & Lease, J. (1998). Functional MRI studies of spatial and nonspatial working memory. *Brain research. Cognitive brain research*, Vol. 7, No. 1, (July 1998), pp. 1-13, ISSN 0926-6410

Dirnagl, U., Villringer, A., Gebhardt, R., Haberl, R.L., Schmiedek, P. & Einhäupl, K.M. (1991). Three-dimensional reconstruction of the rat brain cortical microcirculation in vivo. *Journal of cerebral blood flow & metabolism*, Vol. 11, No. 3, (May 1991), pp. 353-60, ISSN 1559-7016

Duncan, A., Meek, J.H., Clemence, M., Elwell, C.E., Tyszczuk, L., Cope, M. & Delpy, D.T. (1995). Optical pathlength measurements on adult head, calf and forearm and the head of the newborn infant using phase resolved optical spectroscopy. *Physics in medicine and biology*, Vol. 40, No 2, (February 1995), pp. 295-304, ISSN 1361-6560

Dunn, A. K., Devor, A., Dale, A. M. & Boas, D. A. (2005). Spatial extent of oxygen metabolism and hemodynamic changes during functional activation of the rat somatosensory cortex. *Neuroimage*, Vol. 27, No. 2, (August 2005), pp. 279-90, ISSN 1095-9572

Enager, P., Piilgaard, H., Offenhauser, N., Kocharyan, A., Fernandes, P., Hamel, E. & Lauritzen, M. (2009). Pathway-specific variations in neurovascular and neurometabolic coupling in rat primary somatosensory cortex. *Journal of cerebral blood flow & metabolism*, Vol. 29, No. 5 (May 2009), pp. 976-86, ISSN 1559-7016

Franceschini, M.A. & Boas, D.A. (2004). Noninvasive measurement of neuronal activity with near-infrared optical imaging. *Neuroimage*, Vol. 21, No. 1, (January 2004), pp.372-86, ISSN 1095-9572

Frangioni, J.V. (2008). New technologies for human cancer imaging. *Journal of clinical oncology*, Vol. 26, No. 24, (August 2008), pp. 4012-21, ISSN 1527-7755

Freeman, W. (1973). Sexual behavior and fertility after frontal lobotomy. *Biological psychiatry*, Vol. 6, No. 1, (February 1973), pp. 97-104, ISSN 1873-2402

Ferrari, M., Hanley, D.F., Wilson, D.A. & Traystman, R.J. (1990). Redox changes in cat brain cytochrome-c oxidase after blood-fluorocarbon exchange. *The American journal of physiology*, Vol. 258, No. 6 Pt 2, (June 1990), pp. H1706-13, ISSN 0002-9513

Fox, P.T., Raichle, M.E., Mintun, M.A. & Dence, C. (1988). Nonoxidative glucose consumption during focal physiologic neural activity. *Science*, Vol. 241, No. 4864, (July 1988), pp. 462-4, ISSN 1095-9203

Frostig, R.D., Lieke, E.E., Ts'o, D.Y. & Grinvald, A. (1990). Cortical functional architecture and local coupling between neuronal activity and the microcirculation revealed by in vivo high-resolution optical imaging of intrinsic signals. *Proceedings of the National Academy of Sciences of the United States of America*, Vol. 87, No. 16, (August 1990), pp. 6082-6, ISSN 1091-6490

Füchtemeier, M., Leithner, C., Offenhauser, N., Foddis, M., Kohl-Bareis, M., Dirnagl, U., Lindauer, U. & Royl, G. (2010). Elevating intracranial pressure reverses the decrease in deoxygenated hemoglobin and abolishes the post-stimulus overshoot upon somatosensory activation in rats. *Neuroimage* Vol. 52, No. 2, (August 2010), pp. 445-54, ISSN 1095-9572

Gjedde, A., Marrett, S. & Vafaee, M. (2002). Oxidative and nonoxidative metabolism of excited neurons and astrocytes. *Journal of cerebral blood flow & metabolism*, Vol. 22, No. 1, (January 2002), pp. 1-14, ISSN 1559-7016

Goff, D.A., Buckley, E.M., Durduran, T., Wang, J. & Licht DJ. (2010). Noninvasive cerebral perfusion imaging in high-risk neonates. *Seminars in perinatology*, Vol. 34, No, 1, (February 2010), pp. 46-56, ISSN 1558-075X

Gratton, G., Maier, J.S., Fabiani, M., Mantulinm, W.W. & Gratton, E. (1994). Feasibility of intracranial near-infrared optical scanning. *Psychophysiology*, Vol. 31, No. 2, (March 1994), pp. 211-5, ISSN 1540-5958

Gratton, G., Corballis, P.M., Cho, E., Fabiani, M. & Hood, D.C. (1995). Shades of gray matter: noninvasive optical images of human brain responses during visual stimulation. *Psychophysiology*, Vol. 32, No. 5, (September 1995), pp. 505-9, ISSN 1540-5958

Grill-Spector, K., Henson, R. & Martin, A. (2006). Repetition and the brain: neural models of stimulus-specific effects. *Trends in cognitive sciences*, Vol. 10, No. 1, (January 2006), pp. 14-23, ISSN 1879-307X

Gross, P.M., Sposito, N.M., Pettersen, S.E., Panton, D.G. & Fenstermacher, J.D. (1987). Topography of capillary density, glucose metabolism, and microvascular function within the rat inferior colliculus. *Journal of cerebral blood flow & metabolism*, Vol. 7, No 2, (April 1987), pp. 154-60, ISSN 1559-7016

Heekeren, H. R., Kohl, M., Obrig, H., Wenzel, R., von Pannwitz, W., Matcher, S.J. Dirnagl, U., Cooper, C.E. & Villringer, A. (1999). Non-invasive assessment of changes in cytochrome-c oxidase oxidation in human subjects during visual stimulation. *Journal of Cerebral Blood Flow and Metabolism*, Vol. 19, No. 6, (June 1999), pp. 592–603, ISSN 1559-7016

Herrmann, M.J., Huter, T., Plichta, M.M., Ehlis, A.C., Alpers, G.W., Mühlberger, A. & Fallgatter, A.J. (2008). Enhancement of activity of the primary visual cortex during processing of emotional stimuli as measured with event-related functional near-infrared spectroscopy and event-related potentials. *Human Brain Mapping*, Vol. 29, No. 1, (January 2008), pp. 28-35, ISSN 1097-0193

Hikosaka, K. & Watanabe, M. (2000). Delay activity of orbital and lateral prefrontal neurons of the monkey varying with different rewards. *Cerebral Cortex*, Vol. 10, No. 3, (March 2000), pp. 263-71, ISSN 1460-2199

Hill, D.K. & Keynes, R.D. (1949). Opacity changes in stimulated nerve. *The Journal of Physiology*, Vol. 108, No. 3, (May 1949), pp. 278-81, ISSN 1469-7793

Hock, C., Villringer, K., Müller-Spahn, F., Wenzel, R., Heekeren, H., Schuh-Hofer, S., Hofmann, M., Minoshima, S., Schwaiger, M., Dirnagl, U. & Villringer, A. (1997). Decrease in parietal cerebral hemoglobin oxygenation during performance of a verbal fluency task in patients with Alzheimer's disease monitored by means of near-infrared spectroscopy (NIRS)--correlation with simultaneous rCBF-PET measurements. *Brain research*, Vol. 755, No. 2, (May 1997), pp. 293-303, ISSN 1872-6240

Holthoff, K. & Witte, O.W. (1996). Intrinsic optical signals in rat neocortical slices measured with near-infrared dark-field microscopy reveal changes in extracellular space. *The Journal of neuroscience*, Vol.16, No. 8, (April 1996), pp. 2740-9, ISSN 1529-2401

Hoshi, Y. & Tamura, M. (1993). Dynamic multichannel near-infrared optical imaging of human brain activity. *Journal of Applied Physiology*, Vol. 75, No. 4, (October 1993), pp.1842-6, ISSN 1522-1601

Huettel, S.A. & McCarthy, G. (2001). Regional differences in the refractory period of the hemodynamic response: an event-related fMRI study. Neuroimage, Vol. 14, No. 5, (November 1995) pp. 967-76, ISSN 1095-9572

Huppert, T.J., Hoge, R.D., Diamond, S.G., Franceschini, M.A. & Boas, D.A. (2006). A temporal comparison of BOLD, ASL, and NIRS hemodynamic responses to motor stimuli in adult humans. *Neuroimage*, Vol. 29, No. 2, (January 2006), pp. 368-82, ISSN 1095-9572

Izzetoglu, K., Bunce, S., Izzetoglu, M., Onaral, B., Pourrezaei, K. (2004). Functional near-infrared neuroimaging. *Conference proceedings: Annual International Conference of the IEEE Engineering in Medicine and Biology Society*, No. 7, pp. 5333-6, ISSN 1557-170X

Izzetoglu, M., Izzetoglu, K., Bunce, S., Ayaz, H., Devaraj, A., Onaral, B. & Pourrezaei, K. (2005) Functional near-infrared neuroimaging. *IEEE transactions on neural systems and rehabilitation engineering*, Vol. 13, No. 2, (June 2005), pp. 153-9, ISSN 1558-0210

Izzetoglu, M., Bunce, S.C., Izzetoglu, K., Onaral, B., & Pourrezaei, K. (2007). Functional brain imaging using near-infrared technology. *Engineering in medicine and biology magazine*, Vol. 26, No. 4, (July-August 2007), pp. 38-46, ISSN 1937-4186

Jöbsis, F.F. (1977). Non-invasive, infrared monitoring of cerebral and myocardial oxygen sufficiency and circulatory parameters. *Science*, Vol. 198, No. 4323, (December 1977), pp. 1264-7, ISSN 1095-9203

Jones, M., Berwick, J., Hewson-Stoate, N., Gias, C. & Mayhew, J. (2005). The effect of hypercapnia on the neural and hemodynamic responses to somatosensory stimulation. *Neuroimage*, Vol. 27, No. 3, (September 2005), pp. 609-23, ISSN 1095-9572

Keilin, D. (1925). On cytochrome, a respiratory pigment, common to animals, yeast, and higher plants. *Proceedings of the Royal Society of London*, Vol. 98, No. 690, (August 1925), pp. 312–339, ISSN 1471-2954

Klein, B., Kuschinsky, W., Schröck, H. & Vetterlein, F. (1986). Interdependency of local capillary density, blood flow, and metabolism in rat brains. *The American journal of physiology*, Vol. 251, No. 6 Pt 2, (December 1986), pp. H1333-40, ISSN 0002-9513

Kleinfeld, D., Mitra, P.P., Helmchen, F. & Denk, W. (1998). Fluctuations and stimulus-induced changes in blood flow observed in individual capillaries in layers 2 through 4 of rat neocortex. *Proceedings of the National Academy of Sciences of the United States of America*, Vol. 95, No. 26, (December 1998), pp. 15741-6, ISSN 1091-6490

Kleinschmidt, A., Obrig, H., Requardt, M., Merboldt, K.D., Dirnagl, U., Villringer, A. & Frahm, J. (1996). Simultaneous recording of cerebral blood oxygenation changes during human brain activation by magnetic resonance imaging and near-infrared spectroscopy. *Journal of cerebral blood flow & metabolism*, Vol. 16, No. 5, (September 1996), pp. 817-26, ISSN 1559-7016

Krawczyk, D.C. (2002). Contributions of the prefrontal cortex to the neural basis of human decision making. *Neuroscience and biobehavioral reviews*, Vol. 26, No.6, (October 2002), pp. 631-64, ISSN 1873-7528

Kurth, C.D., Steven, J.M. & Nicolson, S.C. (1995). Cerebral oxygenation during pediatric cardiac surgery using deep hypothermic circulatory arrest. *Anesthesiology*. Vol. 82, No, 1, (January 1995), pp. 74-82, ISSN 1528-1175

Leff, D.R., Orihuela-Espina, F., Elwell, C.E., Athanasiou, T., Delpy, D.T., Darzi, A.W. & Yang GZ. (2011). Assessment of the cerebral cortex during motor task behaviours in adults: a systematic review of functional near infrared spectroscopy (fNIRS) studies. *Neuroimage*, Vol. 54, No. 4, (February 2011), pp. 2922-36, ISSN 1095-9572

León-Carrion J., Damas-López, J., Martín-Rodríguez, J.F., Domínguez-Roldán, J.M., Murillo-Cabezas, F., Barroso Y. Martin, J.M. & Domínguez-Morales, M.R. (2008). The hemodynamics of cognitive control: the level of concentration of oxygenated hemoglobin in the superior prefrontal cortex varies as a function of performance in a modified Stroop task. *Behavioural brain research*. Vol. 193, No. 2, (November 2008), pp. 248-56, ISSN 1872-7549

León-Carrión, J., Izzetoglu, M., Izzetoglu, K., Martín-Rodríguez, J.F., Damas-López, J., Barroso y Martin, J.M. & Domínguez-Morales, M.R. (2010). Efficient learning produces spontaneous neural repetition suppression in prefrontal cortex. *Behavioural brain research*, Vol, 208, No. 2, (April 2010), pp. 502-8. ISSN 1872-7549

León-Carrión, J., Martín-Rodríguez, J.F., Damas-López, J., Pourrezai, K., Izzetoglu, K., Barroso y Martin, J.M. & Domínguez-Morales, M.R. (2007$_a$). A lasting post-stimulus activation on dorsolateral prefrontal cortex is produced when processing valence and arousal in visual affective stimuli. *Neuroscience letters*, Vol. 422, No. 3, (July 2007), pp.147-52, ISSN 1872-7972

Leon-Carrion, J., Martín-Rodríguez, J.F., Damas-López, J., Pourrezai, K., Izzetoglu, K., Barroso Y Martin, J.M. & Dominguez-Morales, M.R. (2007$_b$). Does dorsolateral prefrontal cortex (DLPFC) activation return to baseline when sexual stimuli cease? The role of DLPFC in visual sexual stimulation. *Neuroscience letters*, Vol. 416, No. 1, (April 2007), pp. 55-60,

Leon-Carrion, J., Damas, J., Izzetoglu, K., Pourrezai, K., Martín-Rodríguez, J.F., Barroso y Martin, J.M. & Dominguez-Morales, M.R. (2006). Differential time course and intensity of PFC activation for men and women in response to emotional stimuli: a functional near-infrared spectroscopy (fNIRS) study. *Neuroscience letters*, Vol. 403, No. 1-2, (July 2006), pp. 90-5. ISSN 1872-7972

Leon-Carrion, J., Domınguez-Morales, M.R., Barroso y Martın, J.M. & Murillo-Cabezas, F. (2005). Epidemiology of traumatic brain injury and subarachnoid haemorrhage. *Pituitary*, Vol. 8, No. 3-4, pp. 197-202, ISSN 1573-7403

Levy, R.J. & Deutschman, C.S. (2007). Cytochrome c oxidase dysfunction in sepsis. *Critical care medicine*, Vol. 35, No. 9 Suppl, (September 2007), pp. S468-75, ISSN 1530-0293

Lin, A.L., Fox, P. T., Yang, Y., Lu, H., Tan, L.H. & Gao, J.H. (2008). Evaluation of MRI models in the measurement of CMRO2 and its relationship with CBF. *Magnetic resonance in medical sciences*, Vol. 60, No. 2, (August 2008), pp. 380-9, ISSN 1880-2206

Lindauer, U., Royl, G., Leithner, C., Kühl, M., Gold, L., Gethmann, J., Kohl-Bareis, M., Villringer, A. & Dirnagl, U. (2001). No evidence for early decrease in blood oxygenation in rat whisker cortex in response to functional activation. *Neuroimage*, Vol. 13, No. 6 Pt 1, (June 2001), pp. 988-1001, ISSN 1095-9572

Lindauer, U., Gethmann, J., Kühl, M., Kohl-Bareis, M. & Dirnagl, U. (2003). Neuronal activity-induced changes of local cerebral microvascular blood oxygenation in the rat: effect of systemic hyperoxia or hypoxia. *Brain research*, Vol. 975, No. 1-2, (June 2003), pp.135-40, ISSN 1872-6240

Lindauer, U., Leithner, C., Kaasch, H., Rohrer, B., Foddis, M., Füchtemeier, M., Offenhauser, N., Steinbrink, J., Royl, G., Kohl-Bareis, M. & Dirnagl, U. (2010). Neurovascular coupling in rat brain operates independent of hemoglobin deoxygenation. *Journal of cerebral blood flow & metabolism*, Vol. 30, No. 4, (April 2010), pp. 757-68, ISSN 1559-7016

Luria, A.R. (1973) Towards the mechanism of naming disturbance. *Neuropsychologia*, Vol. 11, No. 4, (October 1973), pp. 417-21, ISSN 1873-3514

Logothetis, N.K., Pauls, J., Augath, M., Trinath, T. & Oeltermann, A. (2001). Neurophysiological investigation of the basis of the fMRI signal. Nature, Vol. 412, No. 6843, (July 2001), pp.150-7, ISSN 1476-4687

Lu, C.M., Zhang, Y.J., Biswal, B.B., Zang, Y.F., Peng, D.L. & Zhu, C.Z. (2010). Use of fNIRS to assess resting state functional connectivity. *Journal of neuroscience methods*, Vol. 186, No. 2, (February), pp. 242-9, ISSN

MacVicar, B.A. & Hochman, D. (1991). Imaging of synaptically evoked intrinsic optical signals in hippocampal slices. *The Journal of neuroscience*, Vol. 11, No. 5, (May 1991), pp. 1458-69, ISSN 1529-2401

MacIntosh, B.J., Klassen, L.M. & Menon, R.S. (2003). Transient hemodynamics during a breath hold challenge in a two part functional imaging study with simultaneous nearinfrared spectroscopy in adult humans. NeuroImage, Vol. 20, No. 2, (October 2003), pp. 1246-52, ISSN 1095-9572

Malonek, D. & Grinvald, A. (1996). Interactions between electrical activity and cortical microcirculation revealed by imaging spectroscopy: implications for functional brain mapping. Science, Vol. 272, No. 5261, (April 1996), pp. 551-4, ISSN 1095-9203

Matcher, S.J., Elwell, C.E., Cooper, C.E., Cope, M. & Delpy, D.T. (1995). Performance comparison of several published tissue near-infrared spectroscopy algorithms. *Analytical biochemistry*, Vol. 227, No. 1, (May 1995), pp. 54-68, ISSN 1096-0309

Mayhew, J., Johnston, D., Martindale, J., Jones, M., Berwick, J. & Zheng, Y. (2001). Increased oxygen consumption following activation of brain: theoretical footnotes using spectroscopic data from barrel cortex. *Neuroimage,* Vol. 13, No. 6 Pt 1, (June 2001), pp. 975-87, ISSN 1095-9572

Minagawa-Kawai, Y., Mori, K., Hebden, J.C. & Dupoux, E., (2008). Optical imaging of infants' neurocognitive development: recent advances and perspectives. *Developmental neurobiology.* Vol. 68, No. 6, (May 2008), pp. 712-28, ISSN 1932-846X

Nakahachi, T., Ishii, R., Iwase, M., Canuet, L., Takahashi, H., Kurimoto, R., Ikezawa, K., Azechi, M., Kajimoto, O. & Takeda, M. (2010). Frontal cortex activation associated with speeded processing of visuospatial working memory revealed by multichannel near-infrared spectroscopy during Advanced Trail Making Test performance. *Behavioural brain research,* Vol. 215, No. 1, (December 2010), pp. 21-7, ISSN 1872-7549

Obrig, H., Hirth, C., Junge-Hulsing, J.G., Doge C., Wolf, T., Dirnagl, U. &. Villringer A. (1996_a) Cerebral oxygenation changes in response to motor stimulation. *Journal of applied physiology,* Vol. 81, No. 3, (September 1996), pp. 1174-83, ISSN 1522-1601

Obrig, H., Heekeren, H., Ruben, J., Wenzel, R., Ndayisaba, J. P., Dirnagl, U., and Villringer, A. (1996_b). Continuous spectrum near-infrared spectroscopy approach in functional activation studies in the human adult. SPIE optics & photonics, Vol. 2926, (December 1996), pp. 58–66, ISSN 1818-2259

Obrig, H. & Villringer, A., 2003. Beyond the visible—imaging the human brain with light. . Journal of cerebral blood flow and metabolism, Vol. 23, No. 1, (January 2003), pp. 1-18, ISSN 1559-7016

Offenhauser, N., Thomsen, K., Caesar, K., & Lauritzen, M. (2005). Activity-induced tissue oxygenation changes in rat cerebellar cortex: interplay of postsynaptic activation and blood flow. *The Journal of physiology,* Vol. 565, No. Pt 1, (May 2005), pp. 279-94, ISSN 1469-7793

Owen-Reece, H., Elwell, C. E., Wyatt, J. S. and Delpy, D. T. (1996). The effect of scalp ischaemia on measurement of cerebral blood volume by near-infrared spectroscopy. *Physiological measurement,* Vol. 17, No. 4, (November 1996), pp. 279-86, ISSN 1361-6579

Owen, A.M. (1997). The functional organization of working memory processes within human lateral frontal cortex: the contribution of functional neuroimaging. *The European journal of neuroscience,* Vol. 9, No. 7, (July 1997), pp. 1329-39, ISSN 1460-9568

Owen, A.M. (2000). The role of the lateral frontal cortex in mnemonic processing: the contribution of functional neuroimaging. *Experimental brain research,* Vol. 133, No. 1, (July 2000), pp. 33-43, ISSN 1432-1106

Owen, A.M., McMillan, K.M., Laird, A.R. & Bullmore, E. (2005). N-back working memory paradigm: a meta-analysis of normative functional neuroimaging studies. *Human Brain Mapping,* Vol. 25, No. 1, (May 2005), pp. 46-59, ISSN 1097-0193

Pickrell, A.M., Fukui, H. & Moraes, C.T. (2009). The role of cytochrome c oxidase deficiency in ROS and amyloid plaque formation. *Journal of bioenergetics and biomembranes,* Vol. 41, No. 5, (October 2009), pp. 453-6, ISSN 1573-6881

Rector, D.M., Poe, G.R, Kristensen, M.P. & Harper, R.M. (1997). Light scattering changes follow evoked potentials from hippocampal Schaeffer collateral stimulation. *Journal of neurophysiology,* Vol. 78, No. 3, (September 1997), pp. 1707-13, ISSN 1522-1598

Royl, G., Füchtemeier, M., Leithner, C., Megow, D., Offenhauser, N., Steinbrink, J., Kohl-Bareis, M., Dirnagl, U. & Lindauer, U. (2008). Hypothermia effects on neurovascular coupling and cerebral metabolic rate of oxygen. *Neuroimage*, Vol. 40, No. 4, (May 2008), pp. 1523-32, ISSN 1095-9572

Ruocco, A.C, Medaglia, J.D., Tinker, J.R., Ayaz, H., Forman, E.M., Newman, C.F., Williams, J.M., Hillary, F.G., Platek, S.M., Onaral, B. & Chute, D.L. (2010). Medial prefrontal cortex hyperactivation during social exclusion in borderline personality disorder. *Psychiatry research*, Vol. 181, No. 3, (March 2010), pp. 233-6, ISSN 1872-7123

Seelig, J.M., Becker, D.P., Miller, J.D., Greenberg, R.P., Ward, J.D. & Choi, S.C. (1985). Traumatic acute subdural haematoma: Major mortality reduction in comatose patients treated within four hours. *The New England Journal of Medicine*, Vol. 304, No. 25, (June 1985), pp. 1511-8, ISSN 1533-4406

Smielewski, P., Kirkpatrick, P., Minhas, P., Pickard, J. D. & Czosnyka, M. (1995). Can cerebrovascular reactivity be measured with near-infrared spectroscopy?. *Stroke; a journal of cerebral circulation*, Vol. 26, No. 12, (December 1995), pp. 2285-92, ISSN 1524-4628

Smielewski, P., Czosnyka, M., Zabolotny, W., Kirkpatrick, P., Richards, H. & Pickard, J. D. (1997). A computing system for the clinical and experimental investigation of cerebrovascular reactivity. *International journal of clinical monitoring and computing*, Vol. 14, No. 3, (August 1997), pp. 185-98, ISSN 0167-9945

Stepnoski, R.A., LaPorta, A., Raccuia-Behling, F., Blonder, G.E., Slusher, R.E. & Kleinfeld, D. (1991). Noninvasive detection of changes in membrane potential in cultured neurons by light scattering. *Proceedings of the National Academy of Sciences of the United States of America.*, Vol. 88, No. 21, (November 1991), pp. 9382-6, ISSN 1091-6490

Strangman, G., Boas, D.A. & Sutton, J.P. (2002). Non-invasive neuroimaging using near-infrared light. *Biological psychiatry*, Vol. 52, No.7, (October 2002), pp. 679-93, ISSN 1873-2402

Tagliaferri, F., Compagnone, C., Korsic, M., Servadei, F., & Kraus, J. (2006). Reperfusion of low attenuation areas complicating subarachnoid haemorrhage. *Acta neurochirurgica. Supplement*, Vol. 96, pp. 85-7, ISSN 0065-1419

Terzian, H. & Ore, GD. (1955). Syndrome of Klüver and Bucy; reproduced in man by bilateral removal of the temporal lobes. *Neurology*, Vol. 5, No. 6, (June 1955), pp. 373-80, ISSN 1526-632X

Thompson, J.K., Peterson, M.R. & Freeman, R.D. (2003). Single-neuron activity and tissue oxygenation in the cerebral cortex. *Science*, Vol. 299, No. 5609, (February 2003), pp. 1070-2, ISSN 1095-9203

Totaro, R., Barattelli, G., Quaresima, V., Carolei, A. & Ferrari, M. (1998). Evaluation of potential factors affecting the measurement of cerebrovascular reactivity by near-infrared spectroscopy. *Clinical science*, Vol. 95, No. 4, (October 1998), pp. 497-504, ISSN 1470-8736

Toronov, V.A.W., Choi, J.H., Wolf, M., Michalos, A., Gratton, E. & Hueber, D., (2001). Investigation of human brain hemodynamics by simultaneous near-infrared spectroscopy and functional magnetic resonance imaging. *Medical physics*. Vol. 28, No. 4, (April 2001), pp. 521-7, ISSN 0094-2405

Toronov, V.A.W., Walker, S., Gupta, R., Choi, J.H., Gratton, E., Hueber, D. & Webb, A., (2003). The roles of changes in deoxyhemoglobin concentration and regional cerebral blood volume in the fMRI BOLD signal. *Neuroimage*, Vol. 19, No. 4, (August 2003), pp. 1521-31, ISSN 1095-9572

Uludağ, K., Steinbrink, J., Kohl-Bareis, M., Wenzel, R., Villringer, A. & Obrig, H. (2004). Cytochrome-c-oxidase redox changes during visual stimulation measured by near-infrared spectroscopy cannot be explained by a mere cross talk artefact. *Neuroimage*, Vol. 22, No. 1, (May 2004), pp.109-19, ISSN 1095-9572

Villringer, A., Planck, J., Hock, C., Schleinkofer, L. & Dirnagl, U. (1993). Near infrared spectroscopy (NIRS): a new tool to study hemodynamic changes during activation of brain function in human adults. *Neuroscience letters*, Vol. 154, No. 1-2, (May 1993), pp. 101-4, ISSN 1872-7972

Villringer, A. & Chance, B. (1997). Non-invasive optical spectroscopy and imaging of human brain function. *Trends in Neuroscience*, Vol. 20, No. 10, (October 1997), pp. 435–442, ISSN 1878-108X

Ward, K.R., Ivatury, R.R., Barbee, R.W., Terner, J., Pittman, R., Filho, I.P. & Spiess, B. (2006). Near infrared spectroscopy for evaluation of the trauma patient: a technology review. *Resuscitation*, Vol. 68, No. 1, (January 2006), pp. 27-44, ISSN 1873-1570

Watanabe, M. (1996). Reward expectancy in primate prefrontal neurons. *Nature*, Vol. 382, No. 6592, (August 1996), pp. 629-32, ISSN 1476-4687

Wharton, D.C. & Tzagoloff, A. (1964). Studies on the electron transfer system. LVII. The near infrared absorption band of cytochrome oxidase. *The Journal of biological chemistry*, Vol. 239, (June 1964), pp. 2036-41, ISSN 1083-351X

Williams L.M., Phillips M.L., Brammer M.J., Skerrett D., Lagopoulos J., Rennie C., Bahramali H., Olivieri G., David, A.S. Peduto A. & Gordon, E. (2001). Arousal dissociates amygdala and hippocampal fear responses: evidence from simultaneous fMRI and skin conductance recording, *Neuroimage* Vol. 14, No. 5, (November 2001), pp. 1070-9, ISSN 1095-9572

Wobst, P., Wenzel, R., Kohl, M., Obrig, H. & Villringer, A. (2001). Linear aspects of changes in deoxygenated hemoglobin concentration and cytochrome oxidase oxidation during brain activation. *Neuroimage*, Vol. 13, No. 3, (March 2001), pp. 520-30, ISSN 1095-9572

Wolf, M., Wolf, U., Choi, J.H., Gupta, R., Safonova, L.P., Paunescu, L.A., Michalos, A., & Gratton, E. (2002). Functional frequency-domain near-infrared spectroscopy detects fast neuronal signal in the motor cortex. *Neuroimage*, Vol. 17, No. 4, (December 2002), pp. 1868-75, ISSN 1095-9572

Wolf, M., Ferrari, M. & Quaresima, V. (2007). Progress of near-infrared spectroscopy and topography for brain and muscle clinical applications. *Journal of biomedical optics*. Vol. 12, No. 6, (November-December 2007), pp. 062104, ISSN 1560-2281

Wong Riley, M.T. (1989). Cytochrome oxidase: an endogenous metabolic marker for neuronal activity. *Trends in neurosciences*, Vol. 12, No. 3, pp. (March 1989), pp. 94-101, ISSN 1878-108X

Zabel, T.A. & Chute, D.L. (2002). Educational neuroimaging: a proposed neuropsychological application of near-infrared spectroscopy (nIRS). *The Journal of head trauma rehabilitation*, Vol. 17, No, 5, (October 2002), pp. 477-88, ISSN 1550-509X

Zaramella, P., Freato, F., Amigoni, A., Salvadori, S., Marangoni, P., Suppjei, A., Schiavo, B. & Chiandetti, L. (2001). Brain auditory activation measured by near-infrared spectroscopy (NIRS) in neonates. *Pediatric research*, Vol.49, No.2, (February 2001), pp. 213-9, ISSN 1530-0447

Zygun, D.A., Laupland, K.B., Hader, W.J., Kortbeek, J.B., Findlay, C., Doig, C.J. & Hameed, S.M. (2005). Severe traumatic brain injury in a large Canadian health region. *Canadian Journal of Neurological Sciences*, Vol. 32, No. 1, (February 2005), pp. 87-92, ISSN 0317-1671

4

Measurement of Brain Function Using Near-Infrared Spectroscopy (NIRS)

Hitoshi Tsunashima, Kazuki Yanagisawa and Masako Iwadate
Nihon University
Japan

1. Introduction

Near-infrared spectroscopy (NIRS) has gained attention in recent years (Hoshi et al., 2001; Tamura, 2003). This non-invasive technique uses near-infrared light to evaluate increases or decreases in oxygenated hemoglobin or deoxygenated hemoglobin in tissues below the body surface.

NIRS can detect the hemodynamics of the brain in real time while the subject is moving. Brain activity can therefore be measured in various environments. Recent research has used NIRS to measure brain activity in a train driver (Kojima et al., 2005, 2006). NIRS has also been used to evaluate the mental activity of an individual driving a car in a driving simulator (Shimizu et al., 2009).

Various arguments have focused on interpretation of signals obtained from NIRS, and no uniform signal-processing method has yet been established. Averaging and baseline correction are conventional signal-processing methods used for the NIRS signal. These methods require block design, an experimental technique that involves repeating the same stimuli (tasks) and resting multiple times in order to detect brain activation during a task. However, brain activation has been noted to gradually decline when a subject repeats the same task multiple times (Takahashi et al., 2006).

Fourier analysis, which is frequently used for signal analysis, transforms information in the time domain into the frequency domain through the Fourier transform. However, time information is lost in the course of the transform. As the NIRS signal fluctuates, time-frequency analysis is suitable for the NIRS signal.

The wavelet transform is an efficient method for time-frequency analysis (Mallat, 1998). This approach adapts the window width in time and frequency so that the window width in frequency becomes smaller when the window width in time is large, or the window width in frequency becomes larger when the window width in time is small. Multi-resolution analysis (MRA) (Mallat, 1989) decomposes the signal into different scales of resolution. MRA with an orthonormal wavelet base effectively facilitates complete decomposition and reconstruction of the signal without losing original information from the signal.

Oxygenated hemoglobin and deoxygenated hemoglobin as measured in NIRS are relative values from the beginning of measurement and vary between subjects and parts of the brain. Simple averaging of the NIRS signal thus should not be applied for statistical analysis. To solve this problem, we propose the Z-scored NIRS signal.

The aim of this chapter is to propose a signal processing method suitable for the NIRS signal and applicable for neuroimaging studies. We first describe the principle underlying measurement of brain activity with NIRS in Section 2. We then propose discrete wavelet-based MRA to extract the task-related signal from original NIRS recordings in Section 3.

In Section 4, we describe simultaneous measurement experiments with NIRS and functional magnetic resonance imaging (fMRI) using mental calculation tasks to confirm the validity of the proposed signal processing method. To investigate relationships between brain blood flow and skin blood flow, measurement is carried out using NIRS and the laser Doppler skin blood flow probe. The Z-scored NIRS signal is proposed for statistical analysis.

Two application examples with the proposed method for NIRS signals are shown in Section 5. We demonstrate the possibility of using the proposed method for evaluating brain activity associated with driving a car in a realistic driving environment. Another application is to brain-computer interfaces (BCIs), which are used in actively conducted studies. A BCI is a system that controls machines and devices by extracting neural information from human brain activity. BCIs are expected to become prominent as nursing robotics, such as artificial hands. The proposed method is applied for BCI systems that can control a robot arm using NIRS. We measured brain activity during actual grasping tasks and imagined grasping tasks using the BCI system to demonstrate the validity of the proposed BCI system.

Finally, some conclusions are given in Section 6.

2. Near-infrared Spectroscopy (NIRS)

Using near-infrared rays, NIRS non-invasively measures changes in cerebral blood flow. The principle of measurement was developed by Jöbsis (1977), based on the measurement of hemoglobin oxygenation in the cerebral blood flow.

In uniformly distributed tissue, incident light is attenuated by absorption and scattering. The following expression, a modified Lambert-Beer law, was therefore used:

$$Abs = -\log(I_{out} / I_{in}) = \varepsilon \bar{l} C + S\,. \tag{1}$$

Here, I_{in} is the irradiated quantity of light; I_{out} is the detected quantity of light; ε is the absorption coefficient; C is the concentration; $\bar{l}$ is the averaged path length; and S is the scattering term.

If it is assumed that no scattering changes in brain tissue occur during activation of the brain, the change in absorption across the activation can be expressed by the following expression:

$$\Delta Abs = -\log(\Delta I_{out} / \Delta I_{in}) = \varepsilon \bar{l}\, \Delta C(\Delta X_{oxy}, \Delta X_{deoxy})\,. \tag{2}$$

Furthermore, if the change in concentration (ΔC) is assumed to be proportional to the changes in oxygenated hemoglobin (ΔX_{oxy}) and deoxygenated hemoglobin (ΔX_{deoxy}), the following relational expression can be obtained:

$$\Delta Abs(\lambda_i) = \bar{l}\,[\varepsilon_{oxy}(\lambda_i)\Delta X_{oxy} + \varepsilon_{deoxy}(\lambda_i)\Delta X_{deoxy}]\,. \tag{3}$$

The absorption coefficients of oxygenated hemoglobin and deoxygenated hemoglobin at each wavelength, $\varepsilon_{oxy}(\lambda_i)$ and $\varepsilon_{deoxy}(\lambda_i)$, are known. As a result, $\bar{l}\Delta X_{oxy}$ and $\bar{l}\Delta X_{deoxy}$ can be obtained by performing measurements with near-infrared rays of two different wavelengths and solving Equation 3. However, the quantity obtained here is the product of the change in concentration and the averaged path length. In general, this averaged path length $\bar{l}$ varies greatly from one individual to another, and from one part of the brain to another. Caution must therefore be exercised in evaluating the results.

3. Signal processing methods for NIRS

3.1 Recording of NIRS signal

As mental calculation tasks, a low-level task comprising simple one-digit addition (e.g., 3 + 5) and a high-level task comprising subtraction and division with a decimal fraction (e.g., 234/(0.61 − 0.35)), were set to obtain NIRS signals. Brain activity in the prefrontal lobe was measured using NIRS. The measurement instrument was the OMM-3000 multichannel NIRS system (Shimadzu Corporation, Japan) (Kohno, 2006).

Figure 1 illustrates the arrangement of optical-fiber units and the location of each channel (3×7 matrix, 32 channels). Figure 2 shows the recorded temporal histories of oxygenated hemoglobin (red line, indicated as oxy-Hb) and deoxygenated hemoglobin (blue line, indicated as deoxy-Hb) in channel 20.

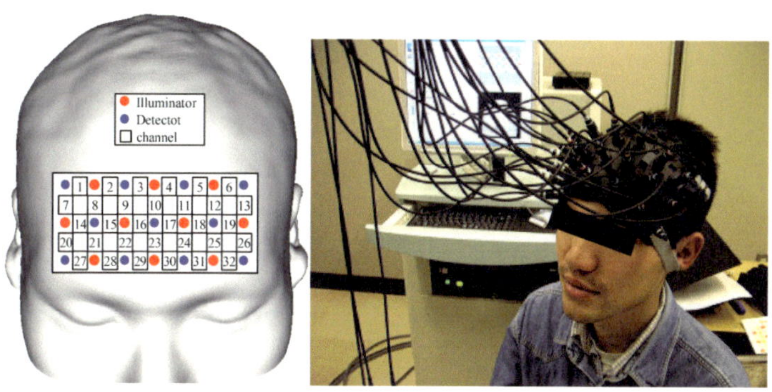

Fig. 1. Position of optical fibers and channels for recording NIRS signals (mental calculation task: matrix, 32 channels)

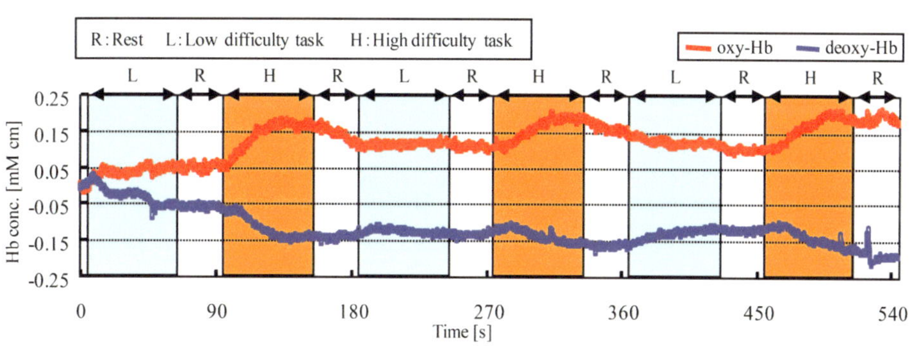

Fig. 2. Temporal history of NIRS signals in mental calculation (channel 20)

3.2 Analysis of NIRS signals

In NIRS signal analysis, brain activity related to a task must be separated from that which is not, since NIRS measures not only signals of brain activity during a task, but also other signals, including measurement noise.

In general, changes in oxygenated hemoglobin and deoxygenated hemoglobin when the brain is activated and restored to the original state exhibit the trend illustrated in Figure 3 (Huettel, 2004). Therefore, if these signals can be extracted from the measured signals, the brain has obviously been activated.

Averaging and baseline correction are conventional signal-processing methods. These methods require block design, an experimental technique that involves repeating the same stimuli (tasks) and resting multiple times in order to detect brain activation during a task.

Averaging is the method by which data are averaged for each task. Randomly generated noise approaches zero with averaging, and only periodic data are left. Averaging is effective when similar reactions are generated repeatedly. However, for cerebral blood flow that shows large variations in reactions to the same stimuli, the reliability of averaged signals is low, and false signals may be created. Furthermore, even significant signals may become undetectable after averaging.

Baseline correction corrects the start and end points of a block to zero to remove gradual trends, based on the assumption that blood flow is restored to its original state during a task block. However, because blood flow involves irregular fluctuations, the reference points are unstable. Therefore, if the whole block is corrected based on those two points alone, signals may be distorted.

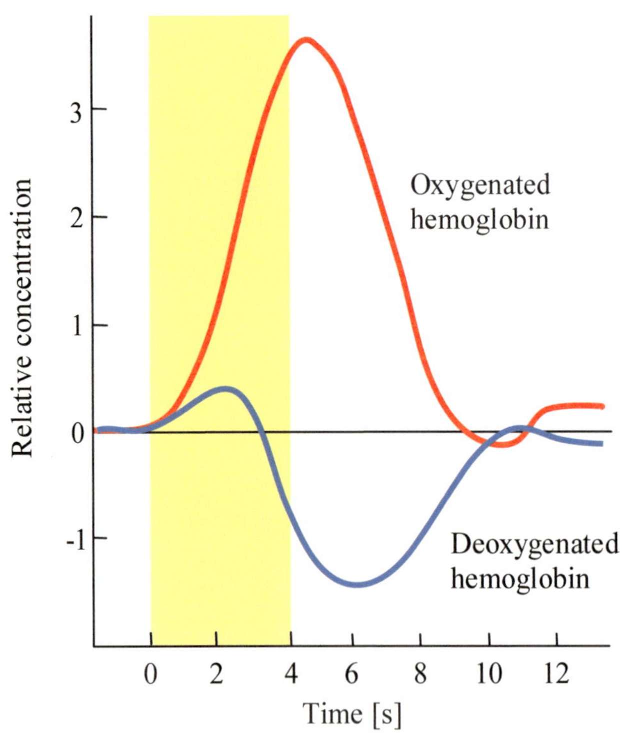

Fig. 3. Schematic of changes in hemoglobin concentration due to neural activity

Figure 4 shows the result of baseline correction applied for NIRS signals (Fig. 2) after removing high-frequency noise using a moving average of 25 data. Figure 5 indicates the functional brain imaging of the frontal lobe. It should be noted that brain activation gradually declines when a subject repeats the same task multiple times.

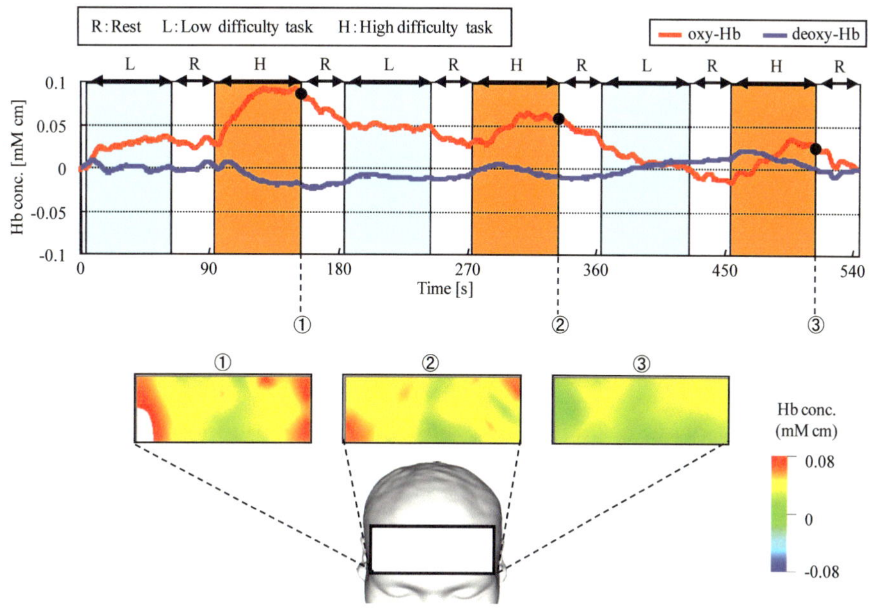

Fig. 4. Results of signal processing with baseline correction and de-noising

3.3 Decomposition and reconstruction of NIRS signals using wavelet transform

3.3.1 Wavelet transform

Fourier analysis, which is frequently used for frequency analysis, transforms information in the time domain into information in the frequency domain through the Fourier transform. However, time information is lost in the course of the transform.

A short-time Fourier transform, or windowed Fourier transform, can be used for time-frequency analysis of signals. However, the detection capacity varies widely, depending on the setting of the window.

In contrast, wavelet transform is an efficient method of time-frequency analysis. This approach adapts the window width in time and frequency so that the window width in frequency becomes smaller when the window width in time is large, or the window width in frequency becomes larger when the window width in time is small.

Wavelet transform expresses the local shape of the waveform to be analyzed, $S(t)$, by shifting and dilating the waveform called the mother wavelet, $\psi(t)$, and then analyzes the waveform.

A wavelet ψ is a function of zero average

$$\int_{-\infty}^{+\infty} \psi(t)dt = 0 \tag{4}$$

which is dilated with a scale parameter a and translated by b as

$$\psi_{a,b}(t) = \frac{1}{\sqrt{a}}\psi(\frac{t-b}{a}). \tag{5}$$

The continuous wavelet transform of signal $S(t)$ is computed with $\psi_{a,b}(t)$ as

$$\tilde{S}(a,b) = \int_{-\infty}^{\infty} S(t)\psi^{*}_{a,b}(t)dt. \tag{6}$$

Here, ψ^{*} denotes the complex conjugate of ψ.

One can construct wavelets ψ such that the dilated and translated function

$$\psi_{m,n}(t) = 2^{-m/2}\psi(2^{-m}t-n) \tag{7}$$

is an orthonormal base. Discrete wavelet transform can be computed by

$$D_m = \int_{-\infty}^{\infty} S(t)\psi_{m,n}(t)dt. \tag{8}$$

In the continuous wavelet transform, information is duplicated, requiring many calculations. Discrete wavelet transform handles a smaller volume of information than continuous wavelet transform, but is able to transform signals more efficiently. Furthermore, use of an orthonormal base facilitates complete reconstruction of original signals without redundancy. The following section describes decomposition and reconstruction of signals using MRA.

3.3.2 Multi-Resolution Analysis (MRA)

MRA decomposes signals into a tree structure using the discrete wavelet transform. In the case of the object time-series signals, $S(t)$, it decomposes the signals into an approximated component (low-frequency component) and multiple detailed components (high-frequency components).

A signal $S(t)$ can be expressed as follows by discrete wavelet transform using an orthonormal base $\psi_{m,n}$ as

$$S(t) = \sum_{n=-\infty}^{\infty} A_{m_0,n}\phi_{m_0,n}(t) + \sum_{m=-\infty}^{m_0}\sum_{n=-\infty}^{\infty} D_{m,n}\psi_{m,n}(t). \tag{9}$$

Here, $\phi_{m,n}(t)$ is the scaling function as defined by the following equation:

$$\phi_{m,n}(t) = 2^{-m/2}\phi(2^{-m}t-n). \tag{10}$$

The coefficient of the approximated component is calculated by

$$A_{m,n} = \int_{-\infty}^{\infty} S(t)\phi_{m,n}(t). \tag{11}$$

The detailed components of the signals on level m can be expressed by

$$d_m = \sum_{n=-\infty}^{\infty} D_{m,n}\psi_{m,n}(t)\,. \tag{12}$$

Thus, signal $S(t)$ can be expressed as

$$S(t) = a_{m_0} + \sum_{m=-\infty}^{m_0} d_m\,. \tag{13}$$

Task-related components can thus be reconstructed from detailed components d_m.
In the wavelet transform, the choice of a mother wavelet $\psi_{m,n}$ is important. We employed a *Daubechies* wavelet (Daubechies, 1992), which is orthonormal base and is a compactly supported wavelet. The vanishing moments of the *Daubechies* wavelet can be changed by an index N. We decided to use a relatively high-order generating index, $N = 7$.

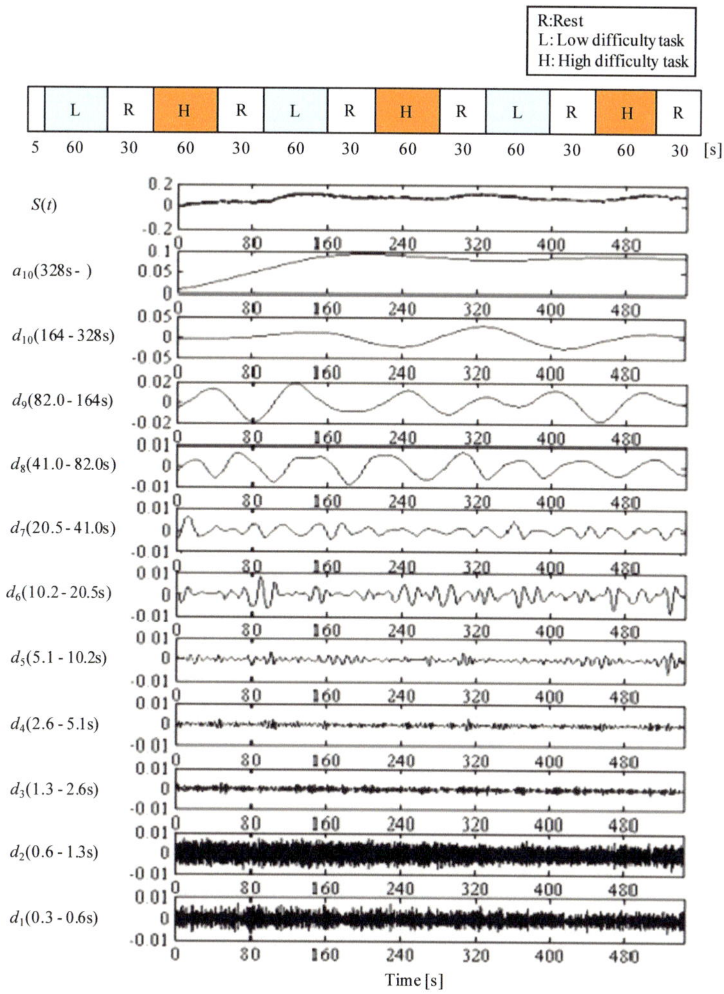

Fig. 5. Decomposition of NIRS signal using a wavelet base (*Daubechie* 7)

Figure 5 presents MRA results for oxygenated hemoglobin in channel 20, where task-related changes were marked. Here, the measured signal was decomposed into ten levels. The trend of the whole experiment was extracted on the approximated component (a_{10}), in the lowest-frequency range.

Here, d_1 and d_2, the highest frequency ranges, showed a relatively large amplitude. It is possible that these ranges represented measurement noise. As the interval for repetition of tasks and rests was 64 s, the d_8 component was the central component of task-related changes. Signals were therefore reconstructed by adding the d_7, d_8, and d_9 components.

Reconstructed signals are illustrated in Figure 6. Of note, the activation pattern of oxygenated hemoglobin and deoxygenated hemoglobin, shown in Figure 3, can be observed very clearly. Comparison between Figure 4 (signal processing with baseline correction and de-noising) and Figure 6 (wavelet-based method) shows the improved performance of the proposed method. Results revealed that oxygenated hemoglobin increased and the brain was activated during mental calculation tasks.

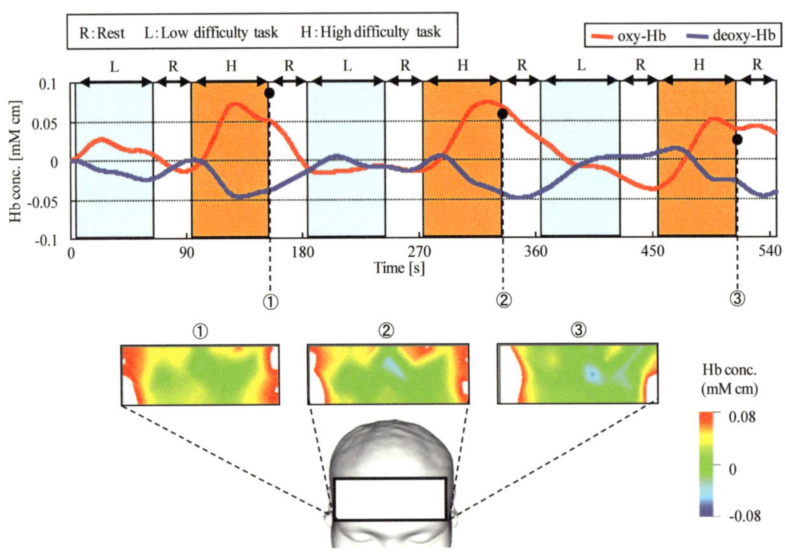

Fig. 6. Results of brain imaging using reconstructed signals

4. Measurement of brain functions under mental workload

4.1 Setting of workload

To confirm the validity of the signal-processing method explained in the previous section, we measured brain functions through simultaneous use of NIRS and fMRI.

To measure brain activity under workload, we used the workload of mental calculation. Mental calculation tasks were set to low, medium, and high levels as follows:

- Low-level task: Simple one-digit addition (e.g., 3 + 5)
- Medium-level task: One-digit addition of three numbers (e.g., 6 + 5 + 9)
- High-level task: Subtraction and division with decimal fraction (e.g., 234/(0.61 – 0.35))

The design of the experiment is presented in Figure 7. Each set was composed of 28 s of task and 36 s of rest, in that order. By arranging three sets for each level in random order, a total of nine sets of experiment were conducted over 592 s.

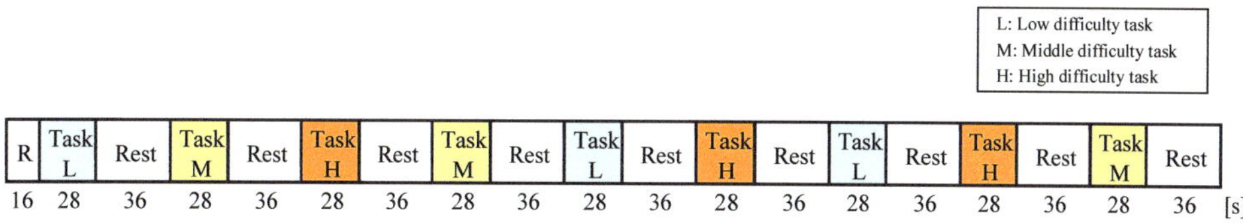

Fig. 7. Experimental design

A 28s task consisted of 14 questions at 2s intervals for the low level, 10 questions at 2.8s intervals for the intermediate level, or two questions at 14s intervals for the high level. The subject answered the questions displayed on the computer monitor without speaking. During the 36s rest time, the subject rested while steadily gazing at a cross mark displayed on the computer monitor.

4.2 NIRS and fMRI signal recording

Brain activity in the prefrontal lobe was measured using NIRS and fMRI simultaneously. NIRS data were collected using the OMM-3000 system (Shimadzu Corporation, Japan) in the MRI scanner.

Data from fMRI (3 mm thickness, 40 slices) were collected using a Siemens Symphony 1.5T (T2*-weighted gradient-echo sequence, TR = 4000 ms, TE = 50 ms, FA = 90 degrees, 64×64 pixels, FOV = 192 mm). Whole-brain images were obtained as T1-weighted images (TR = 2200 ms, TE = 3.93 ms, FA = 15 degrees, TI = 1100 ms, 1 mm^3 voxel, FOV = 256 mm).

Data from fMRI were pre-processed using Statistical Parametric Mapping (SPM99; Welcome Department of Imaging Neuroscience, UK) Normalized contrast images were smoothed with an isotropic Gaussian kernel (FWHM = 12 mm). Regions of interest (ROIs) were defined as clusters of 10 or more voxels in which estimated parameter values differed significantly from zero ($p<0.01$).

Subjects were nine healthy volunteers (nine men, no women). The arrangement of optical fiber units and measurement positions is shown in Figure 1.

4.3 Signal processing

Figure 8 presents measurement results through all channels for Subject A during the first three tasks. During the mental calculation task at the high level (i.e., the third task), oxygenated hemoglobin increased and deoxygenated hemoglobin decreased on both outer sides of the frontal lobe.

Figure 9 presents MRA results for oxygenated hemoglobin in channel 26, where task-related changes were marked. The trend of the whole experiment was extracted on the approximated component (a_{10}). As the interval of repetition of tasks and rests was 64 s, the d_8 component was the central component of task-related changes. Signals were thus reconstructed by adding the d_7, d_8, and d_9 components.

Reconstructed signals from channel 26 are illustrated in Figure 10. Results revealed that oxygenated hemoglobin increased and the brain was activated during mental calculation tasks. Furthermore, such changes became larger as the level of mental calculation task increased.

Figure 11 shows a comparison of functional brain imaging by fMRI and NIRS with the proposed method. The rectangle in the fMRI image indicates the region of measurement with NIRS. NIRS images agree with those for fMRI at a different workload level. This result supports the effectiveness of MRA with the discrete wavelet transform.

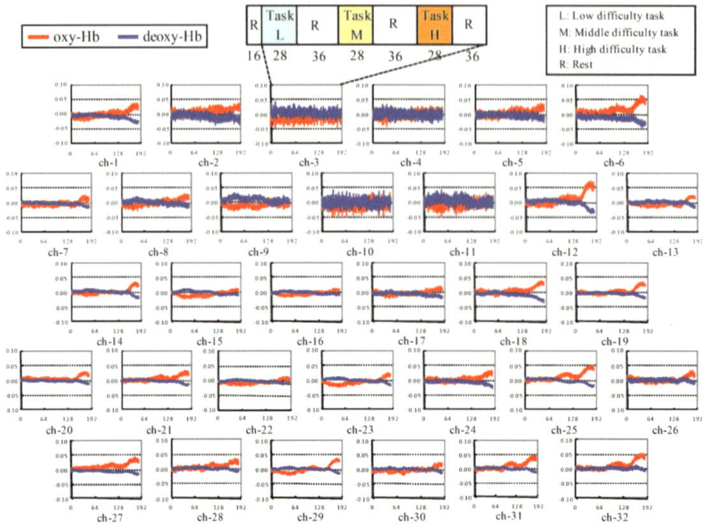

Fig. 8. Hemoglobin concentration changes in frontal lobe

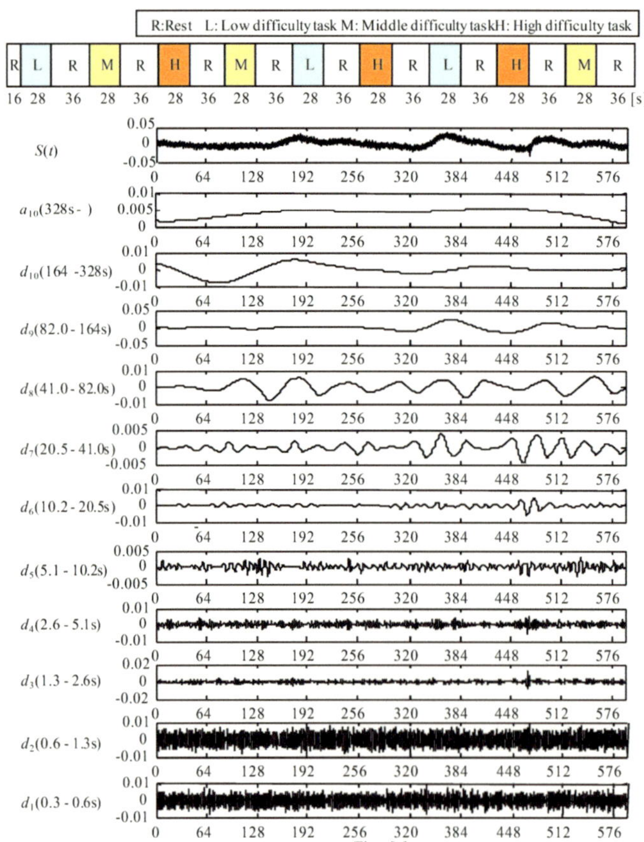

Fig. 9. Decomposition of NIRS signal (channel 26)

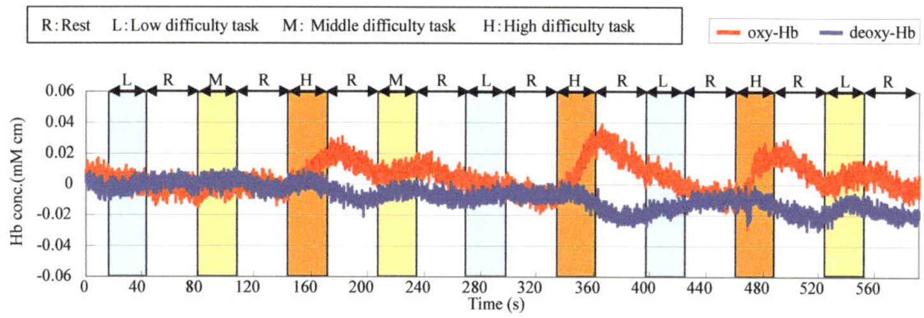

(a) Original signal

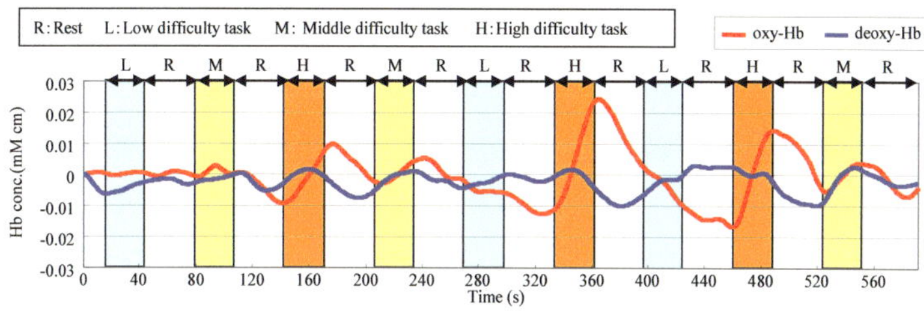

(b) Reconstructed NIRS signal

Fig. 10. Comparison of original signal and reconstructed signal (channel 26)

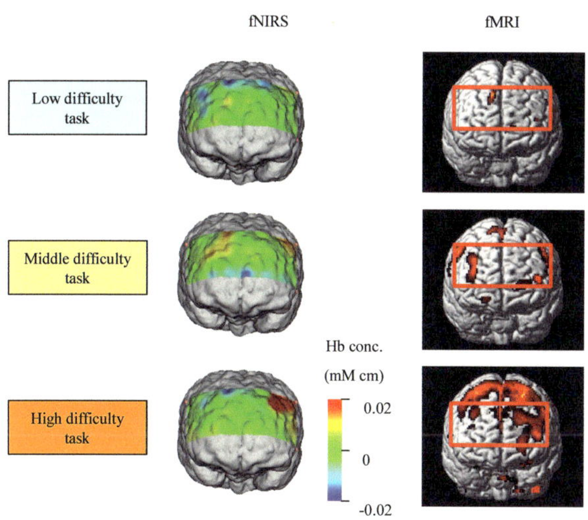

Fig. 11. Functional brain imaging by fMRI and NIRS

4.4 Influence of skin blood flow (SkBF)

To investigate relationships between brain blood flow and SkBF, we took measurements using NIRS and the laser Doppler SkBF probe. The laser Doppler SkBF probe (Advance Corporation, Japan) was placed on the right side of the forehead, 5 cm from the nasal root. The semiconductor laser Doppler velocimeter used a monochromatic light source at 780 nm. Figure 12 shows the comparison of NIRS signal (cerebral blood flow) and SkBF. Oxygenated hemoglobin increased and the brain was activated during mental calculation tasks. Furthermore, such changes became larger as the level of mental calculation task increased. But, SkBF did not increase in relation to task level.

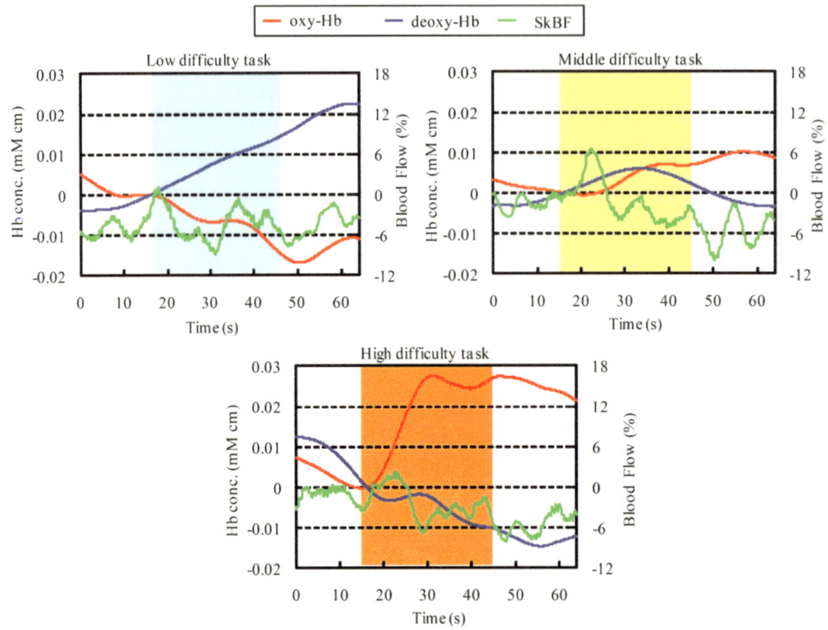

Fig. 12. Comparison of NIRS signal (channel 26) and SkBF

Mean values of oxygenated hemoglobin and SkBF at each task level are shown in Figure 13. The mean value of NIRS (Fig. 13(a)) became higher with higher task level. However, the mean value of SkBF (Fig. 13(b)) did not change in relation to task level. This result confirmed that SkBF did not influence NIRS signals (cerebral blood flow) in the recognition task.

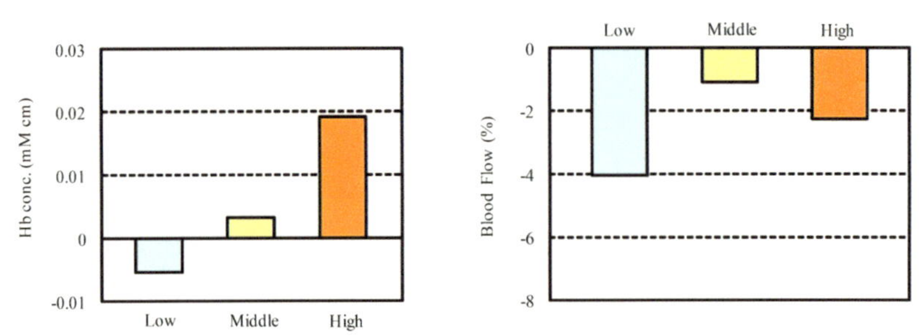

(a) Result of oxy-Hb mean value (b) Result of SkBF mean value

Fig. 13. Averaged result for oxy-Hb and SkBF at each task level

4.5 Statistical analysis

The NIRS signal expresses the quantity of relative changes using the start point as the reference. However, comparisons of measurements between subjects or statistical processing of measurements of all subjects cannot be implemented using this signal as is. Therefore, we propose a method for converting data of oxygenated hemoglobin and deoxygenated hemoglobin reconstructed by MRA into Z-scores using the following expression, so that the mean value is 0 and standard deviation is 1.

$$Z = \frac{X - \mu}{\sigma} \tag{14}$$

Here, x is the signal of oxygenated hemoglobin or deoxygenated hemoglobin reconstructed using MRA; μ is the mean value; and σ is the standard deviation.

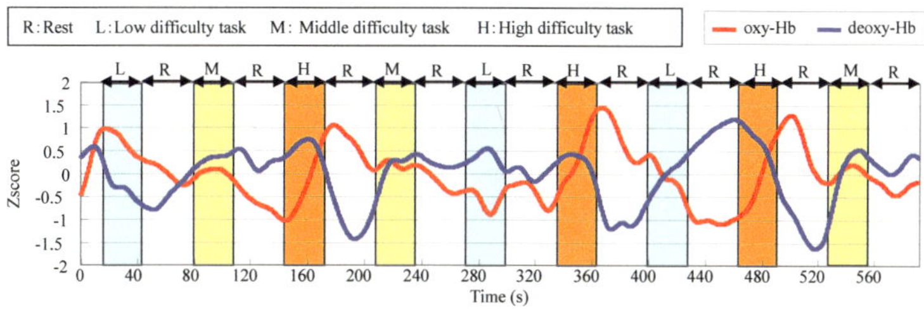

(a) Averaged reconstructed fNIRS signal (channel 26)

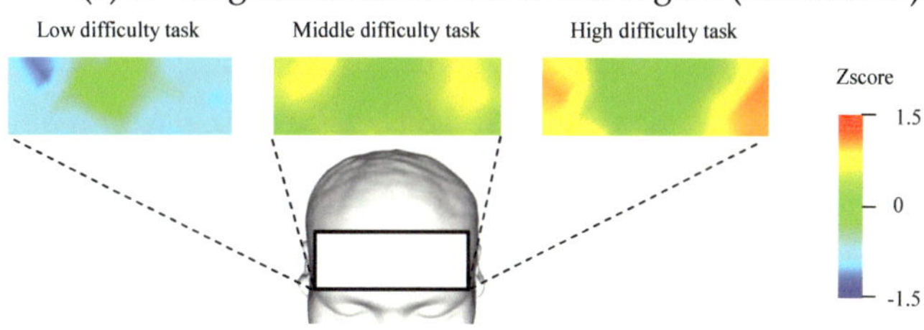

(b) Brain activity imaged by averaged NIRS signals

Fig. 14. Results of group analysis of NIRS signals for nine subjects

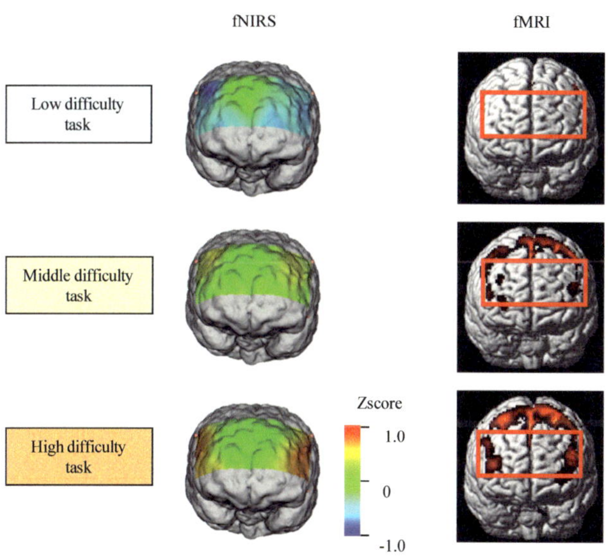

Fig. 15. Functional brain imaging by fMRI and NIRS (group analysis for nine subjects)

Figure 14 shows averaged NIRS signals using Z-score for nine subjects. Of note, the difference in workload level is reflected in the gradient of the oxygenated hemoglobin concentration. Figure 15 shows the results of group analysis for nine subjects. The rectangle in the fMRI image indicates the region of measurement with NIRS. NIRS images agree with results of fMRI regarding different workload levels. This result supports the effectiveness of the proposed method.

4.6 Subjective and objective evaluation of workload

In this experiment, the workload of each subject was measured using the Japanese version of NASA-TLX to evaluate correlations between the workload of mental calculation tasks and the objective evaluation using NIRS. The NASA-TLX is composed of six measures: mental requirements; physical requirements; temporal demand; work performance; effort; and frustration. Before workload evaluation, the subject performed one-to-one comparisons of the importance of elements of the workload involved in task performance.

The weight of each measure was based on the number of times an element was selected as more important during 15 one-to-one comparisons. When evaluating the workload of each task, the subject placed a mark at the appropriate position on the segment drawn between both extremes for each of the six measures.

A weighted workload (WWL) score was obtained by reading the position of each evaluation mark on a scale of 0 to 100 and multiplying by the weight for each measure determined by one-to-one comparison, then averaging all the products. Figure 16 (left) presents the WWL score of Subject A as determined by NASA-TLX. Workload became higher with higher task level.

Figure 16 (right) shows the results for 9 subjects evaluated using the maximum gradient of oxygenated hemoglobin in the task with different workload levels. Multivariate test using the Ryan method was used. Significant differences between high- and low-level tasks, or between high- and medium-level tasks are apparent ($p<0.05$). The results exhibited good correlation with subjective evaluation using NASA-TLX. This result confirms the feasibility of evaluating workload using the signal of cerebral blood flow obtained from NIRS.

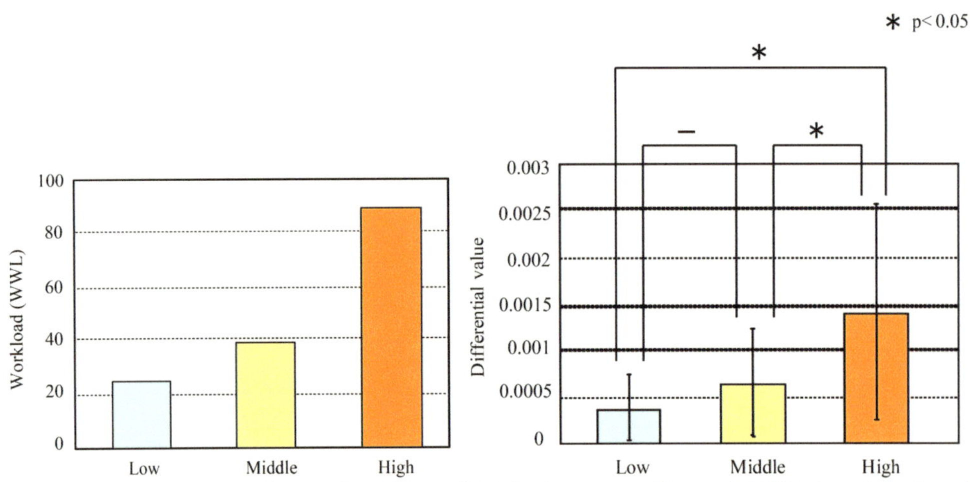

(a) Workload evaluation by NASA-TLX. (b) Maximum gradient of NIRS signal during the task

Fig. 16. Subjective and objective evaluation of workload

5. Application examples

5.1 Measurement of brain functions while driving a car

5.1.1 Background

Car drivers obtain visual information on the surrounding environment, recognize and judge that information suitably and then control their vehicle using the steering wheel, accelerator and brake pedal operations. Human brain activity functions to control all of these processes. In situations where it is necessary to predict unexpected danger, brain activity of the driver is thought to strengthen the cognitive function by spontaneously raising the level of attention. In the course of developing driver support systems, having a clear understanding of human brain activity is important in such driving situations.

In recent years, various driving-assistance systems have been developed to improve safety by reducing driver workloads. Examples include the adaptive cruise control (ACC) system, which maintains a safe distance between the driver's vehicle and the vehicle ahead, and the lane-keeping assistance system, which keeps the car in a lane through steering support.

However, while driver workload is reduced, the attention of the driver may also be reduced, resulting in unexpected accidents. Driver workload thus needs to be examined from the perspectives of cognitive engineering and human physiology. It is necessary to clarify relationships between driver workload and brain activity, which includes recognition and judgment. Driver attention then needs to be evaluated and the relationship between brain activity and driving performance clarified.

A small number of neuroimaging studies have used driving simulators to examine brain activity during driving. In these studies (Uchiyama, 2003; Spiers & Maguire, 2007), fMRI has been used. However, fMRI has many shortcomings in evaluating driving performance, requiring the subject to lie in a narrow cylinder during evaluation and not permitting movement of the body, particularly the head. This situation makes the driving task unrealistic and unnatural.

5.1.2 Driving task

To verify that the reduction in driving workload with ACC could be evaluated from brain activity, we conducted an experiment that involved the use of a driving simulator simulating following a vehicle (Fig. 17).

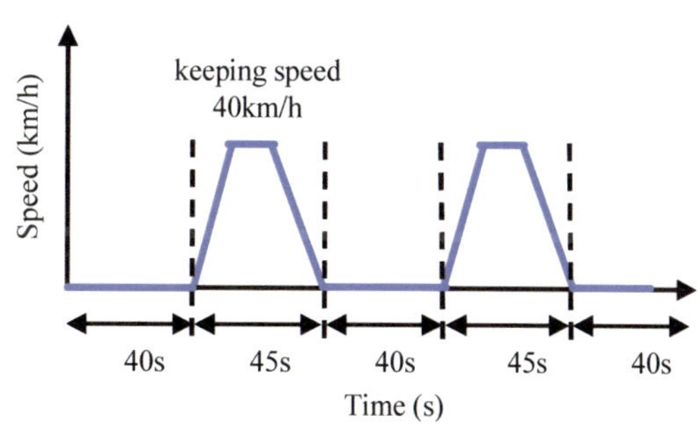

Fig. 17. Speed pattern of leading car

The main specifications of the driving simulator were as follows. Dimensions: 2,440 mm (W) × 2,280 mm (H) × 1,850 mm (D), front view: wide-field (138 degrees) screen projection, DLP projector with a total pixel count of 780,000 (XGA), rear view: 3 mirror independent LCD display 640×480 pixel (VGA), computer graphics: redraw speed, 30-60 frames/s, simulation system: 6-axis motion base system using six electric screw cylinders.

Driving tests were conducted under two conditions: one involved following a vehicle while utilizing the ACC; and the other involved following a vehicle while driving without ACC. The subject performed practice runs to become somewhat skilful in handling the driving simulator and then drove twice under each condition. Brain activity during one condition was compared with that during the other condition.

5.1.3 Measurement method

Brain activity in the frontal lobe was measured using NIRS. Figure 18 depicts the scene of the experiment. The measuring instrument was the OMM-300 near-infrared imaging device (Shimadzu Corporation, Japan). Figure 19 illustrates the arrangement of optical-fiber units (3 × 9 matrix, 42 channels).

Numbers between the light-emitting fiber unit and the light-receiving fiber unit denote the measurement channels; measurements were performed through a total of 42 channels. Furthermore, driving performance was also recorded on the driving simulator while measuring brain activity. Four male subjects in their 20s participated; all were in healthy condition and had ordinary driving licenses.

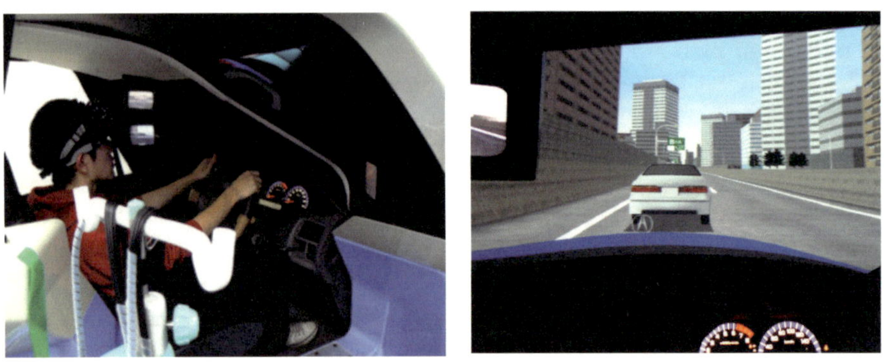

Fig. 18. Experiment with driving simulator (driver follows the proceeding vehicle with and without ACC)

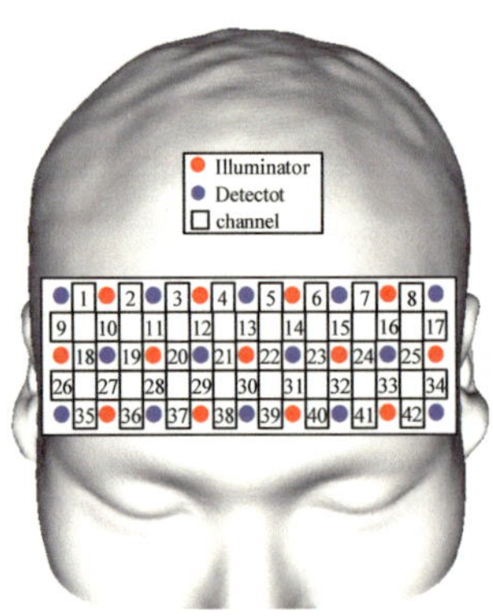

Fig. 19. Position of optical fibers and channels (driving task: 3×9 matrix, 42 channels)

5.1.4 Decomposition and reconstruction of NIRS signals

NIRS signals include signals that are unrelated to brain activity (e.g., noise of the measurement instrument, influences of breathing, and changes in blood pressure). These unrelated signals need to be removed to evaluate brain activity in detail. The measured NIRS signals were thus decomposed through MRA using discrete wavelet transform, and components related to the driving task were reconstructed. Group analysis using Z-score was then conducted for all subjects.

5.1.5 Results

Figure 20 presents the results of group analysis for four drivers without ACC, while Figure 21 presents the results with ACC. Figure 20(a) confirms that oxygenated hemoglobin increased when the subject drove without ACC and exhibited a high value in the latter half of the task. The brain function imaged in Figure 20(b) confirms that, as common brain activity, both outer portions of the frontal lobe became active during the driving task.

Figure 21(a) indicates that oxygenated hemoglobin did not increase while driving with the use of ACC. Also, the brain function image in Figure 21(b) reveals that the frontal lobe was less active than when the subject drove without ACC. This result may reflect the reduction of driving workload by ACC.

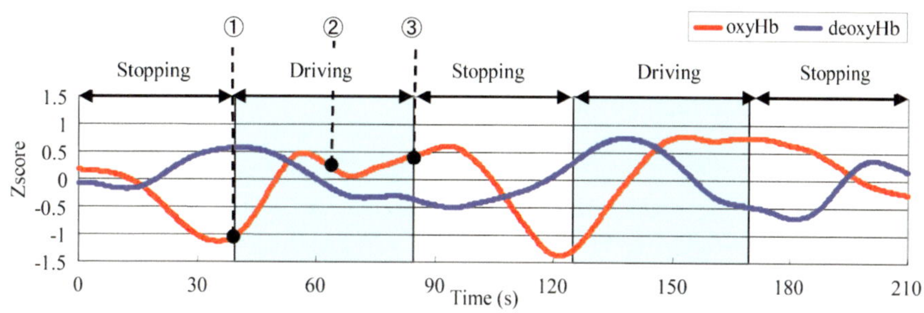

(a) Averaged reconstructed NIRS signal (channel 26)

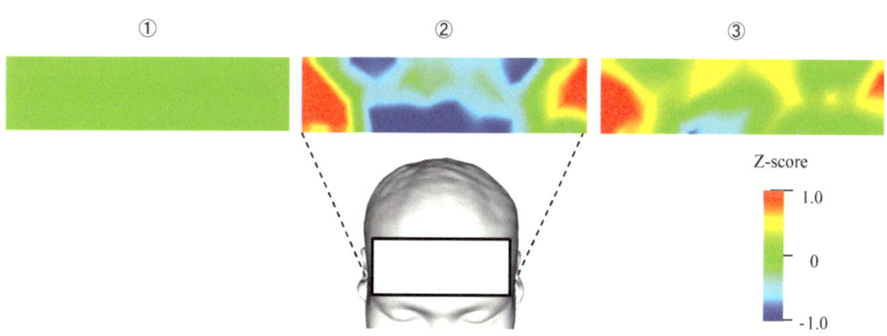

(b) Functional brain imaging

Fig. 20. Results of group analysis for four drivers without ACC system

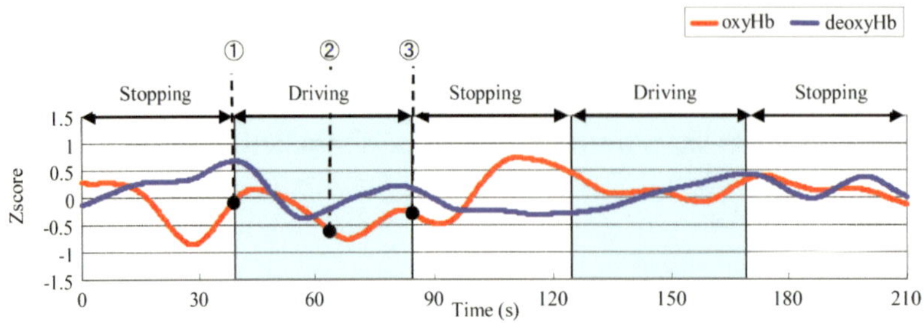

(a) Averaged reconstructed NIRS signal (Channel no. 26)

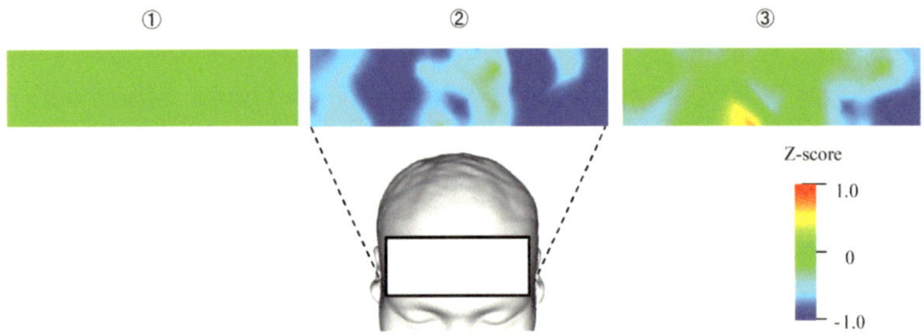

(b) Functional brain imaging

Fig. 21. Results of group analysis for four drivers with ACC system

5.2 Brain-Computer Interface (BCI) using NIRS

5.2.1 Background

Currently, the concept of BCIs is under intense study. BCIs extract activity from the human brain as cranial nerve information and use the information as inputs to control machinery and equipment. If this could enable the operation of machinery and equipment directly from cranial nerve information without the subject moving the hands and feet, such systems could be applied to care-taking robots for physically handicapped individuals.

BCI systems can be divided into two types. The invasive type reads cranial nerve information using electrodes embedded directly into the brain. The non-invasive type reads cranial nerve activity from the surface of the head using NIRS or electroencephalography (EEG). The invasive type offers high signal accuracy, but imposes heavy burdens on the user, such as the need for invasive procedures and the risk of infections after such procedures. The non-invasive form thus seems to have wider applicability.

In a study on the non-invasive type, Matsumura et al. extracted cranial nerve information using EEG and controlled a humanoid robot (Matsumura & Nakagawa, 2006). Many other studies of BCIs have used EEG. However, EEG may be greatly affected by movement of the user's body, and is vulnerable to electronic noise. In contrast, NIRS imposes fewer restrictions on body movement than EEG and is more resistant to electronic noise, so the load imposed on the user is less and electronic devices have no influence. The present study therefore focused on BCIs using NIRS.

In an earlier study, Nagaoka et al. developed an NIRS-BCI rehabilitation system (Nagaoka et al., 2010). In that study, electric stimuli corresponding to cranial nerve information were applied to the biceps brachii muscle of the user by setting a threshold on signals measured from NIRS, in order to cause the elbow joint to move. Signals measured by NIRS are unstable, since signals components that are irrelevant to the subject (e.g., noise of measurement instruments, heartbeat, and respiration) are included. Moreover, no processing method for NIRS signals has yet been established. For these reasons, obtaining a highly accurate operation by merely setting a simple threshold on NIRS signals is difficult.

In this study, we assumed artificial arms for physically handicapped individuals and proposed a BCI system that would enable operation of the robot arms using NIRS to measure cranial nerve information in a non-invasive manner. Furthermore, we applied new signal-processing methods, such as multiresolution analysis with discrete wavelet transform and a brain activity-judging method that uses derivatives of NIRS signals, to achieve highly accurate on/off operations.

In imaging tasks where the subject performs imaging in the brain without moving the body, signal intensity is weak and the presence of brain activity is difficult to judge. We therefore first verified the effectiveness of the system and judging method in grasping tasks, which have high signal intensity, and then verified the identification accuracy of the system from tests that involve imaged grasping tasks, with consideration of applying the system.

5.2.2 A robot arm control using a NIRS-BCI system

Figure 22 depicts a robot arm control system that uses a NIRS-BCI system. This system is composed of a cerebral function measurement section, a feature extraction and recognition section, and a device control section. In the cerebral function measurement section, the oxygenated hemoglobin level of the user is measured using the OMM-3000 multichannel NIRS instrument made by Shimadzu Corporation, Japan. In the feature extraction and recognition section, the threshold is obtained by analyzing the original signal of oxygenated hemoglobin that was measured. When oxygenated hemoglobin after analysis exceeds the threshold obtained in the feature extraction and recognition section, the on signal is sent to the device control section to enable rotation of the joint of the robot arm (MR-999; Elekit, Japan).

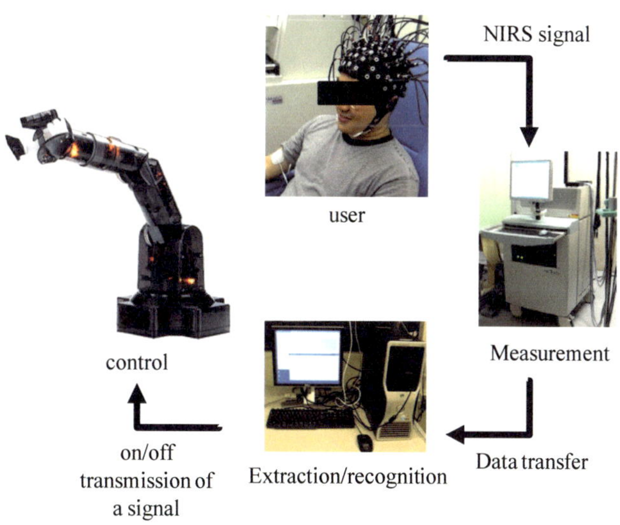

Fig. 22. Robot arm control using the NIRS-BCI system

Experiments were conducted using the robot arm control system depicted in Figure 22. Optical fibers were arranged in 4×4 matrices on the right and left sides to perform measurement, with a total of 48 channels.

Five trials were carried out, with each trial consisting of 10 s of pre-task rest, 30 s of task, and 10 s of post-task rest. The first two trials were defined as the learning stage, where the feature extraction and recognition section learned the fluctuation pattern of the user's oxygenated hemoglobin levels without moving the robot.

In the third and subsequent trials, the robot arm was rotated according to the learned pattern corresponding with oxygenated hemoglobin. Both grasping tasks and imaged grasping tasks were performed. The subject was instructed to rest during the rest time. The motor area was selected as the measurement site.

5.2.3 Judgment of brain activity

Judgment with a simple threshold

In the judgment method that used a simple threshold, the average oxygenated hemoglobin level in the first two trials and the standard deviation were converted to Z-scores, and the moving average was obtained. The threshold was set to 20% of the maximum oxygenated hemoglobin level during the first two trials; judgment was made in the third and subsequent trials, and an "on" state was judged when oxygenated hemoglobin level exceeded this threshold.

Changes in density of oxygenated hemoglobin level and the judgment results for imaged grasping tasks and actual grasping tasks are depicted in Figure 23. In Figure 23(a), "on" judgments were observed in the first and second trials, but not in the third trial. Next, in Figure 23(b), "on" judgments were made in all tasks from the first to third trials, but "on" and "off" judgments alternated within a short time, indicating instability. Furthermore, an "on" judgment was made during the rest period in the second trial, indicating erroneous judgments.

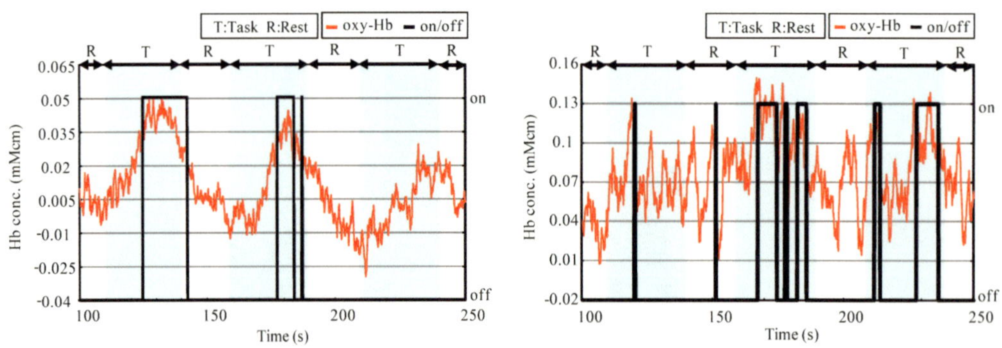

(a) Actual grasping tasks (b) Imagined grasping tasks

Fig. 23. Results for on/off decisions using a simple threshold

Judgment using oxygenated hemoglobin level and its derivative

NIRS can measure both change in density of oxygenated hemoglobin and that of deoxygenated hemoglobin; however, the change in density of oxygenated hemoglobin is highly correlated with the change in regional cerebral blood flow (rCBF) (Hoshi, 2001), and an increase in rCBF reflects an increase in neural activity. We therefore focused on the oxygenated hemoglobin signal.

Furthermore, the derivative of oxygenated hemoglobin is highly correlated with the workload of the task as shown in Section 4.6, so we judged brain activity using two indices: oxygenated hemoglobin; and its derivative. First, NIRS signals include signal components that are irrelevant to brain activity (e.g., noise of measurement instruments, influences of respiration, and fluctuations of blood pressure). Signals were thus decomposed and reconstructed by MRA.

The original oxygenated hemoglobin signal and reconstructed oxygenated hemoglobin signal are depicted in Figure 24(a). In Figure 24(a), oxygenated hemoglobin includes not only brain activity, but also the effects of blood pressure, breathing and measurement noises. However, in Figure 24(b), the reconstructed oxygenated hemoglobin signal can be seen to be smoothed.

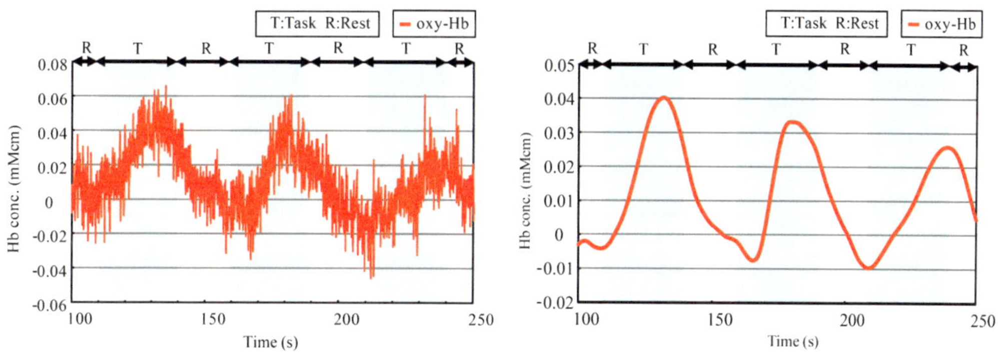

(a) Original oxy-Hb signal (b) Reconstructed oxy-Hb signal

Fig. 24. Changes in original and reconstructed oxygenated hemoglobin signals

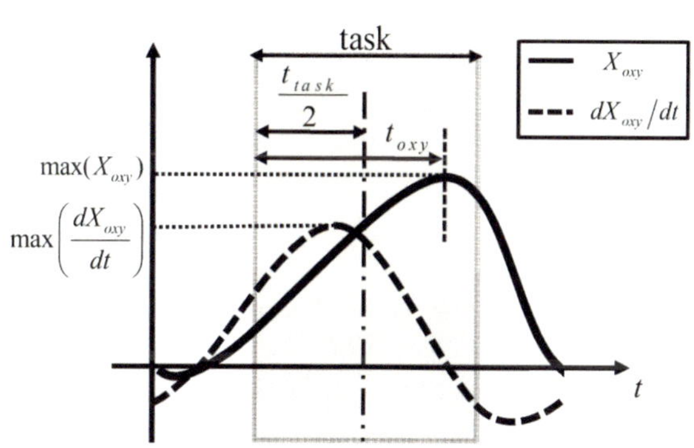

Fig. 25. Oxygenated hemoglobin concentration change due to neural activity

Changes in oxygenated hemoglobin and its derivative when the brain is activated are depicted in Figure 25. Oxygenated hemoglobin was defined as X_{oxy} and its derivative was defined as dX_{oxy}/dt. The threshold of oxygenated hemoglobin (denoted as y_1) and that of the derivative (denoted as y_2) were computed by $y_1 = K_1 \max(X_{oxy})$ and $y_2 = K_2 \max(dX_{oxy}/dt)$. K_1 and K_2 were weight factors that depended on the point where X_{oxy} reached a maximum.

The point where X_{oxy} reached a maximum was defined as $e = (t_{oxy} - t_{task}/2)/(t_{task}/2)$. Here, t_{task} was a time at which tasks were performed and t_{oxy} was a time from start of the task to when X_{oxy} reached a maximum. In this study, K_1 and K_2 were set to $K_1 = 0.8e + 0.2$ and $K_1 = -0.8e + 1$. If X_{oxy} reached maximum in the middle of the task, y_1 was 20% of the maximum value of X_{oxy}. If X_{oxy} reached maximum at the end of the task, y_2 was 20% of the maximum value of dX_{oxy}/dt. The on/off decision (on = 1, off = 0) was made by Y (= 1: $X_{oxy}>y_1$ or $dX_{oxy}/dt>y_2$, = 0: otherwise).
The judgment result for grasping tasks when the proposed judgment method was applied is depicted in Figure 26(a), and that for imaged grasping tasks is depicted in Figure 26(b).

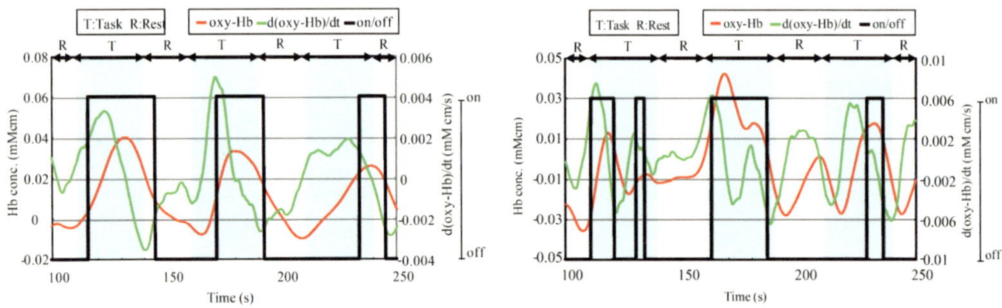

(a) Actual grasping tasks (b) Imagined grasping tasks

Fig. 26. Result of on/off decision using oxygenated hemoglobin and its derivative

In contrast to the judgment method where a simple threshold was imposed on oxygenated hemoglobin in grasping tasks (Fig. 23(a)), "on" judgments were confirmed during the first and all subsequent tasks with the method depicted in Figure 26(a). However, "on" judgments were made continually for 5 s after completion of the task in each trial, indicating that erroneous judgments may be made. The judgment method thus needs further refinement.
In contrast to the judgment method where a simple threshold was imposed on oxygenated hemoglobin in imaged grasping tasks (Fig. 23(b)), more stable judgment was made in Figure 26(b), and the problem of alternating "on" and "off" judgments within a short time was reduced.

6. Conclusions

A signal-processing method to extract task-related components with MRA based on discrete wavelet transform is proposed for NIRS. Integration of data from multiple subjects using Z-scores was then developed for statistical group analysis.
Brain activity of subjects with workloads comprising different levels of mental calculation tasks were measured using NIRS and fMRI. NIRS images constructed using the proposed method agreed with fMRI images at different workload levels. Those results show that the proposed method is effective for evaluating brain activity measured by NIRS.
Comparison between NIRS signal (cerebral blood flow) and skin blood flow showed that skin blood flow does not affect NIRS signal in the recognition task.
Changes in brain activity in connection with workload were compared with the subjective evaluation of workload by NASA-TLX. Good correlation was observed between brain

activity detected by NIRS and workload scores obtained from NASA-TLX. This result indicates the possibility of evaluating workload from cerebral blood flow signals obtained using NIRS.

Whether the reduction of driving workload by ACC can be evaluated from brain activity was evaluated through experiments using a driving simulator. The results revealed that while the outer portions of the frontal lobe were active in connection with driving performance when the subject drove without ACC, no activity related to driving performance was seen with the use of ACC. These results suggest the possibility of evaluating driving-assistance systems through the evaluation of driving workload from measurement of brain activity using NIRS.

We developed MRA using discrete wavelet transform as a real-time post-signal processing for NIRS-BCI system and applied this approach to control of a robot arm. With a judgment method that used a simple threshold, no stable operation could be obtained for grasping tasks or imaged grasping tasks.

We proposed a judgment method that uses two indices (oxygenated hemoglobin and the derivative of oxygenated hemoglobin) for judging brain activity, and adjusts the threshold of oxygenated hemoglobin and its derivative depending on the point of maximum oxygenated hemoglobin during the task. Results indicate that our proposed method enables more accurate judgments than use of a simple threshold. We thus confirmed the feasibility of our proposed method for a NIRS-BCI system.

7. Acknowledgment

This work was supported by the Nihon University Multidisciplinary Research Grant in 2006, 2007 and 2010.

8. References

Hoshi, Y., Kobayashi, N., Tamura, M. (2001). Interpretation of nearinfrared spectroscopy signals, A study with a newly developed perfused rat brain model, *Journal of Applied Physiology*, Vol.90, No.5, pp.1657-1662

Tamura, M. (2003). Functional near-infrared spectoroscopy, *Advances in Neurological Sciences*, Series C, Vol.47, No.6, pp.891-901

Kojima, T., Tsunashima, H., Shiozawa, T., Takada, H. and Sakai, T. (2005). Measurement of Train Driver's Brain Activity by Functional Near-Infrared Spectroscopy (fNIRS), *Optical and Quantum Electronics*, Vol.37, No.13-15, pp. 1319-1338

Kojima, T., Tsunashima, H., Shiozawa, T. (2006). Measurement of train driver's brain activity by functional near-infrared spectroscopy (fNIRS), *COMPUTERS IN RAILWAYS X*, WIT Press

Shimizu, T., Hirose, S., Obara, H., Yanagisawa, K., Tsunashima, H., Marumo, Y., Haji. T. and Taira, M. (2009). Measurement of Frontal Cortex Brain Activity Attribute to the Driving Workload and Increased Attention, *SAE paper* NO. 2009-01-054

Takahashi, K., Watanabe, N. and Harada, T. (2006). Preliminary experiment of the evaluation of a VR based training system using brain activity, *Virtual Reality Society of Japan Annual Conference*, Vol. 11 pp. 354-355, ISSN 1349-5062, Japan, 2006

Mallat, S. (1998). *A Wavelet Tour of Signal Processing*, Academic Press, ISBN 978-0124666061, USA

Mallat, S. (1989). A theory for multiresolution signal decomposition: the wavelet representation, *IEEE Transactions on Pattern Recognition and Machine Intelligence*, Vol.11, No.7, pp.674-693

Jöbsis, FF. (1977). Non-invasive infrared monitoring of cerebral and myocardial oxygen sufficiency and circulatory parameters, *Science*, Vol.198, pp.1264-1267

Kohno, S. , Ishikawa, A., Tsuneishi, S., Amita, T., Shimizu, K. and Mukuta, Y. (2006). Application development of functional near-infrared imaging system, *Shimadzu Review*, Vol. 63, No.3.4, pp.195-200

Huettel, S. A. (2004). *Functional Magnetic Resonance Imaging*, Sinauer Associate, Inc., ISBN 978-0878932887, USA

Daubechies, I. (1992). *Ten Lectures on Wavelets*, CBMS-NSF Regional Conference Series In Applied Mathematics; Society for Industrial and Applied Mathematics, No.61, ISBN 978-0898712742

Mallat, S. (1989). A theory for multiresolution signal decomposition: the wavelet representation, *IEEE Transactions on Pattern Recognition and Machine Intelligence*, Vol.11, No.7, pp.674-693

Uchiyama, Y., Ebe, K., Kozato, A., Okada, T., Sadato, N. (2003). The neural substrates of driving at a safe distance: a functional MRI study, *Neuroscience Letters*, Vol.352-3, pp.199-202

Spiers, H. J. and Maguire, E. A. (2007). Neural substrates of driving behaviour, *Neuro Image*, No.36, pp.245-255

Matsumura, H. and Nakagawa, M. (2006). An EEG-based Humanoid Robot Control System, *The institute of electronics, information and communication engineers*, Vol.106, No.345, pp.63-68, ISSN 09135685

Nagaoka, T., Sakatani, K., Awano, T., Yokose, N., Hoshino, T., Murata, Y., Katayama, Y., Ishikawa, A., Eda, H. (2010). Development of a new rehabilitation system based on a brain-computer interface using near infrared spectroscopy, *Advances in Experimental Medicine and Biology*, Vol.662, pp. 497-503

5

Towards Model-Based Brain Imaging with Multi-Scale Modeling

Lars Schwabe and Youwei Zheng
Adaptive and Regenerative Software Systems
Dept of Computer Science and Electrical Engineering
Universität Rostock, Rostock,
Germany

1. Introduction

Brain imaging has been a key technology in advancing our understanding of the neuronal basis of cognition. However, in order to fully unleash the power of brain imaging it needs to be combined with other sources of information such as gene expression, behavioural performance, as well as with computational models.

In so-called "model-based brain imaging" computational models of how the brain processes information are employed in order to interpret the data. A prominent example is the use of models from reinforcement learning in order to interpret responses in basal ganglia, or frontal cortex. However, while such a model-based brain imaging certainly adds a new level of explanation beyond the mere description of the evoked neuronal activations, it will always be limited by the spatial and temporal resolution of the employed imaging technologies.

Here, we argue that the application of multi-scale modeling, which bridges the gap between the various spatial and temporal scales, is a necessary next step in the analysis of brain imaging data. For example, this way it will be possible to simulate the effects of altered membrane currents under pharmacological manipulation on brain-wide network dynamics and compare simulation results with recorded brain imaging data.

We emphasize that one important benefit of models is to operationalize as many assumptions as possible (Section 2). Then, we summarize the state-of-the-art in Neuroinformatics tool support, which is necessary for multi-scale models in model-based brain imaging. We also argue that even without complete physical models, which bridge the various scales, a data-driven approach using partly phenomenological model can be pursued, but this calls for new Neuroinformatics tools (Section 3). We summarize some of our recent work in network modeling of the visual system, where we performed systematic model comparisons (Section 4), and we close with identifying a challenging test case for multi-scale modeling in model-based brain imaging, namely the investigation of the neuronal basis of the self (Section 5).

2. Two dimensions of theory-dependence of observations in neuroscience

Brain imaging studies are already heavily dependent on various kinds of models. We argue that a key advantage of models in brain imaging (and in the interpretation of neuronal data in general) is to make assumptions explicit in order to deal with the fact that all observations are theory-dependent. Interestingly, we can distinguish two dimensions of theory-dependence in brain imaging (**Figure 1a**): *First*, the dependence on the physical theories upon which the measurement devices like magnetic resonance imaging (MRI) scanners are built; *second*, the dependence on computational theories to derive teleological explanations of brain activity. While the former is shared with other scientific disciplines, the latter is a more recent advancement. Let us consider these two dimensions of theory-dependence in greater detail.

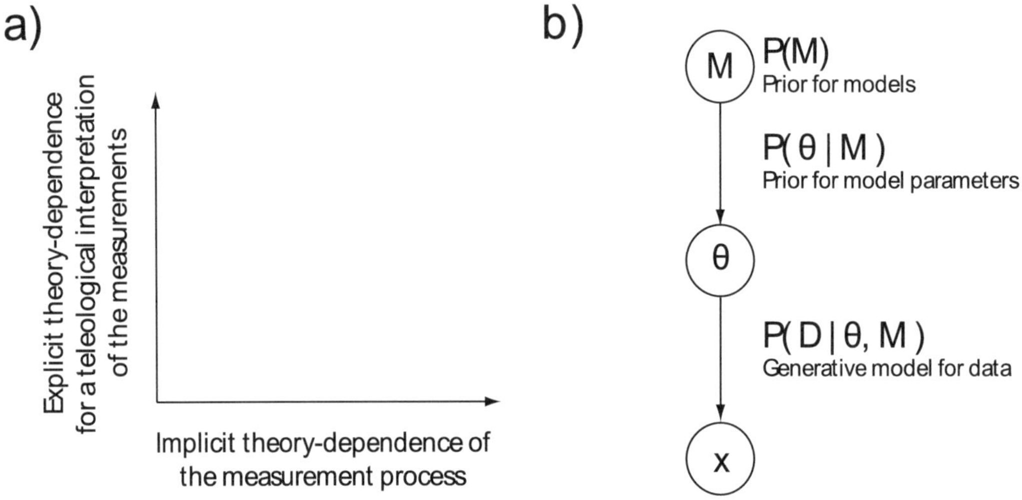

Fig. 1. Theory-dependence of observations and Bayesian model comparison. **a)** In brain imaging one can identify two dimensions of theory-dependence of observations: an implicit dependence on the theories underlying the measurement devices (such as the working of an MRT scanner), and a more recent explicit theory-dependence, where computational theories are used in order to interpret neuronal activations in a teleological manner with formally defined computational theories. **b)** Graphical model for Bayesian model comparison. Models M are parameterized with parameters θ. Once prior distributions $P(\theta \mid M)$ and forward models $P(\mathbf{x} \mid \theta)$ are defined, different models M (each of which is parameterized with a θ) can be compared with each other.

2.1 Theory-dependence of the measurement process

Since the work of Fleck (Fleck, 1979), Kuhn (Kuhn, 1962), and also Popper (Popper, 1972) in the last century we know that all scientific observations are theory-laden, i. e. even the most basic "facts" depend on a certain theoretical background. These ideas have been developed with physics as the main application domain, because in the last century physics experienced many radical changes of its fundamental theories. In brain imaging the theory-dependence of observations becomes most visible when considering the measurement process. For example, it is still not clear how signals from functional magnetic resonance imaging (fMRI) should best be interpreted in terms of neuronal and synaptic activations, and models are needed to ensure a proper interpretation of the measured brain activation in terms of neuronal activity (Almeida and Stetter, 2002). The situation is similar for research in electroencephalography (EEG), where source localization methods aim at solving the inverse problem of estimating the sources of electrical activity inside the head based on the measured EEG activity outside the head. This kind of theory-dependence is usually *implicit*, but can be made explicit in terms of a model for the measurement process as part of the data analysis.

2.2 Theory-dependence of the interpretation of the data

Another more recent kind of theory-dependence in neuroscience is not implicit, but explicit theory-dependence. Here, the neuronal activity in the nervous system is interpreted in terms of a (computational) function for the organism in a teleological manner. Teleological explanations in biology have a long history, but what makes their re-appearance in neuroscience attractive is that nowadays they are often articulated in at least a semi-formal way, but now more often also in an explicit formal manner. A prime example is reward learning. Here, algorithms from reinforcement learning are used to provide a basis for the semantic interpretation of the neuronal activations (Schultz, 2002). In other words, the neuronal circuitry in the brain is considered as a "wetware" on which algorithms are running (with all the associated constraints brought about by the slow processing speed and sluggishness of nervous systems compared to today's computers). Here, the empirical observations are *intentionally* theory-dependent, which we think is noteworthy and a new tool in the methodological toolbox to investigate complex biological systems.

2.3 Models make the theory-dependencies explicit

Both kinds of theory-dependence can be made explicit using models, which then allows for systematic comparisons between competing models on the basis of experimental observations. The approach of Bayesian model comparison is widely accepted as a principled method for comparing different models. **Figure 1b** shows the graphical model (graphical models are marriage of graph and probability theory used artificial intelligence and statistics) for Bayesian model comparison. Different models *M* can be parameterized with a parameter vector θ. Once prior distributions $P(\theta|M)$ are specified, observed data **x** can be used in order to compare different models M_1 and M_2 using the so-called posterior odds $P(M_1|\theta)/P(M_2|\theta)$, or the posterior distributions over model parameters θ for a certain model can be inspected. Performing the necessary calculations, such as evaluating or estimating the integral $\int P(\mathbf{x}|\theta,M)P(\theta|M)d\theta$, is technically demanding and defining the prior distributions $P(\theta|M)$ can be non-trivial. Still, however, this way of model comparison can serve as a general framework for model-based brain imaging even with multi-scale models, i. e. the particular definition of $P(\mathbf{x}|\theta)$ will need to incorporate both kinds of theory-dependence (see Section 3.3).

3. Neuroinformatics support

Neuroinformatics is an emerging discipline, which provides methods and tool support for neuroscience. Prime examples are databases for neuronal data, and tools for modeling and simulation. Let us briefly review selected advances in this field in order to identify ways in which Neuroinformatics could contribute to model-based brain imaging with multi-scale models.

3.1 Neuroinformatics support for sharing and analysis of data

The brain imaging community has always been very progressive in terms of sharing data and tools. While new analysis methods could certainly be developed within a single method-oriented laboratory, it is the community-wide evaluation of new methods, which provides their ultimate test. The free sharing of tools is certainly helpful.

In the field of fMRI studies, the SPM software (http://www.fil.ion.ucl.ac.uk/spm) is probably the most widely used open source software, and comparing models given observed data is a well-developed feature of SPM. It is the tool of choice to apply Dynamic Causal Models (DCMs) to brain imaging data, i. e. performing Bayesian model comparison with Neural Mass Models (NMMs), which are models accounting for averaged population activity in a whole cortical area with a greatly simplified local circuit architecture. Other software packages for specialized tasks such as, for example, multivariate pattern classification exist, but the advantage of a mature platform with a long tradition such as SPM is that one can almost consider it as a "software ecosystem" for data analysis as other tools and toolboxes can easily be integrated into analysis workflows.

In the field of EEG studies, the situation is more diverse. This may be due to the fact that EEG as a brain-imaging modality has been (and still is) in a "renaissance" phase, i. e. it is recognized that new analysis methods can pull out much more information about brain states than plain averaging. Prominent tools for EEG analysis are EEGLAB (Delorme and Makeig, 2004) and the FieldTrip toolbox (Oostenveld et al., 2011), both of which support time-frequency analysis and source localization, namely dipole-based localization and the beamformer algorithm, respectively. EEGLAB is the probably best first choice for applying Independent Component Analysis (ICA) to EEG data (Onton and Makeig, 2006). Even though the application of ICA to EEG is controversial, recent advances suggest that properly adapted variants of ICA can yield physiologically plausible results (Hyvärinen et al., 2010). SPM can also be applied for EEG analysis, and it supports DCMs for EEG data. Another prominent tool for EEG analysis is Cartool (http://brainmapping.unige.ch/cartool), which supports a so-called topographic analysis of event-related potentials (Pascual-Marqui et al., 1995; Murray et al., 2008) as well as distributed source localization. In contrast to the other Matlab-based tools, Cartool is an application for the Windows operating systems with a graphical user interface and currently no possibility for external scripting, i. e. it cannot be part of an automated toolchain.

In terms of data sharing, it is notable that for more than 10 years the fMRI community has the possibility to share the raw data (Editorial, 2000). Initially, this was viewed rather skeptically, but it has facilitated the development of new analysis methods (Van Horn and Ishai, 2007). Unfortunately, it appears that EEG researchers do not typically take such an approach and are still far more protective of "their" data. As of now, this also applies to data sharing in neurophysiology. Only some neurophysiology researchers freely share their data via web pages. However, progress and standardization can be expected from efforts taken by, for example, the International Neuroinformatics Coordination Facility or actions of major funding agencies and publishers.

Taken together, the sharing of tools and data from various imaging modalities (including neurophysiology) is an essential prerequisite for applying multi-scale modeling to model-based brain imaging. Very likely, there will never be a single tool to cover all requirements for data analysis. Instead, a "software ecosystem" with loose coupling between components (such as in terms of specifications for data and file formats and ultimately implementations using service-oriented architectures) appears as a promising solution. The existing Matlab-based tools come closest to such an ecosystem.

3.2 Neuroinformatics support for multi-scale modeling

In order to evaluate the forward model, $P(\mathbf{x}\,|\,\theta)$, for multi-scale models one needs to account for the observed data in terms of the neuronal activity of synaptically coupled neurons. Do we currently have enough knowledge in order to define such models mathematically, not to mention their numerical simulation? For example, for fMRI it is still not clear if the signal reflects pre- or postsynaptic activity (Logothetis, 2008), or excitatory or inhibitory synaptic activity (Lauritzen and Gold, 2003). For EEG forward models, the anisotropy of the conductivities may matter (Güllmar et al., 2010), and linking local field potentials to the spiking/synaptic activity is also a current research topic (Rasch et al., 2009).

For example, we have recently combined NMMs and anisotropic head-models in order to simulate EEG activity (Zimmermann et al., 2011) as an attempt for a multi-scale forward model. Here, we argue that even without a complete physical description of how spiking activity causes, for example, EEG signals one could still pursue model-based brain imaging with multi-scale models, namely by using phenomenological models for those parts of the full model, where a physical description is currently not available. The procedure of Bayesian model comparison is blind to the physical plausibility or "truth" of a model, $P(\mathbf{x}\,|\,\theta)$, but only compares probabilistic models with each other. Thus, by using data from multiple imaging modalities and employing phenomenological models for the boundaries between different scales of modeling, one could iteratively improve these models. Of course, one needs to accept that parts of such multi-scale models are incomplete. From a pragmatic perspective, this shifts the focus from finding a "true" model or physical principle to bridge the gap between different scales to the very practical question: How to simulate forward models, and how to share models?

Sharing models in terms of scripts for established simulators like NEURON, GENESIS or NEST has been a major step towards facilitating the exchange of models. Recently, these efforts have been extended by the development of simulator-independent model descriptions like generating models via Python scripts (Davison et al., 2008), renewed interest in NeuroML (Goddard et al., 2001), or the recent NineML initiative (http://ninml.org). Compared to Systems Biology, however, corresponding efforts in Computational Neuroscience are less developed in terms of model exchange (De Schutter, 2008), because a standard as widely accepted as the Systems Biology Markup Language (SBML) is still missing, but it is actively developed within the Neuroinformatics community. As of now, web portals like ModelDB (http://senselab.med.yale.edu/modeldb) or, for vision science, the Visiome (http:// visiome.neuroinf.jp) are an excellent source of models in terms of scripts for simulators. Hopefully, in the near future, such portals will also host model descriptions (as compared to simulator scripts), similar to the BioModels database for Systems Biology models (http://www.ebi.ac.uk/biomodels). However, we argue that it is essentially the multiplicity of different (spatial and temporal) scales of neuronal models, which makes similar efforts a challenge for Neuroinformatics.

3.3 Is there any Neuroinformatics support for multi-facet modeling?

In addition the different scales, neuronal systems can also be described at different levels of abstractions such as in terms of the neuronal dynamics, but also in terms of the computations carried out by the neuronal "wetware". Marr distinguished between the computational problem, the algorithmic solution, and a "wetware" used to execute the algorithm (Marr, 1982). This distinction is very close to a typical computer science approach, where the algorithms are clearly distinct from the hardware on which they are running. Such an apparently clear separation has been questioned recently, because the algorithms and the neuronal "wetware" may not be as independent as previously thought (Noë, 2005). Computational Neuroscience researchers have produced hypotheses, which aim at bridging the gap between mere mechanistic descriptions and computational properties by essentially proposing transformations from algorithmic descriptions to neuronal circuitry. Is there any Neuroinformatics support for such a multi-facet modeling? Can multi-facet modeling be considered within the framework of Bayesian model comparison?

The answer to the first question is simply "no". As of now, there is no tool support to explicitly formulate such multi-facet models, but we have recently started to address this problem (Ansorg and Schwabe, 2010) by taking inspiration from software engineering. How can such multi-facet models fit into the framework of Bayesian model comparison? One simply needs to define a forward model $P(\mathbf{x}|\theta)$ for the observed data, but for multi-facet models this calls for defining a computational model *and* a transformation into the "wetware". If proper description languages for such multi-facet models and transformations would be available, one could compare different hypothesis about the computations in neuronal circuits in a data-driven way. Readily available candidates for such multi-facet modeling include hypotheses about the role of dopamine in reward learning (Schultz, 2002), or postulates about population codes in sensory systems (Ma et al., 2006).

4. Selected advances in cortical microcircuit models

The NMMs employed in DCMs are a major step beyond the mere statistical models embodied in, for example, effective connectivity analyses. However, these NMMs often assume a simplified cortical architecture. In our modeling of visual cortical networks we also employed mean-field firing rate models as in NMMs (as well as more detailed models with so-called "spiking neurons"). We could show that single neuron responses in primary visual cortex (V1) are best explained when the local cortical microcircuits are assumed to operate in a balance between strong recurrent excitation and inhibition (Mariño et al., 2005a; Stimberg et al., 2009), and that inter-areal feedback into V1 may play a crucial role in "lateral inhibition" (Schwabe et al., 2006a; Ichida et al., 2007; Schwabe et al., 2010). To the best of our knowledge, such and other recent advances in cortical microcircuits models have not yet been implemented into NMMs used in brain imaging. Here we review some of these advances and outline how they could be used in model-based brain imaging with multi-scale models.

4.1 The operating regime of local cortical computations

More than 50 years after the discovery of orientation tuning in V1, there are still controversial discussions about the underlying neuronal circuits (**Figure 2a**). Probably the dominant controversy relates to the question: To what extent is neuronal selectivity in sensory systems determined by the afferent feedforward connections vs. intra-cortical processing (or even feedback from higher visual areas)? Previous theoretical studies already investigated a so-called "balanced regime" of neuronal networks, where excitatory and inhibitory inputs are balanced and largely cancel each other out. We have investigated such an operating regime in joint experimental-modeling studies.

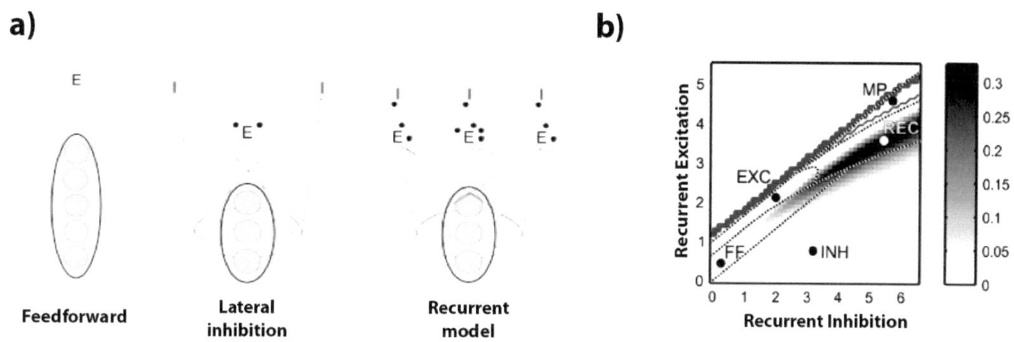

Fig. 2. Orientation tuning models and Bayesian posterior over models. **a)** Illustrations of circuits, which may compute orientation-tuned responses in area V1. **b)** Bayesian posterior for models enumerated in terms of the strength of local recurrent inhibition (x-axis) and excitation (y-axis), given the data reported in (Mariño et al., 2005b). (Figure 2b is taken from Stimberg et al. (2009), by permission of Oxford University Press)

A study by Stimberg et al. (2009) employed a Bayesian approach to investigate data reported first by Mariño et al. (2005b). Most importantly, a class of models was defined, which includes all the different variants shown in **Figure 2a**, by considering the strength of recurrent excitation and inhibition within a network model of an approx. 1mm^2 cortical patch as parameters θ in a forward model $P(\mathbf{x}|\theta)$. Then, using this forward model, the posterior probabilities over the model parameters were computed, given the experimental data (**Figure 2b**). It turned out that a recurrent regime (**Figure 2a**, right icon) is the most probable regime. The details of this calculation and the simulations are given in Stimberg et al. (2009). A few aspects of this study are important to emphasize here: *First*, the data to be explained by the network model was already postprocessed data from multiple experimentally recorded neurons, i. e. it was not aimed at accounting for every recorded spike. *Second*, compared to the NMMs used in DCMs the network model referred to a smaller scale than accessible by current brain imaging studies (<1mm^2). *Third*, this model used parameter values for the model neurons (such as membrane conductances), which are at best good guesses informed by other studies, but way beyond a comprehensive characterization in a single preparation. *Finally,* the class of models was sufficiently restricted so that one could investigate the full posterior distribution.

Hence, this study demonstrates that large-scale network simulations can be used successfully in a Bayesian model comparison (of models within a properly defined class). Note that while the employed model certainly lacks many potentially biophysically relevant details, it is far more realistic than the NMMs used in DCMs. We argue that the most relevant way, in which it goes beyond the NMMs, is *not* the level of biophysical realisms but the fact that it operates the model network in a "balanced" regime. In such a regime, recently termed "inhibition stabilized network" (Ozeki et al., 2009) as recurrent excitation makes the network unstable in the absence of recurrent inhibition, even small external inputs can be amplified via local recurrent connections. The dynamic properties of such strong local recurrent connections have not yet been considered in DCMs, which address inter-areal networks and use greatly simplified local circuit models.

4.2 Contextual effects and "lateral inhibition"

In another series of joint experimental-modeling studies we investigated such inter-areal networks, but we focused on the detailed microcircuits of the inter-areal connections. This is a key question one needs to deal with when interpreting large-scale brain activations in terms of network models. Here, the spatial scales of the connections need to be identified (see Angelucci et al. (2002) for the corresponding anatomy of feedback within the visual system), but network simulations needs to be conducted in order to predict the physiological responses.

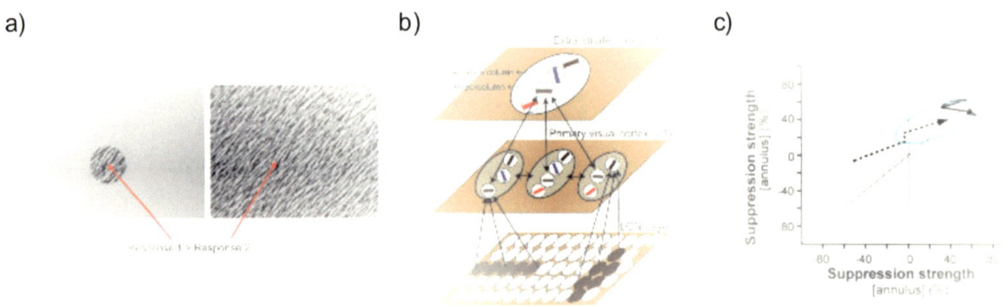

Fig. 3. Surround suppression in network models and data-model comparison. **a)** Illustration of surround suppression: When the surround of a neuron's classical receptive field is also stimulated, then the response is reduced. **b)** Illustration of a recurrent network model of many recurrently coupled orientation hypercolumns in area V1. They receive feedforward inputs from the lateral geniculate nucleus (LGN), are interconnected via long-range horizontal connections within V1 and reciprocally to another retinotopically organized extra-striate visual area (here: area MT). **c)** Summary of surround suppression data from macaque V1 from two experimental conditions (stimulus in the classical receptive field at high, y-axis, and low, x-axis, contrast). The ellipse indicates the 50% confidence region of the measured surround suppression in N=63 cells. The lines show predicted surround suppression of the recurrent network model from Schwabe et al. (2006) for increasing strength of the *inter*-areal feedback connections to local inhibitory cells for moderate (dashed) and strong *intra*-areal (solid) lateral inhibition. (Figure 3c is taken from Schwabe et al.(2010), with permission from Elsevier).

A prominent phenomenon of interest in visual neuroscience is surround suppression. When another stimulus in the surround of a classical receptive field of a neuron is shown, then the response is suppressed compared to the stimulation of only the classical receptive field. **Figure 3a** illustrates this for visually responsive neurons tuned to orientation. The concept of "lateral inhibition" is usually invoked to explain this surround suppression, i. e. recurrent connections between different $1mm^2$ patches implement a competition via mutual suppression. In a modeling study we predicted that feedback from extrastriate areas into V1 (see **Figure 3b** for an illustration of the model architecture) may play a major role in mediating this "lateral inhibition" (Schwabe et al., 2006a), which in this model is an inter-areal inhibition. Interestingly, we also predicted that stimuli with a large separation from the receptive field of the recorded neuron could even facilitate (and not only suppress) the responses when the classical receptive field is stimulated at low contrast. Later we confirmed this prediction experimentally (Ichida et al., 2007). These studies show that stimulus-driven responses and their modulation can depend on the stimulus properties and are mediated by inter-areal connections. Most importantly, such studies could inform the stimulus design in brain-imaging experiments (Harrison et al., 2007). While the models of the $1mm^2$ patches of cortex (see Section 4.1) are currently at the limit of the spatial resolution accessible to fMRI, the spatially more extended models considered in these studies are in principle directly applicable as network models in DCMs, but now with cortical areas explicitly modeled as spatially extended patches of cortex.

In our investigation of inter-areal networks we also performed systematic comparisons between model predictions and the experimentally recorded single neuron responses, but here we did *not* apply a Bayesian approach (Schwabe et al., 2010), and this can serve to highlight an important distinction to be respected for the comparison of network models, namely between the definition of a "noise model" and variability due to true heterogeneity of the recorded neurons. Let $\mathbf{y} = \mathbf{f}(\text{Input};\theta)$ denote the functional dependence between a sensory input into a neuronal network model, parameterized by θ, and a mean output $\mathbf{y}$ predicted by, for example, a NMM. Since the experimental observations $\mathbf{x}$ are usually much more variable than predicted by such a mean output, one could formulate a noise model, such as $\mathbf{x} = \mathbf{y} + \eta$ with η being additive Gaussian noise, for the observations $\mathbf{x}$, which shall account for the observed variability in the data. We have experimentally measured the strength of surround suppression of neurons with an oriented stimulus in the classical field brought about by stimulation at more distant visual field locations (the "far surround"). A summary of the measured surround suppression strengths is shown in **Figure 3c** in terms of the error ellipse (50% confidence) around the estimated mean suppression for two experimental conditions (high contrast stimulus in the center, y-axis, vs. low contrast stimulus, x-axis). Clearly, the measured suppression strengths are variable, but we assumed that this variability is due to the fact that we recorded different types of neurons without being able to distinguish them based on the extracellular recordings. For example, it is conceivable that some neurons were excitatory while others were inhibitory, some neurons may operate in a different local network neighborhood than others, etc. In Schwabe et al. (2010) we hypothesized that this variability is due to different strengths of the intra-areal vs. inter-areal connections (the model parameter θ), and we simulated the network model with different parameter values. As we increased, for example, the strength of the feedback

connections in the model (to local inhibitory neurons in V1) we predict different strengths of surround suppression (see lines in **Figure 3c**). For certain strengths the predicted suppression is within the 50% confidence region while for others it is outside.
This study shows that one can respect the variability in the data in terms of heterogeneity of the underlying microcircuits and still use experimental data with NMM-like network models in order to learn something about the actual microcircuits: Here, we found that *within the class of models we considered* the models with stronger feedback projections to inhibitory neurons in the model V1 produce quantitatively better matches to the measured surround suppression than models with less feedback to these inhibitory neurons; see Schwabe et al. (2010) for more details. Of course, stochastic models respecting heterogeneity in single cell properties and network connections, or models for large-scale simulations could be described with model parameters θ, which capture such heterogeneity and hence would be directly useable within a Bayesian model comparison.

5. The neuronal basis of the self as a test case

Multi-scale models will soon enter model-based brain imaging studies. The method of DCMs can be extended to include cortical circuit models, which take into account, for example, the exquisite balance between excitation and inhibition, or the retinotopy and spatial scales of intra- and inter-areal connections. This could also lead to a re-evaluation of many already published brain imaging studies, where a "neuronal activation" was associated with a certain informally described function. One such discipline, which lacks more formalized models suitable for model-based brain imaging, is the emerging field of "the neuroscience of the self". In other words, we argue that addressing the fundamental question of how the brain organizes self-related computations is a challenging test case for model-based brain imaging with multi-scale models, in particular because of the lack of computational models and the need for microcircuits models to ensure a proper interpretation of the already available imaging data.

5.1 Computational modeling of self-related processing

We argue that investigating self-related processing in the brain in order to determine the neuronal basis of the first-person perspective, or "selfhood" (Blanke and Metzinger, 2009), is a challenging but do-able test case for model-based brain imaging with multi-scale models. Of course, one could ask: Why address such problems, given that we still haven't resolved the circuitry underlying orientation tuning in V1?
What makes investigating the neuronal basis of the self a challenging test case is that we are currently lacking proper computational models for that, but brain-imaging studies suggest that certain brain regions and networks (including the so-called default mode network) may play an important role. It has been shown experimentally that by using incongruent multi-sensory stimulations the apparently hard-wired body scheme and body image of a subject can be disturbed as evident in the so-called "rubber hand illusion" (Botvinick and Cohen, 1998) or an extension of this to the full body (Lenggenhager et al., 2007). By applying computational concepts developed for the visual and sensory-motor system, we proposed computational models for such self-related processing, which do not at all refer to a "self" but only to (multi)sensory signals relevant

for self-related tasks. For example, vestibular signals are likely to be of importance (Schwabe and Blanke, 2008) as well as proper multi-sensory integration in sensory-motor loops (Schwabe and Blanke, 2007; Kannape et al., 2010). We have conceptualized the sense of self as a set of learning and inference algorithms for such self-related sensory signals, in particular vestibular signals, which are running on a neuronal "wetware". Thus, from a computational perspective, the processing of self-related (multi)sensory signals may be very similar to the processing of, say, visual signals in the visual system. Accordingly, such computational theories can be tested in a similar manner, but the main challenge is to control the sensory stimulation. Ideally one would like to exert fine-grained control over the vestibular stimulations, but in fMRI studies this is only possible via caloric or galvanic stimulation, which are far from the stimulation encountered in more natural scenarios. Thus, in order to investigate the self via brain imaging, one shall investigate the brain activity of whole bodies in action. As of now this is only possible with brain-wide intracranial recordings as pursued in, for example, the Neurotycho project (http://neurotycho.org), because EEG in behaving human subjects is very noisy. In the Neurotycho project, the full-body motions of freely behaving monkeys are also recorded. Unfortunately, the vestibular system is widely distributed (Lopez and Blanke, 2011). This makes large-scale recordings necessary so that animal studies may be the method of choice for the foreseeable future. Initiatives such as the Neurotycho project provide valuable data, which can also enter a Bayesian model comparison, where the forward models may now also account for the full-body motions (recorded via motion-capture technology). Of course, simulating such forward models calls for combining models at various scales and coupling them with each other via phenomenological models.

5.2 The function role of the temporoparietal junction

Model-based brain imaging with multi-scale models can be performed in a truly data-driven manner once the model classes are defined. We have argued that it is already applicable even in the absence of a complete physical model for relating, for example, spikes to measured EEG activity (given that proper Neuroinformatics tool support is available). Then, applying such techniques could help to decipher the computational role and network connectivity of those brain areas, where we currently have only a rather limited grasp on their role for cognition. One such area is the temporoparietal junction (TPJ). Very briefly, the TPJ has been implicated in the theory of mind (Young et al., 2010), mental perspective taking and out-of-body experiences (Blanke and Mohr, 2005), and as part of an attention-management network (Corbetta et al., 2008). Having available formal model-descriptions of such theories in computational terms (which is not yet possible as we don't have a proper support for multi-facet modeling), and a proposal for how to transform them into neuronal activations would allow for systematically comparing such theories using data. The need to formally describe such computational theories becomes evident by inspecting the rather descriptive nature of many imaging experiments. As of now, the computational theories imported from, for example, research in the visual and sensory-motor system seem to be the most promising candidates to explain TPJ activations in computational terms, namely as part of a (Bayesian) model a subject is using internally in order to infer the state of another person's mind (Kilner et al., 2007), as part of an attention-management network (Corbetta et al., 2008), or simply as a vestibular error signals in imagined (but not actually carried out) full-body movements in the case of mental perspective taking. In the case of distributed brain activations and in a still rather exploratory phase of investigating self-related brain networks, combining multi-facet modeling and (even phenomenological) multi-scale models may be most fruitful.

6. Conclusion and future research

In summary, we have emphasized that a Bayesian model comparison is the most systematic method to compare different models on the basis of measurements. The explicit use of models makes the theory-dependence of observations explicit and emphasizes that within a Bayesian model comparison we compare only models within a class (or between classes) of models as compared to finding a single "true" model. Our work in modeling orientation tuning and surround suppression further emphasize this: The employed models are certainly more detailed than the NMMs currently employed in brain-imaging, but they are also far too simplistic to account for many biophysical details. Still, our comparison of such network models within a class of models for a given data set is a valuable example of a systematic model comparison.

We also argued that multi-scale modeling, combined with multi-facet modeling, will be an important method for investigating even rather challenging neuroscientific questions such as explaining the neural basis of the self in terms of computational and neuronal models. This can be done even in the absence of a complete multi-level model for relating spikes to macroscopic data from brain imaging, namely by employing phenomenological models. As a consequence, we see the development of supporting Neuroinformatics tools to support the data-driven comparison of multi-scale and multi-facet models as an important step for future research.

7. References

Almeida R, Stetter M (2002) Modeling the link between functional imaging and neuronal activity: synaptic metabolic demand and spike rates. NeuroImage 17:1065-79 Available at: http://www.ncbi.nlm.nih.gov/pubmed/12377179 [Accessed May 4, 2011].

Angelucci A, Levitt JB, Walton EJS, Hupe J-M, Bullier J, Lund JS (2002) Circuits for local and global signal integration in primary visual cortex. The Journal of Neuroscience 22:8633-46 Available at: http://www.ncbi.nlm.nih.gov/pubmed/12351737.

Ansorg R, Schwabe L (2010) Domain-Specific Modeling as a Pragmatic Approach to Neuronal Model Descriptions In Brain Informatics, Lecture Notes in Computer Science (6334) Springer, p. 168-179.

Blanke O, Metzinger T (2009) Full-body illusions and minimal phenomenal selfhood. Trends in cognitive sciences 13:7-13 Available at: http://www.ncbi.nlm.nih.gov/pubmed/19058991.

Blanke O, Mohr C (2005) Out-of-body experience, heautoscopy, and autoscopic hallucination of neurological origin Implications for neurocognitive mechanisms of corporeal awareness and self-consciousness. Brain research. Brain research reviews 50:184-99 Available at: http://www.ncbi.nlm.nih.gov/pubmed/16019077.

Botvinick M, Cohen J (1998) Rubber hands "feel" touch that eyes see. Nature 391:756 Available at: http://www.ncbi.nlm.nih.gov/pubmed/9486643.

Corbetta M, Patel G, Shulman GL (2008) The reorienting system of the human brain: from environment to theory of mind. Neuron 58:306-24 Available at: http://www.ncbi.nlm.nih.gov/pubmed/18466742.

Davison AP, Brüderle D, Eppler J, Kremkow J, Muller E, Pecevski D, Perrinet L, Yger P (2008) PyNN: A Common Interface for Neuronal Network Simulators. Frontiers in Neuroinformatics 2:11 Available at: http://www.pubmedcentral.nih.gov/articlerender.fcgi?artid=2634533&tool=pmcentrez&rendertype=abstract [Accessed September 13, 2010].

De Schutter E (2008) Why are computational neuroscience and systems biology so separate? PLoS computational biology 4:e1000078 Available at: http://www.ncbi.nlm.nih.gov/pubmed/18516226.

Delorme A, Makeig S (2004) EEGLAB: an open source toolbox for analysis of single-trial EEG dynamics including independent component analysis. Journal of Neuroscience Methods 134:9-21 Available at: http://www.ncbi.nlm.nih.gov/pubmed/15102499 [Accessed May 3, 2011].

Editorial (2000) A debate over fMRI data sharing. Nature Neuroscience 3:845-6 Available at: http://www.ncbi.nlm.nih.gov/pubmed/10966604 [Accessed May 3, 2011].

Fleck L (1979) The Genesis and Development of a Scientific Fact T. J. Merton & R. K. Trenn, eds. Chicago: University of Chicago Press.

Goddard NH, Hucka M, Howell F, Cornelis H, Shankar K, Beeman D (2001) Towards NeuroML: model description methods for collaborative modelling in neuroscience. Philosophical Transactions of the Royal Society of London. Series B, Biological Sciences 356:1209-28 Available at: http://www.pubmedcentral.nih.gov/articlerender.fcgi?artid=1088511&tool=pmcentrez&rendertype=abstract [Accessed May 3, 2011].

Güllmar D, Haueisen J, Reichenbach JR (2010) Influence of anisotropic electrical conductivity in white matter tissue on the EEG/MEG forward and inverse solution. A high-resolution whole head simulation study. NeuroImage 51:145-63 Available at: http://www.ncbi.nlm.nih.gov/pubmed/20156576 [Accessed May 3, 2011].

Harrison LM, Stephan KE, Rees G, Friston KJ (2007) Extra-classical receptive field effects measured in striate cortex with fMRI. NeuroImage 34:1199-208 Available at: http://www.ncbi.nlm.nih.gov/pubmed/17169579.

Hyvärinen A, Ramkumar P, Parkkonen L, Hari R (2010) Independent component analysis of short-time Fourier transforms for spontaneous EEG/MEG analysis. NeuroImage 49:257-71 Available at: http://www.ncbi.nlm.nih.gov/pubmed/19699307.

Ichida JM, Schwabe L, Bressloff PC, Angelucci A (2007) Response Facilitation From the "Suppressive" Receptive Field Surround of Macaque V1 Neurons. Journal of Neurophysiology:2168 -2181

Kannape O a, Schwabe L, Tadi T, Blanke O (2010) The limits of agency in walking humans. Neuropsychologia 48:1628-36 Available at: http://www.ncbi.nlm.nih.gov/pubmed/20144893 [Accessed August 4, 2010].

Kilner JM, Friston KJ, Frith CD (2007) The mirror-neuron system: a Bayesian perspective. Neuroreport 18:619-23 Available at: http://www.ncbi.nlm.nih.gov/pubmed/17413668.

Kuhn TS (1962) The Structure of Scientific Revolutions. Chicago: University of Chicago Press.

Lauritzen M, Gold L (2003) Brain Function and Neurophysiological Correlates of Signals Used in Functional Neuroimaging. Neurophysiology 23:3972-3980

Lenggenhager B, Tadi T, Metzinger T, Blanke O (2007) Video ergo sum: manipulating bodily self-consciousness. Science (New York, N.Y.) 317:1096-9 Available at: http://www.ncbi.nlm.nih.gov/pubmed/17717189.

Logothetis NK (2008) What we can do and what we cannot do with fMRI. Nature 453:869-78 Available at: http://www.ncbi.nlm.nih.gov/pubmed/18548064 [Accessed May 3, 2011].

Lopez C, Blanke O (2011) The thalamocortical vestibular system in animals and humans. Brain Research Reviews Available at: http://www.ncbi.nlm.nih.gov/pubmed/21223979 [Accessed March 17, 2011].

Ma WJ, Beck JM, Latham PE, Pouget A (2006) Bayesian inference with probabilistic population codes. Nature Neuroscience 9:1432-8 Available at: http://www.ncbi.nlm.nih.gov/pubmed/17057707.

Mariño J, Schummers J, Lyon DC, Schwabe L, Beck O, Wiesing P, Obermayer K, Sur M (2005)(a) Invariant computations in local cortical networks with balanced excitation and inhibition. Nature Neuroscience 8:194-201 Available at: http://www.ncbi.nlm.nih.gov/pubmed/15665876.

Mariño J, Schummers J, Lyon DC, Schwabe L, Beck O, Wiesing P, Obermayer K, Sur M (2005)(b) Invariant computations in local cortical networks with balanced excitation and inhibition. Nature Neuroscience 8:194-201 Available at: http://www.ncbi.nlm.nih.gov/pubmed/15665876.

Marr D (1982) Vision. W.H.Freeman & Co Ltd.

Murray MM, Brunet D, Michel CM (2008) Topographic ERP analyses: a step-by-step tutorial review. Brain topography 20:249-64 Available at: http://www.ncbi.nlm.nih.gov/pubmed/18347966.

Noë A (2005) Action in Perception. Cambridge, MA: MIT Press.

Onton J, Makeig S (2006) Information-based modeling of event-related brain dynamics. Brain 159:99-120

Oostenveld R, Fries P, Maris E, Schoffelen J-M (2011) FieldTrip: Open source software for advanced analysis of MEG, EEG, and invasive electrophysiological data. Computational Intelligence and Neuroscience 2011:156869 Available at: http://www.pubmedcentral.nih.gov/articlerender.fcgi?artid=3021840&tool=pmcentrez&rendertype=abstract [Accessed April 29, 2011].

Ozeki H, Finn IM, Schaffer ES, Miller KD, Ferster D (2009) Inhibitory stabilization of the cortical network underlies visual surround suppression. Neuron 62:578-92 Available at: http://www.ncbi.nlm.nih.gov/pubmed/19477158.

Pascual-Marqui RD, Michel CM, Lehmann D (1995) Segmentation of brain electrical activity into microstates: model estimation and validation. IEEE Transactions on Biomedical Engineering 42:658-65 Available at: http://www.ncbi.nlm.nih.gov/pubmed/7622149 [Accessed May 3, 2011].

Popper K (1972) Objective Knowledge: An Evolutionary Approach. New York: Oxford University Press.

Rasch M, Logothetis NK, Kreiman G (2009) From neurons to circuits: linear estimation of local field potentials. Journal of Neuroscience 29:13785-96 Available at: http://www.pubmedcentral.nih.gov/articlerender.fcgi?artid=2924964&tool=pmcentrez&rendertype=abstract [Accessed September 14, 2010].

Schultz W (2002) Getting formal with dopamine and reward. Neuron 36:241-63 Available at: http://www.ncbi.nlm.nih.gov/pubmed/12383780.

Schwabe L, Blanke O (2007) Cognitive neuroscience of ownership and agency. Consciousness and cognition 16:661-6 Available at: http://www.ncbi.nlm.nih.gov/pubmed/17920522 [Accessed September 7, 2010].

Schwabe L, Blanke O (2008) The vestibular component in out-of-body experiences: a computational approach. Frontiers in Human Neuroscience 2:17 Available at: http://www.pubmedcentral.nih.gov/articlerender.fcgi?artid=2610253&tool=pmcentrez&rendertype=abstract.

Schwabe L, Ichida JM, Shushruth S, Mangapathy P, Angelucci A (2010) Contrast-dependence of surround suppression in Macaque V1: Experimental testing of a recurrent network model. NeuroImage 1:1-16 Available at: http://www.ncbi.nlm.nih.gov/pubmed/20079853.

Schwabe L, Obermayer K, Angelucci A, Bressloff PC (2006)(a) The role of feedback in shaping the extra-classical receptive field of cortical neurons: a recurrent network model. Journal of Neuroscience 26:9117-29 Available at: http://www.ncbi.nlm.nih.gov/pubmed/16957068.

Schwabe L, Obermayer K, Angelucci A, Bressloff PC (2006)(b) The role of feedback in shaping the extra-classical receptive field of cortical neurons: a recurrent network model. Journal of Neuroscience 26:9117-29 Available at: http://www.ncbi.nlm.nih.gov/pubmed/16957068.

Stimberg M, Wimmer K, Martin R, Schwabe L, Mariño J, Schummers J, Lyon DC, Sur M, Obermayer K (2009) The operating regime of local computations in primary visual cortex. Cerebral Cortex 19:2166-80 Available at: http://www.ncbi.nlm.nih.gov/pubmed/19221143.

Van Horn JD, Ishai A (2007) Mapping the human brain: new insights from FMRI data sharing. Neuroinformatics 5:146-53 Available at: http://www.ncbi.nlm.nih.gov/pubmed/17917125 [Accessed May 3, 2011].

Young L, Camprodon JA, Hauser M, Pascual-Leone A, Saxe R (2010) Disruption of the right temporoparietal junction with transcranial magnetic stimulation reduces the role of beliefs in moral judgments. PNAS 107:6753-8 Available at: http://www.ncbi.nlm.nih.gov/pubmed/20351278.

Zimmermann U, Petersen S, Schwabe L, Rienen U van (2011) Combination of Neural-Mass Models With Anisotropic Head Models to Simulate EEG-Signals In CEM2011 8th Int Conference on Computation in Electromagnetics Warsaw.

6

Functional Brain Imaging Using Non-Invasive Non-Ionizing Methods: Towards Multimodal and Multiscale Imaging

Irene Karanasiou
School of Electrical and Computer Engineering
National Technical University of Athens
Greece

1. Introduction

Current and future trends in functional neuroimaging focus on the combination and synchronous application of imaging modalities by integrating more than one measures of brain function, e.g., hemodynamic and electrophysiological (EEG and fMRI). These multi-modal approaches aim at achieving sufficient temporal and spatial resolution in order to localize neural activity and identify the functional connectivity between different brain regions, hypothesizing that the multi-modal information represents the same neural networks (Laufs et al., 2008).

In parallel, besides the impressive recent advancements in neuroimaging research, arguably even more outstanding advances have been reported in molecular medicine and genetics research. In this context, current and future trends in medical research aim at bridging biomolecular information and neural function through studies in anatomic and functional biomedical imaging, focusing on methods to discover novel markers influencing specific traits in psychiatric and neurological diseases. The new field of imaging genetics uses neuroimaging methods to assess the impact of genetic variance on the human brain. Ideally, several imaging methods are implemented in combination to achieve an optimal characterization of structural and functional parameters. The latter are statistically related to the genotype, resulting in a form of a genetic association study. Such procedures acting as a mediator between genetic polymorphisms and psychiatric disease risk may shed light on the relevant underlying neural processes (Hariri et al. 2006). Although this approach is still relatively novel, the emerging literature and initial results hold great promise that it may contribute to the understanding of the pathophysiology of complex psychiatric and neurological disorders. Importantly, the future trends in neuroimaging envision imaging of the chemical functions of the organ cells and even realtime images of the genes and proteins at work within cells. These will convey sophisticated fingerprints of disease processes and better assessment of the effectiveness of curative procedures. Overall, it is evident that profiling of the molecular changes in disease will also expand the scope of body imaging.

In this scientific and technological milieu, the widely-acknowledged "THz gap" makes this region of the electromagnetic spectrum a scientific frontier, with critical questions in physics, chemistry, biology, and medicine that need answers. All molecules (biological, organic, inorganic, etc) have vibrational and rotational spectra that lie in the Terahertz frequency range with signatures resulting from intra- and inter-molecular interactions. Terahertz technology is considered a viable option for medical imaging (Siegel, 2004), since many biological and chemical substances exhibit signatures in this spectral region. Opportunities for imaging modality development in the Terahertz spectrum range, offers the possibility of understanding complex reactions in which the chemical state of the sample under study changes as time evolves. Nevertheless, despite recent advances, this part of the electromagnetic spectrum, remains unexplored and challenging with respect to medical applications (Siegel, 2004; Sherwin et al., 2004).

The next big challenge in the field of medical imaging and especially neuroimaging is the wide application of functional imaging methods in clinical practice, which will add significant knowledge towards a more holistic comprehension of the mechanisms of neurological and psychiatric diseases. The identification of effective therapeutic strategies, which will have a dramatic impact on the lives of millions of people, as neuropsychiatric disorders (e.g., mood disorders, stroke, epilepsy) are among the most common diseases, will then be the most valuable consequence.

Taking into consideration the aforementioned, the present chapter will focus on the following topics:

a. short review of state-of-the-art of non-invasive, non-ionizing functional neuroimaging techniques,
b. current and future trends in multimodal neuroimaging comprising concurrent measurements during activation of specified brain areas in-vivo via non-invasive and non-ionizing methodologies,
c. current and future trends in neuroimaging genetics with emphasis on the potential identification of new brain biomarkers related to brain functionality both in health and disease through Terahertz biomolecule imaging (ex-vivo) and the newly developed optogenetics method.

2. State-of-the-art of non-ionizing functional brain imaging techniques

The main current common methods for functional neuroimaging are functional magnetic resonance imaging (fMRI), multichannel electroencephalography (EEG), magnetoencephalography (MEG) and near infrared spectroscopic imaging (NIRSI) or functional near infrared spectroscopy (fNIRS). fMRI and fNIRS can measure localized changes in cerebral blood flow related to neural activity. Two other methods which are not actually 3D imaging modalities, but both contain information that, after appropriate post-processing, may result in three-dimensional brain maps of the recorded data, are EEG and MEG.

Local voltage fluctuations or changes in blood flow and volume, are referred to as activations. These activations are monitored and recorded with the various neuroimaging techniques when a subject performs a particular task and it is suggested that local brain activations may be involved in the underlying neural processes which mediate behavior. For instance, in tasks with visual stimulation, extensive activation of the occipital lobe is typically observed. This is explained by the fact that this rear part of the brain receives signals from the retina and is considered to be associated with visual perception.

Different methods present different advantages for research fact that resulted in the design and development of experimental studies that currently focus on a combined concurrent implementation of the various modalities. Several research groups, for example, have reported results of data elicited using synchronous EEG recordings and fMRI during event-related experimental procedures or fNIR and EEG recordings for instance, aiming at achieving sufficient temporal and spatial resolution to clarify the functional connectivity of neural processes, provided that the methodology combinations represent the same neural networks. Before, presenting the current and future trends of the multimodal configurations of the abovementioned techniques, a brief overview of the current state-of-the-art attributes of each methodology is given in the following sections.

2.1 Recent advances in Magnetic Resonance Imaging techniques

Magnetic Resonance Imaging (MRI) is a well known structural imaging modality that is being used in clinical practice to distinguish tumors, inflammatory lesions, and other pathologies from the normal brain anatomy while it has also been proven useful for the diagnosis of demyelinating disorders. Recently, special advanced techniques of magnetic resonance tomography such as diffusion weighted imaging (DWI), functional magnetic resonance (fMRI) and spectroscopy gave new insights to the acquired images, providing also information about the function and chemical metabolites of the brain. Various MRI techniques, also without the use of contrast agents may present venous or arterial angiograms.

More specifically, diffusion-weighted imaging (DWI), diffusion tensor imaging (DTI) and tractography methods constitute an original microarchitectural approach based on water molecule diffusion nearly set to be introduced into clinical practice (Cotten et. Al, 2009). Importantly, the acquisition of diffusion-weighted MRI (DW-MRI) data is multidimensional. Multiple three-dimensional volumes with different diffusion-sensitization scanning parameters are provided by the modality. Following, implementation of appropriate post-processing procedures result in the reconstruction of the features of the three-dimensional diffusion profile of water molecule in each voxel. Depending on the chosen processing technique, different features of the diffusion scatter pattern at voxel level can be estimated.

In this context, many approaches are being proposed for the processing of a set of DW-MRI volumes with diffusion tensor imaging (DTI) being the most popular. Many quantitative measures can be calculated from the diffusion tensor (Pierpaoli et al., 1996) that can be used for in between-subject comparisons, as well as in within-subject follow-up studies.

In parallel, tractography is currently the only tool that allows in an entirely non-invasive manner and in-vivo the reconstruction of white matter anatomical paths. The simplest tractography approaches generate, in a deterministic way, curves that are tangent to the vector field of DTI principal eigenvectors (Basser et al., 2000; Mori et al., 1999). More advanced methods, consider the uncertainty associated with these vectors to produce distributions of curves in a probabilistic framework (Behrens et al., 2003; Parker et al., 2003). Latest approaches utilize frameworks that allow incorporation of information from different MRI modalities to study brain anatomical connectivity that will also allow observations of functional connectivity as well by revealing the way activation of one part of the brain affects and is related to other areas (Sotiropoulos et al., 2010).

Functional magnetic resonance imaging (fMRI) measures the hemodynamic response related to neural activity in the brain, in other words the hemodynamic correlates of neural activity (Cui et al., 2011). It measures the blood oxygen level-dependent (BOLD) response that results from local concentration changes in paramagnetic deoxy-hemoglobin (deoxy-

Hb) (Ogawa et al., 1990a), first discovered the 90s (Ogawa et al., 1990b; Ogawa et al., 1992; Kwong et al., 1992) and is the most common functional magnetic resonance imaging technique. Due mainly to the relatively high spatial resolution provided by this technique fMRI has rapidly become the gold standard for in vivo imaging of human brain activity, (Cui et al., 2011). The main current clinical application of fMRI is presurgical mapping of speech and motor brain areas as well as epilepsy foci (Stippich et al., 2007).

Recently, during rest conditions, functional imaging studies have shown that multiple cortical brain regions are functionally linked forming the so called resting-state networks (Raichle et al., 2001; Greicius et al., 2003; Raichle and Snyder, 2007) and fMRI is suitable to study this functional connectivity of the human brain (Damoiseaux et al., 2006). This finding led to the hypothesis that these regions constitute a network supporting a default mode of brain function. The suggested high level of functional connectivity within resting-state networks implies the existence of direct neuroanatomical connections between the respective functionally linked brain regions to facilitate the ongoing interregional neuronal communication. White matter tracts are the structural highways of our brain, enabling information to travel quickly from one brain region to another (van den Heuvel et al., 2009).

Both functional and diffusion MR images are acquired with fast imaging protocols. The most commonly used fast imaging protocol is echo planar imaging (EPI), which allows the acquisition of an image within a time window of a few milliseconds (Mansfield, 1984; Turner et al., 1990). It should be noted that EPI images suffer from low signal-to-noise-ratio (SNR) a parameter that should be considered when designing experiments.

2.2 Optical methods

The part of the electromagnetic spectrum with wavelengths from approximately 650nm to 950nm, is known as near-infrared (NIR) light and has been described as an "optical window" into biological tissue since it is weakly absorbed by tissue. Due to this property, light of these wavelengths may be detected after having penetrated tissue at a depth of a few centimeters. NIR light eventually interacts with biological tissue and therefore, also, with the human brain tissues. Based on the absorption of different wavelengths of light as it passes through the head, optical methods, such as near infrared spectroscopy (NIRS), have been developed to provide another non-invasive measure of local brain activation (Villringer et al., 1995; Strangman et al., 2002).

Oxyhemoglobin (HbO2) and deoxyhemoglobin (HbR)are the two principal chromophores that are absorbed in the NIR wavelength range and thus constitute two biologically relevant markers for brain activity (Strangman et al., 2002). In other words, near-infrared spectroscopy can provide information on concentrations of oxy-and deoxy-hemoglobin in cortical areas of the brain related to the activation of the brain regions in question. Significant differences in the absorption spectra at near-infrared wavelengths have been observed for other tissue chromophores as well, such as cytochrome oxidase during acquisition of simultaneous data from several wavelengths.

The detection of such hemodynamic markers, as also noted in previous sections, is considered as an indirect measure of brain function. Interestingly, it has been suggested that diffuse optical techniques may simultaneously provide both indirect and even direct measures of neuronal activity monitoring. In this context, supporting data exist to imply that diffuse optical methods may detect cell swelling taking place 50–200 milliseconds after neuronal firing. Although, the spatial interrelations between such signals and hemodynamic ones remain subject to investigation, they could be feasibly recorded by sufficiently high-speed and sensitive detectors (Strangman et al., 2002).

Hence, by measuring the changes in the intensity of diffusely transmitted near-infrared light across a brain tissue volume, in non-invasive manner from sensors placed on the human skull, it is possible to gain well-localized information about haemoglobin oxygenation, cytochrome-c-oxidase redox state, and two types of changes in light scattering reflecting either membrane potential (fast signal) or cell swelling (slow signal) during local brain activation (Strangman et al., 2002). Advantages of the optical methods include biochemical specificity, a temporal resolution in the millisecond range, the potential of measuring intracellular and intravascular events simultaneously and the portability of the devices enabling bedside examinations (Villringer and Chance, 1997).

Based on the above mentioned, it becomes reasonably evident that near-infrared (NIR) imaging techniques have become an increasingly popular research means to study brain activity (Cooper et al., 2009) non-invasively using harmeless non-ionizing radiation (Gibson et al 2005, Hillman 2007). To date fNIRS has been successfully applied in several fields providing interesting and meaningful brain activation related data (Cui et al., 2011). NIRS has been used to investigate and add useful knowledge to the understanding of the physiological mechanisms of the BOLD response (Toronov et al., 2003; Hoge et al., 2005; Kleinschmidt et al., 1996; Schroeter et al., 2006; Emir et al., 2008; Malonek et al., 1997; Huppert et al., 2006, 2007, 2009). After early studies employing single-site near-infrared spectroscopy, first near-infrared imaging devices are being applied successfully for low-resolution functional brain imaging (Strangman et al., 2002; Villringer and Chance, 1997). NIRS is a very portable technique (Atsumori et al., 2009) and has been proposed as a useful technology for non-invasive brain–computer interfaces (Power et al., 2010; Coyle et al., 2004, 2007; Sitaram et al., 2007; Utsugi et al., 2008). NIRS has been used to study brain activity in both event-related tasks and resting states (Boecker et al., 2007; Herrmann et al., 2005; White et al., 2009; Honda et al., 2010; Zhang et al., 2010; Lu et al., 2010). It has been also proposed as useful alternate in experimental paradigms which are difficult to perform in the MRI scanner, such as face-to-face communication (Suda et al., 2010) or driving (Tomioka et al., 2009).

The applications of NIR techniques which improve spatial information by affording two-dimensional imaging of changes in both oxyhaemoglobin (HbO2) and de-oxyhaemoglobin (HHb) during stimuli driven experiments, include optical topography (OT) (Obrig and Villringer 2003; Cooper et al., 2009). This methodology has been broadly used to study the functional activation of the motor (Franceschini et al 2003, Maki et al 1996) and visual (Zeff et al 2007) cortices as well as in experimental procedure investigating language processing and development (Pe˜na et al 2003; see Cooper et al., 2009 for more details).

NIRS instrumentation is a flexible and portable technology and can be made unobtrusive, low-cost, low-power, even robust to motion artifacts (e.g., Totaro et al 1998) or technology enabling such artifacts to be successfully tackled (Izzetoglu et al., 2005; Izzetoglu et al., 2010). It is supported by three main categories of systems, each presenting advantages and drawbacks: time domain, frequency domain and continuous wave systems (Strangman et al., 2002).

Continuous wave fNIRS systems (CW) apply light to tissue with invariable amplitude and measure the attenuation of the amplitude of the incident light (Hoshi, 2003; Izzetoglu et al., 2004; Obrig & Villringer, 2003; Irani et al., 2007). Although it is evident that CW systems provide less information than time or frequency domain systems, they also have several benefits that are important for certain applications: they can be manufactured using light emitting diodes (LEDs) and not necessarily using lasers, thus increasing safety with respect to their possible negative effects on vision (e.g. possible negative effect on eye retinas); their total cost can be significantly lower than time and frequency domain systems, enabling deployment of these systems in clinical settings; minimization of dimensions of these systems is also feasible proving them practical solutions for use in educational or clinical settings (Irani et al., 2007). Laser-based time-resolved or frequency domain systems, on the other hand, provide information on both phase and amplitude, and their use is compulsory experimental setups where more precise quantification of fNIRS signals is crucial to ensure robustness of results taking advantage of the added spatial specificity of time domain instruments and the ability to separate absorption and scattering effects (see Hoshi, 2003; Izzetoglu et al., 2004; Obrig & Villringer, 2003; Irani et al., 2007 for more discussion of these system differences). In general, the selection of the fNIR system architecture is determined by the spatial resolution and sensitivity requirements of the brain area activation related research question (Strangman et al., 2002). For investigations of cortical activation and especially when referenced to an external topographic system (e.g., the international 10/20 system), diffuse optical methods seem to provide opportunities and capabilities unavailable with any other brain functional imaging existing technology (Strangman et al., 2002).

2.3 EEG and MEG

Electroencephalography (EEG) and magnetoencephalography (MEG) are well known widely practiced brain monitoring techniques on the scalp surface of the electromagnetic effects of activation of groups of neurons, but without actually being directly three-dimensional imaging techniques. Nevertheless, they are briefly presented in this chapter, focusing on their main operational principles and on a short overview of the inverse problem solution approaches which result in the 3D mapping of EEG and MEG recording, mainly due to the following: measuring electromagnetic field distributions allows localization of cognitive processing (Haufe et al., 2011); EEG and MEG are used in conjunction with functional imaging modalities in most multimodal emerging settings; based on the aforementioned and taking also into account that both noninvasive localization methodologies can be applied without restriction (as opposed to invasive measurements), it is evident that they are highly significant for neuroscience research and medical diagnosis.
The main advantage of the EEG methodology, besides being entirely harmless, is the high temporal resolution opposed though to the relatively low spatial resolution achieved. The typically low EEG spatial resolution is due to the presence of a multilayered tissue interface, such as the skull, the cerebrospinal fluid and other cortex tissue layers between the electrode and the source of brain activation that is being measured (Cooper et al., 2009). Based on the aforementioned it is obviously derived that the scalp maps, namely the activation pattern distributions, of the corresponding cognitive processes elicited via the EEG/MEG measurement analysis, only afford an estimation of the actual underlying sources (Haufe et al., 2011). These spatial maps are derived by the inverse problem solution, which because of its ill-posedness imposes significant restrictions on the way the inverse solution is derived (Darvas et al., 2004). In other words, this inverse problem is ill-defined since any measurement can be equally well justified by infinitely different source distributions (Haufe et al., 2011).

Various approaches have been developed and discussed in order to evaluate inverse problem procedures and to assess the statistical significance of the subsequent results (for a review on this subject, see Darvas et al., 2004; Haufe et al., 2011). It should be noted though that recent developments in this field include the following: (i) independent components analysis has been relevantly recently considered as a useful means of separating physiological and other noise processes from brain activation, and possibly for also revealing distinct dissociated components of neural activation; (ii) time–frequency analysis application to single trial data has been proven useful to the identification of underlying communication mechanisms between neuronal clusters; (iii) the development of multimodal concurrent data acquisition methodologies reveal the potential of combining the high temporal resolution of electrophysiological data with the higher spatial resolution of hemodynamic effects (e.g. Dale et al., 2000; Darvas et al., 2004).

Magnetoencephalography measures the other component of electromagnetism, the magnetic field outside the head induced by current flow within the brain generated directly by neural current generators (Darvas et al., 2004). These primary currents are activated during an event-related study and are used in solving the inverse problem since they are localized to brain activated areas. Recently, MEG and EEG are mostly considered as complementary modalities and MEG based experiments routinely include concurrent multichannel EEG recording (Darvas et al., 2004).

2.4 Focused Microwave Radiometry

Active imaging is very important in the context of clinical practice and has proven its indisputable contribution to medical diagnosis. Nevertheless, constant research efforts are pursued in order to minimize radiation exposure during medical imaging (e.g., CT, PET) since the number of repetitive scans a person may undergo during a specified period of time in order to ensure patient safety is limited. Considering the above, as well as the wide variety of potentially harmful agents that coexist in contemporary everyday life, entirely passive, non-invasive and painless assessment of brain function in living subjects constitutes a wishful perspective and scientific vision.

Under this rationale, the functional imaging perspective of a novel passive microwave imaging device is being investigated during the past 7 years (Karanasiou et al., 2004, 2008; Karathanasis et al., 2010; Gouzouasis et al., 2010). Microwave radiometry is an important scientific research and application area of microwave sensing because it provides a passive sensing technique for detecting naturally emitted electromagnetic radiation. This technique has been used in biomedical applications mainly for monitoring the temperature distribution in depth inside the human body. The proposed system (Microwave Radiometry Imaging System, MiRaIS), is able to provide real-time temperature and/or conductivity variation measurements. The functional imaging perspective of this system is based on the fact that both local temperature and conductivity variations in the brain have been associated with brain activation.

More specifically, it has been suggested that knowledge of thermal patterns inside the brain may provide useful information about brain activity. Under normal, quiet, resting conditions intrabrain heat production is balanced by heat dissipation from the brain, while under several physiological conditions temperature balance modifications occur and brain temperatures either increase above (hyperthermia) or decrease below (hypothermia) their average resting-state values. Experiments have reported for instance, increase by 1–2 C during the transition from sleep to wakefulness (Abrams and Hammel, 1964; Delgado and Hanai, 1966), in response to various stressful, emotionally arousing, and even simple environmental stimuli (Abrams and Hammel, 1964; Delgado and Hanai, 1966; Moser et al., 1993; Yablonskiy et al., 2000; Kiyatkin 2005; Kiyatkin, 2007). Brain temperature balance may also be affected by pharmacological drugs, which influence brain metabolism and consequently alter heat dissipation to the external environment (Kiyatkin, 2007). Thus, brain temperatures fluctuations that naturally take place may cause significant functional consequences given that most physical and chemical processes that determine neuronal activity are dependent by temperature (Kiyatkin, 2007). Thus, It has been suggested that brain temperature fluctuations reflect neural activation (Kiyatkin et al. 2002). Even empirical data obtained with fMRI suggest that increases in regional cerebral blood flow during functional stimulation can cause local changes in brain temperature and subsequent local changes in oxygen metabolism (Yablonskiy et al. 2000). Nevertheless, brain temperature changes in humans remains generally unknown because of lack of actual direct experimental studies (Kiyatkin, 2007).

In addition, another parameter that has been suggested to change during functional neuronal activity is the electrical conductivity of the brain. It has been hypothesized that an increase of regional cerebral blood volume (rCBV) due to neuronal activity will lead to the decrease of cortical impedance (increase of conductivity) because blood has lower impedance than the surrounding cortex (Geddes and Baker, 1967). During functional activity, there is a predominant impedance decrease as a result of an increase in blood volume. During epilepsy and ischemia, it has also been reported that impedance increases due to cell swelling because this reduces the size of the conductive extra-cellular space (Andrew and MacVicar, 1994). Since brain activation produces changes in regional cerebral blood flow (rCBF), it will also produce conductivity changes in the same direction. These (increased usually) blood-flow changes are associated to increased rCBV. Also, reproducible impedance changes of approximately 0.5% have been measured in humans during visual, or motor activity, using 3-D electrical impedance tomography (EIT) (Tidswell et al., 2001).

As stated above, the MiRaIS system measures temperature and/or conductivity fluctuations at low microwave frequencies. Following the aforementioned rationale, if brain activation related temperature and/or conductivity variation measurements changes can be measured with the proposed method, then it could be used to image brain activity in an entirely passive and non-invasive manner that it is completely harmless and can be repeated as often as necessary without any risk even for sensitive populations. The operation principal of the proposed system is based on the use of an ellipsoidal beamformer providing the necessary focusing on the brain areas of interest. Its main advantage is that it operates in an entirely passive and non - invasive manner. In order to use a diagnostic and device such as the proposed one, it is of great importance to achieve imaging of any arbitrary area inside the human head, placed on the ellipsoid's focal point where maximum peak of radiation is achieved. Previous theoretical results have shown the system's ability to focus on specific areas of human head models with varying depths and positions with respect to the ellipsoidal focal point (Karanasiou et al., 2004; 2008). Also, in an effort to improve the system's focusing properties several configurations using dielectric matching layers on the air - model interface or as filling material inside the ellipsoid chamber were tested both theoretically and experimentally showing promising results for the reduction of the scattering effects on the interface under consideration (Karathanasis et al., 2010; Gouzouasis et al., 2010). Both spatial resolution and detection depth provided by the system have been estimated through detailed theoretical analysis and validation experimental procedures using phantoms and animals (e.g. Karanasiou et al., 2004, 2008; Karathanasis et al., 2010; Gouzouasis et al., 2010). In the range 1.3–3.5 GHz, imaging of the head model areas placed at the ellipsoid's focus is feasible with a variety of detection depths (ranging from 2 to 4.5 cm) and spatial resolution (ranging from less than 1 cm to over 3 cm), depending on the frequency used. The system's temperature resolution ranges from 0.5 ◦C to less than 1 ◦C in phantom and small animal experiments.

Importantly, the system has been used in human experiments in order to explore the possibility of passively measuring brain activation changes that are possibly attributed to local conductivity and/or temperature changes. The results indicate the potential value of using focused microwave radiometry to identify brain activations possibly involved or affected in operations induced by particular psychophysiological tasks (Karanasiou et al. 2004).

3. State-of-the-art and beyond of multimodal neuroimaging

After having reviewed all basic operation principles and attributes of the functional brain imaging methodologies, it is concluded that MEG and EEG differ from fMRI and fNIR, not only in the physiological processes that are measured but also in the properties of the inverse problem solutions that result in the functional images (Darvas et al., 2004).

Thus, in summary, on one hand MEG and EEG signals directly record neuronal activation at the millisecond scale at which they occur whereas fMRI and fNIR measure neuronal activation indirectly through hemodynamic changes detection at the order of 1s. In addition, it is still under investigation whether these neuronal and hemodynamic changes refer to the same brain activated areas. Regarding the solution of the inverse problem of MEG and EEG it is illposed affording estimation solutions based on the imposed constraints and methodologies used whereas fMRI directly provides images of the activated areas. Finally, fNIR is a less expensive and more easily administered than the gold standard fMRI, having also better temporal resolution and providing larger content information (both oxygenated and deoxygenated haemoglobin data). Nevertheless, it is a not a clinically implemented technology yet with inferior spatial resolution and decreased signal-to-noise ratio compared to fMRI (Cooper et al., 2011).

Since each of the non-ionizing non-invasive functional brain imaging techniques has different characteristics as described in the preceding section, in order to acquire the most valuable complementary data in terms of quality and quantity, benefiting from the advantages of the various techniques, combination of two or more techniques is expected (Shibasaki, 2008). The so-called multimodal approach may be achieved either by post-measurement combination and fusion of data or via simultaneous use of hemodynamic and electrophysiological techniques in order to reveal the multifactorial interplay of the underlying mechanisms during brain activation (Shibasaki, 2008).

In this chapter only the latter will be presented whereas the first category holds the disadvantage of uncontrolled background since it is not possible to guarantee the exact same experimental conditions between different measurement sessions (Honda et al., 1998; Shibasaki, 2008).

3.1 Simultaneous fMRI-EEG

Simultaneous fMRI and EEG is the most widely implemented multimodal human brain mapping technique which aims at combining high time and spatial resolution in a signle

modality, affording research of functional cortical activity and neurovascular coupling. Due to technological progress, technical obstacles are constantly superimposed and concurrent fMRI-EEG studies are increasingly and successfully performed in a variety of recent studies (e.g. Horwitz and Poeppel, 2002; Sammer et al., 2005; Otte and Halsband, 2006; Stern, 2006; Horovitz et al., 2008; Shibasaki, 2008; Ritter and Villringer 2006, Mulert et al 2004; Cooper et al., 2009) including cognitive processing, epileptic and seizure activity in children and adults (Gotman, 2008; Vulliemoz et al., 2010; Cooper et al., 2011) and neurovascular coupling (e.g. Kruggel et al 2000, Goldman et al 2002, Gotman et al 2006; Cooper et al., 2010).
The main artefacts that occur in simultaneous fMRI and EEG recordings rise from the interference of the scanner gradients with the EEG and many artefact elimination methods have been developed to manage this drawback (e.g. Ritter et al., 2007). Other artefacts rise from human physiological activity such as electrocardiographic artefacts and relevant removal methods have also been implemented successfully (Nakamura and Shibasaki, 1987; Nakamura et al., 1990; Shibasaki, 2008).
Currently, simultaneous recording of EEG in the MR scanning room is usually pursued in clinical practice for the presurgical evaluation of partial epilepsy patients (Jager et al., 2002; Stern, 2006). In research, EEG and fMRI paradigms are increasingly developed to study the underlying mechanisms of functional processing in a non-invasive manner combining high time resolution neuronal activation measurements with high spatial resolution hemodynamic response imaging (Shibasaki, 2008).

3.2 Simultaneous EEG-fNIR

The complementary information that is acquired by simultaneously measuring electrophysiological and cerebral blood volume changes, besides the combined fMRI-EEG settings, it has also recently been exploited by simultaneous EEG and NIR spectroscopy (Rovati et al 2007, Roche-Labarbe et al 2007; Cooper et al., 2009).
fNIR and other optical methods such as diffuse optical imaging presents several advantages compared to fMRI which have been exploited in recent studies involving neonatals and infants (Cooper et al.,2011, Telkemeyer et al., 2011; Ancora et al., 2009). They are portable, compatible with EEG and relatively insensitive to movement artifacts and therefore suitable to be used on neonatals and infants. Recently, two studies of concurrent assessment of vascular based imaging and electrophysiological responses of neonatal seizure (Cooper et al., 2011) and infant language acquisition (Telkemeyer et al., 2011) have been carried out with combined EEG and fNIR. Other studies of the simultaneous inegrated use of the two methodologies include the measurement of workload states (Hirshfield et al., 2009), mental stress (Ishii et al., 2008), during epileptic discharges (Machado et al., 2011), in auditory sensory gating (Ehlis et al., 2009).

3.3 Simultaneous MEG-fNIR

Besides the combination of EEG with fNIR, recently simultaneous MEG with fNIR measurements are being performed to once more investigate the neurovascular coupling of activated brain areas. After the first feasibility study using nonselective NIRS and DC-MEG recordings (Mackert et al., 2004, Mackert et al., 2008), several studies with simultaneous MEG and fNIR measurements have been realized (e.g. Sander et al., 2007; Mackert et al., 2008; Ou et al., 2009). Recently, during a standard motor task time-resolved multichannel NIRS (trNIRS) has been combined with DC-MEG to analyze simultaneously and quantitatively hemodynamic and neuronal changes in activated brain areas (Mackert et al., 2008).

In another recent study (Ou et al., 2009), by simultaneous implementation of diffuse optical imaging (DOI) and magnetoencephalography (MEG) neurovascular coupling is once more investigated. Interestingly, an event-related and not a block design of the experimental paradigm has been followed to achieve evaluation of the contribution of single neural components to the hemodynamic responses, enabling direct comparison of the elicited results with the significant number of neurovascular coupling findings in animals using invasive recordings (Ou et al., 2009).

3.4 Simultaneous fMRI-fNIRs

Several research efforts of the simultaneous implementation of the fMRI and NIRS methodologies have been reported over the last two decades (Kleinschmidt et al., 1996; Punwani et al., 1998; Toronov et al., 2001; Mehagnoul-Schipper et al., 2002; Strangman et al., 2002; MacIntosh et al., 2003; Huppert et al., 2006; Zhang et al., 2006). These studies provide convincing evidence regarding the effective correlation and combination of the two methodologies towards a more practical implementation (Toyoda et al., 2008). Combined fMRI and NIR methods have also been widely used in animal studies (Zhang et al., 2006).

The main constraint imposed by the integration of the two modalities and actually occurs every time during any experimental design in the MR chamber, is the fact that the use of only non-magnetic material is allowed. In the case of combined fMRI-EEG measurements, research and technological progress have resulted in the construction of MRI-compatible EEG devices, many of which currently exist commercially. Similarly, the optical probe must be designed and constructed to be fully MRI-compatible without causing any MR image distortion. Also, the final setup must afford accurate co-registration of optical and MR images in order to achieve an efficient integration of the two imaging techniques (Zhang et al., 2006). The high spatial resolution is accomplished through structural MR imaging where all optical and functional MR data are co-registered. This procedure also forms the basis of the inverse problem solution and the possibility to superimpose all data on the Talairach space for group studies (Zhang et al., 2006).

3.5 Simultaneous recordings using more than two modalities

As shown in previous sections, current and future trends in functional human brain mapping focus research on implementing multimodal approaches in order to acquire the largest possible set of measurements of correlates of neural activity in a single experimental procedure. It has been shown that there is a strong correlation between mass neuronal activity and localized changes in blood flow and volume and this is the reason why methodologies that measure electrophysiological responses are combined with techniques the measure hemodynamic changes in the multimodal approaches in question. Interestingly, each of these modalities through the so-called steady state measurements reveal brain areas that are functionally and structurally correlated and thus, provide new insights into brain function (Gore et al., 2006). Attempts to integrate more than two modalities are also pursued by combing simultaneous fMRI, NIR and ERP measurements (Gore et al., 2006).

In this context, besides electrophysiological and hemodynamic measurements, feasibility of integrating additional measures, such as non-invasive local temperature and conductivity measurements could also be investigated. Magnetic Resonance Spectroscopy (MRS) can measure temperature noninvasively (e.g. Corbett et al., 1997). It is a well-established technique that uses an MRI scanner to detect certain naturally occurring brain metabolites. By interpreting the relative frequencies of a reference metabolite (N-acetyl aspartate; NAA) and water, it is possible to estimate tissue temperature with precision of approximately +0.5°C (Harris et al., 2008). Microwave Radiometry with the additional advantage of being completely passive maybe used for estimating temperature and/or conductivity changes non-invasively in the brain.

Taking all of the above into consideration, research efforts focus on integrating MiRaIs with EEG and fNIR (Karanasiou et al., 2009). A customized head cap for simultaneous mounting of EEG electrodes and the proposed fNIR system according to the 10-20 system that is also MiRaIS-compatible and appropriate post-processing software tools, focusing on fNIR/EEG image reconstruction are being developed. Therefore, the resulting multi-modal measurements will comprise electrical activity (EEG), blood flow (fNIR), as well as temperature and conductivity variations (MiRaIS) in activated cortical areas.

4. State-of-the-art and beyond of neuroimaging genetics: THz imaging and optogenetics

Besides multimodal functional imaging and the indisputable advances in this field, current and future trends in neuroscience research aim at bridging neural function and biomolecular information and studying microscopic processes at the molecule level. This scope is pursued through studies both in anatomic and functional biomedical imaging, integrating the rapidly advancing research fields of medical imaging/neuroimaging and molecular medicine/genetics. In this context, research has emphasized new methods for discovering novel markers that may have an influence on specific features in psychiatric and neurological diseases, expecting to also take advantage of next-generation imaging technologies that will potentially afford the monitoring of the chemical processes of the cells within the organs and produce real-time images of biomolecules, such as genes and proteins functioning within cells.

In this scientific and technological milieu, the widely acknowledged 'THz gap', including the complete frequency range from 100 GHz up to 30 THz, makes this region of the electromagnetic spectrum a scientific frontier holding great promise not only for identifying and classifying biomolecules, but also for understanding the underlying molecular dynamics. All molecules (biological, organic, inorganic, etc) have inherent vibrational and rotational spectra that lie in the terahertz frequency regime with spectral signatures resulting from intra- and inter-molecular interactions. Specific proteins for instance, absorb certain characteristic t-ray frequencies leading to a distinct terahertz 'fingerprint' for each biomolecule; sensors that can detect this absorption may reveal the identity of the protein. To this end, THz technology can serve as a viable option for medical imaging envisaging the expansion of current knowledge on biomolecular information and its correlation with neural function.

The THz "gap" became the subject of research for the past 8 years approximately and its application in biomedicine is considered very promising (Bakopoulos et al., 2009). Considerable effort has been invested in the development of applications of the THz frequency regime (0.1–5 THz) for the detection and characterization of biological material focusing on their interaction with THz radiation (e.g. Siegel, 2004; Woolard et al., 2005) as well as for the detection of cancer by developing novel THz imaging systems (Woodward et al., 2005; Wahaia et al., 2010). Nevertheless, THz waves is a state-of-the-art research field exhibiting constant technological progress and as such the interaction of biological materials with THz radiation is not completely known and still under investigation: the THz response of biological samples is considerably affected by the specific radiation properties, the experimental configuration as well as the sample preparation and measurement procedures. THz technology may add significant knowledge to the understanding of brain function in health and disease by providing biochemical profiling of various neurotransmitters in various conditions. Recent findings support the abovementioned claims; a novel study on the use of terahertz (THz) spectroscopy to distinguish between healthy and diseased snap-frozen tissue samples obtained from three regions of the human brain has been recently reported (Png et al., 2009). The research team based their work on the fact that as protein structures have been successfully marked using THz radiation, the group vibrational modes of protein plaques could be also probed in the THz frequency range. With this view, they used tissue samples with Alzheimer's disease; the latter were neuropathologically diagnosed to comprise abnormal high quantity of protein plaques consistent with the disease in question. Results showed that a rough classification between healthy and diseased tissue was accomplished based on their THz absorption spectra, which could be attributed to pathological changes in the diseased tissue (Png et al., 2009).

Recently, a few more studies have been reported towards the same research direction (Abbas et al., 2009; Treviño-Palacios et al., 2010). A new approach including the development of integrated THz circuits for the detection of biochemical events was implemented to the detection of nitric oxide synthase (NOS) activity (Abbas et al., 2009). The authors designed and fabricated a BioMEMS (Biological MicroElectro-Mechanical System) compatible with microfluidic circulation and electromagnetic propagation which they successfully used to detect NOS activity ex vivo. Real-time THz spectroscopy was used to detect biomolecule processes associated with neurodegenerative phenomena (Abbas et al., 2009). Another group, classify healthy and cancerous tissue using the non-ionizing water absorption to terahertz radiation. This seems to be a somewhat complementary reciprocal classification methodology since one of main drawbacks that THz radiation is not being currently widely considered for in-vivo body imaging is the large absorption by body water content (Treviño-Palacios et al., 2010).

In parallel, in the broader field of genetic imaging, the use of a novel combination of fMRI with a recently developed state-of-the-art technique called optogenetics (Boyden et al., 2005), holds great promise to reveal direct evidence that the fMRI signal is a compelling measure of brain activity. Moreover, combining functional imaging with a technique that controls subpopulations of neurons using light, will result in the enhancement of the basis of neuroscience research and lead new ways to understanding the mechanisms and treatment of brain injury and disease (Lee et al., 2010). The researchers support that the new functional genetic imaging technique, the integrated optogenetics and BOLD-fMRI (ofMRI) will enable the observation of the big picture of the causal connectivity of neurons in specific brain regions without of course suggesting that absence of a BOLD signal would prove the absence of such connectivity. ofMRI aims at further probing and defining the causal generation of BOLD signals and most importantly at enabling the causal connectivity mapping of cells which are genetically and anatomically- by circuit topology -defined (Lee et al., 2010). Nevertheless, this approach being significantly novel and recent is also followed by reservations and some doubts; the validity of the technique itself as well as the interpretation of the fMRI data is still being questioned and under constant debate (Logothetis 2010).

5. Conclusion

Functional neuroimaging has had a huge impact in cognitive neurosciences and in our understanding of the healthy human brain. The next big challenge in this field is the wide application of functional imaging methods in a clinical context, which will help us understand the mechanisms of neurological and psychiatric diseases and to identify effective therapeutic strategies, which will have a dramatic impact in the lives of millions of people, as neuropsychiatric disorders (e.g., mood disorders, stroke, epilepsy) are among the most common diseases.

More precise assessment of the underlying biophysics of the measured signals and especially of their interrelations will be extremely important for the better understanding of the healthy and diseased brain. The proposed unprecedented concurrent assessment of multiple biophysical correlates of neural activation (blood flow, volume and oxygenation, conductivity and temperature) will allow detailed correlation studies that will further elucidate the nature of brain activation measurement and the neurovascular coupling.

The current decade may be remembered in the future for the progress of neuroscience beyond the level of basic and clinical, into a field of innovative and challenging research applications. The development of new tools and methodologies and pursuing integrated approaches focus on revealing not only the underlying mechanisms of the measured neural correlates of local brain activation but also on leading the way to the global mapping of their interrelations, connectivity and causal activation.

Functional brain imaging research in conjunction with the rapidly expanding knowledge in genetics, offers not only the promise of dramatic cures and amelioration of mental health, but also a profound understanding of the brain's functionality.

6. Acknowledgment

The author would like to thank Dr. Stamatis Sotiropoulos for his insightful comments and suggestions on MRI advanced techniques and DTI analysis, Dr. Nikolaos Pleros and Dr. Paraskevas Bakopoulos for their enlightening clarifications on the technical issues of THz imaging.

7. References

Abbas, A., Dargent, T., Croix, D., Salzet, M., & Bocquet, B. (2009). Ex-vivo detection of neural events using THz BioMEMS. Medical Science Monitor, 15(9), MT121-MT125

Abrams R, Hammel HT (1964) Hypothalamic temperature in unanesthetized albino rats during feeding and sleeping. Am J Physiol 206:641–646

Ancora Gina, Eugenia Maranella, Chiara Locatelli, Luca Pierantoni, Giacomo Faldella, Changes in cerebral hemodynamics and amplitude integrated EEG in an asphyxiated newborn during and after cool cap treatment, Brain and Development, vol. 31, no 6, pp. 442-444, June 2009

Andrew R. and B. Mac Vicar, "Imaging cell volume changes and neuronal excitation in the hippocampal slice," Neuroscience, vol. 62, pp. 371–383, 1994.

Atsumori, H., Kiguchi, M., Obata, A., Sato, H., Katura, T., Funane, T., Maki, A., 2009. Development of wearable optical topography system for mapping the prefrontal cortex activation. Rev. Sci. Instrum. 80, 043704.

Bakopoulos P, I Karanasiou, P. Zakynthinos, N. Pleros, H. Avramopoulos N. Uzunoglu "A tunable continuous wave (CW) and short-pulse optical source for THz brain imaging applications," Meas Sci Technol, vol. 20, 104001,2009.

Basser PJ, Pajevic S, Pierpaoli C, Duda J, Aldroubi A. In vivo fiber tractography using DT-MRI data. Magnetic Resonance in Medicine 44, 625-632, 2000.

Behrens T E, M W Woolrich, M Jenkinson, H Johansen-Berg, R G Nunes, S Clare, P M Matthews, J M Brady, and S M Smith Characterization and propagation of uncertainty in diffusion-weighted MR imaging. Magnetic Resonance in Medicine 50, 1077-1088, 2003.

Boecker, M., Buecheler, M.M., Schroeter, M.L., Gauggel, S., 2007. Prefrontal brain activation during stop-signal response inhibition: an event-related functional nearinfrared spectroscopy study. Behav. Brain Res. 176, 259–266.

Boyden, E.S., Zhang, F., Bamberg, E., Nagel, G., Deisseroth, K. Millisecond-timescale, genetically targeted optical control of neural activity (2005) Nature Neuroscience, 8 (9), pp. 1263-1268.

Cooper R. J., N. L. Everdell, L. C. Enfield, A. P. Gibson, Alan Worley, and Jeremy C. Hebden Design and evaluation of a probe for simultaneous EEG and near-infrared imaging of cortical activation Phys Med Biol. 2009 April 7; 54(7): 2093–2102

Cooper R. J., R. Eames, J. Brunker, L. C. Enfield, A. P. Gibson, and Jeremy C Hebden A tissue equivalent phantom for simultaneous near-infrared optical tomography and EEG Biomed Opt Express. 2010 September 1; 1(2): 425–430.

Cooper, R. J., Hebden, J. C., O'Reilly, H., Mitra, S., Michell, A. W., Everdell, N. L., et al. (2011). Transient haemodynamic events in neurologically compromised infants: A simultaneous EEG and diffuse optical imaging study. NeuroImage, 55(4), 1610-1616.

Corbett RJ, Laptook A, Weatherall P., Noninvasive measurements of human brain temperature using volume-localized proton magnetic resonance spectroscopy. J Cereb Blood Flow Metab. 1997;17:363–369.

Cotten Anne, Erwan Kermarrec, Antoine Moraux, Jean-Francois Budzik, New MRI Sequences, Joint Bone Spine, Volume 76, Issue 6, December 2009, Pages 588-590

Coyle, S., Ward, T., Markham, C., McDarby, G., 2004. On the suitability of near-infrared (NIR) systems for next-generation brain–computer interfaces. Physiol. Meas. 25, 815–822.

Coyle, S.M., Ward, T.E., Markham, C.M., 2007. Brain–computer interface using a simplified functional near-infrared spectroscopy system. J. Neural Eng. 4, 219–226.

Cui Xu, Signe Bray, Daniel M. Bryant, Gary H. Glover, Allan L. Reiss, A quantitative comparison of NIRS and fMRI across multiple cognitive tasks, NeuroImage, Volume 54, Issue 4, 14 February 2011, Pages 2808-28

Dale, A., Liu, A., Fischl, B., Buckner, R., Belliveau, J., Lewine, J., Halgren, E., 2000. Dynamic statistical parametric mapping: combining fMRI and MEG for high-resolution imaging of cortical activity. Neuron 26, 55–67.

Damoiseaux J. S., S. A. R. B. Rombouts, F. Barkhof, P. Scheltens, C. J. Stam, S. M. Smith, and C. F. Beckmann Consistent resting-state networks across healthy subjects Proc Natl Acad Sci U S A. 2006 September 12; 103(37): 13848–13853.

Darvas F., D. Pantazis, E. Kucukaltun-Yildirim, R.M. Leahy, Mapping human brain function with MEG and EEG: methods and validation, NeuroImage, Volume 23, Supplement 1, Mathematics in Brain Imaging, 2004, Pages S289-S299

Delgado JMR, Hanai T (1966) Intracerebral temperatures in free-moving cats. Am J Physiol 211:755–769

Dwight L. Woolard, Elliott R. Brown, Michael Pepper, And Michael Kemp, Terahertz Frequency Sensing and Imaging : A Time of Reckoning Future Application ?, Proceedings of The IEEE, 93(10), (2005),1722-1743.

Ehlis A.-C., T.M. Ringel, M.M. Plichta, M.M. Richter, M.J. Herrmann, A.J. Fallgatter, Cortical correlates of auditory sensory gating: A simultaneous near-infrared spectroscopy event-related potential study, Neuroscience, vol. 159, no 3, pp. 1032-1043, March 2009

Emir, U.E., Ozturk, C., Akin, A., 2008. Multimodal investigation of fMRI and fNIRS derived breath hold BOLD signals with an expanded balloon model. Physiol. Meas. 29, 49–63.

Franceschini M A, Fantini S, Thompson J H, Culver J P and Boas D A 2003 Hemodynamic evoked response of the sensorimotor cortex measured noninvasively with near-infrared optical imaging Psychophysiology 40 548–60

Geddes L. A. and L. E. Baker, "The specific resistance of biological material: A compendium of data for the biomedical engineer and physiologist," Med. Biol. Eng., vol. 5, pp. 271–293, 1967.

Gibson A P, Hebden J C and Arridge S R 2005 Recent advances in diffuse optical imaging Phys.Med. Biol. 50 R1–43

Gore John C., Silvina G. Horovitz, Christopher J. Cannistraci, Pavel Skudlarski, Integration of fMRI, NIROT and ERP for studies of human brain function, Magnetic Resonance Imaging, Volume 24, Issue 4, May 2006, Pages 507-513

Gouzouasis I.A., K.T. Karathanasis, I.S. Karanasiou, N.K. Uzunoglu, "Contactless Passive Diagnosis for Brain Intracranial Applications: A Study Using Dielectric Matching Materials", Bioelectromangetics 2010, DOI 10.1002/bem.20572.

Greicius MD, Krasnow B, Reiss AL, Menon V. Functional connectivity in the resting brain: a network analysis of the default mode hypothesis. Proc Natl Acad Sci U S A 100, 253-258, 2003.

Hariri A.R., E.M. Drabant and D.R. Weinberger, Imaging Genetics: Perspectives from Studies of Genetically Driven Variation in Serotonin Function and Corticolimbic Affective Processing, Biol. Psych. 59 (2006), 888-897

Harris BA, Andrews PJD, Marshall I, Robinson TM, Murray GD. Forced convective head cooling device reduces human cross-sectional brain temperature measured by magnetic resonance: a non-randomized healthy volunteer pilot study. Br J Anaesth 2008; 100: 365–72.

Haufe Stefan, Ryota Tomioka, Thorsten Dickhaus, Claudia Sannelli, Benjamin Blankertz, Guido Nolte, Klaus-Robert Muller, Large-scale EEG/MEG source localization with spatial flexibility, NeuroImage, Vol. 54, no 2, pp. 851-859, January 2011

Herrmann, M.J., Ehlis, A.C., Wagener, A., Jacob, C.P., Fallgatter, A.J., 2005. Near-infrared optical topography to assess activation of the parietal cortex during a visuo-spatial task. Neuropsychologia 43, 1713–1720.

Hillman E M C 2007 Optical brain imaging in vivo: techniques and applications from animal to man J. Biomed. Opt. 12 051402

Hirshfield, Leanne, Chauncey, Krysta, Gulotta, Rebecca, Girouard, Audrey, Solovey, Erin, Jacob, Robert, Sassaroli, Angelo, Fantini, Sergio, Combining Electroencephalograph and Functional Near Infrared Spectroscopy to Explore Users' Mental Workload Editors Schmorrow, Dylan, Estabrooke, Ivy, Grootjen, Marc, Book Title: Foundations of Augmented Cognition. Neuroergonomics and Operational Neuroscience, Lecture Notes in Computer Science, 2009, Springer Berlin / Heidelberg, 239-247, Volume: 5638

Hoge, R.D., Franceschini, M.A., Covolan, R.J.M., Huppert, T., Mandeville, J.B., Boas, D.A., 2005. Simultaneous recording of task-induced changes in blood oxygenation, volume, and flow using diffuse optical imaging and arterial spin-labeling MRI. Neuroimage 25, 701–707.

Honda, Y., Nakato, E., Otsuka, Y., Kanazawa, S., Kojima, S., Yamaguchi, M.K., Kakigi, R., 2010. How do infants perceive scrambled face? A near-infrared spectroscopic study. Brain Res. 1308, 137–146.

Hoshi, Y. (2003). Functional near-infrared optical imaging: Utility and limitations in human brain mapping. Psychophysiology, 40(4), 511–520.

Huppert, T.J., Allen, M.S., Benav, H., Jones, P.B., Boas, D.A., 2007. A multicompartment vascular model for inferring baseline and functional changes in cerebral oxygen metabolism and arterial dilation. J. Cereb. Blood Flow Metab. 27, 1262–1279.

Huppert, T.J., Allen, M.S., Diamond, S.G., Boas, D.A., 2009. Estimating cerebral oxygen metabolism from fMRI with a dynamic multicompartment Windkessel model. Hum. Brain Mapp. 30, 1548–1567.

Huppert, T.J., Hoge, R.D., Diamond, S.G., Franceschini, M.A., Boas, D.A., 2006b. A temporal comparison of BOLD, ASL, and NIRS hemodynamic responses to motor stimuli in adult humans. Neuroimage 29, 368–382.

Irani, Farzin, Platek, Steven M., Bunce, Scott, Ruocco, Anthony C. and Chute, Douglas , (2007) 'Functional Near Infrared Spectroscopy (fNIRS): An Emerging Neuroimaging Technology with Important Applications for the Study of Brain Disorders', The Clinical Neuropsychologist, 21:1, 9 - 37

Ishii Yoshikazu,; Hajime Ogata,; Hidenori Takano,; Hidenori Ohnishi,; Toshiharu Mukai,; Tohru Yagi,; Study on mental stress using near-infrared spectroscopy, electroencephalography, and peripheral arterial tonometry Engineering in Medicine and Biology Society, 2008. EMBS 2008. 30th Annual International Conference of the IEEE, 20-25 Aug. 2008, 4992 - 4995

Izzetoglu Meltem, Prabhakar Chitrapu, Scott Bunce, and Banu Onaral Motion artifact cancellation in NIR spectroscopy using discrete Kalman filtering Biomed Eng Online. 2010; 9: 16.

Izzetoglu, K., Bunce, S. B. O., Pourrezaei, K., & Chance, B. (2004). Functional optical brain imaging using NIR during cognitive tasks [special issue]. International Journal of Human–Computer Interaction, 17, 211–227.

Izzetoglu, M., Devaraj, A., Bunce, S., & Onaral, B. (2005). Motion artifact cancellation in NIR spectroscopy using Wiener filtering. IEEE Transactions on Biomedical Engineering, 52(5), 934–938.

Karanasiou I. S., N. K. Uzunoglu, and C. Papageorgiou, "Towards functional non-invasive imaging of excitable tissues inside the human body using Focused Microwave Radiometry," IEEE Trans. Microw. Theory Tech., vol. 52, no. 8, pp. 1898–1908, Aug. 2004.

Karanasiou I.S., K.T. Karathanasis, A. Garetsos, N.K. Uzunoglu, "Development and Laboratory Testing of a Noninvasive Intracranial Focused Hyperthermia System", IEEE Trans Microw. Theory. Tech., vol., 56, pp. 2160-2171, 2008.

Karanasiou, I.S. Combined functional data from multispectral non-ionizing and non-invasive brain imaging, Page(s): 1 - 4, Proceedings of ITAB 2009, Digital Object Identifier : 10.1109/ITAB.2009.5394312

Karathanasis K. T., I. A. Gouzouasis, I. S. Karanasiou, M. I. Giamalaki, G. Stratakos, and N. K. Uzunoglu, "Noninvasive Focused Monitoring and Irradiation of Head Tissue Phantoms at Microwave Frequencies", IEEE Trans. on Inf. Tech in Biomedicine, vol. 14, no 3, pp.657-663, 2010

Kiyatkin E. A., "Brain temperature fluctuations during physiological and pathological conditions," Eur. J. Appl. Physiol., vol. 101, pp. 3–17, 2007.

Kiyatkin E. A., P. L. Brown, and R. A. Wise, "Brain temperature fluctuation: a reflection of functional neural activation," Eur. J. Neurosci., vol. 16, pp. 164–168, 2002.

Kiyatkin EA (2005) Brain hyperthermia as physiological and pathological phenomena. Brain Res Rev 50:27–56

Kleinschmidt, A., Obrig, H., Requardt, M., Merboldt, K.D., Dirnagl, U., Villringer, A., Frahm, J., 1996. Simultaneous recording of cerebral blood oxygenation changes during human brain activation by magnetic resonance imaging and near-infrared spectroscopy. J. Cereb. Blood Flow Metab. 16, 817–826.

Kwong KK, Belliveau JW, Chesler DA, Goldberg IE, Weisskoff RM, Poncelet BP, Kennedy DN, Hoppel BE, Cohen MS, Turner R, et al. Dynamic Magnetic Resonance Imaging of Human Brain Activity During Primary Sensory Stimulation. PNAS 89: 5951–55, 1992.

Laufs H., J. Daunizeau, D.W. Carmichael, A. Kleinschmidt, Recent advances in recording electrophysiological data simultaneously with magnetic resonance imaging, Neuroimage 40 (2008), 515-528

Lee, J.H., Durand, R., Gradinaru, V., Zhang, F., Goshen, I., Kim, D.-S., Fenno, L.E., Ramakrishnan, C., Deisseroth, K. Global and local fMRI signals driven by neurons defined optogenetically by type and wiring (2010) Nature, 465 (7299), pp. 788-792.

Logothetis, N.K. Bold claims for optogenetics (2010) Nature, 468 (7323), pp. E3-E4.

Lu, C.M., Zhang, Y.J., Biswal, B.B., Zang, Y.F., Peng, D.L., Zhu, C.Z., 2010. Use of fNIRS to assess resting state functional connectivity. J. Neurosci. Meth. 186, 242–249.

Machado A., J.M. Lina, J. Tremblay, M. Lassonde, D.K. Nguyen, F. Lesage, C. Grova, Detection of hemodynamic responses to epileptic activity using simultaneous Electro-EncephaloGraphy (EEG)/Near Infra Red Spectroscopy (NIRS) acquisitions, NeuroImage, Vol. 56, no 1, pp. 114-125, May 2011

Mackert Bruno-Marcel, Stefanie Leistner, Tilmann Sander, Adam Liebert, Heidrun Wabnitz, Martin Burghoff, Lutz Trahms, Rainer Macdonald, Gabriel Curio, Dynamics of cortical neurovascular coupling analyzed by simultaneous DC-magnetoencephalography and time-resolved near-infrared spectroscopy, NeuroImage, Vol. 39, no 3, pp. 979-986, February 2008

Mackert, B.M.,Wubbeler, G., Leistner, S., Uludag, K., Obrig, H., Villringer, A., Trahms, L., Curio, G., 2004. Neurovascular coupling analyzed noninvasively in the human brain. NeuroReport 15, 63–66.

Maki A, Yamashita Y, Watanabe E and Koizumi H 1996 Visualizing human motor activity by using non-invasive optical topography Front. Med. Biol. Eng. 7 285–97

Malonek, D., Dirnagl, U., Lindauer, U., Yamada, K., Kanno, I., Grinvald, A., 1997. Vascular imprints of neuronal activity: relationships between the dynamics of cortical blood flow, oxygenation, and volume changes following sensory stimulation. Proc. Natl Acad. Sci. USA 94, 14826–14831.

Mansfield P Real-time echo-planar imaging by NMR. British Medical Bulletin 40, 187-190, 1984.

Mori, S., Crain, B. J., Chacko, V. P. and Van Zijl, P. C. M. (1999), Three-dimensional tracking of axonal projections in the brain by magnetic resonance imaging. Annals of Neurology, 45: 265–269.

Moser E, Mathiesen I, Andersen P (1993) Association between brain temperature and dentate field potentials in exploring and swimming rats. Science 259:1324–1326

Obrig, H. & Villringer, A. (2003). Beyond the visible—imaging the human brain with light. Journal of Cerebral Blood Flow and Metabolism, 23(1), 1–18.

Ogawa S, D W Tank, R Menon, J M Ellermann, S G Kim, H Merkle, and K Ugurbil Intrinsic signal changes accompanying sensory stimulation: Functional brain mapping with magnetic resonance imaging. PNAS 89: 5675–79, 1992.

Ogawa S, Lee TM, Nayak AS, Glynn P. Oxygenation-sensitive contrast in magnetic resonance image of rodent brain at high magnetic fields. Magnetic Resonance in Medicine 14: 68–78, 1990b.

Ogawa, S., Lee, T.M., Kay, A.R., Tank, D.W., 1990a. Brain magnetic resonance imaging with contrast dependent on blood oxygenation. Proc. Natl Acad. Sci. USA 87, 9868–9872.

Opportunities in THz Science, Report of a DOE-NSF-NIH Workshop, Ed. by M. S. Sherwin, C. A. Schmuttenmaer, and P. H. Bucksbaum, February 2004, Arlington, VA

Ou Wanmei, Ilkka Nissila, Harsha Radhakrishnan, David A. Boas, Matti S. Hamalainen, Maria Angela Franceschini, Study of neurovascular coupling in humans via simultaneous magnetoencephalography and diffuse optical imaging acquisition, NeuroImage, Volume 46, Issue 3, 1 July 2009, Pages 624-632

Parker GJ, Haroon HA, Wheeler-Kingshott CA. A framework for a streamline-based probabilistic index of connectivity (PICo) using a structural interpretation of MRI diffusion measurements. J Magn Reson Imaging 18, 242-254, 2003.

Pe˜na M, Maki A, Kovaˇci´c D, Dehaene-Lambertz G, Koizumi H, Bouquet F and Mehler J 2003 Sounds and silence: an optical topography study of language recognition at birth Proc. Natl. Acad. Sci. USA. 100 11702–5

Pierpaoli C, Jezzard P, Basser PJ, Barnett A, Di Chiro G. Diffusion tensor MR imaging of the human brain. Radiology 201, 637-648, 1996.

Png, G. M., Flook, R., Ng, B. W. -., & Abbott, D. (2009). Terahertz spectroscopy of misfolded proteins in bio-tissue. Paper presented at the 34th International Conference on Infrared, Millimeter, and Terahertz Waves, IRMMW-THz 2009)

Power, S.D., Falk, T.H., Chau, T., 2010. Classification of prefrontal activity due to mental arithmetic and music imagery using hidden Markov models and frequency domain near-infrared spectroscopy. J. Neural Eng. 7, 026002

Raichle Marcus E., Abraham Z. Snyder, A default mode of brain function: A brief history of an evolving idea, NeuroImage, Volume 37, Issue 4, 1 October 2007, Pages 1083-1090

Raichle Marcus E., Ann Mary MacLeod, Abraham Z. Snyder, William J. Powers, Debra A. Gusnard and Gordon L. Shulman Proceedings of the National Academy of Sciences of the United States of America A default mode of brain function. Proc Natl Acad Sci U S A.;98(2):676-82, 2001.

Schroeter, M.L., Kupka, T., Mildner, T., Uludag, K., von Cramon, D.Y., 2006. Investigating the post-stimulus undershoot of the BOLD signal–a simultaneous fMRI and fNIRS study. Neuroimage 30, 349–358.

Shibasaki Hiroshi Human brain mapping: hemodynamic response and electrophysiology. Clin Neurophysiol. 2008 April; 119(4): 731–743.

Siegel P.H., "THz Technology in Biology and Medicine," IEEE Trans. Microwave Theory and Techniques, vol. 52, no. 10, pp. 2438-2448, Oct. 2004.

Siegwart, R. (2001). Indirect Manipulation of a Sphere on a Flat Disk Using Force Information. *International Journal of Advanced Robotic Systems,* Vol.6, No.4, (December 2009), pp. 12-16, ISSN 1729-8806

Sitaram, R., Zhang, H.H., Guan, C.T., Thulasidas, M., Hoshi, Y., Ishikawa, A., Shimizu, K., Birbaumer, N., 2007. Temporal classification of multichannel near-infrared spectroscopy signals of motor imagery for developing a brain–computer interface. Neuroimage 34, 1416–1427.

Sotiropoulos Stamatios N., Li Bai, Paul S. Morgan, Cris S. Constantinescu, Christopher R. Tench, Brain tractography using Q-ball imaging and graph theory: Improved connectivities through fibre crossings via a model-based approach. Neuroimage, 49(3),2444-2456, 2010

Stippich C, Rapps N, Dreyhaupt J, Durst A, Kress B, Nennig E, Tronnier VM, Sartor K. Localizing and lateralizing language in patients with brain tumors: feasibility of routine preoperative functional MR imaging in 81 consecutive patients Radiology. 243(3), 828-36, 2007.

Strangman G., D. A. Boas, J. P. Sutton, Non-Invasive Neuroimaging Using Near-Infrared Light, Biological Psychiatry 52 (2002), 679–693

Suda, M., Takei, Y., Aoyama, Y., Narita, K., Sato, T., Fukuda, M., Mikuni, M., 2010. Frontopolar activation during face-to-face conversation: an in situ study using near-infrared spectroscopy. Neuropsychologia 48, 441–447.

Telkemeyer Silke ,Rossi Sonja ,Nierhaus Till ,Steinbrink Jens ,Obrig Hellmuth ,Wartenburger Isabell, Acoustic processing of temporally modulated sounds in infants: evidence from a combined near-infrared spectroscopy and EEG study, Frontiers in Psychology, 2, 2011

Tidswell T., A. Gibson, R. H. Bayford, and D. S. Holder, "Three-dimensional electrical impendance tomography of human brain activity," NeuroImage, vol. 13, pp. 283–294, 2001

Tomioka, H., Yamagata, B., Takahashi, T., Yano, M., Isomura, A.J., Kobayashi, H., Mimura, M., 2009. Detection of hypofrontality in drivers with Alzheimer's disease by nearinfrared spectroscopy. Neurosci. Lett. 451, 252–256.

Toronov, V., Walker, S., Gupta, R., Choi, J.H., Gratton, E., Hueber, D., Webb, A., 2003. The roles of changes in deoxyhemoglobin concentration and regional cerebral blood volume in the fMRI BOLD signal. Neuroimage 19, 1521–1531.

Totaro R, Barattelli G, Quaresima V, Carolei A, Ferrari M (1998): Evaluation of potential factors affecting the measurement of cerebrovascular reactivity by near-infrared spectroscopy. Clin Sci (Colch) 95:497–504.

Toyoda Hiroshi, Kenichi Kashikura, Tomohisa Okada, Satoru Nakashita, Manabu Honda, Yoshiharu Yonekura, Hideo Kawaguchi, Atsushi Maki, Norihiro Sadato, Source of nonlinearity of the BOLD response revealed by simultaneous fMRI and NIRS, NeuroImage, Vol. 39, no 3, pp. 997-1013, February 2008

Treviño-Palacios, C. G., Celis-López, M. A., Lárraga-Gutiérrez, J. M., García-Garduño, A., Zapata-Nava, O. J., Orduña Díaz, A., et al. (2010). Brain imaging using T-rays instrumentation advances. AIP Conference Proceedings, vol. 1310, pp. 146-149 Eleventh Mexican Symposium on Medical Physics, December 7, 2010

Turner R, Le Bihan D, Maier J, Vavrek R, Hedges LK, Pekar J. Echo-planar imaging of intravoxel incoherent motion. Radiology 177, 407-414, 1990

Utsugi, K., Obata, A., Sato, H., Aoki, R., Maki, A., Koizumi, H., Sagara, K., Kawamichi, H., Atsumori, H., Katura, T., 2008. GO-STOP control using optical brain–computer interface during calculation task. IEICE Trans. Commun. E91-B, 2133–2141.

van den Heuvel MP, Mandl RC, Kahn RS, Hulshoff Pol HE. Functionally linked resting-state networks reflect the underlying structural connectivity architecture of the human brain. Human Brain Mapping, 30: 3127–3141, 2009.

Villringer A., B. Chance, Non-invasive optical spectroscopy and imaging of human brain function, Trends in Neirosciences 20 (1997), 435-442.

Villringer A., U. Dirnagl, Coupling of brain activity and cerebral blood flow: basis of functional neuroimaging. Cerebrovasc Brain Metab Rev 7 (1995), 240-276

Wahaia, F., Valusis, G., Bernardo, L. M., Oliveira, A., Macutkevic, J., Kasalynas, I., et al. (2010). Detection of colon and rectum cancers by terahertz techniques. Paper presented at the Progress in Biomedical Optics and Imaging - Proceedings of SPIE, , 7715

White, B.R., Snyder, A.Z., Cohen, A.L., Petersen, S.E., Raichle, M.E., Schlaggar, B.L., Culver, J.P., 2009. Resting-state functional connectivity in the human brain revealed with diffuse optical tomography. Neuroimage 47, 148–156.

Woodward R M et al 2003 Terahertz pulsed imaging of skin cancer in the time and frequency domain J. Biol. Phys. 29 257

Yablonskiy DA, Ackerman JH, Raichle ME (2000) Coupling between changes in human brain temperature and oxidative metabolism during prolonged visual stimulation. Proc Natl Acad Aci 97:7603–7608

Zeff B W, White B R, Dehghani H, Schlaggar B L and Culver J P 2007 Retinotopic mapping of adult human visual cortex with high-density diffuse optical tomography Proc. Natl. Acad. Sci. 104 12169–74

Zhang, H., Zhang, Y.J., Lu, C.M., Ma, S.Y., Zang, Y.F., Zhu, C.Z., 2010. Functional connectivity as revealed by independent component analysis of resting-state fNIRS measurements. Neuroimage 51, 1150–1161.

Zhang, X., Toronov, V.Y., Webb, A.G. Integrated measurement system for simultaneous functional magnetic resonance imaging and diffuse optical tomography in human brain mapping (2006) Review of Scientific Instruments, 77 (11), art. no. 114301

7

Diffusion Tensor Imaging: Structural Connectivity Insights, Limitations and Future Directions

Linda J. Lanyon
University of British Columbia
Canada

"The brain is a monstrous, beautiful mess. Its billions of nerve cells-called neurons-lie in a tangled web that displays cognitive powers far exceeding any of the silicon machines we have built to mimic it"
William F. Allman

1. Introduction

Almost 40 years since the invention of magnetic resonance imaging (MRI)(Lauterbur, 1973) and just over 25 years since the first use of diffusion imaging (Le Bihan et al., 1986; Merboldt, Hanicke, & Frahm, 1985; Taylor & Bushell, 1985), the pace of advance of these fields and rate of publication of findings are still increasing. MRI neuroimaging delivers enticing insights into the function of the human brain. Elucidation of the networks in the brain that allow information to be processed in a hugely parallel and adaptive manner is crucial to the understanding of brain function. Functional MRI (Kwong et al., 1992; Ogawa et al., 1992) has shown that the brain is a modularised highly distributed system with components specialising in one or more types of information processing (Kanwisher, 2010), such as the network of cortical regions involved in the visual processing of faces (C. J. Fox, Iaria, & Barton, 2008; Haxby, Hoffman, & Gobbini, 2000; Ishai, Schmidt, & Boesiger, 2005; Kanwisher, McDermott, & Chun, 1997; Rossion et al., 2003). Investigation of the large-scale interconnectivity of these modules will lead to better understanding of how these functional building blocks cooperate to confer human cognition, behaviour, memory and conscious thought. Diffusion tensor imaging (DTI) is a non-invasive MRI method used to visualize white matter pathways by identifying the location and orientation of large white matter bundles, at the millimetre-level of 3D visualization. The remarkable advantage of this technique is that it provides the first opportunity to non-invasively investigate this structural connectivity *in vivo* in human beings.
The aim of this chapter is to provide an accessible outline of DTI methods and their use in elucidating large-scale brain connectivity. We will review the field discussing results from human DTI in health and disease, using examples to demonstrate the use of DTI in providing an indication of the structural integrity of cortical white matter, and correlation of individual structure and behavioural performance. We will describe the principles of DTI

tractography and show how this is used to investigate and visualize white matter pathways in healthy and pathological brains. Finally, we will discuss future developments in the field, in particular directions of research that aim to overcome some of the current limitations of the technique. We begin with the principles of diffusion-weighted MRI.

2. Foundations of the field: DW-MRI and the diffusion tensor

DTI employs diffusion-weighted MRI (DW-MRI) scanning. MRI techniques generally observe properties of hydrogen nuclei, which consist of a single proton, and are the most dominant atom in the human body due to the abundance of water molecules. DW-MRI observes the displacement of these protons due to random Brownian motion (diffusion). Specifically, the technique measures the probability density function of proton displacements over a fixed time interval. In the presence of a strong magnetic field inside the MRI scanner, water protons are excited and begin to precess (spin), in similar fashion to a series of gyroscopes, in phase with each other. For functional MRI, a T2-weighted scan measures the time taken in different media for this precession to relax, following excitation. When molecules are able to move freely, this relaxation tends to take longer, so areas of cerebral spinal fluid (CSF) tend to appear brighter than white or grey matter and white matter tends to appear darker than grey matter. Similarly, in DW-MRI, differences in the homogeneity of the precession of water molecules are used to confer information about media type. In these scans a dephasing gradient pulse field is used to dephase the precession of molecules. The extent of dephasing varies along the gradient, as shown in figure 1. A subsequent rephasing gradient of opposite polarity restores phase to all molecules that have not moved. Molecules that have moved in the time between the two gradient pulses will not have their phase fully refocused by the rephasing pulse. By applying this pair of gradients between MRI excitation and data collection, the image is sensitised to the motion of water molecules by diffusion (or flow). The strength of diffusion-weighting is often expressed as a *b* value, which is proportional to the product of the square of the gradient strength and the time interval between the two pulses. The extent of signal decay depends on the diffusion constants of the medium. Signal from CSF decays faster and, therefore, produces a darker image than that for the rest of the brain. The signal from white matter decays the slowest and, therefore, white matter appears as the darkest regions of the image. Simple scalar *apparent diffusion constant* (ADC) images reflect this overall signal-loss and the acute stage of stroke can be detected from these images because swelling restricts diffusion and so the affected region appears bright (Moseley et al., 1990).

In anisotropic media such as brain white matter, a single scalar measurement of diffusion (ADC) is insufficient because the measured diffusivity depends on the orientation of the tissue. A symmetric **diffusion tensor** (Basser, Mattiello, & LeBihan, 1994; Crank, 1975) is used to characterise diffusion in 3 dimensions. The tensor is usually visualised as an elliptical Gaussian. MRI scanners can measure diffusion along any desired angular direction by using in combination three independent gradient units that are orthogonal to each other. In order to create a diffusion tensor, information must be acquired from gradients applied at a minimum of 6 independent angular directions (Basser, et al., 1994), typically more are used, in addition to an image acquired without diffusion weighting (known as a b0 image). In regions where diffusion of water molecules is unhindered, such as in CSF, molecules are able to diffuse equally in all directions producing an isotropic distribution. In this case, the diffusion tensor is isotropic, depicted as a sphere. In contrast, in white matter, fiber membranes restrict diffusion in the direction perpendicular to the fibers. In fact, water

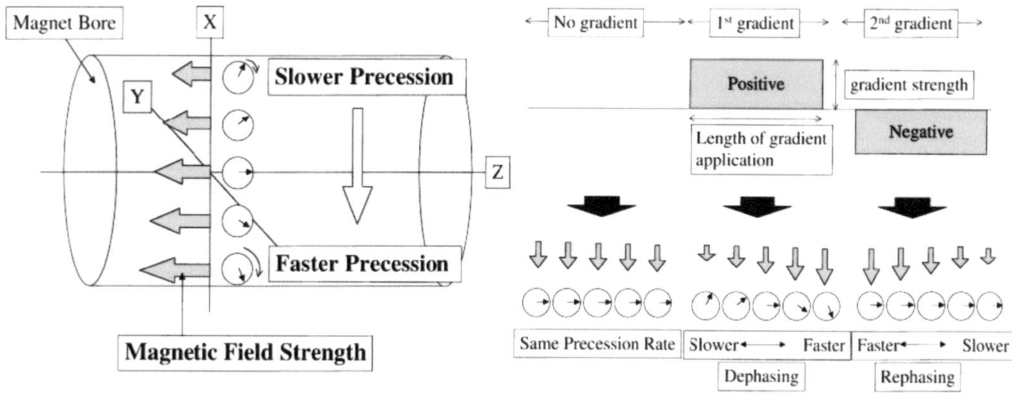

Fig. 1. Illustration of DW-MRI, from Mori and Barker (1999) figures 5 & 6. First, a dephasing gradient pulse is applied (as shown on the left). This causes protons to lose their uniform phase (dephase) because each proton starts to precess at different rates depending on its position in space. The gradient shown on the left is applied (shown here in the x direction), introducing a linear magnetic field inhomogeneity with a specified time period, magnitude, and direction. The length of grey arrows indicates the strength of the magnetic field that is non-uniform during the application of the gradients. The direction along the magnet bore (the strong static magnetic field to which the main magnetic field aligns) is defined as z. Following application of the gradient field, precession rates vary according to position of the protons within the field, as shown. After a time delay, a rephrasing gradient pulse of opposite magnitude polarity is applied (see diagram on right) and the system restores uniform phase (rephase). This rephasing is complete only when protons did not move by Brownian motion (i.e. diffuse) during the time between the application of the first and second gradients. The less complete the rephasing, the more signal loss results. *(Figures reproduced with permission from John Wiley and Sons)*

diffuses 3-7 times more rapidly along the length of axons aligned in white matter tracts than in the direction perpendicular to the axons (Le Bihan, 2003; Pierpaoli, Jezzard, Basser, Barnett, & Di Chiro, 1996). This results in a tensor that is elongated, anisotropic in shape, such that the longest principle axis of the tensor reflects the main direction of diffusion in the voxel. While unmyelinated axonal membranes are sufficient to produce anisotropic diffusion (Beaulieu & Allen, 1994), the presence of myelin further modulates anisotropy (Beaulieu, 2002) and this leads the technique to be suitable to detect a range of diseases that affect myelin. Anisotropy is higher in white than grey matter, and in adult brains compared to those of newborns. In fact, DTI has been used to quantify the development of major white matter pathways in premature infants in whom indices of anisotropy increase with age (Berman et al., 2005). The presence and direction of fiber tracts can be inferred from the diffusion tensor but, given the size of imaged voxels (typically 1-4mm for DTI) compared to the size of an axon (<10μm, white matter packing density $10^{11}m^{-2}$), many collinear fibers must be present to influence overall diffusion anisotropy across the voxel. This is why DTI tractography, discussed later, typically describes the path of major white matter fiber bundles in the brain. The reader is referred to Basser and Jones (2002), Hagmann et al. (2006) and Mori and Barker (1999) for further explanation of DW-MRI.

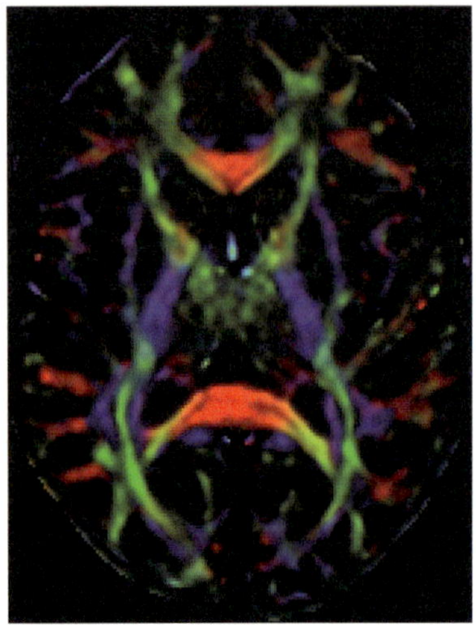

Fig. 2. Directionality-coloured anisotropy map, axial slice view. Voxels with anisotropic diffusion in the superior-inferior direction are shown in blue, anterior-posterior in green and left-right in red (for example, part of the corpus callosum)

Various scalar indices can be derived from the diffusion tensor to describe the profile of diffusion within an imaged voxel. **Mean diffusivity** (MD), a scalar invariant to the direction of anisotropy, describes the overall mean-squared displacement of molecules. MD has been shown to increase in certain disease states, for example in Alzheimer's disease (Agosta et al., 2011), likely reflecting a loss of white matter integrity. Of the diffusion anisotropy indices, the most commonly used is **fractional anisotropy** (FA), which ranges from 0 for isotropic diffusion to 1 for anisotropic diffusion. FA values across the brain are typically plotted in a colour-coded manner to form a directionality-coloured FA map, such as the one shown in figure 2. It can be seen that tensor information alone somewhat delineates white matter structure in the brain because it shows the locations and orientation of areas of high anisotropy. However, this information is based on local anisotropy in each imaged voxel. Tractography techniques, described later, consolidate this information to form a description of the pathways.

3. Correlating structure & behaviour

3.1 Individual variation in the healthy population

DTI can be used as an index of individual structural variation within the human population. Differences in DTI indices have been shown to correlate with measures of behavioural performance in both health and disease. For example, correlation between FA and behavioural performance has been found in cognitive domains such as reading ability (Klingberg et al., 2000), visuo-spatial attention (Tuch et al., 2005) and mental rotation (Wolbers, Schoell, & Buchel, 2006). We compared FA value in the human hippocampal region with healthy individual behavioural performance during a spatial navigation task in a virtual environment (Iaria, Lanyon, Fox, Giaschi, & Barton, 2008). The ability to spatially orient within an environment varies greatly between individuals (Ohnishi, Matsuda, Hirakata, & Ugawa, 2006). In our experiment subjects first had to navigate within a computerised virtual environment to form a "cognitive map" (Tolman, 1948), a spatial memory of the environment. Next, they were asked to navigate to a specified landmark as quickly as possible using the shortest route. The task, therefore, involved both learning and retrieval components. Subjects underwent MRI scanning to obtain a high-resolution structural scan and diffusion-weighted scans using 32 gradient directions. Using these images we draw a region of interest (ROI) in the region of each subject's hippocampus, as shown in figure 3, and obtained the mean FA value within this ROI (using DTI Studio software (Hiang & Mori)). The results revealed a statistically significant correlation between the FA in the right hippocampus and the time spent by the participants performing both the learning and retrieval tasks. Subjects with higher FA values in the area of the right hippocampus required less time to form a cognitive map (figure 4a) and were more efficient in using the map during navigation in the subsequent retrieval task (figure 4b). No similar correlations were found in the left hemisphere.

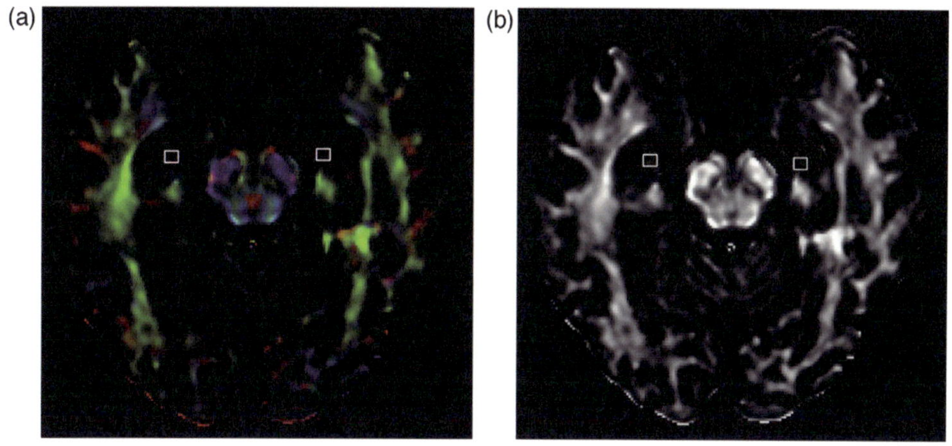

Fig. 3. Region of interest drawn in hippocampal area, from Iaria et al. (2008) figure 2. ROIs in the bilateral hippocampal regions are shown overlaid on diffusion images: (a) the color-coded directionality maps (directions: red=left-right, green=anterior-posterior direction, blue=inferior-superior) and (b) monochromatic FA maps.

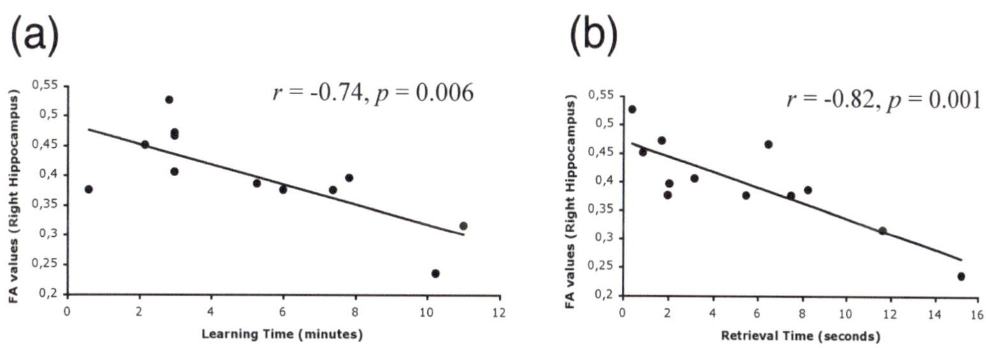

Fig. 4. FA value correlates with spatial navigation performance in healthy individuals, from Iaria et al. (2008) figure 3. A negative correlation was found between FA values of the right hippocampus and (a) the time spent by the participants to form a cognitive map of the environment (the learning task) and (b) the average time they spent to reach the target locations (the retrieval task).

3.2 Structural variation with age

Diffusivity properties of cerebral white matter change across the lifespan of healthy individuals, likely reflecting developmental and aging-related changes in tract morphology (Bennett, Madden, Vaidya, Howard, & Howard, 2010; Davis et al., 2009; Kochunov et al., 2010; Madden et al., 2009; Madden et al., 2007). Aging causes increases in MD and decreases in FA, presumably due to deterioration in the integrity of white matter tracts due to demyelination (Abe et al., 2002; Yoon, Shim, Lee, Shon, & Yang, 2008). Recent studies have established an anterior-posterior gradient of age-related deterioration amongst healthy

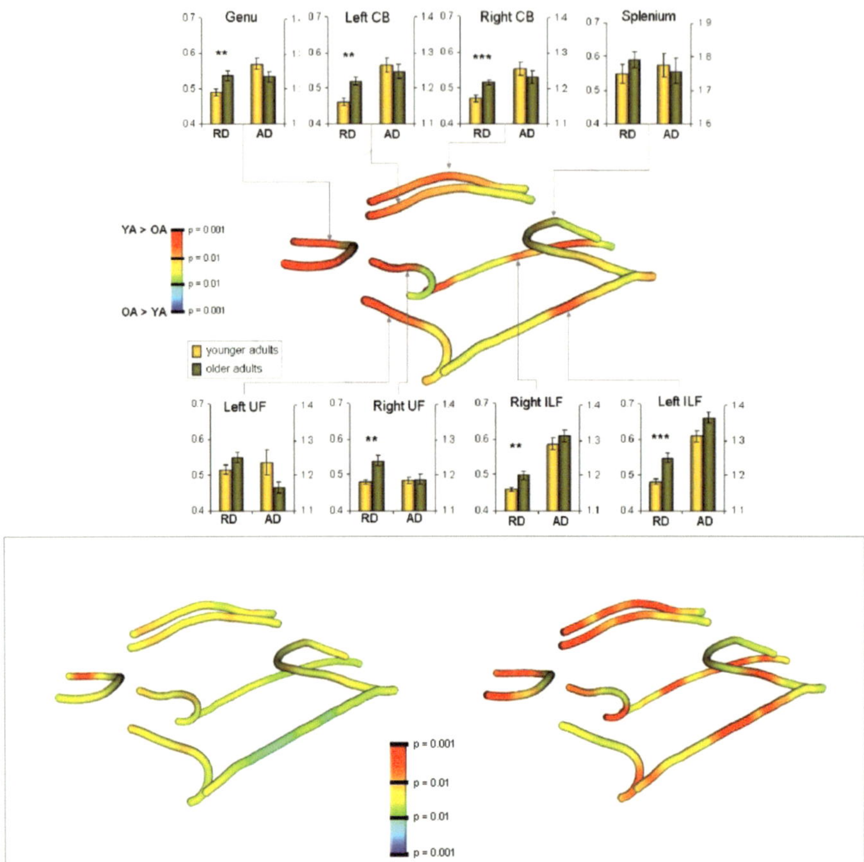

Fig. 5. Age-related differences in fractional anisotropy (FA), radial diffusivity (RD) and axial diffusivity (AD) for specific tracts, from Davis et al. (2009) figures 2 & 3.
Top, FA differences are shown along a tract; FA data were smoothed with a 6mm kernel and displayed upon mean tracts from a representative subject for the genu, uncinate fasciculi, cingulum bundle, inferior longitudinal fasciculi, and splenium. RD and AD differences are displayed in graphs corresponding to specific tracts. Metric dimensions: AD, RD: 10^{-3} mm^2/s; * = $P < 0.01$; ** = $P < 0.005$; *** = $P < 0.001$. YA = younger adults; OA = older adults.
Below, differences in AD (left) and RD (right) are represented upon the same tracts, demonstrating greater age-related effects for RD than AD. Colour scales for RD have been reversed such that OA > YA differences are reflected by warmer colors.
(Figures reproduced with permission from Elsevier)

adults, such that indices of diffusivity show anterior regions of cortex are affected more, or perhaps sooner, than posterior regions (Bennett, et al., 2010; Davis, et al., 2009; Madden, et al., 2007; Yoon, et al., 2008). This anterior-posterior gradient of age impact is the reverse of the gradient observed in the childhood development of white and grey matter, where anterior regions have a more protracted development course than posterior regions (Eluvathingal, Hasan, Kramer, Fletcher, & Ewing-Cobbs, 2007; Giedd et al., 1999; Paus et al., 1999; Sowell et al., 2004; Sowell, Trauner, Gamst, & Jernigan, 2002). A current trend in DTI aging research is to examine radial diffusivity (RD) and axial diffusivity (AD), indices of diffusion in the primary and perpendicular directions of the diffusion tensor, which contribute to FA. AD describes the principal eigenvector of the diffusion tensor and is assumed to indicate the integrity of axons (Glenn et al., 2003) or changes in extra-axonal/extracellular space (Beaulieu & Allen, 1994). RD describes an average of the eigenvectors that are perpendicular to the principal diffusion direction and is assumed to reflect changes associated with myelination or glial cell morphology (Song et al., 2003; Song et al., 2002; Song et al., 2005). Such techniques provide a unique insight into normal cortical changes across the lifespan that can also be correlated with associated behavioural changes.

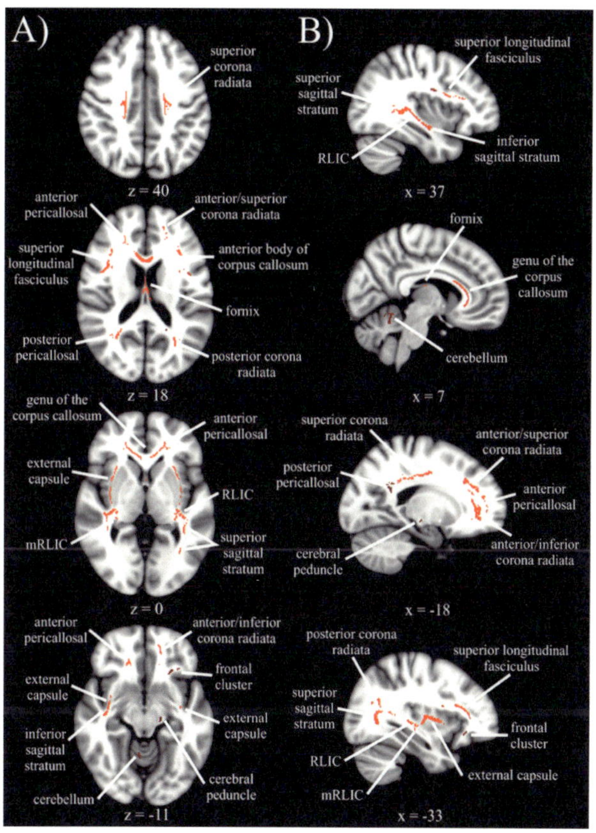

Fig. 6. FA differences across the brain related to aging, from Bennett et al. (2010) figure 1. Shown in red are white matter clusters where FA was significantly greater in younger compared to older adults, across four axial and four sagittal slices. Axial slices are presented in radiological orientation (right = left). RLIC = retrolenticular part of the internal capsule. *(Figure reproduced with permission from John Wiley and Sons)*

A recent study (Davis, et al., 2009) used streamline tractography (described later) to establish the location of several major white matter pathways in each individual's brain. Reconstructed tracts were then averaged to form a mean position for each pathway in each individual, and then combined into two groups: younger (mean age 20 years) and older (mean age 69 years) adults. In 10mm segments along each pathway, mean FA, AD and RD values were examined. Age-related differences were apparent in all three indices but especially the FA and AD. Consistent with the anterior-posterior model of FA changes with aging, the greatest age-related changes in FA occurred in anterior segments of longitudinal fibers that traversed the frontal lobe (see figure 5). In particular, examination of the cingulum bundle and uncinate fasciculus showed that age effects increase gradually from the posterior to anterior brain, likely due to myelodegeneration. In all cases age differences were greater for radial than axial diffusivity. In contrast, an age-related study (Bennett, et al., 2010) that examined FA changes throughout the brain rather than those within specified tracts, found that reduced FA values in older adults (as shown in figure 6) were caused by either an increase in RD only, increases in both RD and AD, or an increase in RD with a corresponding decrease in AD, depending on region of the brain. Again, the largest changes were observed in frontal regions. The frontal cortex seems to be susceptible to early deterioration in dementia also. Changes in AD in tracts projecting to the frontal cortex have been associated with cases of amnestic mild cognitive impairment, a pre-cursor to Alzheimer's disease, with changes in diffusivity in all directions, and widespread FA decrease, apparent in cases of Alzheimer's disease (Agosta, et al., 2011).

3.3 DTI in disease

In addition to comparisons within the healthy population, DTI indices have been used to detect structural differences, and provide an index of disease state, in a range of neuropsychiatric and neurological diseases, for example multiple sclerosis (Sigal, Shmuel, Mark, Gil, & Anat, 2010), Huntington's disease (Rosas et al., 2010), schizophrenia (Manoach et al., 2007), obsessive-compulsive disorder (Cannistraro et al., 2007), bipolar disorder (Adler et al., 2004; Beyer et al., 2005), Alzheimer's disease (Hanyu et al., 1997; Pievani et al., 2010), amnestic mild cognitive impairment (Agosta, et al., 2011), and in presymptomatic groups at risk of developing Alzheimer's disease (Gold, Powell, Andersen, & Smith, 2010). Since anisotropy is modulated by the presence of myelin, diffusion indices have been used to demonstrate changes in white matter integrity in many diseases that involve myelin degeneration and, recently, as a way to measure neuroprotective therapies (R. J. Fox et al., 2011).

We used FA value to detect white matter deterioration in Niemann-Pick Type C (NPC) disease (Scheel, Abegg, Lanyon, Mattman, & Barton, 2010). NPC is a fatal autosomal recessive neurodegenerative disorder resulting from mutations in the NPC1 or NPC2 genes (Vanier & Millat, 2003) that leads to impaired intracellular lipid trafficking and consequent excess lysosomal storage of glycosphingolipids and cholesterol in multiple tissues. In the central nervous system, the storage material results in dysfunction and death of Purkinje and other select neuronal cells (Karten, Peake, & Vance, 2009). The disorder affects the entire brain but some regions are particularly susceptible, with cerebellar degeneration leading to gait ataxia (a lack of coordination of muscle movements), dysarthria (motor speech disorder) and dysphagia (difficulty swallowing), and cortical degeneration leading to dementia and seizures. An early characteristic sign of the disease is vertical supranuclear gaze palsy, meaning that patients find it extremely difficult to make vertical eye movements, while their horizontal eye movements are nearer normal. These eye movement deficits are reflected in more severe cell loss in the rostral interstitial nucleus of the medial longitudinal fasciculus (riMLF), the nucleus linked to the generation of vertical eye movements, compared to the paramedian pontine reticular formation (PPRF), the nucleus linked to the generation of horizontal eye movements (Solomon, Winkelman, Zee, Gray, & Buttner-Ennever, 2005). Standard clinical MR sequences are relatively insensitive to changes in the early stages of NPC. However, DTI, which measures the integrity of myelinated axons, is a plausible technique to identify early NPC changes, given the impaired lipid storage associated with the disease.

We examined FA values across the brain of a young early-stage NPC patient in comparison with a group of healthy control subjects. We found significantly lower FA in the patient compared to controls, particularly in white matter regions, as shown in figure 7. A voxelwise analysis, using a voxel-by-voxel statistical contrast (tract based spatial statistics tool of FSL: Smith et al., 2006) revealed some clusters of local FA differences. Of particular interest was a region of reduced FA in the dorsal midbrain because of the involvement of this region (riMLF) in the generation of vertical eye movements. Another prominent cluster was found in the superior cerebellar peduncle, a possible cause of the patient's cerebellar ataxia. After one year of treatment, areas of reduced FA persisted but there were significantly fewer voxels with lower FA and the cerebellar peduncle cluster was reduced in size, which might have been linked with the patient's improved tremor and dysarthria, and reports of fewer falls. Also, the midbrain cluster was not apparent after treatment, possibly correlating with the patient's slight improvement in making vertical eye movements.

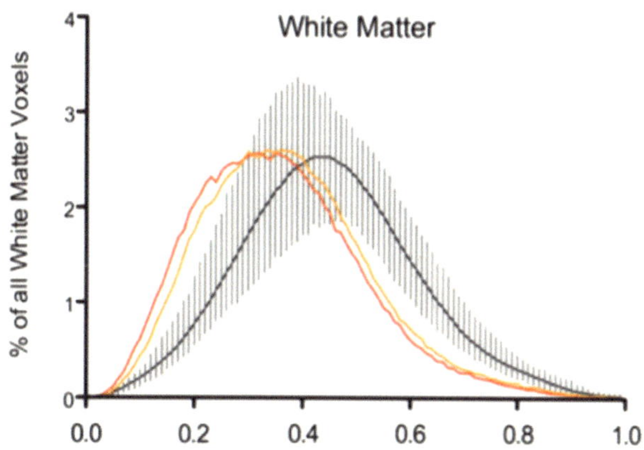

Fig. 7. Histogram of FA values for white matter regions, from Scheel et al. (2010) figure 2. Mean healthy FA value is shown as the black line with vertical errors bars representing the range of values. The NPC patient's FA value before treatment is shown (red line), and after 1 year of treatment with Miglustat (orange line). The patient's white matter has significantly lower FA value than that of healthy controls. The mean FA in the patient's white matter (0.359) was more than 6 standard deviations from the control's mean (0.452 ± 0.016). After treatment, the FA value improved to 0.377, but was still 5 standard deviations from the control's mean. *(Figure reproduced with permission from Elsevier)*

This example demonstrates the use of FA as an early marker of disease state (before abnormalities were evident in standard clinical MRI), revealing local changes that correlate with specific clinical signs. FA was also used as an objective structural index to track disease progression and assess the effects of treatment.

4. Visualising tracts

Assuming that the largest principal axis of the diffusion tensor aligns with the predominant fiber orientation in the MRI voxel, a vector field is created that reflects the orientation of fibers at all voxels throughout the brain. **Tractography** is the 3D reconstruction of tract trajectories from these vector fields. At the resolution of MRI voxels (typically 1-4mm for DTI), reconstructed tracts reflect the orientation of large white matter bundles present in the brain. The technique does not permit the tracking of individual axons or dendrites (whose typical size is <10μm). Hence, tractography models large-scale connectivity within the brain. It has provided insights into *in vivo* white matter morphology in health and disease/lesion. Methods of DTI tractography generally seek to propagate a line through the field using a deterministic algorithm based on tensor information at each stage of the propagation[1]. This is known as *streamline tractography* (Mori & Barker, 1999; Mori, Crain, Chacko, & van Zijl, 1999; Mori & van Zijl, 2002). Simply, the vector field is converted into a continuous number field and a line is propagated through this field with a small step size, using the distance-averaged vector information, as depicted in figure 8. This algorithm is known as fiber assignment by continuous tracking (FACT) and was used for the first successful tract reconstruction, performed for a fixed rat brain (Mori, et al., 1999; Xue, van Zijl, Crain, Solaiyappan, & Mori, 1999). From a starting *seed* voxel or ROI, tractography commences and lines are propagated while the FA value indicates high anisotropy (typically a threshold of 0.2 is chosen because voxels with lower FA value tend to be in grey matter or CSF). An example of fibers tracked from the striate cortex (area V1) is shown in figure 9.

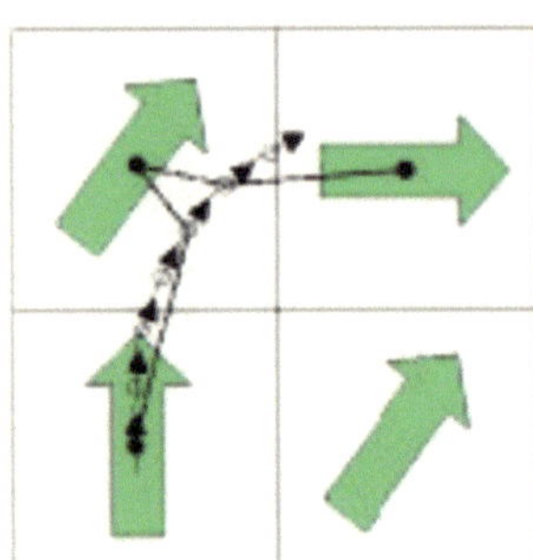

Fig. 8. FACT streamline technique for tractography, from Mori and van Zijl (2002).
(Figure reproduced with permission from John Wiley and Sons)

[1] An alternative approach to propagating a line thorough the tensor vector field is to use energy maximisation techniques (Parker, 2000). These techniques use principles of global energy minimisation to find the energetically most favourable path by which two points are connected. So far this approach has been less extensively adopted than streamline tractography and probabilistic methods.

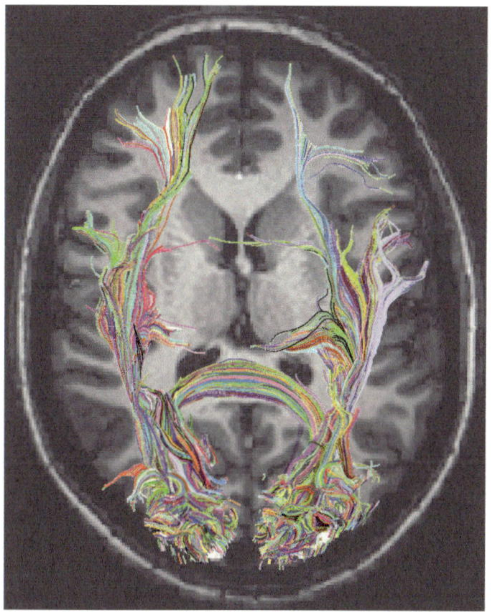

Fig. 9. Streamline tractography using primary visual cortex (area V1) as an ROI. An oval seed ROI was drawn over the occipital pole and streamline tractography performed in DTI Studio (Hiang & Mori). Reconstructed tracts are shown in 3 dimensions overlaid on a 2 dimensional axial brain slice. Tracts forming part of the optic radiation and corpus callosum are some of the pathways shown. Note each tracked 'fiber' represents a line that has been tracked through the tensor vector field so each line represents multiple real axons and dendrites.

Once the tractography encounters a region of low anisotropy it ceases. An issue with this approach is that a DTI voxel is a few millimetres in size and more than one bundle of oriented tracts might be present, i.e. tracts of different orientations may cross within the voxel. If there are two predominant fiber directions within the voxel, the tensor may appear 'pancake-shaped' (see Mori & van Zijl, 2002, for review) and, with higher numbers of directions the overall diffusion may appear isotropic. If the tractography is unable to determine the onward fiber direction, due to tensor isotropy, it stops at that voxel. Hence, tractography is difficult in regions of complex fiber architecture. Nonetheless, streamline tractography results are robust for major pathways and have been shown to have good correspondence with known neuroanatomy (Kang, Zhang, Carlson, & Gembris, 2005; Mori & van Zijl, 2002). To illustrate the potential and limitations of tractography, we will now discuss two studies where this form of deterministic streamline tractography was used to investigate pathways for visual perception in healthy humans.

4.1 Pathways for visual motion perception

Patients who sustain a loss of the primary visual cortex (striate area V1) are rendered blind in the respective part of their visual field. Most of these cortically blind patients have no residual visual perception. However, some "blindsight" patients (Weiskrantz, 1998) retain residual visual abilities such as the ability to make perceptual discriminations or perform associated visuomotor control at better than chance levels, while denying conscious awareness of stimuli in their blind visual fields (Blythe, Kennard, & Ruddock, 1987; Corbetta, Marzi, Tassinari, & Aglioti, 1990; Perenin & Jeannerod, 1975; Perenin, Ruel, &

Hecaen, 1980). Several reports suggest that V1 is necessary for conscious visual perception (Celesia, Bushnell, Toleikis, & Brigell, 1991; Cowey & Stoerig, 1997; Merigan, Nealey, & Maunsell, 1993). However, some degraded conscious "blindsight" vision may remain, particularly if structures like the superior colliculus, LGN and extrastriate cortex are not directly affected. Conscious perception of visual motion seems to be particularly likely to be spared (Barbur, Watson, Frackowiak, & Zeki, 1993; Blythe, et al., 1987; Giaschi et al., 2003; Mestre, Brouchon, Ceccaldi, & Poncet, 1992; Morland et al., 1999; Perenin, 1991; Ptito, Lepore, Ptito, & Lassonde, 1991; Riddoch, 1917; Schoenfeld, Heinze, & Woldroff, 2002), and motion perception has even been reported in a case where the striate cortex was completely congenitally absent (Giaschi, et al., 2003). Many cortical regions exhibit motion sensitivity, but key areas are the middle temporal area (MT), medial superior temporal cortex (MST) and the fundus of the superior temporal cortex (FST), known collectively in humans as the V5/MT complex, or V5/MT+ (Zeki et al., 1991). The main route by which V5/MT+ receives visual inputs from the retina is via the lateral geniculate nucleus (LGN) of the thalamus, which projects to V1 which, in turn, projects to V5/MT+. If this were the sole pathway by which visual motion is perceived, damage to any part of this path should render the person blind to visual motion. Human and animal studies suggest that there may be direct projections, perhaps from LGN, pulvinar or superior colliculus, to V5/MT+ that bypass V1 (Cowey & Stoerig, 1991; Rodman, Gross, & Albright, 1989; Stoerig & Cowey, 1997). Such pathways might be responsible for the residual visual abilities observed in some cortically blind patients.

We used a combined functional magnetic resonance imaging (fMRI) and streamline tractography approach to investigate the presence of sub-cortical connections to V5/MT+ in 10 healthy human subjects (Lanyon, Giaschi et al., 2009). DTI data were collected using 32 gradient directions. We first localised V5/MT+ in each subject using fMRI (because the exact anatomical location of this area is subject to individual variation (Dumoulin et al., 2000; Watson et al., 1993) and then used this region as the seed for tractography. We performed all analyses in each subject's native space, without conversion to a standard brain template, in order to retain individual differences in tract morphology. Tracts extending to area V1 were eliminated from the analysis. We found individual variation in the results of tractography: direct connections between V5/MT+ and sub-cortical locations were found in 4 of our 10 subjects. All 4 of these subjects had fibers connecting V5/MT+ with the pulvinar, 2 had fibers connecting with the superior colliculus and 1 subject had fibers connecting with the region of the LGN. An example of fibers tracked to the pulvinar in one subject is given in figure 10. Further examples are given in Lanyon, Giaschi et al. (2009). Consistent with known feedback connections from V5/MT+ to the pons in monkeys (Boussaoud, Desimone, & Ungerleider, 1992; Maunsell & van Essen, 1983), fibers were found extending inferiorly in the brain stem through the pons in 3 of the 4 subjects, and a small number proceeded into the medulla.

Since the outputs of tractography are computationally-derived it is important to validate findings with other forms of evidence. Our tractography findings are supported by studies in monkeys: feedforward thalamic and collicular projections to V5/MT+ have been described (Boussaoud, et al., 1992; Cowey & Stoerig, 1991, 1997; Cusick, Scripter, Darensbourg, & Weber, 1993; Lin & Kaas, 1980; Rockland, Andresen, Cowie, & Robinson, 1999; Sincich, Park, Wohlgemuth, & Horton, 2004; Stoerig & Cowey, 1997); MST and FST have been shown to be reciprocally connected to the pulvinar, and to project to the pons (Boussaoud, et al., 1992); and feedback connections have been found from area MT to the pulvinar, LGN, the superior colliculus and the pons (Maunsell & van Essen, 1983; Wall, Symonds, & Kaas, 1982). DTI tractography can only confirm the presence of a hypothesised fiber tract, it does not provide information about the direction of axonal projections. Hence, the pathways we have identified could represent feedforward connections from thalamus to V5/MT+, or feedback from V5/MT+, or both. The evidence from monkeys supports both forms of connection.

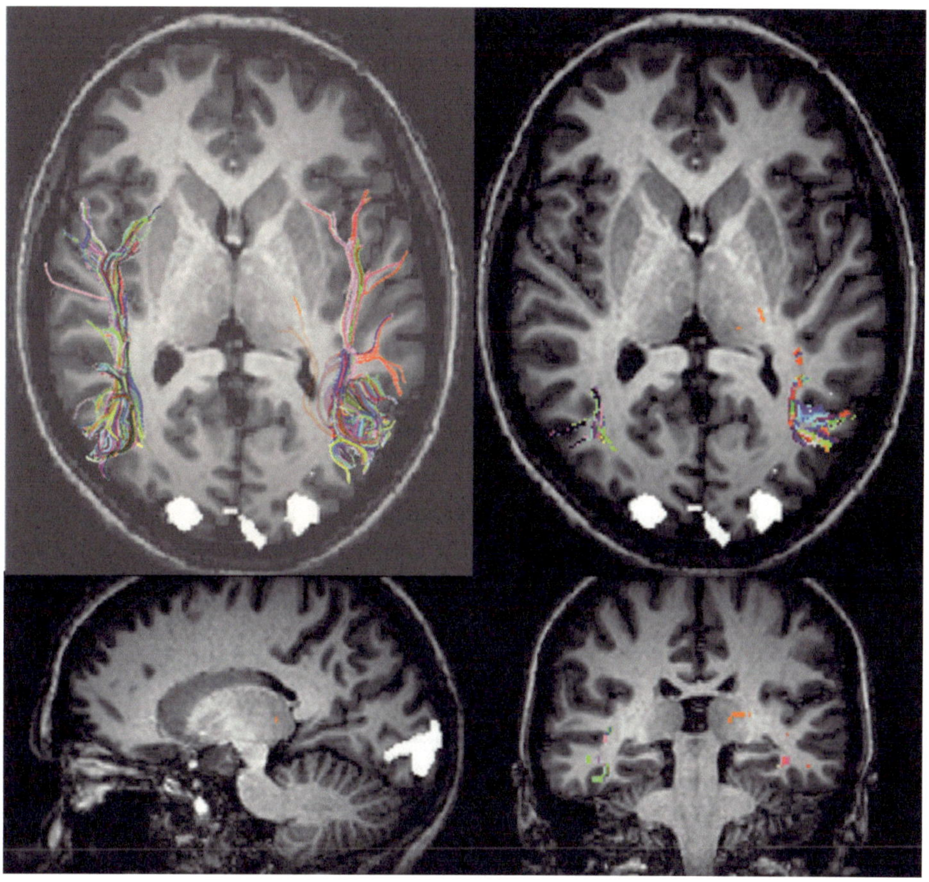

Fig. 10. Streamline tractography using functionally-defined visual cortical area V5/MT+ as an ROI, with fibers extending to area V1 eliminated.
Fibers extend from V5/MT+ to the pulvinar nucleus of the thalamus in the left hemisphere (orange line). The panels show output from DTI Studio (Hiang & Mori). Top left: reconstructed tracts are shown in 3 dimensions overlaid on a 2 dimensional axial brain slice. In the other panels only the fibers present in that slice are shown (top right: axial, bottom left: sagittal, bottom right: coronal views). Images are displayed in radiological convention (right = left). White regions denote the location of functional activation in V1 and V5/MT+.

An example of a subject in which tractography did not connect V5/MT+ with subcortex is shown in figure 11. This inter-subject variability could be due to the technical limitations of DTI tractography in terms of resolving crossing fibers within a voxel, particularly since we were tracking through regions of complex fiber structure. However, the diversity in our results could also reflect true inter-subject anatomical variability of pathways, as suggested by others (Leh, Johansen-Berg, & Ptito, 2006). Finding a direct pathway between subcortical structures and V5/MT+ in less than half our healthy subjects is consistent with the fact that only a minority of patients with cortical visual loss retain residual visual abilities (Barton & Sharpe, 1997; Kasten, Wuest, & Sabel, 1998; Scharli, Harman, & Hogben, 1999).

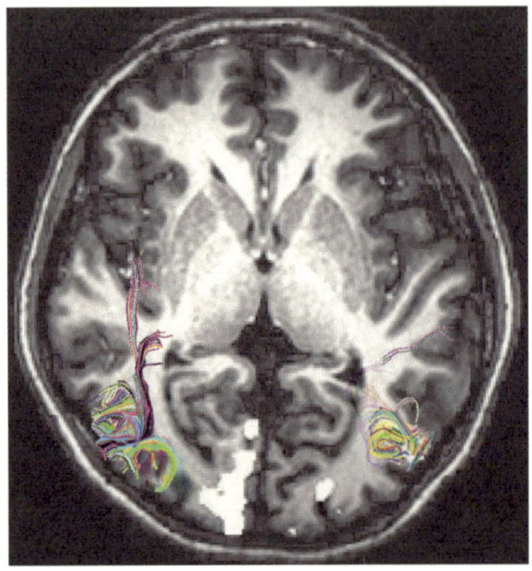

Fig. 11. Tractography in a subject for whom fibers did not connect V5/MT+ with subcortex.

4.2 The network for face perception

Functional MRI studies have identified multiple cortical regions that are involved in face perception, a key visuosocial skill (Gobbini & Haxby, 2007; Haxby, et al., 2000; Ishai, et al., 2005; Rossion, et al., 2003). Current models divide these into a core system, which is predominantly involved in the processing of facial stimuli, and an extended system which, though not solely involved in face processing, contributes to it (Gobbini & Haxby, 2007; Haxby, et al., 2000). The core system consists of the occipital face area (OFA), located on the inferior occipital gyrus; the fusiform face area (FFA), located on the lateral fusiform gyrus; and a face-selective region in the posterior superior temporal sulcus (pSTS) (Haxby, et al., 2000; Ishai, et al., 2005; Kanwisher, et al., 1997). These regions consistently show increased activity in fMRI studies that contrast activity to faces over other objects, with the right hemisphere being dominant for face processing. Damage to component parts of face processing cortical network can result in face processing deficits, a condition known as prosopagnosia (Barton, 2003; Rossion, et al., 2003). Patients with prosopagnosia are typically unable to recognize faces, a major social impediment. Prosopagnosia is a selective visual agnosia and the ability to recognize other objects is usually unimpaired. Prosopagnosia can take a developmental form, where onset occurs prior to the development of normal face recognition abilities (either due to genetic causes or acquired in early childhood), or be acquired in later life through cortical damage due to illness or injury. Various cortical lesion locations have been associated with the condition (see C. J. Fox et al., 2008, for a review). While loss of one or more of the functional components of the core face network is an obvious cause in some patients, for example a lesion in the area of the OFA in patient PS (Rossion, et al., 2003), other patients have robust fMRI activation in the three cortical areas of the core network. It has been suggested that some cases of prosopagnosia could be due to damage to the connectivity of the face processing network (C. J. Fox, et al., 2008).

In order to better understand interconnectivity of the cortical face-processing network we performed DTI tractography in 5 healthy subjects and examined fibers tracked from OFA, FFA and pSTS, which were defined by fMRI. For the fMRI face-selective region localiser we contrasted activity invoked by presentation of static pictures of neutral and emotionally expressive faces with that evoked by presentation of static pictures of non-living objects (see C. J. Fox, Iaria, & Barton, 2009, for fMRI methods). A threshold of $p<0.05$, Bonferonni corrected, was used to determine the extent of activation and this became the seed region for DTI tractography. DTI data were collected using 32 gradient directions. Structural, functional and DTI images were co-registered and streamline tractography was performed in Brain Voyager QX (www.brainvoyager.com, Brain Innovation) for each subject. All fMRI and DTI analysis were performed in each subject's own native brain space, without conversion to a standard template. Figure 12 shows fibers tracked from the regions of the core network in an example subject. Fibers from right OFA and FFA interconnected these regions and fibers from these posterior regions travelled anteriorally along the inferior longitudinal fasciculus toward the inferior temporal cortex (a region which forms part of the extended network, possibly contributing facial memories). We found a lack of fibers connecting right OFA, FFA and the right anterior temporal lobe in a prosopagnosic patient who had a right amygdalohippocampectomy for epilepsy that resulted in lesion of the anterior part of the inferior longitudinal fasciculus (Lanyon, Scheel, Fox, Iaria, & Barton, 2009). Contrary to current models of the core cortical network for face perception (Haxby, et al., 2000), our tractography did not reveal a connection between pSTS and either FFA or OFA. However, we cannot rule out the existence of a connection between pSTS and these posterior regions because tractographic technical difficulty may have prevented fibers traversing this region, since it contains the intersection of several major fiber pathways.

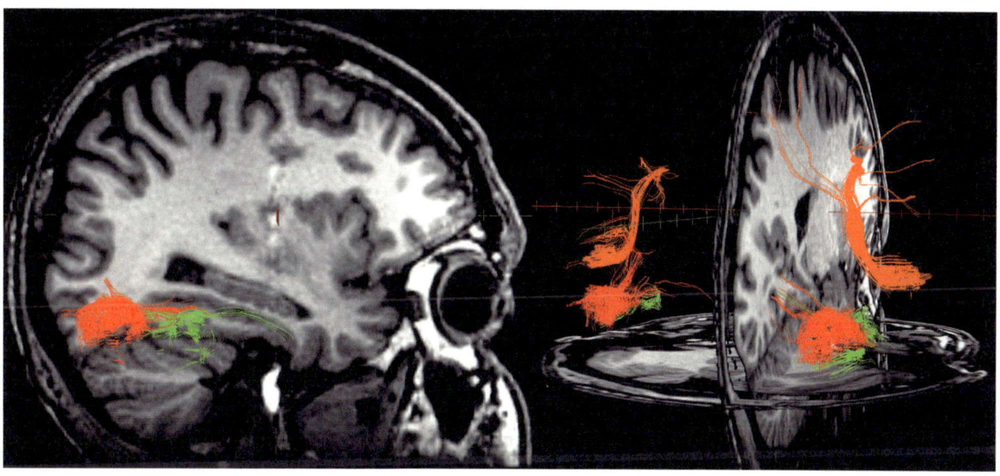

Fig. 12. Results of tractography showing fibers extending from core face-selective areas. The core network was defined by fMRI and then tractography performed using these areas as seed regions. OFA (red) FFA (green) and pSTS (orange) fibers in a healthy subject are shown. In the right hemisphere, fibers from OFA and FFA interconnect these two regions and extend along the inferior longitudinal fasciculus towards the inferior temporal cortex, as shown on the left. The three dimensional view on the right shows that the pSTS is not connected with OFA or FFA in our tractographic analysis. OFA = occipital face area; FFA = fusiform face area; pSTS = face-selective region in the posterior superior temporal sulcus.

4.3 Limitations and alternatives to the tensor model

The tensor model of diffusion provided the first and currently most popular technique to map fiber orientations in the brain. It has proved to be a powerful model that has stimulated much research in the field of DW-MRI and adoption of these techniques. This has led to many insights into human neuroanatomy with visualisation of major fiber pathways in the brain. However, in fitting a Gaussian distribution of diffusion to each voxel, the tensor model assumes there is a single predominant orientation of fibers travelling within the voxel, and this results in the major limitation of DTI. In voxels containing complex fiber architecture, the tensor model cannot describe more than one dominant fiber orientation. Current research is attempting to provide models and tractography approaches that better account for the distribution of diffusion in voxels that contain crossing fibers. Many solutions rely on measuring diffusion over a higher number of angular directions. These techniques are referred to as *high angular resolution diffusion imaging* (HARDI). These high-resolution methods aim to provide richer information about the direction of fibers in voxels that contain numerous fiber orientations.

4.3.1 Diffusion Spectrum Imaging (DSI)

DSI Diffusion spectrum imaging (DSI)(Wedeen, Hagmann, Tseng, Reese, & Weisskoff, 2005; Wedeen et al., 2008) is a high angular technique that reconstructs a full account of fiber orientations by transforming data directly from the DW-MRI measurements. The result is an *orientation distribution function* (ODF). An ODF may be considered a deformed sphere whose radius in a given direction is proportional to the sum of values of the diffusion probability density function in that direction. The ODF has peaks in the directions in which the probability density function has most mass, which DSI assumes are the fiber directions. DSI is a superior technique to DTI in that DSI is able to resolve multiple fiber orientations. However, DSI is very time intensive during acquisition, because several hundreds of image volumes are required (compared to a minimum of 6 in DTI), and this has hindered its widespread use because it is often not well tolerated by subjects.

4.3.2 Multi-compartmental models

Models of diffusion that account for the multi-compartmental nature of matter within the voxel attempt to overcome the limitation of DTI imposed by the fitting of the single orientation Gaussian. Such models assume that each voxel comprises a discrete number of compartments reflecting particular fiber directions and extra-axonal components (Assaf, Freidlin, Rohde, & Basser, 2004; Behrens et al., 2003). Hence, these models are an extension of DTI in which the tensor model is simply generalised to account for more than one fiber orientation, for example the single Gaussian model is replaced with a mixture of Gaussian densities. A problem with this approach is in deciding how many fiber orientations should be fitted, since selecting two or more can result in a loss of accuracy in voxels that contain a single predominant fiber orientation. A prominent model by Behrens et al. (2003) replaces the Gaussian model with a tensor that has only one nonzero eigenvalue and a Gaussian distribution in all other directions. Hence, a single fiber direction combined with isotropic diffusion in all other directions is modelled. Behrens et al. also take a probabilistic approach in which the likelihood of various fiber orientations is considered. This local probability distribution is then used to confer global probability estimations when determining whether two regions connect. This probabilistic tractography approach uses a sampling technique to draw samples based on the probability estimate of fibre direction at each voxel. Samples are generated from each voxel within the seed region and a connectivity distribution results in which the probability of a pathway passing through a voxel is reflected in the number of samples passing through it. Connections are visualised by applying a threshold to view only the most likely pathways from all calculated possible connection paths. Hence, local and global probability information is used to determine the likelihood of connections. Whereas streamline tractography traces fibers through regions of high anisotropy where uncertainty is low, these methods chose to model the uncertainty of fiber direction at each local voxel. Hence, it is claimed that this approach offers an advantage over streamline methods when tracking through regions of crossing fibers and orientation uncertainty. Typically tracts are converted to a standard anatomical template for group analysis and this carries some disadvantage in terms of a loss of individual information, given the high level of individual variation in morphology of both white and grey matter[2].

4.3.3 Estimators of the Orientation Distribution Function (ODF)

A new generation of multiple-orientation fiber reconstruction algorithms is emerging. These attempt to combine the benefits of DTI (speed of acquisition) with the sophistication of the high angular DSI approach in estimating multiple fiber orientations. A distribution of fiber orientations within a voxel is assumed, rather than the discrete number assumed in the multi-compartmental approaches. Hence, these methods do not suffer from the problem of model selection since it is not required to know the number of fiber orientations in advance. Data is acquired using the spherical sampling scheme typical of DTI and the ODF is approximated by estimating the angular structure of the proton displacement probability density function directly from the MRI measurements. Examples of these approaches are q-ball imaging (Tuch, Reese, Wiegell, & Wedeen, 2003), spherical deconvolution (Tournier, Calamante, Gadian, & Connelly, 2004) and PASMRI (Jansons & Alexander, 2003). These algorithms produce results in regions of fiber crossings that are in good agreement with DSI: see Alexander (2005) for a review of current approaches. However, these methods are currently computationally and acquisition-time heavy, and many still require implementation in software with a simple user interface to facilitate widespread adoption.

4.4 Validation of results

The outputs of tractography are very compelling and aesthetically interesting but results should be interpreted with some caution since tracked fibers are computational constructs and not imaged directly from the brain unlike chemically traced fibers, for example. Hence, it is normal practise for the results of DTI tractography to be compared with known findings from "gold standard" techniques such as chemical tract tracing in animal models and histological staining of brain slices. There will not necessarily be an exact correspondence of results, however, since DTI provides a level of macroscopic information that is difficult to obtain using chemical tracers in individual axons. DTI tractography then provides information that forms part of the converging evidence about brain connectivity. For

[2] The issue of group analysis applies in general to all methods of tractography if fiber tracking is based upon ROIs defined by a group-level fMRI analysis since the location of these functionally-defined regions will extend into different regions of white matter in each individual and, hence, result in tracts being selected that would not be derived from an individual analysis.

example, our tractographic identification of a pathway for visual motion perception is consistent not only with other DTI studies using alternative tractography techniques (Leh, Chakravarty, & Ptito, 2008) but with the thalamic projections described in many histological and tracing studies, discussed above. Overall, tractography has proved to be remarkably accurate in reconstructing major fiber pathways in the human brain thought to exist based on evidence from post-mortem studies and animal models (Mori, et al., 1999).

5. Conclusion

Understanding how neural network connectivity confers human behaviour in health and disease is one of the most important challenges facing neuroscientists in the 21st century. DTI affords the ability to investigate the structure of large white matter pathways *in vivo*, offering profound insights into living human neural anatomy. In addition to its use in neuroscientific research, DTI as a method for detecting and monitoring certain disease states seems certain to become established in normal clinical practice. In this chapter we described a case of early Niemann-Pick Type C disease in which DTI revealed significant white matter structural changes which were not evident on standard clinical MRI structural imaging (Scheel, et al., 2010).

DTI offers an important contribution to the emerging array of scientific methods that aim to reveal insights into large-scale connectivity in the brain. Methods of fMRI *functional connectivity* (see Rogers, Morgan, Newton, & Gore, 2007, for a review) confer information about connectivity between functionally active regions of the brain by examining temporal correlations in the fMRI signals in the active regions. Methods of *effective connectivity* additionally provide information about causal relationships, i.e. the direction of influence of one area upon another. Whereas DTI reveals structural connectivity in the brain, functional and effective connectivity methods show how these networks change under different stimulus or task conditions. Hence, DTI and functional/effective connectivity together can provide converging evidence about neural networks, from both a structural and a conditional (task- or stimulus-related) perspective. Such insights into structural and functional neural connectivity have not previously been possible *in vivo*. In addition, computational neuroscience models based on these empirical findings will provide a theoretical grounding for understanding neural network connectivity, as well as provoking further empirical investigation to answer questions deriving from these models.

Foremost amongst the key challenges in the development of DW-MRI methods is the development of algorithms capable of elucidating fiber directions in regions of complex structural architecture whilst being computationally tractable and remaining feasible in terms of acquisition times. The immediate future of DW-MRI research centres on improving methods for high angular resolution diffusion imaging so that acquisition and computation times are feasible. Techniques that exploit the full orientation distribution function of diffusion within each voxel will ultimately lead to better definition of fiber orientation in complex matter and, hence, provide more reliable descriptions of neural connectivity. To allow widespread adoption of these evolving technologies, it is necessary for the algorithms to be implemented in software platforms that can be readily used by medical and other researchers. As these new methods become more accessible in terms of acquisition times, computational tractability and general usability, DW-MRI will become an increasingly important method and even more pervasive in neuroscience research and in medical diagnosis and monitoring. DTI is just the beginning of this important field.

"The human brain, then, is the most complicated organization of matter that we know"
Isaac Asimov

6. Acknowledgments

This work was supported by a Post-doctoral Fellowship from the Michael Smith Foundation for Health Research. Many thanks to my co-authors of various studies described in this chapter: Jason Barton MD PhD (to whom I extend additional thanks for providing the environment to study DTI), Debbie Giaschi PhD, Kevin Fitzpatrick BSc, Simon Au Young MSc, Giuseppe Iaria PhD, Michael Scheel MD, Mathias Abegg MD PhD, Christopher Fox PhD, Bruce Bjornson MD, Lu Diao, Andre Mattman MD.

7. References

Abe, O., Aoki, S., Hayashi, N., Yamada, H., Kunimatsu, A., Mori, H., et al. (2002). Normal aging in the central nervous system: quantitative MR diffusion-tensor analysis. *Neurobiology of Aging, 23*(3), 433-441.

Adler, C. M., Holland, S. K., Schmithorst, V., Wilke, M., Weiss, K. L., Pan, H., et al. (2004). Abnormal frontal white matter tracts in bipolar disorder: a diffusion tensor imaging study. *Bipolar Disorders, 6*(3), 197-203.

Agosta, F., Pievani, M., Sala, S., Geroldi, C., Galluzzi, S., Frisoni, G. B., et al. (2011). White matter damage in Alzheimer disease and its relationship to gray matter atrophy. *Radiology, 258*(3), 853-863.

Alexander, D. C. (2005). Multiple-fiber reconstruction algorithms for diffusion MRI. *Annals of the New York Academy of Sciences, 1064*, 113-133.

Assaf, Y., Freidlin, R. Z., Rohde, G. K., & Basser, P. J. (2004). New modeling and experimental framework to characterize hindered and restricted water diffusion in brain white matter. *Magnetic Resonance in Medicine, 52*(5), 965-978.

Barbur, J. L., Watson, J. D., Frackowiak, R. S., & Zeki, S. (1993). Conscious visual perception without V1. *Brain, 116 (Pt 6)*, 1293-1302.

Barton, J. J. (2003). Disorders of face perception and recognition. *Neurologic Clinics, 21*(2), 521-548.

Barton, J. J., & Sharpe, J. A. (1997). Smooth pursuit and saccades to moving targets in blind hemifields. A comparison of medial occipital, lateral occipital and optic radiation lesions. *Brain, 120 (Pt 4)*, 681-699.

Basser, P. J., & Jones, D. K. (2002). Diffusion-tensor MRI: theory, experimental design and data analysis - a technical review. *NMR in Biomedicine, 15*(7-8), 456-467.

Basser, P. J., Mattiello, J., & LeBihan, D. (1994). Estimation of the effective self-diffusion tensor from the NMR spin echo. *Journal of Magnetic Resonance, Series B, 103*(3), 247-254.

Beaulieu, C. (2002). The basis of anisotropic water diffusion in the nervous system - a technical review. *NMR in Biomedicine, 15*(7-8), 435-455.

Beaulieu, C., & Allen, P. S. (1994). Determinants of anisotropic water diffusion in nerves. *Magnetic Resonance in Medicine, 31*(4), 394-400.

Behrens, T. E., Woolrich, M. W., Jenkinson, M., Johansen-Berg, H., Nunes, R. G., Clare, S., et al. (2003). Characterization and propagation of uncertainty in diffusion-weighted MR imaging. *Magnetic resonance in medicine, 50*(5), 1077-1088.

Bennett, I. J., Madden, D. J., Vaidya, C. J., Howard, D. V., & Howard, J. H., Jr. (2010). Age-related differences in multiple measures of white matter integrity: A diffusion tensor imaging study of healthy aging. *Human Brain Mapping, 31*(3), 378-390.

Berman, J. I., Mukherjee, P., Partridge, S. C., Miller, S. P., Ferriero, D. M., Barkovich, A. J., et al. (2005). Quantitative diffusion tensor MRI fiber tractography of sensorimotor white matter development in premature infants. *NeuroImage, 27*(4), 862-871.

Beyer, J. L., Taylor, W. D., MacFall, J. R., Kuchibhatla, M., Payne, M. E., Provenzale, J. M., et al. (2005). Cortical white matter microstructural abnormalities in bipolar disorder. *Neuropsychopharmacology, 30*(12), 2225-2229.

Blythe, I. M., Kennard, C., & Ruddock, K. H. (1987). Residual vision in patients with retrogeniculate lesions of the visual pathways. *Brain, 110*, 887-905.

Boussaoud, D., Desimone, R., & Ungerleider, L. G. (1992). Subcortical connections of visual areas MST and FST in macaques. *Visual Neuroscience, 9*(3-4), 291-302.

Cannistraro, P. A., Makris, N., Howard, J. D., Wedig, M. M., Hodge, S. M., Wilhelm, S., et al. (2007). A diffusion tensor imaging study of white matter in obsessive-compulsive disorder. *Depression and Anxiety, 24*(6), 440-446.

Celesia, G. G., Bushnell, D., Toleikis, S. C., & Brigell, M. G. (1991). Cortical blindness and residual vision: is the "second" visual system in humans capable of more than rudimentary visual perception? *Neurology, 41*(6), 862-869.

Corbetta, M., Marzi, C. A., Tassinari, G., & Aglioti, S. (1990). Effectiveness of different task paradigms in revealing blindsight. *Brain, 113*, 603-616.

Cowey, A., & Stoerig, P. (1991). The neurobiology of blindsight. *Trends in Neurosciences, 14*(4), 140-145.

Cowey, A., & Stoerig, P. (1997). Visual detection in monkeys with blindsight. *Neuropsychologia, 35*(7), 929-939.

Crank, J. (1975). *The Mathematics of Diffusion*. Oxford: Oxford University Press.

Cusick, C. G., Scripter, J. L., Darensbourg, J. G., & Weber, J. T. (1993). Chemoarchitectonic subdivisions of the visual pulvinar in monkeys and their connectional relations with the middle temporal and rostral dorsolateral visual areas, MT and DLr. *The Journal of Comparative Neurology, 336*(1), 1-30.

Davis, S. W., Dennis, N. A., Buchler, N. G., White, L. E., Madden, D. J., & Cabeza, R. (2009). Assessing the effects of age on long white matter tracts using diffusion tensor tractography. *NeuroImage, 46*(2), 530-541.

Dumoulin, S. O., Bittar, R. G., Kabani, N. J., Baker, C. L., Jr., Le Goualher, G., Bruce Pike, G., et al. (2000). A new anatomical landmark for reliable identification of human area V5/MT: a quantitative analysis of sulcal patterning. *Cerebral Cortex, 10*(5), 454-463.

Eluvathingal, T. J., Hasan, K. M., Kramer, L., Fletcher, J. M., & Ewing-Cobbs, L. (2007). Quantitative diffusion tensor tractography of association and projection fibers in normally developing children and adolescents. *Cerebral Cortex, 17*(12), 2760-2768.

Fox, C. J., Iaria, G., & Barton, J. J. (2008). Disconnection in prosopagnosia and face processing. *Cortex, 44*(8), 996-1009.

Fox, C. J., Iaria, G., & Barton, J. J. (2009). Defining the face processing network: optimization of the functional localizer in fMRI. *Human Brain Mapping, 30*(5), 1637-1651.

Fox, R. J., Cronin, T., Lin, J., Wang, X., Sakaie, K., Ontaneda, D., et al. (2011). Measuring myelin repair and axonal loss with diffusion tensor imaging. *American Journal of Neuroradiology, 32*(1), 85-91.

Giaschi, D., Jan, J. E., Bjornson, B., Young, S. A., Tata, M., Lyons, C. J., et al. (2003). Conscious visual abilities in a patient with early bilateral occipital damage. [Case Reports]. *Developmental Medicine & Child Neurology, 45*(11), 772-781.

Giedd, J. N., Blumenthal, J., Jeffries, N. O., Castellanos, F. X., Liu, H., Zijdenbos, A., et al. (1999). Brain development during childhood and adolescence: a longitudinal MRI study. *Nature Neuroscience, 2*(10), 861-863.

Glenn, O. A., Henry, R. G., Berman, J. I., Chang, P. C., Miller, S. P., Vigneron, D. B., et al. (2003). DTI-based three-dimensional tractography detects differences in the pyramidal tracts of infants and children with congenital hemiparesis. *Journal of Magnetic Resonance Imaging, 18*(6), 641-648.

Gobbini, M. I., & Haxby, J. V. (2007). Neural systems for recognition of familiar faces. *Neuropsychologia, 45*(1), 32-41.

Gold, B. T., Powell, D. K., Andersen, A. H., & Smith, C. D. (2010). Alterations in multiple measures of white matter integrity in normal women at high risk for Alzheimer's disease. *NeuroImage, 52*(4), 1487-1494.

Hagmann, P., Jonasson, L., Maeder, P., Thiran, J. P., Wedeen, V. J., & Meuli, R. (2006). Understanding diffusion MR imaging techniques: from scalar diffusion-weighted imaging to diffusion tensor imaging and beyond. *RadioGraphics, 26*, S205-223.

Hanyu, H., Shindo, H., Kakizaki, D., Abe, K., Iwamoto, T., & Takasaki, M. (1997). Increased water diffusion in cerebral white matter in Alzheimer's disease. *Gerontology, 43*(6), 343-351.

Haxby, J. V., Hoffman, E. A., & Gobbini, M. I. (2000). The distributed human neural system for face perception. *Trends in Cognitive Sciences, 4*(6), 223-233.

Hiang, H., & Mori, S. Retrieved from http://lbam.med.jhmi.edu/DTIuser/DTIuser.asp.

Iaria, G., Lanyon, L. J., Fox, C. J., Giaschi, D., & Barton, J. J. (2008). Navigational skills correlate with hippocampal fractional anisotropy in humans. *Hippocampus, 18*(4), 335-339.

Ishai, A., Schmidt, C. F., & Boesiger, P. (2005). Face perception is mediated by a distributed cortical network. *Brain Research Bulletin, 67*(1-2), 87-93.

Jansons, K. M., & Alexander, D. C. (2003). Persistent Angular Structure: new insights from diffusion MRI data. *Information Processing in Medical Imaging 2003. Proceedings of the 18th International Conference* (Vol. 18, pp. 672-683). Ambleside, United Kingdom.

Kang, N., Zhang, J., Carlson, E. S., & Gembris, D. (2005). White matter fiber tractography via anisotropic diffusion simulation in the human brain. *IEEE Transactions on Medical Imaging, 24*(9), 1127-1137.

Kanwisher, N. (2010). Functional specificity in the human brain: a window into the functional architecture of the mind. *Proceedings of the Nationall Academy of Science of the United States of America, 107*(25), 11163-11170.

Kanwisher, N., McDermott, J., & Chun, M. M. (1997). The fusiform face area: a module in human extrastriate cortex specialized for face perception. *The Journal of Neuroscience, 17*(11), 4302-4311.

Karten, B., Peake, K. B., & Vance, J. E. (2009). Mechanisms and consequences of impaired lipid trafficking in Niemann-Pick type C1-deficient mammalian cells. *Biochimica et Biophysica Acta, 1791*(7), 659-670.

Kasten, E., Wuest, S., & Sabel, B. A. (1998). Residual vision in transition zones in patients with cerebral blindness. *Journal of Clinical and Experimental Neuropsychology, 20*(5), 581-598.

Klingberg, T., Hedehus, M., Temple, E., Salz, T., Gabrieli, J. D., Moseley, M. E., et al. (2000). Microstructure of temporo-parietal white matter as a basis for reading ability: evidence from diffusion tensor magnetic resonance imaging. *Neuron, 25*(2), 493-500.

Kochunov, P., Williamson, D. E., Lancaster, J., Fox, P., Cornell, J., Blangero, J., et al. (2010). Fractional anisotropy of water diffusion in cerebral white matter across the lifespan. *Neurobiology of Aging, In Press.*

Kwong, K. K., Belliveau, J. W., Chesler, D. A., Goldberg, I. E., Weisskoff, R. M., Poncelet, B. P., et al. (1992). Dynamic magnetic resonance imaging of human brain activity during primary sensory stimulation. *Proceedings of the Nationall Academy of Science of the United States of America, 89*(12), 5675-5679.

Lanyon, L. J., Giaschi, D., Young, S. A., Fitzpatrick, K., Diao, L., Bjornson, B. H., et al. (2009). Combined functional MRI and diffusion tensor imaging analysis of visual motion pathways. *Journal of Neuro-Ophthalmology, 29*(2), 96-103.

Lanyon, L. J., Scheel, M., Fox, C. J., Iaria, G., & Barton, J. J. S. (2009). Disconnection of cortical face network in prosopagnosia revealed by diffusion tensor imaging *Journal of Vision, 9*(8), 482.

Lauterbur, P. C. (1973). Image formation by induced local interactions - examples employing nuclear magnetic-resonance. *Nature, 242*(5394), 190-191.

Le Bihan, D. (2003). Looking into the functional architecture of the brain with diffusion MRI. *Nature Reviews Neuroscience, 4*(6), 469-480.

Le Bihan, D., Breton, E., Lallemand, D., Grenier, P., Cabanis, E., & Laval-Jeantet, M. (1986). MR imaging of intravoxel incoherent motions: application to diffusion and perfusion in neurologic disorders. *Radiology, 161*(2), 401-407.

Leh, S. E., Chakravarty, M. M., & Ptito, A. (2008). The connectivity of the human pulvinar: a diffusion tensor imaging tractography study. *International Journal of Biomedical Imaging, 2008*, 789539.

Leh, S. E., Johansen-Berg, H., & Ptito, A. (2006). Unconscious vision: new insights into the neuronal correlate of blindsight using diffusion tractography. *Brain, 129*(Pt 7), 1822-1832.

Lin, C. S., & Kaas, J. H. (1980). Projections from the medial nucleus of the inferior pulvinar complex to the middle temporal area of the visual cortex. *Neuroscience, 5*(12), 2219-2228.

Madden, D. J., Spaniol, J., Costello, M. C., Bucur, B., White, L. E., Cabeza, R., et al. (2009). Cerebral white matter integrity mediates adult age differences in cognitive performance. *Journal of Cognitive Neuroscience, 21*(2), 289-302.

Madden, D. J., Spaniol, J., Whiting, W. L., Bucur, B., Provenzale, J. M., Cabeza, R., et al. (2007). Adult age differences in the functional neuroanatomy of visual attention: A combined fMRI and DTI study. *Neurobiology of Aging, 28*(3), 459-476.

Manoach, D. S., Ketwaroo, G. A., Polli, F. E., Thakkar, K. N., Barton, J. J., Goff, D. C., et al. (2007). Reduced microstructural integrity of the white matter underlying anterior

cingulate cortex is associated with increased saccadic latency in schizophrenia. *NeuroImage, 37*(2), 599-610.
Maunsell, J. H., & van Essen, D. C. (1983). The connections of the middle temporal visual area (MT) and their relationship to a cortical hierarchy in the macaque monkey. *The Journal of Neuroscience, 3*(12), 2563-2586.
Merboldt, K. D., Hanicke, W., & Frahm, J. (1985). Self-diffusion NMR imaging using stimulated echoes. *Journal of Magnetic Resonance, 64*(3), 479-486.
Merigan, W. H., Nealey, T. A., & Maunsell, J. H. (1993). Visual effects of lesions of cortical area V2 in macaques. *The Journal of Neuroscience, 13*(7), 3180-3191.
Mestre, D. R., Brouchon, M., Ceccaldi, M., & Poncet, M. (1992). Perception of optical-flow in cortical blindness - a case report. *Neuropsychologia, 30*(9), 783-795.
Mori, S., & Barker, P. B. (1999). Diffusion magnetic resonance imaging: its principle and applications. *The Anatomical Record, 257*(3), 102-109.
Mori, S., Crain, B. J., Chacko, V. P., & van Zijl, P. C. (1999). Three-dimensional tracking of axonal projections in the brain by magnetic resonance imaging. *Annals of Neurology, 45*(2), 265-269.
Mori, S., & van Zijl, P. C. (2002). Fiber tracking: principles and strategies - a technical review. *NMR in Biomedicine, 15*(7-8), 468-480.
Morland, A. B., Jones, S. R., Finlay, A. L., Deyzac, E., Le, S., & Kemp, S. (1999). Visual perception of motion, luminance and colour in a human hemianope. *Brain, 122 (Pt 6)*, 1183-1198.
Moseley, M. E., Kucharczyk, J., Mintorovitch, J., Cohen, Y., Kurhanewicz, J., Derugin, N., et al. (1990). Diffusion-weighted MR imaging of acute stroke: correlation with T2-weighted and magnetic susceptibility-enhanced MR imaging in cats. *American Journal of Neuroradiology, 11*(3), 423-429.
Ogawa, S., Tank, D. W., Menon, R., Ellermann, J. M., Kim, S. G., Merkle, H., et al. (1992). Intrinsic signal changes accompanying sensory stimulation: functional brain mapping with magnetic resonance imaging. *Proceedings of the Nationall Academy of Science of the United States of America, 89*(13), 5951-5955.
Ohnishi, T., Matsuda, H., Hirakata, M., & Ugawa, Y. (2006). Navigation ability dependent neural activation in the human brain: an fMRI study. *Neuroscience Research, 55*(4), 361-369.
Parker, G. J. (2000). *Tracing fiber tracts using fast marching.* Paper presented at the International Society of Magnetic Resonance, Denver, CO.
Paus, T., Zijdenbos, A., Worsley, K., Collins, D. L., Blumenthal, J., Giedd, J. N., et al. (1999). Structural maturation of neural pathways in children and adolescents: in vivo study. *Science, 283*(5409), 1908-1911.
Perenin, M. T. (1991). Discrimination of motion direction in perimetrically blind fields. *NeuroReport, 2*(7), 397-400.
Perenin, M. T., & Jeannerod, M. (1975). Residual vision in cortically blind hemifields. *Neuropsychologia, 13*(1), 1-7.
Perenin, M. T., Ruel, J., & Hecaen, H. (1980). Residual visual capacities in a case of cortical blindness. *Cortex, 16*(4), 605-612.
Pierpaoli, C., Jezzard, P., Basser, P. J., Barnett, A., & Di Chiro, G. (1996). Diffusion tensor MR imaging of the human brain. *Radiology, 201*(3), 637-648.

Pievani, M., Agosta, F., Pagani, E., Canu, E., Sala, S., Absinta, M., et al. (2010). Assessment of white matter tract damage in mild cognitive impairment and Alzheimer's disease. *Human Brain Mapping, 31*(12), 1862-1875.

Ptito, A., Lepore, F., Ptito, M., & Lassonde, M. (1991). Target detection and movement discrimination in the blind field of hemispherectomized patients. *Brain, 114*, 497-512.

Riddoch, G. (1917). Dissociation of visual perceptions due to occipital injuries, with especial reference to appreciation of movement. *Brain, 40*, 15-57.

Rockland, K. S., Andresen, J., Cowie, R. J., & Robinson, D. L. (1999). Single axon analysis of pulvinocortical connections to several visual areas in the macaque. *The Journal of Comparative Neurology, 406*(2), 221-250.

Rodman, H. R., Gross, C. G., & Albright, T. D. (1989). Afferent basis of visual response properties in area MT of the macaque. I. Effects of striate cortex removal. *The Journal of Neuroscience, 9*(6), 2033-2050.

Rogers, B. P., Morgan, V. L., Newton, A. T., & Gore, J. C. (2007). Assessing functional connectivity in the human brain by fMRI. *Magnetic Resonance Imaging, 25*(10), 1347-1357.

Rosas, H. D., Lee, S. Y., Bender, A. C., Zaleta, A. K., Vangel, M., Yu, P., et al. (2010). Altered white matter microstructure in the corpus callosum in Huntington's disease: Implications for cortical "disconnection". *NeuroImage, 49*(4), 2995-3004.

Rossion, B., Caldara, R., Seghier, M., Schuller, A. M., Lazeyras, F., & Mayer, E. (2003). A network of occipito-temporal face-sensitive areas besides the right middle fusiform gyrus is necessary for normal face processing. *Brain, 126*(Pt 11), 2381-2395.

Scharli, H., Harman, A. M., & Hogben, J. H. (1999). Blindsight in subjects with homonymous visual field defects. *Journal of Cognitive Neuroscience, 11*(1), 52-66.

Scheel, M., Abegg, M., Lanyon, L. J., Mattman, A., & Barton, J. J. (2010). Eye movement and diffusion tensor imaging analysis of treatment effects in a Niemann-Pick Type C patient. *Molecular Genetics and Metabolism, 99*(3), 291-295.

Schoenfeld, M. A., Heinze, H. J., & Woldroff, M. G. (2002). Unmasking motion-processing activity in human brain area V5/MT+ mediated by pathways that bypass primary visual cortex. *NeuroImage, 17*(2), 769-779.

Sigal, T., Shmuel, M., Mark, D., Gil, H., & Anat, A. (2010). Diffusion tensor imaging of corpus callosum integrity in multiple sclerosis: Correlation with disease variables. *Journal of Neuroimaging, in press. Epub ahead of print doi:10.1111/j.1552-6569.2010.00556.x.*

Sincich, L. C., Park, K. F., Wohlgemuth, M. J., & Horton, J. C. (2004). Bypassing V1: a direct geniculate input to area MT. *Nature Neuroscience, 7*(10), 1123-1128.

Smith, S. M., Jenkinson, M., Johansen-Berg, H., Rueckert, D., Nichols, T. E., Mackay, C. E., et al. (2006). Tract-based spatial statistics: Voxelwise analysis of multi-subject diffusion data. *NeuroImage, 31*(4), 1487-1505.

Solomon, D., Winkelman, A. C., Zee, D. S., Gray, L., & Buttner-Ennever, J. (2005). Niemann-Pick type C disease in two affected sisters: ocular motor recordings and brain-stem neuropathology. *Annals of the New York Academy of Sciences, 1039*, 436-445.

Song, S. K., Sun, S. W., Ju, W. K., Lin, S. J., Cross, A. H., & Neufeld, A. H. (2003). Diffusion tensor imaging detects and differentiates axon and myelin degeneration in mouse optic nerve after retinal ischemia. *NeuroImage, 20*(3), 1714-1722.

Song, S. K., Sun, S. W., Ramsbottom, M. J., Chang, C., Russell, J., & Cross, A. H. (2002). Dysmyelination revealed through MRI as increased radial (but unchanged axial) diffusion of water. *NeuroImage, 17*(3), 1429-1436.

Song, S. K., Yoshino, J., Le, T. Q., Lin, S. J., Sun, S. W., Cross, A. H., et al. (2005). Demyelination increases radial diffusivity in corpus callosum of mouse brain. *NeuroImage, 26*(1), 132-140.

Sowell, E. R., Thompson, P. M., Leonard, C. M., Welcome, S. E., Kan, E., & Toga, A. W. (2004). Longitudinal mapping of cortical thickness and brain growth in normal children. *The Journal of Neuroscience, 24*(38), 8223-8231.

Sowell, E. R., Trauner, D. A., Gamst, A., & Jernigan, T. L. (2002). Development of cortical and subcortical brain structures in childhood and adolescence: a structural MRI study. *Developmental Medicine & Child Neurology, 44*(1), 4-16.

Stoerig, P., & Cowey, A. (1997). Blindsight in man and monkey. *Brain, 120*, 535-559.

Taylor, D. G., & Bushell, M. C. (1985). The spatial mapping of translational diffusion coefficients by the NMR imaging technique. *Physics in Medicine and Biology, 30*(4), 345-349.

Tolman, E. C. (1948). Cognitive maps in rats and men. *Psychological Review, 55*, 189-208.

Tournier, J. D., Calamante, F., Gadian, D. G., & Connelly, A. (2004). Direct estimation of the fiber orientation density function from diffusion-weighted MRI data using spherical deconvolution. *NeuroImage, 23*(3), 1176-1185.

Tuch, D. S., Reese, T. G., Wiegell, M. R., & Wedeen, V. J. (2003). Diffusion MRI of complex neural architecture. *Neuron, 40*(5), 885-895.

Tuch, D. S., Salat, D. H., Wisco, J. J., Zaleta, A. K., Hevelone, N. D., & Rosas, H. D. (2005). Choice reaction time performance correlates with diffusion anisotropy in white matter pathways supporting visuospatial attention. *Proceedings of the National Academy of Sciences of the United States of America, 102*(34), 12212-12217.

Vanier, M. T., & Millat, G. (2003). Niemann-Pick disease type C. *Clinical Genetics, 64*(4), 269-281.

Wall, J. T., Symonds, L. L., & Kaas, J. H. (1982). Cortical and subcortical projections of the middle temporal area (MT) and adjacent cortex in galagos. *The Journal of Comparative Neurology, 211*(2), 193-214.

Watson, J. D., Myers, R., Frackowiak, R. S., Hajnal, J. V., Woods, R. P., Mazziotta, J. C., et al. (1993). Area V5 of the human brain: evidence from a combined study using positron emission tomography and magnetic resonance imaging. *Cerebral Cortex, 3*(2), 79-94.

Wedeen, V. J., Hagmann, P., Tseng, W. Y. I., Reese, T. G., & Weisskoff, R. M. (2005). Mapping complex tissue architecture with diffusion spectrum magnetic resonance imaging. *Magnetic Resonance in Medicine, 54*(6), 1377-1386.

Wedeen, V. J., Wang, R. P., Schmahmann, J. D., Benner, T., Tseng, W. Y., Dai, G., et al. (2008). Diffusion spectrum magnetic resonance imaging (DSI) tractography of crossing fibers. *NeuroImage, 41*(4), 1267-1277.

Weiskrantz, L. (1998). Consciousness and commentaries *Toward a Science of Consciousness II - Second Tucson Discussions and Debates 1996* (pp. 371-377). University of Arisona, Tucson, AZ, USA: MIT Press, Cambridge, MA.

Wolbers, T., Schoell, E. D., & Buchel, C. (2006). The predictive value of white matter organization in posterior parietal cortex for spatial visualization ability. *NeuroImage, 32*(3), 1450-1455.

Xue, R., van Zijl, P. C., Crain, B. J., Solaiyappan, M., & Mori, S. (1999). In vivo three-dimensional reconstruction of rat brain axonal projections by diffusion tensor imaging. *Magnetic Resonance in Medicine, 42*(6), 1123-1127.

Yoon, B., Shim, Y. S., Lee, K. S., Shon, Y. M., & Yang, D. W. (2008). Region-specific changes of cerebral white matter during normal aging: a diffusion-tensor analysis. *Archives of Gerontology and Geriatrics, 47*(1), 129-138.

Zeki, S., Watson, J. D., Lueck, C. J., Friston, K. J., Kennard, C., & Frackowiak, R. S. (1991). A direct demonstration of functional specialization in human visual cortex. *The Journal of Neuroscience, 11*(3), 641-649.

8

A Triangulation-Based MRI-Guided Method for TMS Coil Positioning

Jamila Andoh and Jean-Luc Martinot
[1]*Montreal Neurological Institute, McGill University*
[2]*International Laboratory for Brain, Music, and Sound (BRAMS), Montreal*
[3]*INSERM- CEA Research Unit 1000 "Neuroimaging & Psychiatry"; Univ Paris-Sud, and Univ. Paris Descartes; SHFJ, and Maison de Solenn - Cochin Hospital; Orsay – Paris*
[1,2]*Canada*
[3]*France*

1. Introduction

1.1 From lesions to functional neuroimaging

The first model about the cerebral organization of cognitive functions was based on lesion observation. This consisted in inferring association between a particular deficit of the language (e.g., word production) and a brain lesion observed post-mortem (Wernicke, 1874; Broca, 1861). Brain imaging techniques (e.g., functional Magnetic Resonance Imaging) provide complementary but different types of information regarding brain-behavior relationships. By providing indirect measures of cerebral activity such as blood flow or oxygen consumption, neuroimaging techniques enable one to establish a relationship between the activities of different brain areas and the cognitive processes being performed (Bestmann et al. 2003; Frith 1997). For instance, the combination of functional magnetic resonance imaging (fMRI) with language tasks has shown that language-related areas have a more complex role than the ones attributed by lesion studies, e.g. Broca's area in the left inferior frontal gyrus has been involved in speech production as well as in speech comprehension, and Wernicke's area located in the left temporoparietal area has been involved in language comprehension as well as phoneme discrimination (Friederici 2002; Luke et al. 2002). In addition, brain imaging studies showed that language processing is not restricted to Broca's and Wernicke's areas as shown by lesion studies, but requires a network of different brain areas which may be interconnected (Catani, Jones, and ffytche 2005; Behrens et al. 2003). However, the measures of brain activity implicate rather than demonstrate the critical contribution of a brain area to behavior, which can lead to misinterpretations.

1.2 Basic principles of TMS

During the last two decades, transcranial magnetic stimulation (TMS) has rapidly become a valuable method to investigate the human brain noninvasively (Siebner et al. 2009; Walsh and Rushworth 1999). TMS is based on electromagnetic induction: a change in electric current generates a magnetic field, which in turn induces a current in a second conductor brought into the magnetic field (Figure 1).

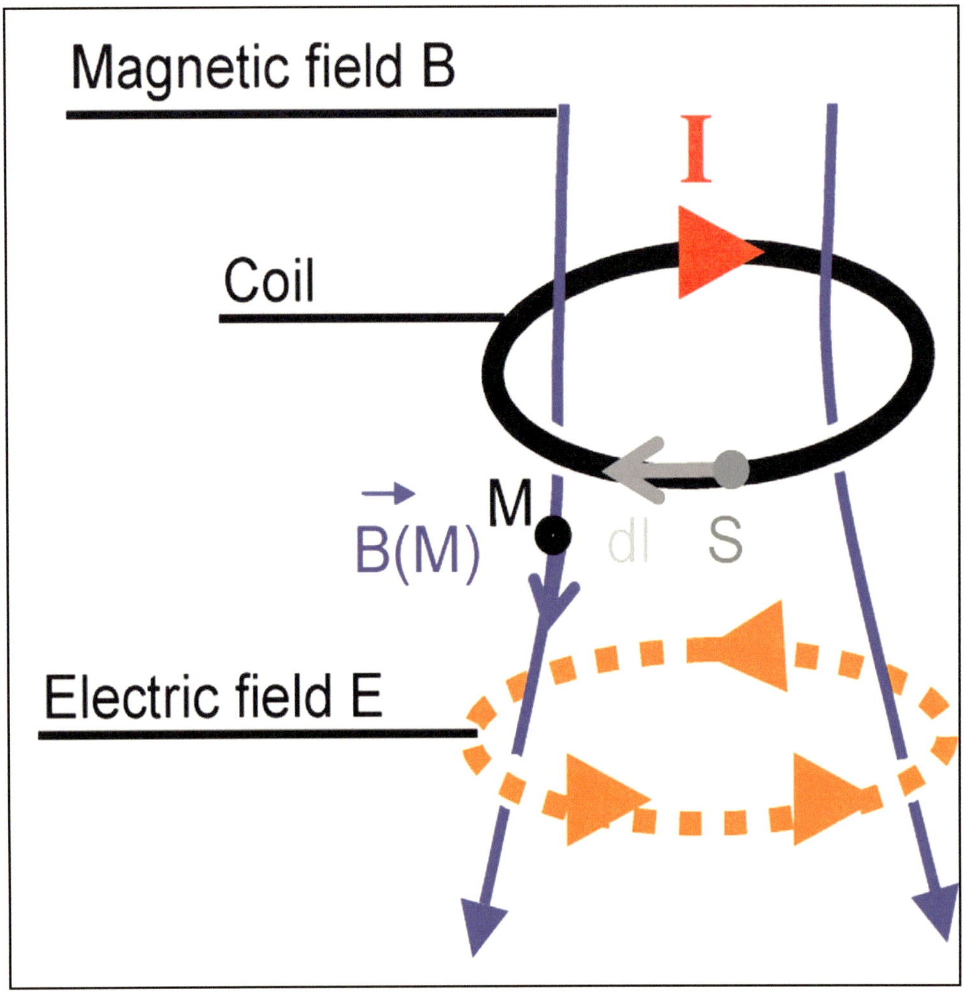

Fig. 1. an electric current (I) flowing through a coil of wire generates a magnetic field (B), which in turns induces electrical current in a secondary conductor.

The focality of stimulation with TMS depends on many factors such as the coil geometry (size and shape), the stimulus intensity or other external parameters such as the electrical properties of the cortex under the coil (Amassian et al., 1992; Cohen et al., 1990; Maccabee et al., 1993). The magnetic field induced by the TMS coil can be defined by the Biot-Savart law (see equation). The integration is performed with the vector *d***l** along the coil windings *Coil* and μ0 is the permeability of free space (see Figure 1).

$$\vec{B}(M)=\frac{\mu_0}{4\pi}\oint_{Coil}\frac{\vec{I}d\vec{l}\wedge \vec{SM}}{\left\|\vec{SM}\right\|^3}$$

The most common coils are the circular coil and the 8-shaped coil (see Figure 2), but recently developed coils (e.g. iron-core, Hesed or stereotactic) provide a more efficient and a deeper stimulation (Epstein and Davey 2002; Roth, Zangen, and Hallett 2002).

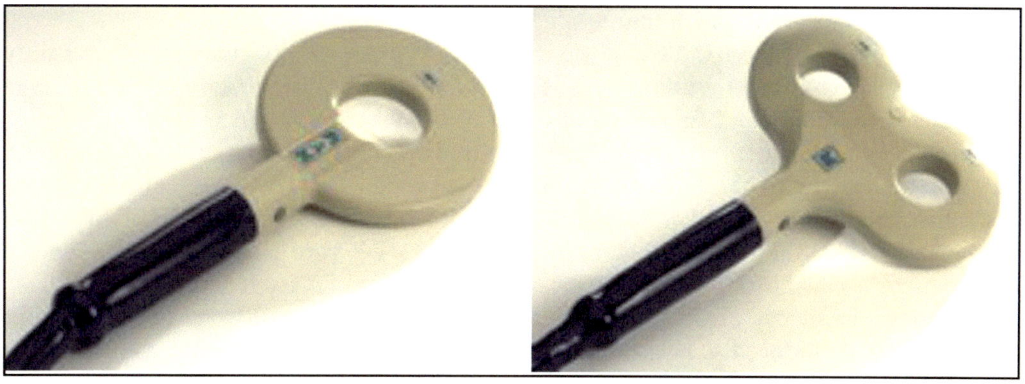

Fig. 2. The two most common TMS coils: (left) the circular coil and (right) the 8-shaped coil.

With a circular TMS coil (see Figure 2, left), the maximum electric field induced in the brain lies in an annulus under the coil (Figure 3). The 8-shaped coil is more focal than the circular coil (around 2 cm and 10 cm respectively) but in practice the circular coil is sometimes preferred over the 8-shaped coil because motor responses can be rapidly evoked without need for accurate coil positioning.

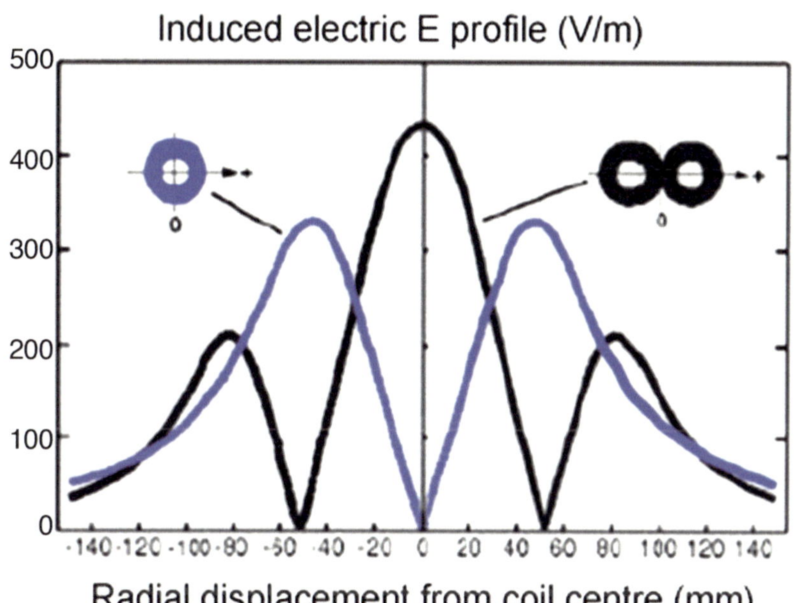

Fig. 3. Focality of the induced electric field for the circular coil (in blue) and for the 8-shaped coil (black). Data from constructor (Magstim Ltd., Wales, UK).

The focality and the strength of stimulation depend on the coil size and on the distance from the coil, both degrading quickly with increasing depth. As an indication, the field at a distance of 4 cm may be only about 30% of that at the coil surface as measured by Bohning et al. (1997) using fMRI and an MR-compatible TMS coil to map the magnetic field induced by the TMS coil in human volunteers.

1.3 TMS and interference with function

By inducing a local electric field, TMS creates a "virtual lesion" that may transiently interfere with cognitive processing. This 'perturb and measure' approach provides a direct link between anatomy and function and could also infer causality in neural connectivity. When TMS is applied over the motor cortex, an immediate motor response is obtained and can be measured by motor evoked potentials. Depending on the frequency of stimulation, TMS has been reported either to excite or to inhibit cortical motor excitability. Low frequency rTMS (<1Hz) on the motor cortex has been shown to result in an inhibition of corticomotor excitability (Chen et al. 1997; Muellbacher et al. 2000; Muellbacher et al. 2002), whereas high frequency rTMS (>1Hz) has been associated with facilitation of corticomotor excitability. TMS-induced effects on cognitive functions can be quantified using indirect measures such as changes in behavioral performance during a cognitive task (e.g. response time or error rate). For example, Andoh et al. (2006, 2008)) applied rTMS over the left temporoparietal area (TMP) of Wernicke and showed a reduced RT during an auditory task of word detection compared with rTMS applied over the left inferior frontal gyrus (IFG, pars opercularis). The authors attributed their findings to the modulation of the semantic processing associated with the left TMP and not with the left IFG. TMS-induced effects can also be directly quantified using fMRI or positron emission tomography (PET) to detect the changes in cerebral blood flow or metabolism respectively. For instance, in a consecutive study, Andoh and Paus (2011) carried out an fMRI scan before and after a series of TMS stimulations applied off-line over the left TMP area (i.e. TMS applied outside of the scanner bore). The comparison of fMRI data pre- and post-rTMS showed a local decrease of the neural activity in the left TMP area, and an increased neural activity in the contralateral right TMP. The authors hypothesized a mechanism of interhemispheric compensation for preserving behavior after a neural interference (for review Andoh and Martinot 2008)). Similar change in activity in language-related network was found by Thiel et al. (2006) reporting a CBF decrease in the stimulated left IFG and a CBF increase in the homologous (contralateral) right IFG during a verb-generation task. In addition, Ilmoniemi et al. (1997) reported comparable results using EEG. The authors showed that stimulation over visual or motor cortex elicits EEG responses around the site of stimulation within a few milliseconds of TMS, followed by responses from a secondary area of activity in the homotopic region of the contralateral hemisphere. These studies show that rTMS effects are not focal and confined to the site of stimulation, but spreads via pre-existing neuronal connections in a network, therefore making TMS a useful tool to investigate functional connectivity and plasticity in the normal brain (Paus et al. 1997; Siebner and Rothwell 2003) as well as in clinical population (Hampson and Hoffman 2010).

1.4 TMS as a clinical treatment

TMS has been investigated as a treatment tool in many neurological and psychiatric diseases, including epilepsy, Parkinson's disease, schizophrenia, or treatment-resistant depression. Because of its ability to modulate neural activity, rTMS has been used to excite or to inhibit certain brain functions reported to be "abnormal" in these patients. For instance, anatomic and functional dysfunctions in brain areas underlying speech generation and perception have been shown in schizophrenic patients prone to auditory hallucinations (Copolov et al. 2003; Shergill et al. 2000). Low frequency rTMS has been applied over the temporoparietal area of Wernicke; and this was shown to decrease its activity and to reduce auditory hallucinations in those patients (Hoffman et al. 2003). Regarding patients with treatment-resistant depression, neuroimaging studies have shown a reduced metabolism in the dorsolateral prefrontal cortex (DLPFC) in comparison with normal volunteers (George et al. 1995). In order to increase the DLPFC activity, TMS has been applied at high frequency (i.e. 10Hz) and results have shown an improvement in some patients. However, results vary among patients and across studies (Hoffman et al. 2003; O'Reardon et al. 2007, 2010). Different factors can account for this variability, such as the parameters of stimulation (frequency, intensity, duration), as well as differences between patients in anatomical and functional localization of areas stimulated.

1.5 Importance of TMS coil placement

The placement of the TMS coil above the proper site of the cortex is critical and several methods have been developed to control the positioning of the TMS coil. For example, some clinical studies have targeted the dorsolateral prefrontal cortex (DLPFC), Brodman's area (BA) 9 and 46, by positioning the coil 5 cm rostrally in the parasagittal plane from the motor cortex (Herwig et al. 2001; Pascual-Leone, Catala, and Pascual-Leone Pascual 1996), see Figure 4A. However, the DLPFC location using the "5-cm method" was found to correspond to Brodman's area (BA) 6 (premotor cortex) or BA 8 (frontal eye field) in 15/22 participants and only 7/22 were correctly targeted for the stimulation of the DLPFC. As this was the method used to locate the left DLPFC in most studies, the high degree of variability in the stimulated target must surely affect clinical results (Herwig et al. 2001). Nauczyciel et al. (2010) evaluated the different sources of variability of this standard "5-cm method" and showed that interindividual anatomical variability and interexpert variability were the two main sources of error. In addition, Rusjan et al. (2010) developed a neuronavigational method based on a standard template and compared the location of the DLPFC with the "5-cm method" and the 10-20 EEG electrode system and found that the neuronavigational method and the 10-20 EEG electrode are superior to the "5-cm method" in reducing inter-subject variability.

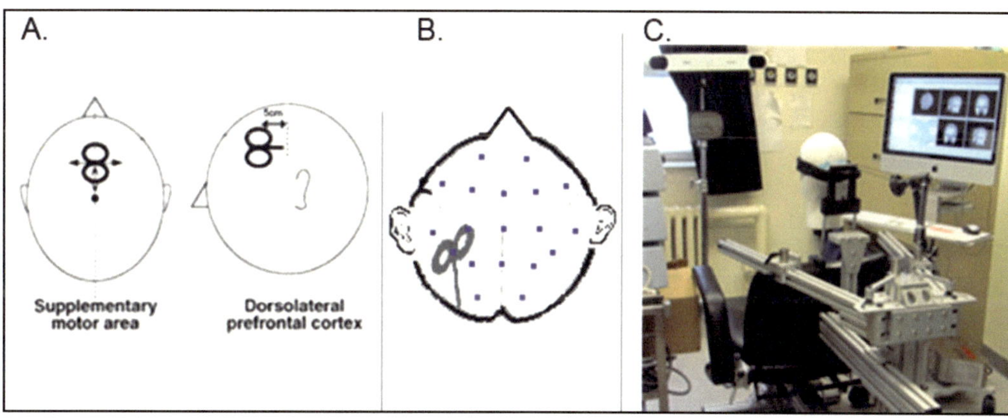

Fig. 4. Examples of methods used to localize the target for TMS. A. The DLPFC was targeted by moving the coil 5 cm forward from the motor cortex. B. Localization of the temporoparietal area of Wernicke using the 10-20 EEG system. C. Frameless stereotaxic system uses data from Magnetic Resonance Imaging to provide online monitoring of the TMS coil position on the participant's head (Rogue Research Inc.).

Other studies used cranial coordinates in the international 10-20 electrode system (i.e. CP5) to localize Wernicke's area (Sparing et al. 2001), see Figure 4B. However, this standardized system does not take into account interindividual anatomo-functional variability of language organization, which depends on the side and degree of language lateralization (Knecht et al. 2000). To reduce the influence of such anatomo-functional variabilities between patients, frameless stereotaxic systems, used in conjunction with functional neuroimaging have been developed to target individual areas according to well-defined anatomo-functional landmarks (Figure 4C). These frameless stereotaxic systems offer a relatively high accuracy of coil positioning over targeted areas (of about 10mm) (Gugino et al. 2001; Lancaster et al. 2004). However, such systems are expensive, heavy and difficult to use in a clinical setting. A recent study compared the accuracy of neuronavigations systems and the 10-20 electrode system while targeting the right intraparietal sulcus (electrode P4) and found that 9 and 47 participants, respectively were sufficient to obtain significant behavioral results.

2. Triangulation-based MRI-guided method

More recently, some new methods have been developed to reliably and inexpensively position the TMS coil manually over the participant's head. Those MRI-guided methods are based on MRI data in order to take into account individual specificity in head size and shape, as well as in anatomical and functional differences between participants. We will describe a triangulation-based MRI-guided method that we have developed and validated (Andoh et al. 2009). We have evaluated its accuracy with the target of the motor cortex because its stimulation produces a measurable muscle twitch quantifiable with motor evoked potentials (MEPs). We also evaluated the reproducibility of the target positioning across operators while targeting the motor cortex and a target in the parietal cortex localized using fMRI during a mental rotation task. This method was recently used in a PET study investigating the influence of prefrontal target region on the efficacy of repetitive TMS in depressive patients resistant to treatment. The authors used a TMS target based on prefrontal hypometabolic regions defined for each patient using individual PET images (Paillere Martinot et al. 2010). In addition, this method was also used in an fMRI study investigating the TMS modulation of temporal areas during language processing (Andoh et al. 2006) or investigating the role of the frequency of TMS stimulation applied over temporoparietal areas (Andoh et al. 2008).

2.1 Description of the MRI-guided method

The MRI-guided method is included in Brainvisa software, freely available online (http://brainvisa.info/) that contains many image processing tools (segmentation of T1-weighted MR images, grey/white classification, meshes of hemisphere surface, etc.). Some of these tools were used in this paper to provide realistic and accurate 3D representations of the head surface and the brain, which enables easy definition of anatomic and functional landmarks in each subject (Riviere et al. 2002). In the following section, we will describe the procedure of the MRI-guided method, and then we will present the MRI protocol, which provides anatomical and functional MR images acquired during a simple motor task in order to individually define the target of the motor cortex onto the subject's head surface. A manual describing the step-by-step procedure is also provided at ftp://ftp.cea.fr/pub/dsv/anatomist/documents/TMS/Andoh_TMS-positioning.pdf.

2.2 Basis of the triangulation-based MRI-guided method

The approach of the MRI-guided method is based on the triangulation (*or "trilateration"*), consisting in determining the relative position of a target (T) using the known locations of two or more reference points (A, B, C) and the distance between the target and each reference point d_i (i=A, B, C). When measurement error is introduced, if we know that the distance from the target T to a reference point i (=A, B or C) lies within a range of distance [d_i + dr], then the third point lies in a circular band between the circles of those two radii. If we know a range for another point, we can take the intersection, which will be either one or two areas bounded by circular arcs (Figure 5). A third point will narrow it down to a smaller area, which therefore limits the variability of the target positioning (Snyman 2005).

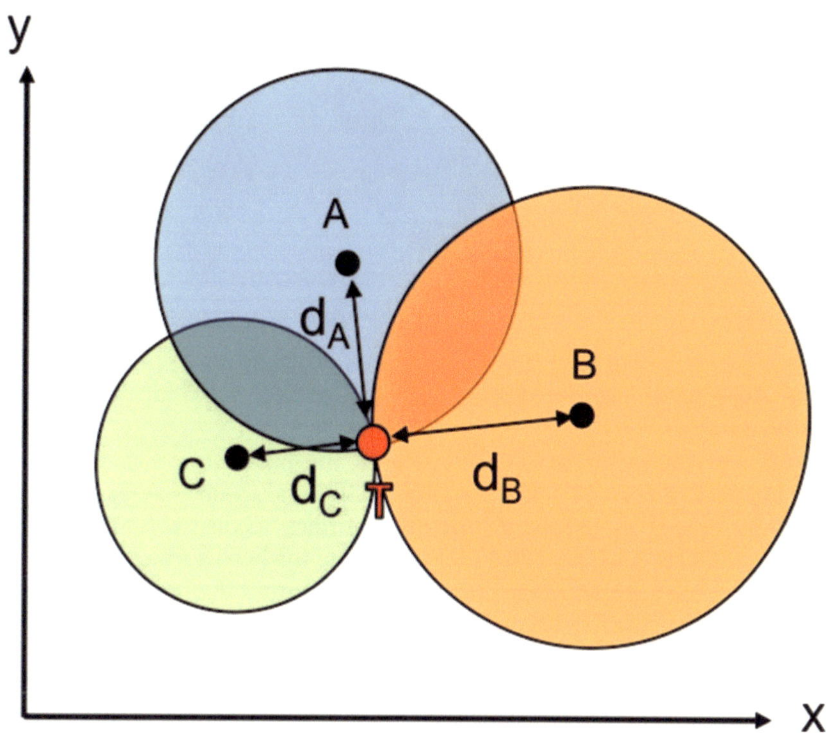

Fig. 5. Determination of the relative position of a target (T) using the known locations of three reference points (A, B, C) and the distance between the target and each reference point (d_A, d_B, d_C).

2.3 Procedure of the MRI-guided method

Some preprocessing steps need to be carried out on the MR anatomical images before using the MRI-guided procedure. First, a "bias analysis" is carried out to correct the standard inhomogeneities in MR images using a bias estimation for each subject (http://www.brainvisa.info/doc/brainvisa/en/processes/VipBiasCorrection.html).

Second, the *"histogram analysis"* leads to estimations of the gray and white matter mean and standard deviations. It relies on a scale-space analysis of the histogram, which is robust to modifications of the MR sequence (Mangin, Coulon, and Frouin 2005). Third, the "*brain segmentation*" uses the parameters given by the previous step to segment the brain (Mangin et al. 2004). The segmentation of the head surface was carried out and MR images were thresholded from the intensity histogram. Then, a morphologic closing was applied to fill up cavities and holes on the head reconstruction and the resulting mesh object was smoothed using a marching-cube algorithm (Figure 6. A, B).

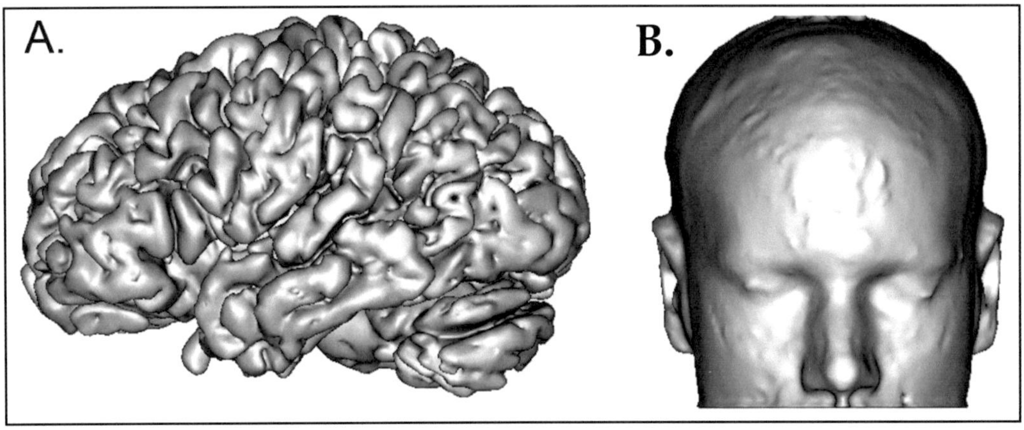

Fig. 6. Segmentation of the brain and head providing 3D reconstruction of A/ the brain and B/ head surfaces.

Once those steps have been processed, the MRI-guided procedure can be carried out following three steps:

1. The first step "target projection" consists in the projection of a cortical target (e.g. maximum peak of cortical activation) onto a 3D head mesh (see Figure 7). This step is particularly crucial as inaccuracy in head surface reconstruction may induce local geometric artefacts, and the target projection onto the head surface may be confounded. To obtain a robust projection of the cortical target onto the head surface, we used the centre of gravity of the (N=10) closest head mesh nodes (Andoh et al. 2006).

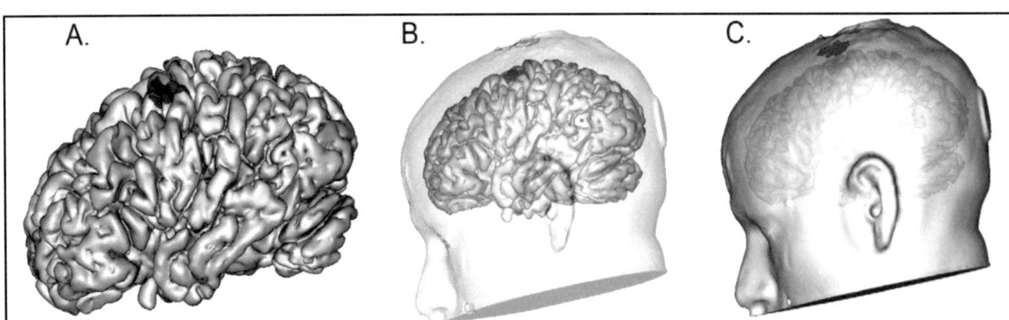

Fig. 7. 3D visualization of a functional target on A/ a brain mesh, B/ a brain mesh with the transparent head surface, and C/ projection of the functional target onto a 3D head surface.

2. The next step consists in computing the geodesic distances (i.e. tangent to the head surface) between the projected target on the head mesh surface and some landmarks on

the subject's head (nose bridge, tragus of both ears, Figure 8). This was done using an algorithm available in Brainvisa software (see manual for more information, ftp://ftp.cea.fr/pub/dsv/anatomist/documents/TMS/Andoh_TMS-positioning.pdf). Three geodesic distances (in mm) were obtained from the target to the nasion, and from the target to the left and right tragi of both ears providing three distances for the triangulation.

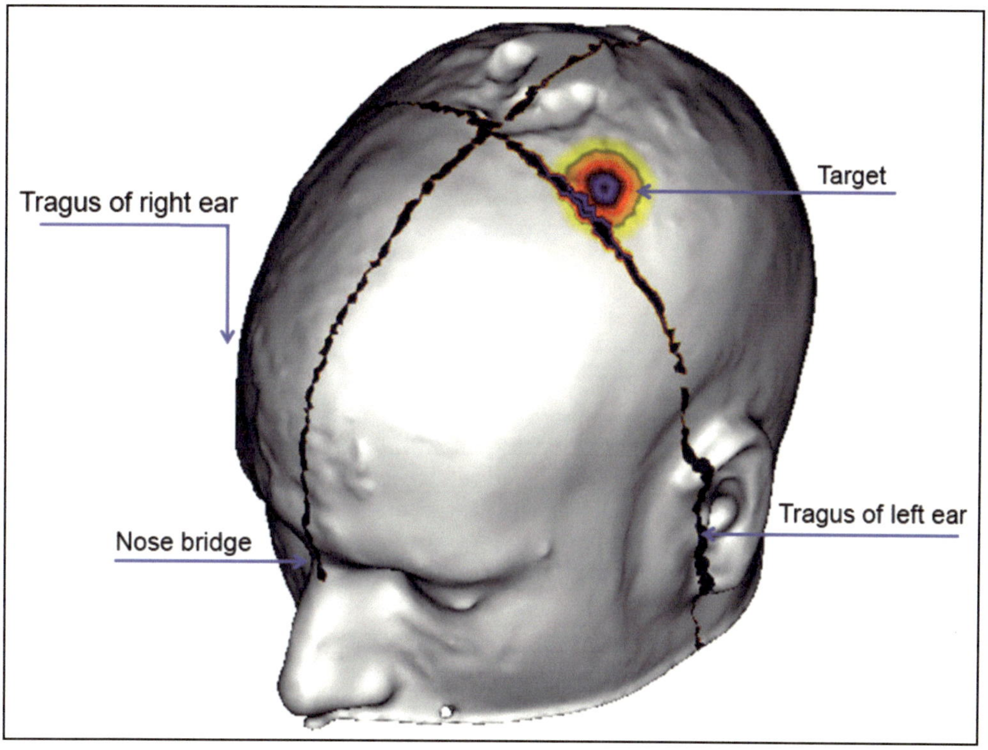

Fig. 8. Positioning of the three head landmarks on the 3D head reconstruction relative to the target location (nose bridge, tragi of both ears).

3. The final step consists in using these three geodesic distances to localize the cortical target onto the participant's head. The point of intersection of the three distances provides the target in order to position the TMS coil; and this position was marked physically on the cap of each participant (Figure 9). The triangulation was done manually, by the same investigator (JA) for all subjects, using three tied threads of lengths equal to the three geodesic distances.

2.4 Accuracy of the method

To assess the accuracy of the method, we used the cortical target of the hand motor area as its stimulation with TMS provides quantitative responses with motor-evoked potentials (Boroojerdi et al. 1999). The cortical target of the hand motor area was defined by the peak of task-related activity while participants were pressing left and right buttons inside an MR scanner. The difference between right and left thumb motor responses provided the location of the left motor cortical area (Figure 10).

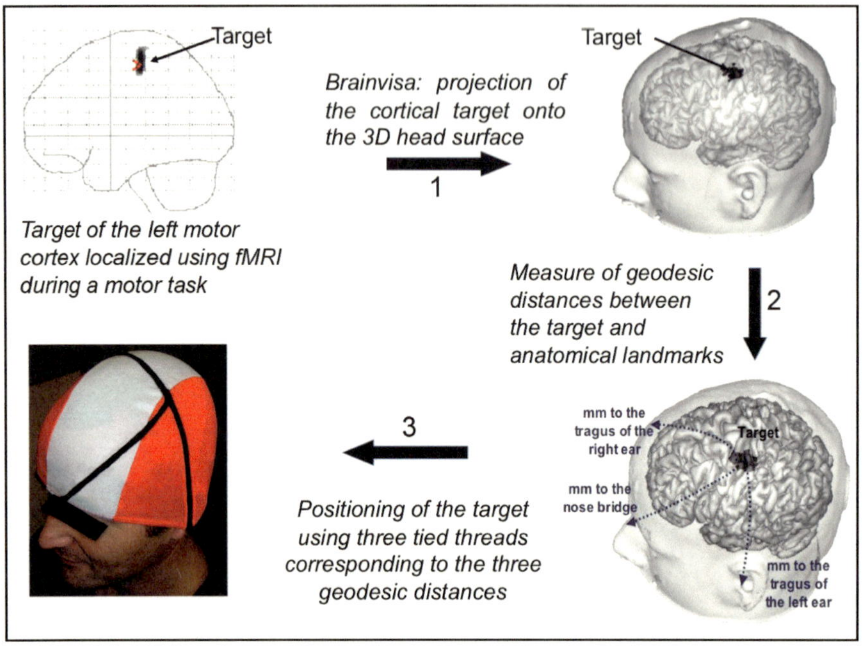

Fig. 9. Illustration of the three steps composing the MRI-guided method. 1/ projection of the cortical target of the motor cortex on a 3D head rendering. 2/ Measure of the geodesic distances (tangent to head surface) between the target and some landmarks on the subject's head (e.g. nose bridge and tragus of both ears). 3/ Positioning of the geodesic distances on the participant's head using three tied threads corresponding to the three distances. The intersection of the three tied threads provided the target location for TMS coil positioning.

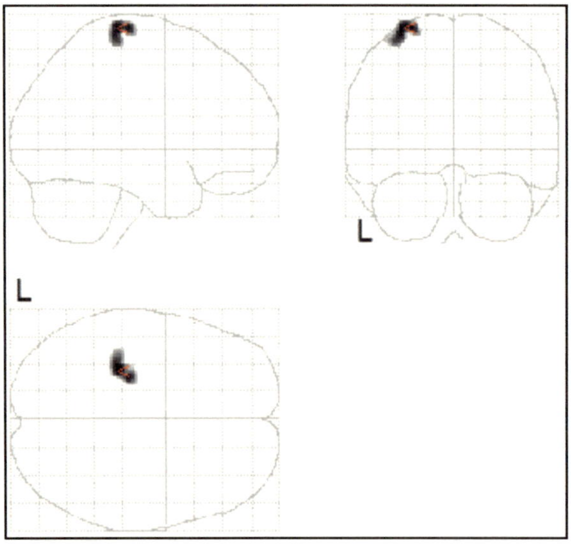

Fig. 10. Definition of the cortical target of the left motor cortical area. The target was defined by the peak of activation resulting from the contrast between right and left thumb motor responses (FWE-corrected; cluster size threshold $p<0.001$).

The accuracy of the method was determined by comparing the coil position over the right thumb motor target obtained from the MRI-guided method (fMRI-target) and the coil position subsequently obtained, where reproducible thumb motor-evoked potentials (MEPs) were elicited from TMS (MEP-target). The 3D coordinates of the two positions (fMRI-target and MEP-target) were obtained with an optical tracking system included in Brainsight™ Frameless. For each participant, the location of the fMRI- and MEP-targets was determined using individual coordinates in native space. Those coordinates were then transformed in standard space for group comparisons.

2.5 Measures of motor-evoked potentials in motor cortex with TMS

The MEP target (the target position that elicits MEPs in response to magnetic stimulation) was defined by the motor threshold criteria (MT), namely the lowest intensity of stimulation for evoking at least five MEPs in a total of ten stimulations with amplitude superior to 50 μV. A surface electromyogram EMG (Keypoint Portable, Medtronic) was used to record MEP amplitude from the relaxed right abductor pollicis brevis (Pascual-Leone et al. 1993; Rossini et al. 1995; Rothwell et al. 1999), see Figure 11. Magnetic stimulation was applied with a MagPro Stimulator (http://www.medtronic.com). Stimulus intensity started at 50% of the stimulator output and was increased in steps of 1% stimulator output.

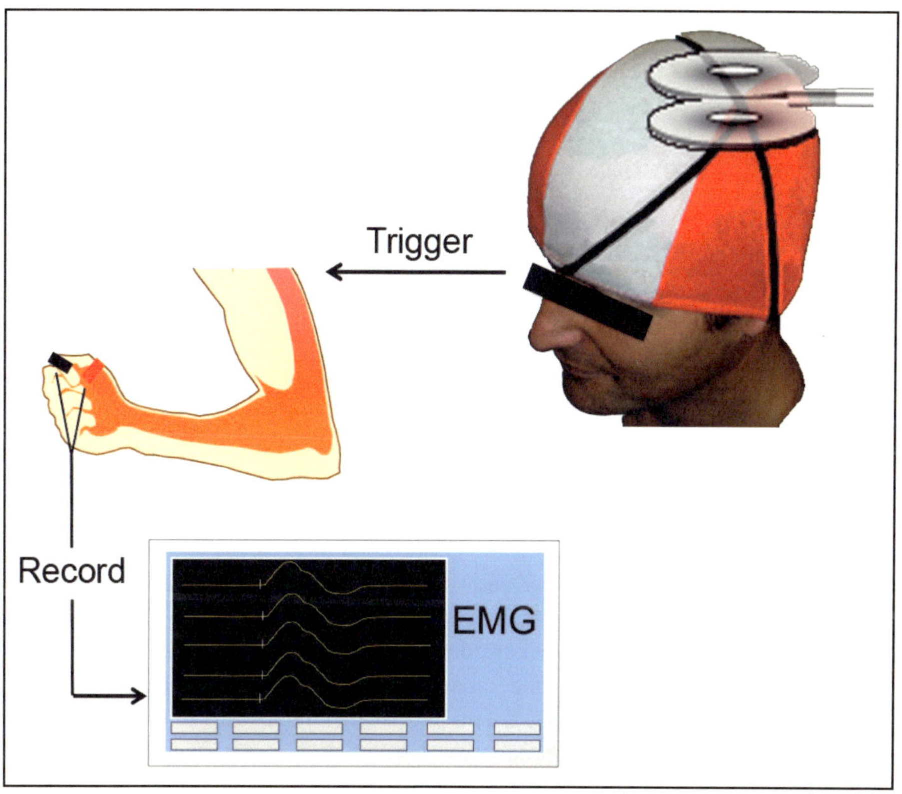

Fig. 11. Recording of motor evoked potentials (MEPs) in response to TMS using an electromyogram (EMG). The MEP target was defined by the lowest intensity of stimulation that induces at least five MEP with an amplitude > 50μV in a total of ten stimulations.

We compared the coil position over the right thumb motor target obtained from the MRI-guided method (fMRI-target) with the coil position obtained subsequently, eliciting reproducible MEPs with stimulation (MEP-target), see Figure 12. For each subject, the coordinates of the coil positions over the fMRI-target (x_{fMRI}, y_{fMRI}, z_{fMRI}) and the MEP-target (x_{MEP}, y_{MEP}, z_{MEP}) were recorded using an optical tracking system and compared using the mean Euclidean distance (D):

$$D= [(x_{fMRI} - x_{MEP})^2 + (y_{fMRI}- y_{MEP})^2 + (z_{fMRI}- z_{MEP})^2]^{1/2} = [D_x^2 + D_y^2 + D_z^2]^{1/2}.$$

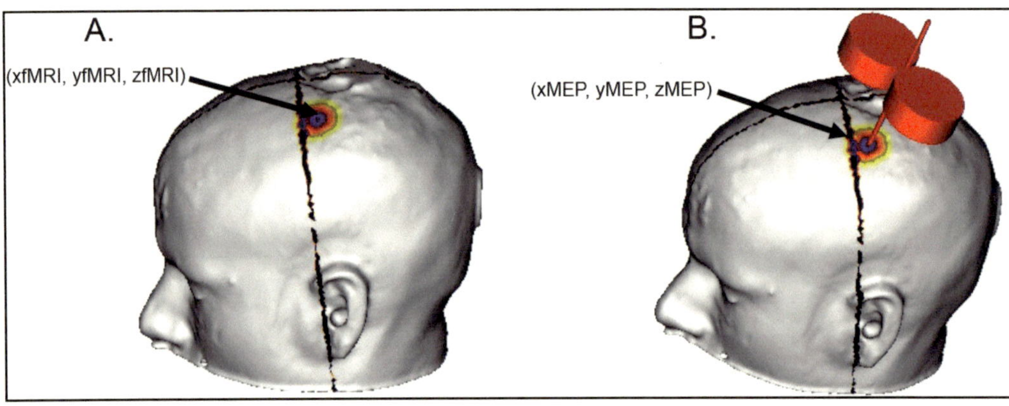

Fig. 12. Locations of A/ the fMRI-target (xfMRI, yfMRI, zfMRI) and B/ the MEP-target (xMEP, yMEP, zMEP) on a 3D head surface. The coordinates of both locations were recorded using an optical tracking system and compared using the mean Euclidean distance.

2.6 Reproducibility

The reproducibility of the target positioning was evaluated between operators by localizing the target of the motor cortex (see section above) and another target, located more posteriorly in the right parietal cortex. This target was functionally defined using a mental rotation task similar to the one used by Cooper and Shepard (1973). The mental rotation task consisted in displaying visually presented asymmetrical alphabetic characters (L, G, a), which had to be judged either normal or mirror image after rotation at different angular orientations. A "resting" condition was added in which subjects were asked to maintain their gaze on a small centrally located crosshair. The contrast between the task-related activity during the mental rotation task, and the resting condition enabled us to find the location of the right parietal cortex in each participant (Figure 13). Two operators used the MRI-guided method blindly and independently to position consecutively the targets of the motor cortex and the right parietal area over the cap of each subject's head. The difference between the locations determined by the two operators was measured by the mean Euclidean distance (see section above).

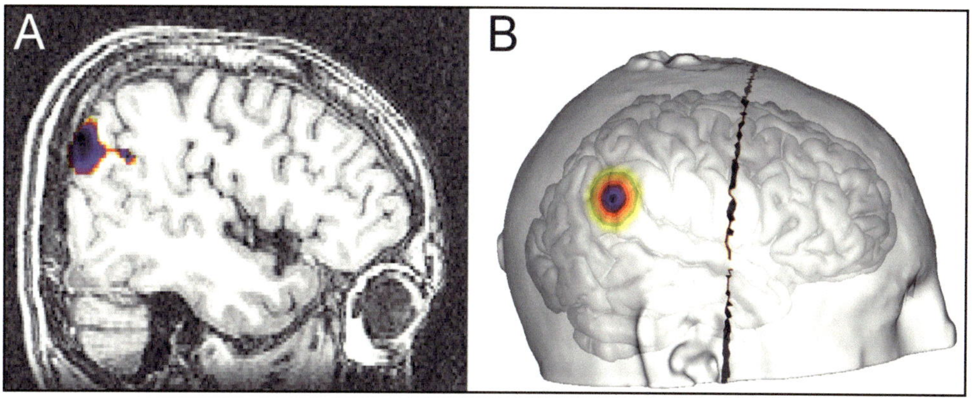

Fig. 13. Definition of a target in the right parietal cortex localized using fMRI during a mental rotation task. A/ location of the task-related activity on a 2D transverse view, and B/ projection of the target onto a 3D head reconstruction.

3. Results

3.1 Accuracy

The mean Euclidean distance (mean ± SD) between the fMRI and the MEP targets was measured for ten participants in their individual spaces and was then transformed in the standard space (MNI, Montreal Neurological Institute) for group analysis (Table 1). The cortical target derived from fMRI during the motor task allowed for determination of the motor threshold in two subjects with an MEP amplitude > 50 μV in 6 out of 10 trials. The mean Euclidean distance (mean ± SD) between the fMRI and the MEP targets was D_m=10.1 ± 2.9 mm, ranging from 5.2 to 14.0 mm. The components of this distance in the x, y, and z-axes were D_x= 4.0 ± 2.2 mm (range 0.6 - 7.7 mm), D_y= 5.0 ± 2.5 mm (range 1.3 - 8.0 mm) and D_z= 7.1 ± 3.0 mm (range 2.8 - 11.1 mm).

Subjects	Euclidean distances (MNI space, mm)			D_m (mm)	Motor threshold (%SO)
	D_x	D_y	D_z		
S1	7.0	4.9	5.4	10.1	50
S2	1.8	5.7	3.2	6.7	58
S3	3.7	5.1	10.0	11.9	58
S4	4.0	8.1	8.8	12.6	51
S5	3.9	7.8	9.1	12.6	60
S6	3.2	1.3	3.9	5.2	65
S7	7.7	1.8	2.8	8.4	56
S8	5.4	6.7	11.1	14.0	61
S9	0.6	6.9	9.3	11.6	56
S10	3.2	1.8	7.3	8.2	63

Table 1. Euclidean distances between the fMRI target and the MEP target in the x axis (D_x), y axis (D_y), and z axis (D_z). D_m is the mean Euclidean distance for each participant averaged across x, y and z axes. The last column is the motor threshold expressed in percentage of stimulator output (%SO).

3.2 Reproducibility

The results of the repositioning of the motor cortex target across two different operators showed a mean Euclidean distance of 6.7 ± 1.4 mm, ranging from 5.4 to 8.3 mm. In all subjects, the MRI-guided method allowed operators to induce a motor response. The results of the repositioning over the right parietal target across operators was determined on four subjects, and showed a mean Euclidean distance of 6.0 ± 3.2 mm, ranging from 1.4 to 8.7 mm.

4. Limitations

Different sources of variability should be considered in the evaluation of this method. First the definition of the tragi of both ears and the nose bridge are anatomic structures on the order of 1 cm diameter, and is therefore operator-dependent. Second, the coil positioning over the target cannot be controlled because once the coil is positioned, we cannot verify the location of the centre of coil. In addition, despite our results are interpreted as evidencing distance differences between the two methods (fMRI and MEP), it is also possible that results reflect the fact that the motor-related response obtained by fMRI and the motor evoked responses induced by TMS are not directly comparable (Lotze et al., 2003; Herwig et al., 2002). Indeed, TMS is activating all excitable circuits within the volume reached by the induced current, whereas fMRI measures increased oxygen supply in capillaries adjacent to neural firing. Since the responses probably do not involve the exact same tissue area, it is possible that they do not imply the same exact spatial representation in the primary motor cortex. Another limiting factor is the assumption that the induced electrical field is the strongest at the center of the figure of eight coil, however the depolarized neurons may not be directly beneath the center of the coil as has been indicated in other studies (Siebner et al., 2009; George et al., 2003), therefore introducing a variability in the concordance of the validation methods.

More recently, similar methods have been developed, showing the crucial need for relatively cheap and straightforward image-guided systems that can be used in the absence of neuronavigation. For instance, Rusjan et al. (2010) developed a manual method based on a standard template to target the left dorsolateral prefrontal cortex in each participant. They reported that the 'neuronavigational method' for localizing the DLPFC provided less inter-subject variability compared with the '5-cm method' or the '10-20 method'. In addition, Weiduschat et al. (2009) developed a surface distance measurements (SDM) method and evaluated its accuracy by comparison with a neuronavigation system. They reported a mean Euclidean distance of 8.3 mm between their method and the neuronavigation system while targeting Broca's area. However, similarly to our method, these methods do not provide an online guiding of TMS coil positions.

5. Conclusions

The MRI-guided method provides a relatively accurate and a low cost solution for TMS coil positioning. We found an accuracy of 10 ± 3 mm for positioning the target of the motor cortex, which is comparable to the accuracy of neuronavigation systems, for instance 10 ± 8 mm (Gugino et al. 2001), 10 ± 3 mm (Lancaster et al. 2004). This accuracy is also consistent with the focality of the TMS coil (e.g. 2 - 3 cm^2, (Thielscher and Kammer 2004). In comparison to neuronavigation systems, the MRI-guided method is relatively inexpensive and does not require any additional setup, which makes it particularly useful for therapeutic protocols conducted at more than one medical center. In addition, the present method is user-friendly and only needs Brainvisa, a software free available on-line. Moreover, a major advantage of this method is its ability to target cortical landmarks anywhere in the whole brain, whereas neuronavigation systems are limited by the field of view of the tracking cameras and cannot localize targets in the occipital cortex. We also showed that this method is reproducible across operators to localize a target in the parietal cortex, with a mean reproducibility of 7 ± 1 mm. However, a main limitation of our method is its inability to provide an online monitoring of TMS coil shifts and orientations, particularly useful for long period of stimulations.

6. Acknowledgment

JA was supported by the French Foundation for Medical Research. We thank R.M. Comeau (Rogue Research Inc., Montreal, Ca; http://www.rogue-research.com) for advice regarding the plugging of the neuronavigation system with Brainvisa software.

7. References

Andoh, J., E. Artiges, C. Pallier, D. Riviere, J. F. Mangin, A. Cachia, M. Plaze, M. L. Paillere-Martinot, and J. L. Martinot. 2006. Modulation of language areas with functional MR image-guided magnetic stimulation. *Neuroimage* 29 (2):619-27.

Andoh, J., E. Artiges, C. Pallier, D. Riviere, J. F. Mangin, M. L. Paillere-Martinot, and J. L. Martinot. 2008. Priming frequencies of transcranial magnetic stimulation over Wernicke's area modulate word detection. *Cereb Cortex* 18 (1):210-6.

Andoh, J., and J. L. Martinot. 2008. Interhemispheric compensation: a hypothesis of TMS-induced effects on language-related areas. *Eur Psychiatry* 23 (4):281-8.

Andoh, J., D. Riviere, J. F. Mangin, E. Artiges, Y. Cointepas, D. Grevent, M. L. Paillere-Martinot, J. L. Martinot, and A. Cachia. 2009. A triangulation-based magnetic resonance image-guided method for transcranial magnetic stimulation coil positioning. *Brain Stimulation* 2 (3):123-131.

Behrens, T. E., M. W. Woolrich, M. Jenkinson, H. Johansen-Berg, R. G. Nunes, S. Clare, P. M. Matthews, J. M. Brady, and S. M. Smith. 2003. Characterization and propagation of uncertainty in diffusion-weighted MR imaging. *Magn Reson Med* 50 (5):1077-88.

Bestmann, S., J. Baudewig, H. R. Siebner, J. C. Rothwell, and J. Frahm. 2003. Is functional magnetic resonance imaging capable of mapping transcranial magnetic cortex stimulation? *Supplements to Clinical neurophysiology* 56:55-62.

Bohning, D. E., A. P. Pecheny, C. M. Epstein, A. M. Speer, D. J. Vincent, W. Dannels, and M. S. George. 1997. Mapping transcranial magnetic stimulation (TMS) fields in vivo with MRI. *Neuroreport* 8 (11):2535-8.

Boroojerdi, B., H. Foltys, T. Krings, U. Spetzger, A. Thron, and R. Topper. 1999. Localization of the motor hand area using transcranial magnetic stimulation and functional magnetic resonance imaging. *Clin Neurophysiol* 110 (4):699-704.

Broca, P.M., 1861. Remarques sur le siège de la faculté de langage articulé, suivies d'une observation d'aphémie (perte de parole). *Bull. Mem. Soc. Anat.* Paris 36, 330–357.

Catani, M., D. K. Jones, and D. H. ffytche. 2005. Perisylvian language networks of the human brain. *Annals of neurology* 57 (1):8-16.

Chen, R., J. Classen, C. Gerloff, P. Celnik, E. M. Wassermann, M. Hallett, and L. G. Cohen. 1997. Depression of motor cortex excitability by low-frequency transcranial magnetic stimulation. *Neurology* 48 (5):1398-403.

Cooper, A.N., and R.N. Shepard. 1973. The time required to prepare for a rotated stimulus. *Memory & Cognition* 1:246-250.

Copolov, D. L., M. L. Seal, P. Maruff, R. Ulusoy, M. T. Wong, H. J. Tochon-Danguy, and G. F. Egan. 2003. Cortical activation associated with the experience of auditory hallucinations and perception of human speech in schizophrenia: a PET correlation study. *Psychiatry research* 122 (3):139-52.

Epstein, C. M., and K. R. Davey. 2002. Iron-core coils for transcranial magnetic stimulation. *Journal of clinical neurophysiology: official publication of the American Electroencephalographic Society* 19 (4):376-81.

Friederici, A. D. 2002. Towards a neural basis of auditory sentence processing. *Trends in cognitive sciences* 6 (2):78-84.

Frith, C.D. & Friston K.J. 1997. Studying brain function with neuroimaging. *Cognitive Neuroscience* ed. M.D.Rugg (Psychology Press: Hove UK.):169–195.

George, M. S., E. M. Wassermann, W. A. Williams, A. Callahan, T. A. Ketter, P. Basser, M. Hallett, and R. M. Post. 1995. Daily repetitive transcranial magnetic stimulation (rTMS) improves mood in depression. *Neuroreport* 6 (14):1853-6.

George ,M.S., Z. Nahas, S. H. Lisanby, T. Schlaepfer, F. A. Kozel, B. D. Greenberg. 2003. Transcranial magnetic stimulation. *Neurosurg Clin N Am* 14:283-301.

Gugino, L. D., J. R. Romero, L. Aglio, D. Titone, M. Ramirez, A. Pascual-Leone, E. Grimson, N. Weisenfeld, R. Kikinis, and M. E. Shenton. 2001. Transcranial magnetic stimulation coregistered with MRI: a comparison of a guided versus blind stimulation technique and its effect on evoked compound muscle action potentials. *Clinical neurophysiology: official journal of the International Federation of Clinical Neurophysiology* 112 (10):1781-92.

Hampson, M., and R. E. Hoffman. 2010. Transcranial magnetic stimulation and connectivity mapping: tools for studying the neural bases of brain disorders. *Frontiers in systems neuroscience* 4.

Herwig, U., F. Padberg, J. Unger, M. Spitzer, and C. Schönfeldt-Lecuona. 2001. Transcranial magnetic stimulation in therapy studies: examination of the reliability of "standard" coil positioning by neuronavigation. *Biological psychiatry* 50 (1):58-61.

Herwig U., K. Kolbel, A.P. Wunderlich, A. Thielscher, C. von Tiesenhausen, M. Spitzer and C. Schönfeldt-Lecuona. 2002. Spatial congruence of neuronavigated transcranial magnetic stimulation and functional neuroimaging, *Clin. Neurophysiol.* 113:462–468.

Hoffman, R. E., K. A. Hawkins, R. Gueorguieva, N. N. Boutros, F. Rachid, K. Carroll, and J. H. Krystal. 2003. Transcranial magnetic stimulation of left temporoparietal cortex and medication-resistant auditory hallucinations. *Archives of general psychiatry* 60 (1):49-56.

Ilmoniemi, R. J., J. Virtanen, J. Ruohonen, J. Karhu, H. J. Aronen, R. Naatanen, and T. Katila. 1997. Neuronal responses to magnetic stimulation reveal cortical reactivity and connectivity. *Neuroreport* 8 (16):3537-40.

Knecht, S., M. Deppe, B. Drager, L. Bobe, H. Lohmann, E. Ringelstein, and H. Henningsen. 2000. Language lateralization in healthy right-handers. *Brain* 123 (Pt 1):74-81.

Lancaster, J. L., S. Narayana, D. Wenzel, J. Luckemeyer, J. Roby, and P. Fox. 2004. Evaluation of an image-guided, robotically positioned transcranial magnetic stimulation system. *Human brain mapping* 22 (4):329-40.

Lotze, M., R.J. Kaethner, M. Erb, L.G. Cohen, W. Grodd, and H. Topka. 2003. Comparison of representational maps using functional magnetic resonance imaging and transcranial magnetic stimulation, *Clin. Neurophysiol.* 114:306–312.

Luke, K. K., H. L. Liu, Y. Y. Wai, Y. L. Wan, and L. H. Tan. 2002. Functional anatomy of syntactic and semantic processing in language comprehension. *Human brain mapping* 16 (3):133-45.

Mangin, J. F., D. Riviere, A. Cachia, E. Duchesnay, Y. Cointepas, D. Papadopoulos-Orfanos, P. Scifo, T. Ochiai, F. Brunelle, and J. Regis. 2004. A framework to study the cortical folding patterns. *NeuroImage* 23 Suppl 1:S129-38.

Mangin, J.F., O. Coulon, and V. Frouin. 2005. Robust brain segmentation using histogram scale-space analysis and mathematical morphology. *In Proc. 1st MICCAI, LNCS-1496, MIT, Boston,*:1230-1241.

Muellbacher, W., U. Ziemann, B. Boroojerdi, and M. Hallett. 2000. Effects of low-frequency transcranial magnetic stimulation on motor excitability and basic motor behavior. *Clinical neurophysiology: official journal of the International Federation of Clinical Neurophysiology* 111 (6):1002-7.

Muellbacher, W., U. Ziemann, J. Wissel, N. Dang, M. Kofler, S. Facchini, B. Boroojerdi, W. Poewe, and M. Hallett. 2002. Early consolidation in human primary motor cortex. *Nature* 415 (6872):640-4.

Nauczyciel, C., P. Hellier, X. Morandi, S. Blestel, D. Drapier, J. C. Ferre, C. Barillot, and B. Millet. 2010. Assessment of standard coil positioning in transcranial magnetic stimulation in depression. *Psychiatry research.*

O'Reardon, J. P., H. B. Solvason, P. G. Janicak, S. Sampson, K. E. Isenberg, Z. Nahas, W. M. McDonald, D. Avery, P. B. Fitzgerald, C. Loo, M. A. Demitrack, M. S. George, and H. A. Sackeim. 2007. Efficacy and safety of transcranial magnetic stimulation in the acute treatment of major depression: a multisite randomized controlled trial. *Biological psychiatry* 62 (11):1208-16.

Repeated Author. 2010. Reply regarding "efficacy and safety of transcranial magnetic stimulation in the acute treatment of major depression: a multisite randomized controlled trial". *Biological psychiatry* 67 (2):e15-7.

Paillere Martinot, M. L., A. Galinowski, D. Ringuenet, T. Gallarda, J. P. Lefaucheur, F. Bellivier, C. Picq, P. Bruguiere, J. F. Mangin, D. Riviere, J. C. Willer, B. Falissard, M. Leboyer, J. P. Olie, E. Artiges, and J. L. Martinot. 2010. Influence of prefrontal target region on the efficacy of repetitive transcranial magnetic stimulation in patients with medication-resistant depression: a [(18)F]-fluorodeoxyglucose PET and MRI study. *The international journal of neuropsychopharmacology / official scientific journal of the Collegium Internationale Neuropsychopharmacologicum* 13 (1):45-59.

Pascual-Leone, A., M. D. Catala, and A. Pascual-Leone Pascual. 1996. Lateralized effect of rapid-rate transcranial magnetic stimulation of the prefrontal cortex on mood. *Neurology* 46 (2):499-502.

Pascual-Leone, A., C. M. Houser, K. Reese, L. I. Shotland, J. Grafman, S. Sato, J. Valls-Sole, J. P. Brasil-Neto, E. M. Wassermann, L. G. Cohen, and et al. 1993. Safety of rapid-rate transcranial magnetic stimulation in normal volunteers. *Electroencephalography and clinical neurophysiology* 89 (2):120-30.

Paus, T., R. Jech, C. J. Thompson, R. Comeau, T. Peters, and A. C. Evans. 1997. Transcranial magnetic stimulation during positron emission tomography: a new method for studying connectivity of the human cerebral cortex. *The Journal of neuroscience : the official journal of the Society for Neuroscience* 17 (9):3178-84.

Riviere, D., J. F. Mangin, D. Papadopoulos-Orfanos, J. M. Martinez, V. Frouin, and J. Regis. 2002. Automatic recognition of cortical sulci of the human brain using a congregation of neural networks. *Medical image analysis* 6 (2):77-92.

Rossini, P. M., M. D. Caramia, C. Iani, M. T. Desiato, G. Sciarretta, and G. Bernardi. 1995. Magnetic transcranial stimulation in healthy humans: influence on the behavior of upper limb motor units. *Brain Res* 676 (2):314-24.

Roth, Y., A. Zangen, and M. Hallett. 2002. A coil design for transcranial magnetic stimulation of deep brain regions. *Journal of clinical neurophysiology: official publication of the American Electroencephalographic Society* 19 (4):361-70.

Rothwell, J. C., M. Hallett, A. Berardelli, A. Eisen, P. Rossini, and W. Paulus. 1999. Magnetic stimulation: motor evoked potentials. The International Federation of Clinical Neurophysiology. *Electroencephalogr Clin Neurophysiol Suppl* 52:97-103.

Rusjan, P. M., M. S. Barr, F. Farzan, T. Arenovich, J. J. Maller, P. B. Fitzgerald, and Z. J. Daskalakis. 2010. Optimal transcranial magnetic stimulation coil placement for targeting the dorsolateral prefrontal cortex using novel magnetic resonance image-guided neuronavigation. *Human brain mapping* 31 (11):1643-52.

Shergill, S. S., M. J. Brammer, S. C. Williams, R. M. Murray, and P. K. McGuire. 2000. Mapping auditory hallucinations in schizophrenia using functional magnetic resonance imaging. *Archives of general psychiatry* 57 (11):1033-8.

Siebner, H. R., T. O. Bergmann, S. Bestmann, M. Massimini, H. Johansen-Berg, H. Mochizuki, D. E. Bohning, E. D. Boorman, S. Groppa, C. Miniussi, A. Pascual-Leone, R. Huber, P. C. J. Taylor, R. J. Ilmoniemi, L. De Gennaro, A. P. Strafella, S. Kahkonen, S. Kloppel, G. B. Frisoni, M. S. George, M. Hallett, S. A. Brandt, M. F. Rushworth, U. Ziemann, J. C. Rothwell, N. Ward, L. G. Cohen, J. Baudewig, T. Paus, Y. Ugawa, and P. M. Rossini. 2009. Consensus paper: Combining transcranial stimulation with neuroimaging (vol 2, pg 58, 2009). *Brain Stimulation* 2 (3):182-182.

Siebner, H. R., and J. Rothwell. 2003. Transcranial magnetic stimulation: new insights into representational cortical plasticity. *Experimental brain research. Experimentelle Hirnforschung. Experimentation cerebrale* 148 (1):1-16.

Siebner, H. R., G. Hartwigsen, T. Kassuba, J. C. Rothwell. 2009. How does transcranial magnetic stimulation modify neuronal activity in the brain? Implications for studies of cognition. *Cortex.* 45, (9):1035-1042.

Snyman, J. A. 2005. Practical Mathematical Optimization: An Introduction to Basic Optimization Theory and Classical and New Gradient-Based Algorithms. *Springer Publishing.*

Sparing, R., F. M. Mottaghy, M. Hungs, M. Brugmann, H. Foltys, W. Huber, and R. Topper. 2001. Repetitive transcranial magnetic stimulation effects on language function depend on the stimulation parameters. *J Clin Neurophysiol* 18 (4):326-30.

Thiel, A., B. Habedank, K. Herholz, J. Kessler, L. Winhuisen, W. F. Haupt, and W. D. Heiss. 2006. From the left to the right: How the brain compensates progressive loss of language function. *Brain Lang* 98 (1):57-65.

Thielscher, A., and T. Kammer. 2004. Electric field properties of two commercial figure-8 coils in TMS: calculation of focality and efficiency. *Clin Neurophysiol* 115 (7):1697-708.

Walsh, V., and M. Rushworth. 1999. A primer of magnetic stimulation as a tool for neuropsychology. *Neuropsychologia* 37 (2):125-35.

Weiduschat, N., B. Habedank, B. Lampe, J. Poggenborg, A. Schuster, W. F. Haupt, W. D. Heiss, and A. Thiel. 2009. Localizing Broca's area for transcranial magnetic stimulation: Comparison of surface distance measurements and stereotaxic positioning. *Brain stimulation* 2 (2):93-102.

Wernicke, C., 1874. Der Aphasische Symptomenkomplex. Cohn and Weigert, Breslau.

9

Biocytin-Based Contrast Agents for Molecular Imaging: An Approach to Developing New *In Vivo* Neuroanatomical Tracers for MRI

Anurag Mishra[1,4] et al.*
[1]*Department for Physiology of Cognitive Processes, Max-Planck Institute for Biological Cybernetics, Tübingen,*
[4]*Department of Chemistry, Durham University, South Road, Durham*
[1]*Germany*
[4]*England*

1. Introduction

One of the most striking characteristic of the brain is its profuse neuronal connectivity. Not surprisingly, the function of the nervous system critically depends on the spatiotemporal pattern of intercommunication between different regions of the brain. Both macro- and microscopic aspects of the wiring diagrams of brain circuits are relevant and need to be understood in order to cope with the complexity of the brain function. In this way, for instance, the long-range connections that carry the functional specification of cortical territories need to be studied together with the detailed microcircuits inside a cortical column. Moreover, the temporal dimension of these wiring diagrams must be investigated since neuronal networks are dynamic structures exhibiting context-dependent changes in synaptic weights (Canals et al., 2009) and numbers (Chklovskii et al., 2004). Investigations over the last decades strongly suggest that stimulus or task related neural activity is distributed over large parts of the brain, covering different cortical and sub-cortical areas. For a detailed understanding of brain function, it is of prime importance to understand the organization of the neuronal connections. To chart the anatomical connections between the various components of brain networks, the neuronal tract tracing technique has been proved to be very useful. Thus, experimental tools that allow the exploration of brain circuits at

*Kirti Dhingra[1,5], Ritu Mishra[2,6], Almut Schüz[1], Jörn Engelmann[2], Michael Beyerlein[1], Santiago Canals[1,7] and Nikos K. Logothetis[1,3]
[1]*Department for Physiology of Cognitive Processes, Max-Planck Institute for Biological Cybernetics, Tübingen, Germany*
[2]*High-Field MR Center, Max-Planck Institute for Biological Cybernetics, Tübingen, Germany*
[3]*Imaging Science and Biomedical Engineering, University of Manchester, Manchester, England*
[4]*Department of Chemistry, Durham University, South Road, Durham, England*
[5]*Case Center for Imaging Research, Department of Radiology, Case Western Reserve University, Cleveland, OH, USA*
[6]*School of Biological & Biomedical Sciences, Durham University, South Road, Durham, England*
[7]*Instituto de Neurociencias CSIC-UMH, Campus de San Juan, San Juan de Alicante, Spain*

diverse organizational levels are mandatory for the understanding of brain intercommunication and information processing.

Magnetic Resonance Imaging (MRI) has great potential for mapping brain connectivity (Koretsky and Silva, 2004). It is a noninvasive volume imaging technique that can be applied longitudinally to the same subject, capturing the temporal dimension of brain connections and providing complete descriptions of large-scale three-dimensional (3-D) neuronal networks. The main limitation of MRI is its low sensitivity. To compensate for weak signals in MRI, efforts have been focused on the development of MR contrast agents. Recently, the paramagnetic ion manganese (Mn^{2+}) has been introduced as a MR-contrast agent for investigating *in vivo* neuronal connectivity (Canals et al., 2008; Pautler et al., 1998). Following the general mechanism of other classical anterograde tracers, Mn^{2+} is taken up by neurons and transported to the distant synaptic terminals where it accumulates and reveals the projection fields (Canals et al., 2008; Leergaard et al., 2003; Murayama et al., 2006; Pautler et al., 1998; Saleem et al., 2002; Sloot and Gramsbergen, 1994; Tjalve et al., 1995; Van der Linden et al., 2002; Watanabe et al., 2004), thus delineating brain connectivity. In contrast to classical tracers, which require processed fixed tissue for data analysis, neuronal tracing with Mn^{2+} as an MR tracer is performed *in vivo*.

However, cellular toxicity is an important drawback that challenges the applicability of Mn^{2+}-enhanced MRI (MEMRI). It has been shown that Mn^{2+} can be cytotoxic at concentrations used for neural tracing (Canals et al., 2008; Chandra et al., 1981; McMillan, 1999; Pal et al., 1999). Additional disadvantages of this technique are its high diffusion at the injection site, which challenge the specificity of the resulting projections, and its incompatibility with other visualization systems (Canals et al., 2008). If Mn^{2+} toxicity is not counteracted, it generates such perturbations in the neuronal circuits under study that eliminate the advantage of using Mn^{2+} as an *in vivo* neuronal tracer. In addition, at the end of an *in vivo* connectivity experiment using a paramagnetic tracer, it could be very informative to analyze the laminar and subcellular distribution of the neuronal connections. Such an experiment cannot be performed by using current MEMRI methods. New non-toxic paramagnetic tracers with anterograde, but also retrograde capabilities (i.e. when the tracer moves from the terminal ends to the soma identifying the origin of a synaptic contact) are desirable, particularly for functional studies, for quantitative 3-D analysis of connectivity, or for repetitive applications investigating the same pathway dynamically over time.

Here we report a strategy to produce neuronal tract tracers with paramagnetic properties, biochemical stability and biocompatibility. The new tracers are imbued with double functionality in a single molecule that allows both *in vivo* longitudinal brain connectivity studies by means of MRI and postmortem subcellular investigation in the same experimental animal. Therefore, the macro- and microscopic aspects of a brain circuit can be simultaneously investigated.

As a proof of concept we focused on the well-known neuroanatomical tracer biocytin which is taken up by neurons and transported in both antero- and retrograde directions (King et al., 1989). Several characteristics make biocytin a good tracer model. It has been used in numerous tracing studies, both after intracellular or extracellular application, and much is known about its biophysical properties (Horikawa and Armstrong, 1988). Due to its high affinity to avidin, it can be visualized by using a host of avidin conjugated markers at the light- and electron microscopic level. Extracellular application of biocytin results in very well localized injection sites with no uptake by fibers of passage or glial cells. These two last characteristics result in a high specificity of biocytin tracings (Kita and Armstrong, 1991; Lapper and Bolam, 1991; Wirsig-Wiechmann, 1994).

Structurally, biocytin consists of D-Biotin and L-lysine connected via an amide bond which is susceptible to cleavage by biotinidase enzyme. Biotinidase is the enzyme mainly responsible for recycling of the vitamin biotin by cleaving biocytin and biotinylated peptides/proteins (Hymes and Wolf, 1996; Mock et al., 1999; Wilbur et al., 1996). Biotinidase plays an important role in brain function (Pispa, 1965; Suchy et al., 1985). A deficiency in the biotinidase enzyme has been linked to several neurological disorders (Heller et al., 2002; Tsao and Kien, 2002; Zaffanello et al., 2003). For this reason, biocytin has relatively small half life *in vivo*, which forces short post injection survival times and increases the probability of only partial reconstruction of neuronal projections. Using the same strategy, we recently introduced two new biocytin-based neuroanatomical tracers [*aminopropyl-biocytin* and *serine-biocytin*; Scheme 1] with improved enzymatic stability (Mishra et al., 2009). The *in vivo* results for these two derivatives of biocytin demonstrated that they are biochemically stable conjugates, retain full tracing capabilities and more importantly these molecules allow longer post-injection survival times due to the improved stability and therefore, provide more detailed and complete connectivity information. The commercial biocytin was totally degraded 96 h postinjection, however, these improved neuronal tracers still stained neuronal cell bodies and fibers at the injection site and remote terminal fields. These improved neuronal tracers present an edge over conventional histological procedures, as their better stability could reduce the problems related to the endogenous degradation of the tracer molecule before the animal is sacrificed. As was suggested in the previous work (Mishra et al., 2009), the applicability of these new agents could be further diversified by coupling with different reporter moieties and utilized for multimodal tracing. For instance, the combination of reported molecules with MR reporters could serve as a tool for magnetic resonance imaging and, hence, be used for visualizing brain connectivity *in vivo*.

Here in, we have followed up our previous investigations and developed two novel and structurally distinct gadolinium (Gd^{3+}) containing biocytin-based multimodal neuronal tracers ([**Gd.L^1**] and [**Gd.L^2**]) (Scheme 1). The backbone of these structures were functionalized by covalently linking the kinetically stable gadolinium caged organic macrocyclic moiety [DOTA and DO3A-serine] as MR reporters to perform *in vivo* longitudinal brain connectivity studies by means of MRI, leaving α-position of lysine moiety free for internalization in neurons and biotin moiety free for avidin binding for subsequent visualization with postmortem microscopic histological methods.

The first MR tracer **[Gd.L^1]** was derived from the recently published stable biocytin variant *aminopropyl-biocytin* (Mishra et al., 2009), whereby [Gd.DOTA] was coupled to *aminopropyl-biocytin* via an amide bond. The second MR tracer, **[Gd.L^2]** consists of a new precursor [Gd.DO3A-serine] which has an orthogonal amine and a carboxylate group on the fourth nitrogen of [Gd.DO3A] for the coupling of biotin and lysine, respectively. By replacing [Gd.DOTA] with FITC in **[Gd.L^1]** fluorescently labeled *aminopropyl-biocytin* **[Fluo.L^1]** was obtained for fluorescence microscopy studies.

We present data that demonstrate the validity of the approach by showing cortical connectivity *in vivo* applying T_1-weighted MR-imaging. In addition, the corresponding subcellular details, fibers and neuronal morphology under light microscopy were investigated in the same experimental animals by means of avidin-biotin interactions and conventional histological techniques.

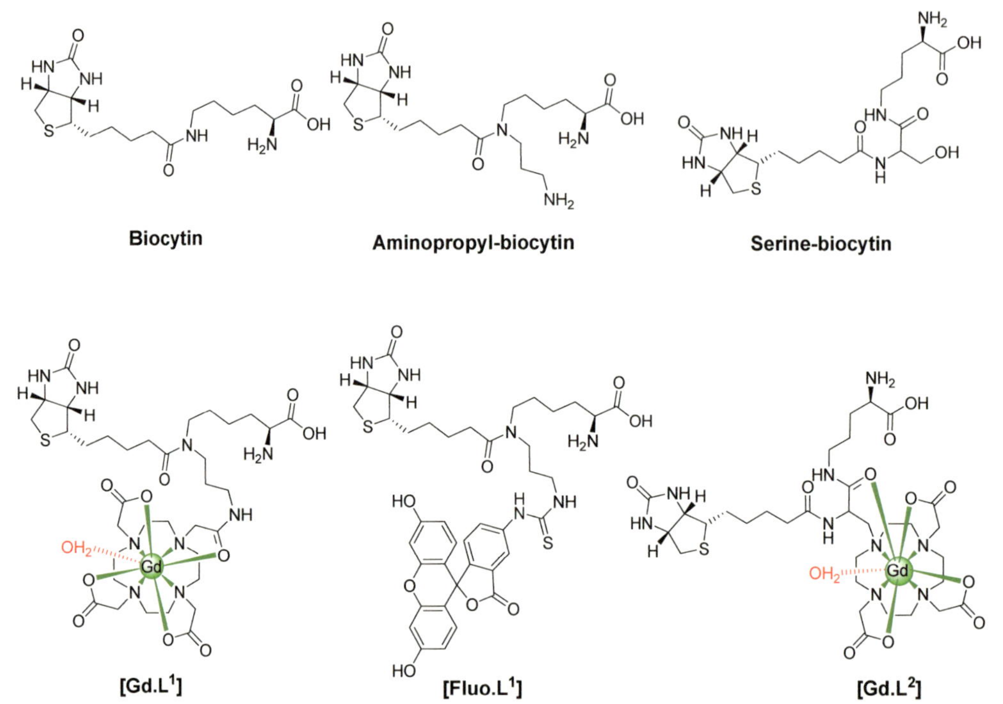

Scheme 1. Structures of studied biocytin-derived neuroanatomical tracers.

2. Results and discussion

2.1 Synthesis of ligands and complexes

Two structurally different Gd^{3+} complexing neuroanatomical tracers (**[Gd.L^1]** and **[Gd.L^2]**; Scheme 1) were designed and synthesized. These conjugates enclosed the [Gd.DO3A] construct as an MR reporter and biotin to be used for microscopic visualization by means of histological techniques.

The first MR tracer **[Gd.L^1]** was derived from stable biocytin variant, propylamine-biocytin (Mishra et al., 2009), where [Gd.DOTA] was coupled to aminopropyl-biocytin via amide bond. **[Gd.L^1]** was synthesised in seven steps prior to complexation with Gd^{3+} (Scheme 2). Propylamine-biocytin **6** was synthesized in three steps, starting with the reaction of acrylonitrile on $^{\alpha}$*N*-carbobenzyloxy-L-lysine methyl ester giving cyano compound **4**. Propinonitrile derivative **5** was obtained after coupling acid D-biotin with the secondary amine of **4** by using PyBroP as a coupling reagent and diisopropylethylamine as the base in anhydrous CH_2Cl_2. Subsequent selective reduction of nitrile groups in the presence of Ra-Ni, H_2, 7M NH_3/MeOH yielded amine intermediate **6**. The macrocycle intermediate **3** (tris-*tert*-butyl-DOTA) was obtained in two steps by stepwise alkylation of tris-*tert*-butyl-DO3A, **1**, with benzylbromoacetate in acetonitrile generating **2,** and following deprotection of benzyl groups produced the corresponding acid **3** in high yield (Pope et al., 2003). Then, tetra-ester **7** was synthesized by coupling of amine **6** and acid **3** [EDC/HOBt/NMM] in anhydrous DMF, from which **L^1** was obtained by successive deprotections (benzylcarbamate removal by hydrogenation using Pd-C as the catalyst, methyl group with LiOH and *tert*-butyl groups with neat TFA).

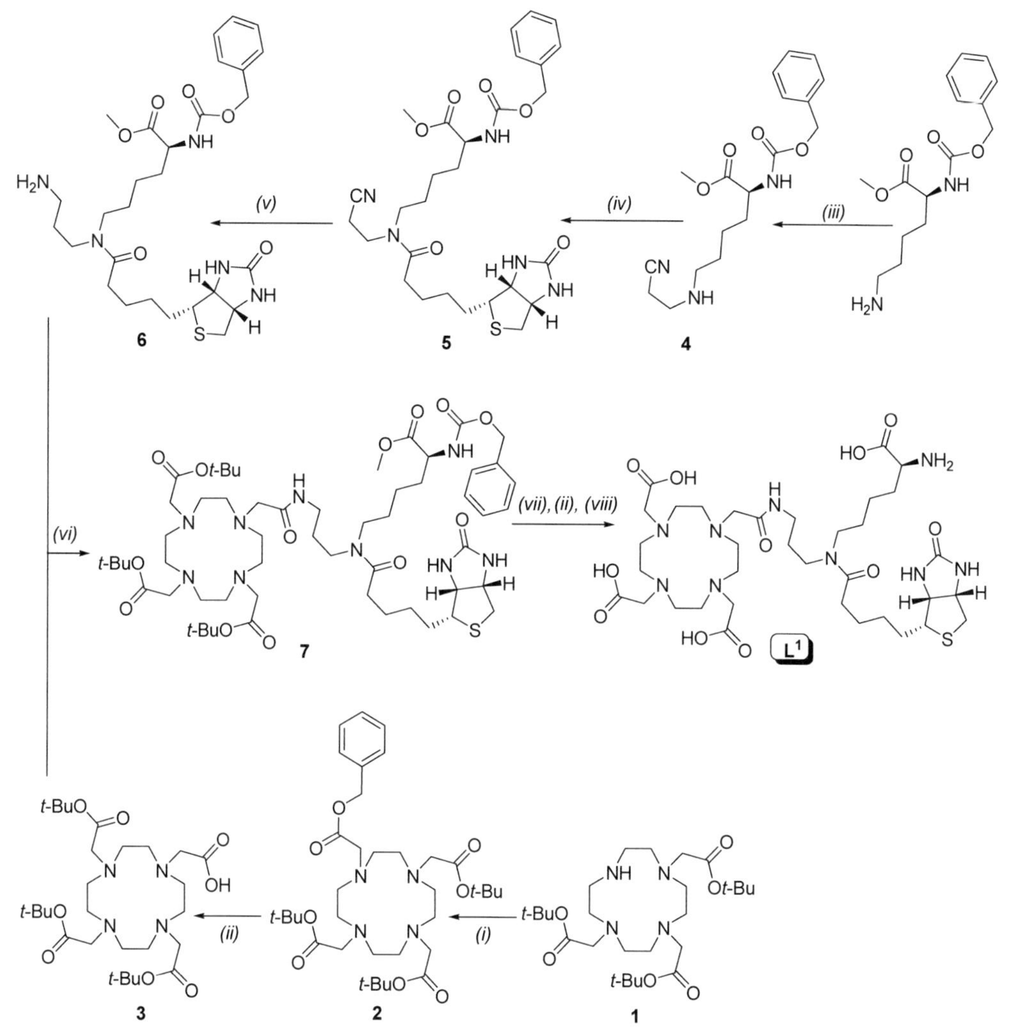

Scheme 2. Reagents and conditions: *(i)* benzylbromoacetate, MeCN, K_2CO_3, 100°C; *(ii)* Pd-C (10%), H_2, MeOH, 50 psi; *(iii)* acrylonitrile, TEA, MeOH; *(iv)* Biotin, PyBroP/DIPEA/CH_2Cl_2; *(v)* Ra-Ni, H_2, 7 M NH_3/MeOH, 50 psi; *(vi)* NMM/EDC/HOBt/DMF; *(vii)* LiOH, THF:MeOH:water (3:2:2); *(viii)* TFA (neat).

The second MR tracer, **[Gd.L²]** consists [Gd.DO3A-serine] which has an orthogonal amine and a carboxylate group available on the fourth nitrogen of [Gd.DO3A] for the coupling of biotin and lysine, respectively. **[Gd.L²]** was synthesized in 9 steps prior to complexation with Gd^{3+} (Scheme 3). Bromination on the hydroxyl group of *N*-carbobenzyloxy-L-serine methyl ester yielded **8**. The bromination reaction was run for no more than 30 min. This avoided the formation of allyl analogues of the product by elimination of bromine. The most reasonable route to synthesize ligand **10** was by alkylation of **8** on **1** but the elimination of the bromine group under highly basic conditions resulted in starting compound together with allyl side product. An alternative route was taken to obtain **10** where monoalkylated intermediate **9** was generated by alkylation of excess cyclen with **8** in anhydrous toluene, which was further alkylated by *tert*-butylbromoacetate yielding **10**. Mono-acid **11** was obtained by mild hydrolysis of the methyl ester in the presence of LiOH, which was further coupled to amine of Boc-Lys-OMe [EDC/HOBt/NMM] in anhydrous DMF to produce **12**. The benzylcarbamate was hydrogenated over Pd/C to yield the secondary amine **13** which was coupled to acid D-biotin [EDC/HOBt/NMM] in anhydrous DMF to give tetra-ester **14**.

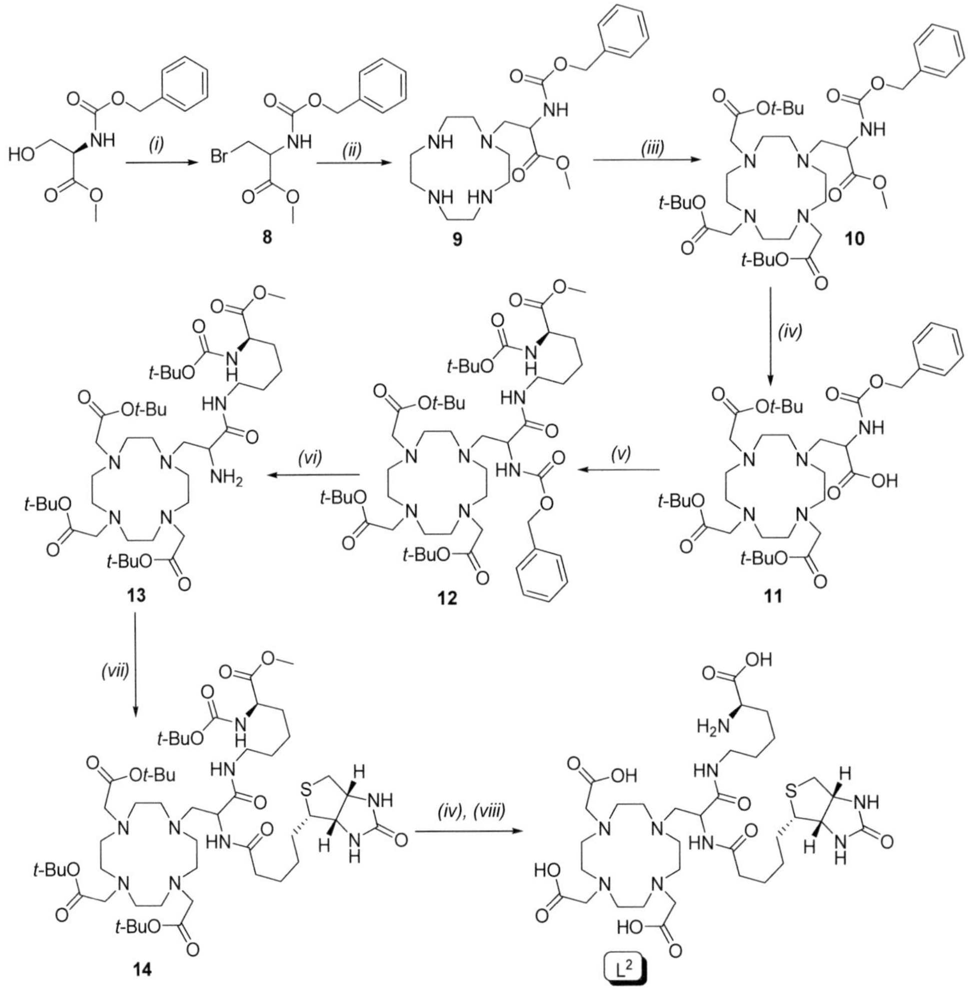

Scheme 3. Reagents and conditions: *(i)* NBS/PPh_3/DMF; *(ii)* cyclen/toluene; *(iii)* *tert*-butyl bromoacetate/Na_2CO_3/MeCN; *(iv)* LiOH, THF:MeOH:H_2O (3:2:2); *(v)* Boc-Lys-OMe, NMM/HOBt/EDC/DMF; *(vi)* Pd-C (10%), H_2, MeOH, 50 psi; *(vii)* biotin, HATU/DIPEA/DMF; *(viii)* TFA (neat).

Carboxylic acid derivative **L²** was obtained by successive deprotections (first the methyl group with LiOH and then *tert*-butyl groups with neat TFA).

Ligands, **L¹** and **L²**, were purified by RP-HPLC and loaded with Gd^{3+} using $GdCl_3.6H_2O$ in water at pH 6.5. The final concentration of Gd^{3+} was determined by inductively-coupled plasma optical emission spectrophotometry (ICP-OES).

2.2 Proton relaxivity modulation of [Gd.L[1]] and [Gd.L[2]] by biotin-avidin interaction

The extensive applications of biotin-avidin interactions have been found attractive in biomolecule detection, medical diagnostics, immunoassays and nanoscience (Bickel et al., 2001; Cao et al., 2003; Caswell et al., 2003; Rivera et al., 2003; Weizmann et al., 2003). Due to the high affinity of biotin to tetrameric avidin, biotinylated compounds can be visualized by light microscopy in postmortem tissues using avidin-conjugated markers. To investigate and quantify the binding behavior of the two contrast agents (CAs) to avidin which is important for the histological detection, we performed MRI experiments at 7T (300 MHz) [phosphate buffered saline (PBS), 7.4 pH, 23°C] with increasing concentrations of avidin proportional to constant concentrations of CAs (0.25 mM) and measured the proton longitudinal relaxivities (r_{1p}).

The proton longitudinal relaxivities (r_{1p}) of **[Gd.L[1]]** and **[Gd.L[2]]** at 7T (300 MHz) [phosphate buffered saline (PBS), 7.4 pH, 23°C] were found to be 5.52±0.08 mM^{-1} s^{-1} and 7.27±0.13 mM^{-1} s^{-1}, respectively. As anticipated, **[Gd.L[1]]** shows similar relaxivity to [Gd.DOTA] complexes. However **[Gd.L[2]]** shows higher relaxivity than that reported in the literature for Gd-DO3A derivatives in such a physiological solution (Caravan et al., 1999). The observed higher relaxivity in solution is explained by the high molecular volume and a significant second-sphere contribution through amide moieties close to the paramagnetic proximity present in the molecule (Aime et al., 1996; Botta, 2000).

Complexes	r_{1p} ($mM^{-1}s^{-1}$)		Change (%)
	[Gd.L[n]]	**[Gd.L[n]]:avidin**	
[Gd.L[1]]	5.52±0.08	6.10±0.11	+11
[Gd.L[2]]	7.27±0.13	6.65±0.09	-9

Table 1. Relaxivity (r_{1p}, $mM^{-1}s^{-1}$) for **[Gd.L[1]]/[Gd.L[2]]** and **[Gd.L[1]]/[Gd.L[2]]:avidin** complexes (23°C, 7T (300 MHz), pH 7.4, PBS, 0.25 mM complex).

Inevitable, r_{1p} of **[Gd.L[1]]** was slightly increased (11%) in contrast to **[Gd-L[2]]** (9% decreased) upon binding to avidin (Table 1). This is in reference to the Solomon–Bloembergen–Morgan theory envisaging that at high magnetic fields, the longitudinal proton relaxivity changes with the opposite of molecular rotational correlation time (τ_R) suggesting that relaxivity change should be expected upon binding of the CAs to macromolecules (Livramento et al., 2006). The saturation in r_{1p} at a ratio approximately at 2:1 (assuming a 2:1 stoichiometry of interaction) for the **[Gd-L[1]]/[Gd-L[2]]:avidin** adduct was obtained which clearly indicating similar steric hindrance of both CAs. These results suggest that **[Gd.L[1]]** and **[Gd.L[2]]** block the adjacent binding sites of biotin but evidently fit into two opposite binding pockets of avidin. The complexes {**[Gd.L[1]]/[Gd.L[2]]:avidin**} (2:1) binding stoichiometry reveal that **[Gd.L[1]]** and **[Gd.L[2]]** could be visualized by binding with avidin via histological techniques. However, an improved visualisation is expected if binding occurred to all pockets of avidin in a 4:1 ratio.

2.3 *In vitro* cell culture studies

It is well known from the literature that biocytin is a low molecular weight compound which has excellent uptake and transport capability in neuronal cells. Biocytin could be used as antero- as well as retrograde neuronal tract-tracer after intra- and extracellular injection in the brain (Kobbert et al., 2000). However, the uptake mechanism of biocytin at higher concentrations is not well known. A rapid and sodium/potassium-dependent high affinity uptake of biocytin in NB2a neuroblastoma cells was reported by Baur et al. This uptake was

very specific and selective to NB2a neuroblastoma cells as compared to C6 astrocytoma cells (Baur et al., 2002). Saturation kinetic of biocytin in a low concentration range was reported. However, the biocytin concentration in the brain is well below the reported concentration at half maximal saturation (K_m) of the biocytin uptake under physiological conditions (Baur et al., 2002). In contrast, after pressure or iontophoretic injection, local concentrations exceed the physiological concentration of biocytin manifold. Thus, the uptake mechanism under such conditions is not yet established.
The Gd-chelated macrocyclic modified biocytin molecules, **[Gd.L^1]** and **[Gd.L^2]**, are high molecular weight compounds as compared to biocytin alone. We investigated the cellular internalization of these compounds and their ability to enhance the MR contrast *in vitro*. For these studies murine N18 neuroblastoma cells were used as cellular model. In order to induce more neuronal metabolic and morphologic features in these tumor cells, serum deprivation was used to differentiate the cells (Marchisio et al., 1979). During the slow stepwise reduction of FBS content in the culture medium to 0.625% the growth rate slowed down and cells started to show a neuronal morphology with a network of neurite-like cellular processes which were completely absent at 10% FBS. Similar *in vitro* studies were also performed with the FITC containing *aminopropyl-biocytin* **[Fluo.L1]**. All cell incubations were performed in HBSS/10 mM HEPES buffer for 6 hours.

2.3.1 *In vitro* studies of cellular toxicity on N18 murine neuroblastoma cells

We first tested whether the contrast agents would have an adverse effect on differentiated N18 cells. For this purpose cells were incubated with **[Gd.L^1]** or **[Gd.L^2]** for 6 h in HBSS/10 mM HEPES and the number of cells were determined by fluorescence spectroscopy using the DNA dye Bisbenzimid Hoechst 33342. Only **[Gd.L^2]** showed a significant cytotoxic effect at 50 μM (Figure 1). Thus, all further experiments were done at concentrations below this level (40 and 20 μM for **[Gd.L^1]** and **[Gd.L^2]**).

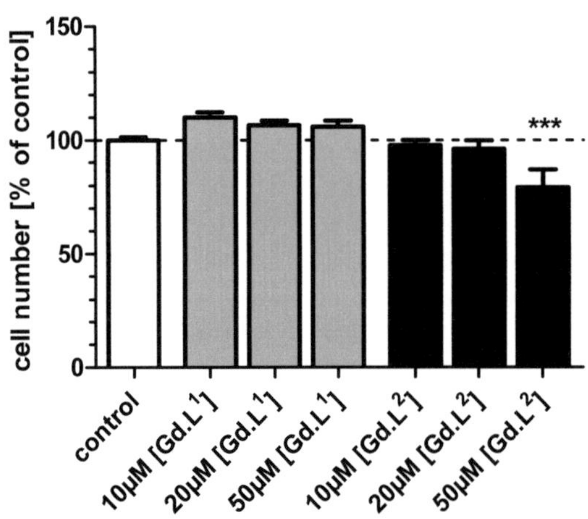

Fig. 1. Evaluation of the acute short term toxicity of **[Gd.L^1]** and **[Gd.L^2]**. Differentiated N18 neuroblastoma cells were incubated with the indicated concentration of **[Gd.L^1]** or **[Gd.L^2]** in HBSS/10 mM HEPES for 6h. Afterwards DNA dye Bisbenzimide Hoechst 33342 was added for 30 min in complete cell culture medium to determine the number of cells by the fluorescence of the dye/DNA conjugate (Ex 355nm/Em 465 nm). Values represent mean±SEM (n=6-12). ***p< 0.001, statistically different compared to control (ANOVA, Dunnett´s multiple comparison test).

2.3.2 Fluorescence microscopy to detect internalization and subcellular distribution

Since the intracellular distribution of **[Gd.L¹]** and **[Gd.L²]** cannot be directly detected by MRI, the fluorophore containing analogue to **[Gd.L¹]**, **[Fluo.L¹]** was used. Fluorescence microscopy of living cells displayed a detectable uptake of the compound into morphologically differentiated N18 cells. Figure 2 shows the cellular localization of **[Fluo.L¹]** after incubation with 50 μM for 12 h and subsequent washing and quenching of remaining extracellular fluorescence by Trypan Blue. **[Fluo.L¹]** (green fluorescence of the covalently linked FITC) was internalized very quickly and mainly accumulated in vesicles in the perinuclear region (nuclei counterstained in blue) of the cells. Green fluorescence of **[Fluo.L¹]** could also be detected in the projections of the cells. These results indicate a predominantly endosomal uptake of **[Fluo.L¹]** into morphologically differentiated neuroblastoma cells. The optical evidence that **[Fluo.L¹]** was also detected along the processes of the cells set grounds for possible application of synthesized compounds as tract tracers.

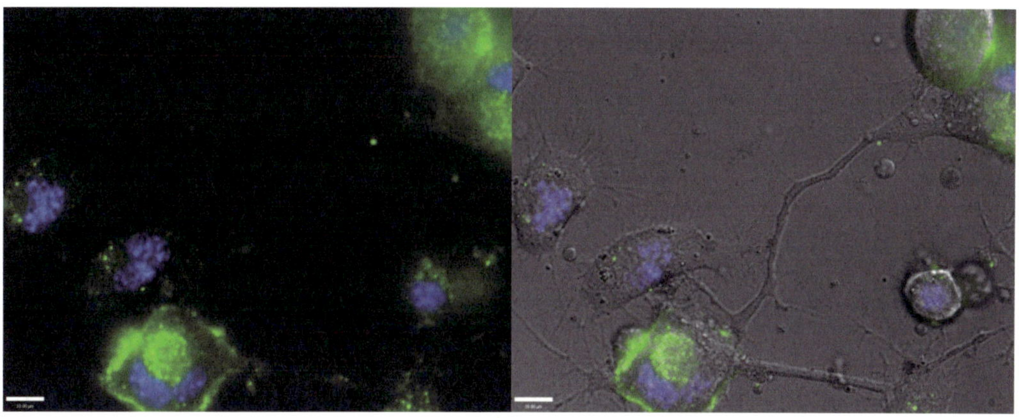

Fig. 2. Optical evidence for intracellular localization of **[Fluo.L¹]** in N18 neuroblastoma cells. Cells were incubated with 50 μM of **[Fluo.L¹]** for 6 h in HBSS/10 mM HEPES as described in materials and methods. Overlay of green (FITC in **[Fluo-L¹]**) and blue fluorescence (DNA dye Hoechst 33342) (left) and in addition of the phase contrast image (right).

2.3.3 MRI studies on N18 murine neuroblastoma cells

After proving the cellular uptake, the ability of **[Gd.L¹]** and **[Gd.L²]** to enhance contrast in MR images of labeled cells was tested. For this purpose differentiated N18 cells were incubated with either 20 or 40 μM of **[Gd.L¹]** or **[Gd.L²]**, respectively. After removal of the incubation medium of all samples the labeled cells were extensively washed with buffer. A constant number of treated cells were transferred into 0.5 mL Eppendorf tubes and cells were allowed to settle down. T_1-weighted images were taken and the values of longitudinal (T_1) relaxation times were measured in an axial slice of cell pellets and supernatant at 3T and room temperature.

Figure 3 shows representative examples of T_1-weighted images achieved after incubation with 20 or 40 μM of **[Gd.L¹]** or 40 μM of **[Gd.L²]**. A significant contrast enhancement could be observed in the images for both compounds compared to control cells incubated in the absence of contrast agent. The determination of apparent cellular relaxation rate $R_{1,cell}$

(=1/$T_{1,cell}$) in the cell pellet confirmed these results (Figure 4). The significance levels here were lower since averages of independent experiments were taken.

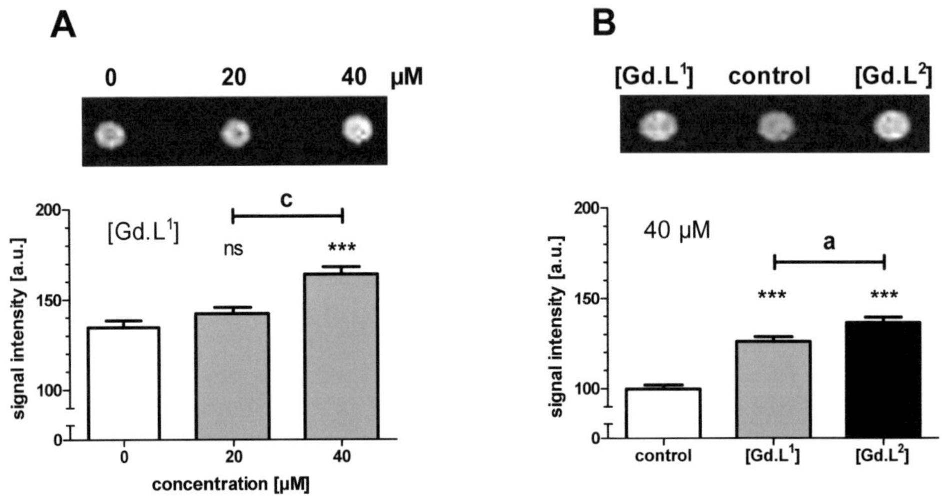

Fig. 3. Examples of T_1-weighted MR images of differentiated N18 neuroblastoma cells and analysis of the signal intensities in these images. Cells were incubated with 20 or 40 µM [**Gd.L**[1]] (A) or 40 µM of [**Gd.L**[1]] and [**Gd.L**[2]] (B) for 6 h in HBSS/10 mM HEPES. Cells were washed, trypsinized and resuspended in fresh culture medium (without CA) at a cell density of 1×10^7 cells/500 µL and transferred into 0.5 mL tubes. Cells were allowed to settle prior to MR experiments for imaging and determination of T_1 values in an axial slice through the cell pellet. Parameters for MRI are given in the experimental part. The bar graphs resulted from the pixelwise evaluation of signal intensity in the corresponding images. Values represent mean±SD (n=37 (A) and 44 (B)); ***, $p>0.001$, significantly different to control, a, $p<0.05$ and c, $p>0.001$, significant difference between 20 µM, 40 µM and [**Gd.L**[1]], [**Gd.L**[2]], respectively (ANOVA, Tukey´s multiple comparison test).

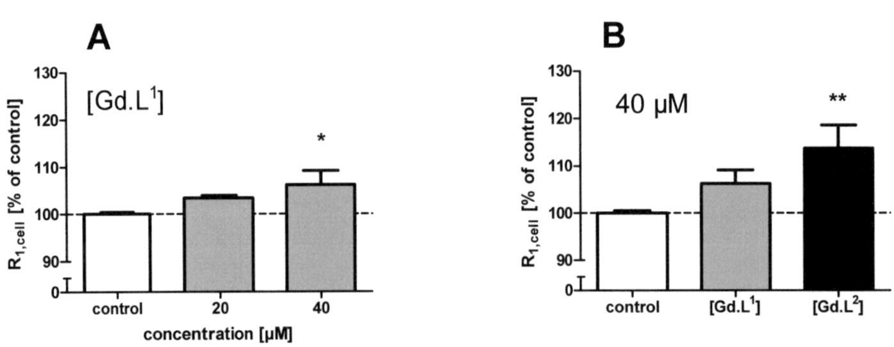

Fig. 4. Cellular relaxation rate $R_{1,cell}$ of differentiated N18 neuroblastoma cells. Values represent mean±SEM (n=2-5); **, $p>0.01$, *, $p>0.05$ significantly different to control (ANOVA, Dunnett´s multiple comparison test).

2.4 *In vivo* uptake and transport: MR and histology studies of [Gd.L^1] and [Gd.L^2] in rat brain

In the final step, we investigated the tracing abilities of these newly synthesized imaging probes, **[Gd.L^1]** and **[Gd.L^2]**, by means of MRI and classical histological methods in the same experimental animal. We performed a series of pressure and iontophoretic injections into the primary motor cortex (M1) of anaesthetized albino rats (Sprague Dawley) and evaluated the transport of these compounds at 24 and 48 h post-injection (see methods section for technical details). After the local injection of **[Gd.L^1]** in the primary motor cortex of the rat, the target area was visualized in T_1-weighted MRI as a large increase in signal (due to the decrease of the T_1 relaxation time; Figure 5A). Statistical analysis comparing baseline images (acquired either before or immediately after the injection) with images acquired after 24 and 48 h revealed a significant increase in T_1-weighted signal intensity in various brain regions

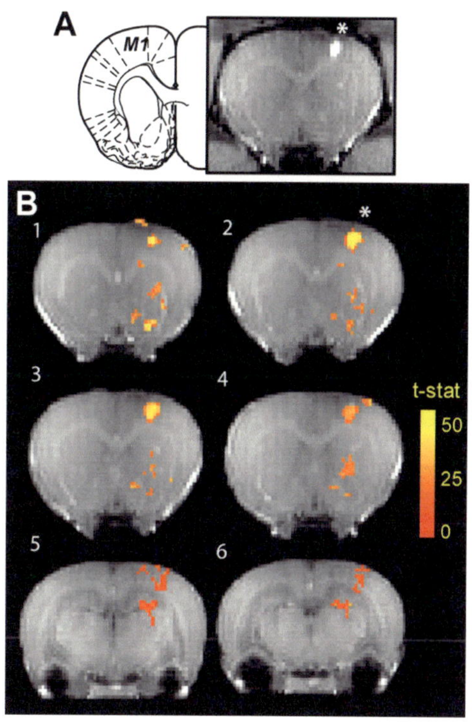

Fig. 5. *In vivo* neuronal tract tracing with **[Gd.L^1]**. Neuronal connections of the primary motor cortex M1 of the rat were investigated. (A) Coronal T_1-weighted images acquired 30 min after the injection of **[Gd.L^1]** in M1. Note the enhanced signal (asterisk) at the injection site. The inset shows a representative scheme of rat brain anatomy at the coordinates of the injection (Paxinos and Watson, 2007). (B) Shown are six coronal MR images illustrating the distribution of **[Gd.L^1]** signal in the brain after an injection in M1. The presence of signal is shown as statistical maps (unpaired t test; $p<0.01$) comparing the baseline (pre-injection scans) and scans acquired 48 h later, superimposed on the anatomical images. The results demonstrate local increases in signal due to **[Gd.L^1]** injection and long-range neuronal tract-tracing after 48 h in the striatum (1-4) and thalamus (5-6). After the last MRI session, the animal was euthanized and the histology is shown in Figure 6.

far away from the injection site. For instance, statistically significant increases in signal intensity were detected in the thalamus and the homologous contralateral M1 cortex (Figure 5B), areas that are well known to be connected with M1, suggesting that the tracer has actually been taken up by neurons *in vivo* and transported in the axons. This result corroborates the neuronal-tracing ability of **[Gd.L¹]** and its suitability for *in vivo* studies of brain connectivity. The MRI results obtained with **[Gd.L²]**, after injection into the M1 cortex, showed a comparable pattern of neural connections as in **[Gd.L¹]** (data not shown).

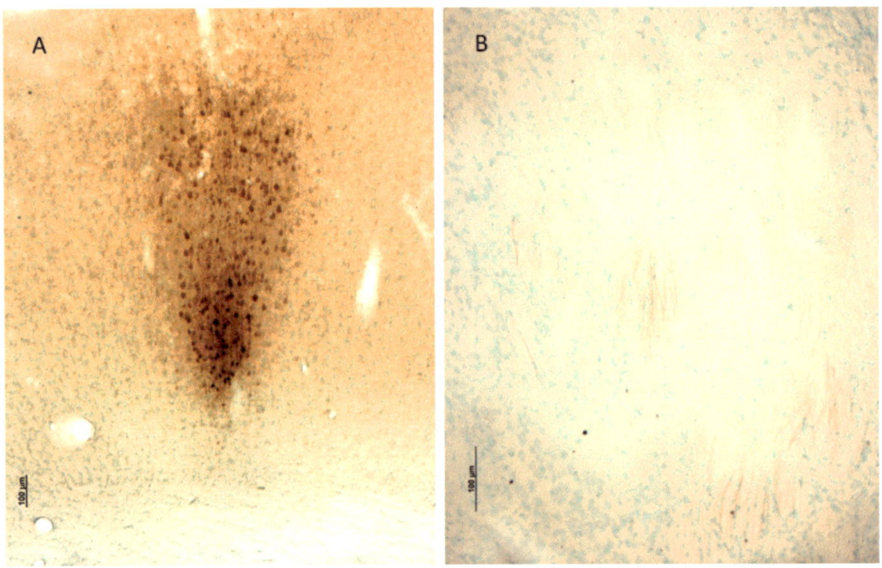

Fig. 6. Histological stain of the same brain as shown in Fig. 5, 48 h after an iontophoretic injection with **[Gd.L¹]**. Neurons at the injection site (A) have been stained. (B) Slightly stained fibres in the striatum bundles. The sections were counterstained with methyl green, visualizing cell bodies in the background. Bars: 100 µm.

Biocytin is a powerful tracer for visualizing connections with histological techniques. In a previous paper (Mishra et al., 2009) we have shown that both kinds of modified biocytin, aminopropyl and serine biocytin, are well suited for tracing and have, in addition, the advantage of being considerably more stable than the biocytin itself. We further investigated the post-mortem tissue sections of the same MR experimental animals. However, no stain could be seen in the case of **[Gd.L²]**, and in case of **[Gd.L¹]** the stain was restricted to places where the concentration is usually strongest, i.e. to the injection site and the striatum bundles (Figure 6). This could be explained by an impaired reaction with the avidin peroxidase-DAB (3,3'-Diaminobenzidine) cocktail, necessary for histological staining. This can be concluded from the fact that our *in vitro* uptake studies on N18 murine neuroblastoma cells clearly revealed that these probes were taken up well by neurons even at low concentrations. The lower modulation of proton longitudinal relaxivity upon avidin binding of **[Gd.L¹]** and **[Gd.L²]** (assuming a 2:1 stoichiometry of interaction) suggested that the interaction with avidin was strongly impaired. To further rule out the lack of uptake and/or transport and support the MRI findings, similar behavior was obtained after *in vivo* injections of **[Fluo.L¹]** into the primary motor cortex (M1) of anaesthetized albino rats and evaluation of the transport of this compound 24 h post-injection. We observed by fluorescence microscopy that [**Fluo.L**[1]] had been taken up by neurons (Figure 7), but we could not detect any stain in the same section using the staining technique depending on the biotin-avidin peroxidase-DAB (3,3'-Diaminobenzidine) cocktail.

It is conceivable that the modifications introduced in the model modified biocytin (aminopropyl and serine biocytin) described above, together with the significant increase in molecular weight by about a factor of 2.5, sterically hinder the staining with avidin peroxidase-DAB cocktail in cells substantially, but retain the uptake and transport properties of the resulting contrast agent.

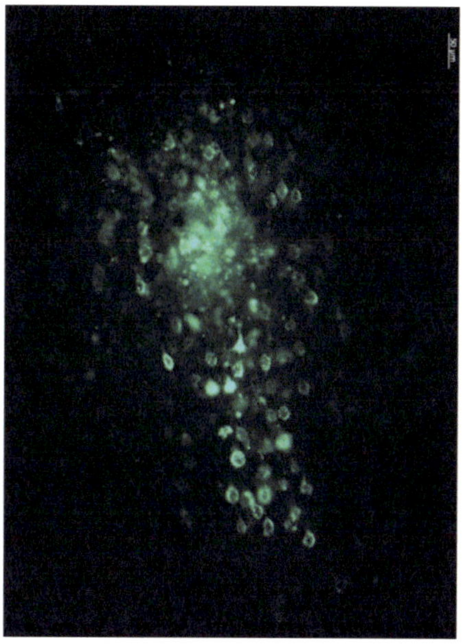

Fig. 7. Injection site in the motor cortex of a rat, 24 h after injection with [**Fluo.L**[1]].
It can be seen that the neurons have taken up the tracer. Under transmission light, no stain could be seen, although the same section had undergone an avidin-biotin reaction. Bar 50 μm.

3. Conclusion

In summary, we present data on the functionalization of biocytin, a well known neuronal tract tracer, and demonstrate the validity of the approach by showing cortical connectivity in live rats with the help of MRI. Our study offers a new platform for the development of multimodal molecular imaging tools for brain connectivity studies *in vivo*.

4. Materials and methods

4.1 Chemicals

All solvents and reagents were purchased at analytical grade from commercial suppliers (Acros, Aldrich, Fluka, Merck, Strem and VWR) and were used without further purification unless otherwise stated. All air- or water-sensitive chemicals were stored under an inert atmosphere. Ultra pure de-ionised water (18 MΩ cm^{-1}) was used throughout.

4.2 Chromatography

Flash column chromatography was performed using flash silica gel 60 (70-230 mesh) from Merck. Thin layer chromatography (TLC) was performed on aluminum sheet silica gel plates with 0.2 mm thick silica gel 60 F_{254} (E. Merck) using different mobile phases. The compounds were visualized by UV irradiation (254 nm) or iodine staining. Reverse phase HPLC was performed at room temperature on a Varian PrepStar Instrument, equipped with PrepStar SD-1 pump heads. UV absorbance was measured using a ProStar 335 photodiode array detector at 214 nm. Analytical RP-HPLC was performed in a stainless steel Chromsep (length 250 mm, internal diameter 4.6 mm and particle size 8 μm) C_{18} column and semi-preparative RP-HPLC was performed on a stainless steel Chromsep (length 250 mm, internal diameter 21.2 mm and particle size 5 μm) C_{18} column (Varian). The compounds were purified using one of the following two methods. Method A: gradient with the mobile phase starting from 95% solvent A (H_2O) and 5% of solvent B (MeOH) to 70% B in 10 min, 90% B in 18 min, 90% B isocratic till 24 min and decreased to 5% B in 28 min. Method B: 95% solvent A (H_2O, 0.1% HCOOH) and 5% solvent B (acetonitrile, 0.1% HCOOH) to 70% solvent B in 10 min and then to 100% in the next 8 min running isocratic for 12 min and then back to 5% solvent B in the next 2 min. The flow rate generally used for analytical HPLC was 1 mL/min and for semi-preparative HPLC 15 mL/min. All the HPLC-grade solvents for HPLC were filtered through a nylon-66 Millipore filter (0.45 μm) prior to use.

4.3 Spectroscopy

^{1}H NMR and ^{13}C NMR spectra were recorded on Bruker DRX250 and DRX400 spectrometers at room temperature. The ^{1}H NMR chemical shifts were adjusted to the residual protons of the solvent peaks which were referenced to TMS (0.0 ppm), and ^{13}C NMR chemical shifts were referenced to $CDCl_3$ (77.0 ppm).
Electrospray ionization mass spectra (ESI-MS in positive and negative ion mode) were performed on an ion trap SL 1100 system (Agilent) and High Resolution (HR) mass spectra were measured on Bruker Daltonics Apex II FT-ICR-MS (Bruker).
Inductively coupled plasma optical emission spectrometry (ICP-OES) for the evaluation of the Gd^{3+} concentration was performed using a Jobin–Yvon Ultima 2 spectrometer.

4.4 *In vitro* MR tube measurements

Longitudinal and transverse relaxation times (T_1 and T_2) of the [**Gd.L^1**] and [**Gd.L^2**] were examined using a vertical 7T (300 MHz)/60-cm diameter bore magnet (Bruker BioSpin). Four different concentrations (1 mM, 0.75 mM, 0.5 mM, 0.25 mM) of [**Gd.L^1**] and [**Gd.L^2**] were prepared in Phosphate-Buffered-Saline (PBS) in 1.5 mL Eppendorf tubes at physiological pH to measure relaxivity. Each tube was filled with 400 µl of the CA solution. The y-axis intercept of the linear regression plot of the relaxation rate obtained for these tubes with the corresponding concentration of CA gave the diamagnetic relaxation rate ($1/T_d$).
To measure the changes in r_1 and r_2 upon binding to avidin, MRI experiments were performed with increasing concentrations of avidin proportional to a constant concentration of [**Gd.L^1**] and [**Gd.L^2**] (0.25 mM) incubated for 1 h at 37°C. The stock solution of avidin (1 mM) was prepared in PBS at pH 7.4.

Axial images were obtained for the set of tubes at 7T and the T_1/T_2 values were then calculated.
Relaxivity at different concentrations of avidin was then calculated using equation [1].

$$r_{1,obs} = (1/T_{1,obs}-1/T_{1,d}) \ / \ [Gd.L^n] \qquad (1)$$

where $T_{1,obs}$ is the measured T_1, $T_{1,d}$ is the diamagnetic contribution of the solvent (calculated to be 2400 - 2700 ms) and [GdL^n] is the concentration in mmol/L of the appropriate Gd(III) complex (n = 1-2).

4.5 Synthesis of ligands and tracers

(*S*)-methyl 3,15-dioxo-10-(5-((3a*R*,4*R*,6a*S*)-2-oxo-hexahydro-1*H*-thieno[3,4-*d*]imidazol-4-yl)pentanoyl)-1-phenyl-16-(4,7,10-tris(2-*tert*-butoxy-2-oxoethyl)-1,4,7,10-tetraazacyclododecan-1-yl)-2-oxa-4,10,14-triazahexadecane-5-carboxylate (7). A solution of compound **6** (0.3 g, 0.52 mmol), NMM (0.12 mL, 1.0 mmol) and HOBt (0.11 g, 0.57 mmol) in anhydrous DMF (15 mL) was stirred at 0-5°C for 15 min and then EDC (0.08 g, 0.57 mmol) was added. The reaction mixture was stirred overnight at room temperature. Completion of the reaction was verified by ESI-MS, the solution was poured into water (50 mL) and extracted with EtOAc (3 x 50 mL). The combined organic layers were dried over anhydrous Na_2SO_4, filtered and the filtrate evaporated under reduced pressure. The residue was purified by column chromatography (silica gel, 10% MeOH in CH_2Cl_2, R_f = 0.15) to give **7** as a yellow gum (0.28 g, 48%). ^{1}H NMR ($CDCl_3$, 250 MHz), δ (ppm): 1.10-1.30 (m, 2H); 1.42 (s, 18H); 1.52 (s, 10H); 1.60-1.95 (m, 12H); 2.03 (br s, 2H); 2.34 (br s, 3H); 2.62-2.99 (m, 6H); 3.32-3.94 (m, 20H); 3.76 (br s, 6H); 3.94-3.98 (m, 2H); 4.23-4.43 (m, 2H); 4.47-4.63 (m, 1H); 5.12 (s, 2H); 5.48-5.77 (m, 1H); 7.29-7.43 (m, 5H). ESI-MS (+): calcd $C_{56}H_{93}N_9O_{13}S$: m/z 1133.5 $(M+H)^+$; found 1133.2 $(M+H)^+$.

[4,7-Bis-carboxymethyl-10-(2-(3-(*N*-((*S*)-5-amino-5-carboxypentyl)-5-((3a*R*,4*R*,6a*S*)-2-oxo-hexahydro-1H-thieno[3,4-d]imidazol-4-yl)pentanamido)propylamino)-2-oxoethyl)-1,4,7,10-tetraaza-cyclododec-1-yl]-acetic acid (L^1). A solution of compound **7** (0.25 g, 0.22 mmol), 10% Pd-C (0.07 g) and H_2 (50 psi) in MeOH (20 mL) was stirred at room temperature in Parr-apparatus for 8 h. Completion of the reaction was verified by ESI-MS, the solution was filtered through a G-4 sintered funnel, and the filtrate was evaporated under reduced pressure. This crude product was further dissolved in TFA (20 mL) and stirred overnight at room temperature. TFA was evaporated under reduced pressure. A solution of crude product in THF:MeOH:water (3:2:2) (10 mL) was stirred at 0-5°C for 15 min and then LiOH (0.11 g, 4.7 mmol) was added. The reaction mixture was stirred for 2 h at room temperature. Completion of the reaction was verified by ESI-MS, the solvent was evaporated under reduced pressure and the residue was purified by preparative HPLC (t_R = 3.8 min). After lyophilization, L^1 was obtained as a light yellow sticky solid (0.1 g, 56%). ^{1}H NMR (D_2O, 250 MHz), δ (ppm): 1.20-2.16 (m, 16H); 2.47 (t, *J*=7.0 Hz, 2H); 2.70-3.90 (br. m, 32H); 4.40-4.53 (m, 1H); 4.24-4.28 (m, 1H). ^{13}C NMR (D_2O, 62.9 MHz), δ (ppm): 24.9; 27.8; 28.2; 30.5; 30.9; 32.8; 35.0; 39.7; 42.4; 46.2; 47.9; 48.4; 50.7; 50.9; 51.2; 53.2; 53.8; 57.1; 58.1; 58.6; 63.0; 64.8; 164.2; 165.3; 167.2; 177.1; 178.0; 178.8. ESI-MS (+): calcd $C_{35}H_{61}N_9O_{11}S$: m/z 816.4 $(M+H)^+$; found 816.3 $(M+H)^+$.

Methyl 2-(benzyloxycarbonylamino)-3-bromopropanoate (8). *N*-carbobenzyloxy-L-serine methyl ester (2 g, 8 mmol) and PPh_3 (4 g, 16 mmol) were added in 50 ml anhydrous DMF.

Finally *N*-bromosuccinimide (2.8 g, 16 mmol) was added in small aliquots to the reaction mixture. The mixture was stirred for 30 minutes at 50 °C. Heating bath was removed and 2 ml of MeOH was added to quench the reaction. 100 ml of ether was added and the reaction mixture was extracted with 100 ml water. The organic layer was dried over anhydrous Na_2SO_4, concentrated under vacuum and purified by column chromatography (silica gel, 30% EtOAc in n-hexane) to give **8** as a yellow gum (2.1 g, 84%). ^{1}H NMR ($CDCl_3$, 400 MHz), δ (ppm): 3.40-3.70 (m, 5H); 4.57-4.62 (m, 1H); 4.91 (s, 2H); 5.49-5.58 (m, 1H); 7.07-7.28 (m, 5H). ^{13}C NMR ($CDCl_3$, 100 MHz), δ (ppm) 33.6; 53.0; 54.2; 67.2; 128.0; 128.2; 128.4; 139.5; 159.5; 169.2. ESI-MS (+): calcd $C_{12}H_{14}BrNO_4$: m/z 317.1 $(M+H)^+$ and found 317.3 $(M+H)^+$.

Methyl 2-(benzyloxycarbonylamino)-3-(1,4,7,10-tetraazacyclododecan-1-yl)propanoate (9). Compound **8** (0.6 g, 1.9 mmol) in 25 ml of toluene was added dropwise to the solution of cyclen (2g, 11.6 mmol) in 100 ml of toluene at room temperature. The reaction mixture was refluxed for 18 h. The reaction mixture was cooled, filtered through a G-4 sintered funnel; filtrate was evaporated under reduced pressure, dissolved in 200 ml CH_2Cl_2, extracted from the water (4x100 ml). The organic layers were combined, dried over anhydrous Na_2SO_4 and then concentrated under vacuum to obtain the product with cyclen. The residue was purified by column chromatography (silica gel, 10% MeOH in CH_2Cl_2) to give **9** as colorless oil (0.34 g, 44%). ^{1}H NMR ($CDCl_3$, 250 MHz), δ (ppm): 2.20-3.02 (m, 18H); 3.69 (s, 3H); 4.36 (br s, 1H); 5.02 (s, 2H); 5.07-5.25 (m, 4H); 7.25-7.40 (m, 5H). ^{13}C NMR ($CDCl_3$, 62.9 MHz), δ (ppm) 43.5; 52.5; 53.2; 53.7; 53.9; 55.0; 59.9; 66.3; 127.7; 128.9; 132.1; 134.2; 161.4; 176.8. ESI-HRMS (+): calcd $C_{20}H_{33}N_5O_4$: m/z 408.2605 $(M+H)^+$; found 408.2607 $(M+H)^+$.

[4,7-Bis-butoxycarbonylmethyl-10-(2-(benzyloxycarbonylamino)-3-methoxy-3-oxopropyl - 1,4,7,10-tetraaza-cyclododec-1-yl]-acetic acid *tert*-butyl ester (10). A solution of compound **9** (4.1 g, 10.1 mmol) and sodium carbonate (6.4 g, 60.0 mmol) was added in 70 ml MeCN (dry) and heated at 60 °C for 1 h. The reaction mixture was cooled and *tert*–butylbromoacetate (5.29 ml, 27.1 mmol) in MeCN (25 ml) was added dropwise. The mixture was then refluxed for 6 h. It was then filtered through a G-4 sintered funnel, washed with MeCN and concentrated under vacuum. The obtained residue was taken in CH_2Cl_2 (100 ml) and extracted with water (2x50 ml). The organic layer was dried over anhydrous Na_2SO_4 and concentrated to yellow oil. The residue was purified by column chromatography (silica gel, 5% MeOH in CH_2Cl_2) to give **10** as light yellow solid (3.5 g, 72%). ^{1}H NMR ($CDCl_3$, 250 MHz), δ (ppm): 1.32 (s, 9H); 1.39 (s, 18H); 1.83-2.56 (m, 8H); 2.60-3.50 (m, 16H); 3.66 (s, 3H); 4.47 (br s, 1H); 4.71 (br s, 1H); 5.24 (s, 2H); 7.16-7.42 (m, 5H). ^{13}C NMR ($CDCl_3$, 62.9 MHz), δ (ppm): 27.8; 28.0; 50.3; 50.5; 51.3; 52.3; 52.6; 53.3; 55.5; 56.1; 56.5; 66.9; 82.1; 82.4; 127.7; 127.9; 128.3; 135.9; 157.0; 171.8; 172.7; 173.1. ESI-HRMS (+): calcd $C_{38}H_{63}N_5O_{10}$: m/z 750.4647 $(M+H)^+$; found 751.4641 $(M+H)^+$.

2-(benzyloxycarbonylamino)-3-(4,7,10-tris(2-*tert*-butoxy-2-oxoethyl)-1,4,7,10-tetraazacyclododecan-1-yl)propanoic acid (11). A solution of compound **10** (0.1 g, 0.13 mmol) was stirred in 7 mL of THF:MeOH:water (3:2:2) at 0-5°C for 15 min and then LiOH (6.5 mg, 0.27 mmol) was added. The reaction mixture was stirred for 2 h at room temperature. The progress of the reaction was checked by ESI-MS. After completion, the reaction mixture was concentrated under reduced pressure and **11** was obtained as white powder (0.76 g, 64%). ^{1}H NMR ($CDCl_3$, 250 MHz), δ (ppm): 1.32 (s, 9H); 1.39 (s, 18H); 1.83-2.56 (m, 8H); 2.60-3.50 (m, 16H); 4.47 (br s, 1H); 4.71 (br s, 1H); 5.24 (s, 2H); 7.16-7.42 (m, 5H). ^{13}C NMR ($CDCl_3$, 62.9 MHz), δ (ppm): 27.8; 28.0; 50.3; 50.5; 52.3; 52.6; 53.3; 55.5; 56.1; 56.5; 66.9; 82.1; 82.4; 127.7; 127.9; 128.3; 135.9; 157.0; 171.8; 172.7; 173.1. ESI-MS (+): calcd $C_{37}H_{61}N_5O_{10}$: m/z 736.9 $(M+H)^+$; found 737.1 $(M+H)^+$.

[4,7-Bis-butoxycarbonylmethyl-10-(2-(benzyloxycarbonylamino)-3-((*R*)-5-(*tert*-butoxycarbonylamino)-6-methoxy-6-oxohexylamino)-3-oxopropyl-1,4,7,10-tetraaza-cyclododec-1-yl]-acetic acid *tert*-butyl ester (12). Compound 11 (0.29 g, 0.4 mmol) was dissolved in DMF (5 ml, dry) and NMM (0.1 ml, 0.9 mmol), EDC (0.086 g, 0.44 mmol) and (*R*)-methyl 6-amino-2-(*tert*-butoxycarbonylamino)hexanoate (0.16 mmol, 0.6 mmol) were added under N_2 atmosphere. The reaction mixture was stirred at 60°C for 1h. Thereafter, HOBt (0.06 g, 0.44 mmol) was added and the heating was continued for 3 h. DMF was evaporated under reduced pressure and the obtained residue was dissolved in EtOAc. The organic layer was washed with water, dried under anhydrous Na_2SO_4, and concentrated under reduced pressure to obtain crude yellowish residue. This was purified by column chromatography (silica gel, 5% MeOH in CH_2Cl_2) to obtain 12 as yellowish solid (46%, 0.18 g). ^{1}H NMR (300 MHz, $CDCl_3$), δ (ppm): 1.20 - 1.54 (m, 38 H), 1.54 - 1.88 (m, 5 H), 1.87 - 2.65 (m, 9 H), 2.64 - 3.12 (m, 8 H), 3.12 - 3.52 (m, 6 H), 3.69 - 3.81 (m, 3 H), 4.15 - 4.32 (m, 1 H), 4.67 (br. s., 1 H), 4.91 - 5.37 (m, 2 H), 7.19 - 7.44 (m, 5 H). ^{13}C NMR (75 MHz, $CDCl_3$), δ (ppm): 22.7, 27.8, 27.9, 28.0, 28.2, 28.8, 31.9, 38.8, 49.9, 52.0, 53.3, 53.5, 55.4, 56.3, 56.4, 66.1, 79.4, 81.8, 81.9, 82.3, 127.3, 127.4, 128.1, 136.8, 155.4, 157.0, 171.8, 172.0, 173.3. ESI-MS (+): calcd $C_{49}H_{83}N_7O_{13}$: *m/z* 978.6 $(M+H)^+$; found 978.5 $(M+H)^+$.

[4,7-Bis-butoxycarbonylmethyl-10-(2-amino-3-((*R*)-5-(*tert*-butoxycarbonylamino)-6-methoxy-6-oxohexylamino)-3-oxopropyl-1,4,7,10-tetraaza-cyclododec-1-yl]-acetic acid *tert*-butyl ester (13). Compound **12** (0.05 g, 0.05 mmol) was dissolved in ethanol (10 ml) and Pd-C (0.005 g, 10% w/w) was suspended. The mixture was stirred in a Parr aparatus under H_2 atmosphere (3 atm) for 4 h. The solvent was evaporated under reduced pressure to obtain the product **13** as yellowish oil in quantitative yield. ^{1}H NMR (300 MHz, $CDCl_3$), δ (ppm): 1.18 - 1.36 (m, 5 H), 1.36 - 1.41 (m, 11 H), 1.41 - 1.46 (m, 23 H), 1.49 - 1.58 (m, 2 H), 1.58 - 1.67 (m, 1 H), 1.69 - 1.85 (m, 1 H), 1.93 - 2.35 (m, 4 H), 2.42 - 2.77 (m, 6 H), 2.76 - 3.02 (m, 6 H), 3.08 - 3.39 (m, 7 H), 3.40 - 3.53 (m, 1 H), 3.68 (s, 3 H), 4.15 - 4.21 (m, 1 H). ^{13}C NMR (75 MHz, $CDCl_3$), δ (ppm): 22.7, 27.9, 28.1, 28.3, 28.8, 32.0, 39.3, 49.9, 51.2, 52.2, 53.5, 55.4, 56.8, 57.8, 79.6, 81.6, 81.9, 82.5, 155.5, 167.67, 167.75, 170.7, 173.4. ESI-MS (+): calcd $C_{41}H_{77}N_7O_{11}$: *m/z* 844.6 $(M+H)^+$; found 844.5 $(M+H)^+$.

[4,7-Bis-carboxymethyl-10-(3-((*R*)-5-amino-5-carboxypentylamino)-3-oxo-2-(5-((3a*S*,4*S*,6a*R*)-2-oxo-hexahydro-1*H*-thieno[3,4-*d*]imidazol-4-yl)pentanamido)propyl)-1,4,7,10-tetraaza-cyclododec-1-yl]-acetic acid (L^2). Compound **13** (0.045 g, 0.053 mmol) was dissolved in anhydrous DMF (2 ml) and HATU (0.022 g, 0.058 mmol) and DIPEA (0.019 ml, 0.1 mmol) were added under inert atmosphere. The reaction mixture was stirred at room temperature for 18 h. The formation of **14** was confirmed by ESI-MS, the solvent was evaporated under reduced pressure and the residue was redissolved in ethylacetate and washed with water. The collected organic layer was dried with anhydrous Na_2SO_4 and evaporated under reduced pressure till dry. The residue was subjected to global deprotection. Methyl ester hydrolysis was carried out by LiOH (0.13 mmol, 0.005 g) in THF:MeOH:H_2O (3:3:2) for 2h. The solvent was evaporated and the residue dissolved in TFA (10 ml, neat) to hydrolyze *tert*-Bu-ester and deprotect the Boc group. TFA was evaporated under reduced pressure to obtain a yellowish residue. The residue was redissolved in water, the pH was increased to 7 and thereafter purified by RP-HPLC (t_R = 4.8) to obtain the product, $\mathbf{L^2}$, as a yellow sticky solid. ^{1}H NMR (300 MHz, D_2O), δ (ppm): 1.33 (br. s., 4 H), 1.42 - 1.60 (m, 5 H), 1.60 - 1.72 (m, 1 H), 1.74 - 1.92 (m, 2 H), 2.16 - 2.38 (m, 2 H), 2.65 - 2.96 (m, 6 H), 2.98 - 3.36 (m, 13 H), 3.41 - 3.60 (m, 3 H), 3.62 (s, 1 H), 3.64 - 3.82 (m, 4 H), 3.84 - 4.03 (m, 3 H), 4.25 - 4.33 (m, 1 H), 4.36

(dd, J=7.88, 4.58 Hz, 1 H), 4.53 (dd, J=7.63, 5.09 Hz, 1 H). ^{13}C NMR (75 MHz, D_2O), δ (ppm): 20.8, 20.9, 23.9, 24.0, 26.9, 27.2, 27.3, 29.0, 34.0, 38.1, 38.9, 46.8, 48.5, 49.9, 51.5, 52.4, 52.8, 53.2, 54.58, 54.68, 55.1, 55.8, 59.4, 61.2, 149.9, 164.5, 173.0, 176.8. Compound 14: ESI-MS (+): calcd $C_{51}H_{91}N_9O_{13}S$: m/z 1070.6 $(M+H)^+$; found 1070.5 $(M+H)^+$. Compound L^2: ESI-MS (-): calcd $C_{33}H_{57}N_9O_{11}S$: m/z 786.4 $(M-H)^-$; found 786.4 $(M-H)^-$.

General Preparation of Gadolinium Complexes of L^1 and L^2. Gadolinium complexes of **L^1** and **L^2** were prepared from corresponding solutions of the ligands (1 eq) and solutions of $GdCl_3.6H_2O$ (1.1 eq). The reaction mixture was stirred at 60°C for 20 h. The pH was periodically checked and adjusted to 6.5 using solutions of NaOH (1 M) and HCl (1 N) as needed. After completion, the reaction mixture was cooled and passed through chelex-100 to trap free Gd^{3+} ions, and the Gd-loaded complexes were eluted. The absence of free Gd^{3+} was checked with xylenol orange indicator. The fractions were lyophilized to obtain off-white solids. These complexes were characterized by ESI-MS in positive and negative mode and the appropriate isotope pattern distributions for Gd^{3+} were recorded.

[Gd.L^1]. ESI-MS (+): calcd $C_{35}H_{58}{}^{155}GdN_9O_{11}S$: m/z 971.3 $[M+H]^+$; found 971.4 $[M+H]^+$, r_{1p} = 5.52 [$mM^{-1}s^{-1}$] at 300 MHz.

[Gd.L^2]. ESI-MS (+): calcd $C_{33}H_{54}{}^{155}GdNaN_9O_{11}S$: m/z 965.2 $[M+Na]^+$; found 965.3 $[M+Na]^+$, r_{1p} = 7.27 [$mM^{-1}s^{-1}$] at 300 MHz.

4.6 *In vitro* cell studies of [Gd.L^1], [Gd.L^2] and [Fluo-L^1]

4.6.1 Cell culture

N18 mouse neuroblastoma cells (kind gift of Prof. Bernd Hamprecht, University of Tübingen, Germany) were cultured as a monolayer at 37°C with 5% CO_2 in antibiotic free Dulbecco's Modified Eagle's Medium (DMEM) supplemented with 10% fetal bovine serum (FBS) and 4 mM L-glutamine, (all purchased from Biochrom AG). Cells were passaged by trypsinization with trypsin/EDTA 0.05/0.02% (w/v) in phosphate-buffered saline (PBS; Biochrom AG, Germany) for 5 minutes every second to third day. Prior to experiments the serum content was stepwise reduced to 0.625% to induce morphological differentiation.

4.6.2 Preparation of labeling solutions

CA were dissolved in water and the concentration was determined by BMS measurement for **[Gd.L^1]** and **[Gd.L^2]** or by absorbance of fluorescein for **[Fluo.L^1]**. For each experiment, dilutions from these stocks were freshly made in incubation medium and thoroughly mixed at indicated concentrations.

4.6.3 Live cell imaging

Microscopy was done in single channel Ibidi slides (Ibidi GmbH, Germany) by inoculation of N18 cells (3 x 10^5 cells/ml) cultured in Dulbecco's Modified Eagle's Medium supplemented with 0.625% fetal bovine serum and 4 mM L-glutamine (all purchased from Biochrom AG). After reaching 70-80% confluency, cells were incubated with 50 μM of **[Fluo.L^1]** for 12 hours. Before washing cells were incubated with nuclear stain Bisbenzimid 33342 (Hoechst 33342) for 5 min. Afterwards, extracellular fluorescence was quenched by the addition of ice-cold Trypan Blue for 3 min (Rennert et al.). After repeated cell washings with Hank's buffered saline solution (HBSS, Biochrom AG, Germany), fluorescence microscopy was performed on a Zeiss Axiovert 200M (Carl Zeiss AG, Germany) with a Plan-Apochromat 63X objective to observe the cellular localization of **[Fluo.L^1]**. The imaging conditions were kept constant for the observation of different samples. Cellular localization and distribution of **[Fluo.L¹]** was determined by irradiating with blue light (470 nm) and observing at 525 nm, and nuclear labeling by Hoechst was imaged at 460 nm. Also phase contrast images with Differential Interference Contrast (DIC) of the same area were made to detect if the cells maintain their normal morphology in the presence of compound.

4.6.4 MR measurement in cells

For MR imaging, serum deprived N18 cells (1.25% FBS) were cultured in 175 cm^2 tissue culture flasks and labeled with 20 or 40 μM of **[Gd.L¹]** or **[Gd.L²]** in HBSS/10mM HEPES for 6h. After incubation samples of the treatment solution were collected, if required centrifuged, and 500 μl were used for determination of R_1 and R_2. Cells were repeatedly washed with HBSS, trypsinized, centrifuged and re-suspended in 0.5 ml Eppendorf tubes at a cell density of 1 x 10^7/500μl in complete medium. Cells were allowed to settle before MR measurements. Tubes with medium only and cells without CA were used as controls. Two tubes of treatment solutions, HBSS/10 mM HEPES as well as of cells for each condition were used. Experiments were done at least twice.

MR imaging of the cell pellets at room temperature (~21 °C) was performed in a 3 T (123 MHz) human MR scanner (MAGNETOM Tim Trio, Siemens Healthcare, Germany), using a 12-channel RF Head coil and slice selective measurements from a slice with a thickness of 1 mm positioned through the cell pellet.

T_1 was measured using an inversion-recovery sequence, with an adiabatic inversion pulse followed by a turbo-spin-echo readout. Between 10 and 15 images were taken, with the time between inversion and readout varying from 23 ms to 3000 ms. With a repetition time of 10 s, 15 echoes were acquired per scan and averaged six times. For T_2, a homewritten spin-echo sequence was used with echo times varying from 18 ms to 1000 ms in about 10 steps and a repetition time of 8 s. Diffusion sensitivity was reduced by minimizing the crusher gradients surrounding the refocusing pulse. All experiments scanned 256^2 voxels in a field-of-view of 110 mm in both directions resulting in a voxel volume of 0.43 × 0.43 × 1 mm^3.

Data analysis was performed by fitting to relaxation curves with self-written routines under MATLAB 7.1 R14 (The Mathworks Inc., United States). The series of T_1 relaxation data were fitted to the following equation.

T_1 series with varying $t = T_I$: $S = S_0 (1 - \exp(-t / T_1) + S_{(TI = 0)} \exp(-t / T_1)$.

Nonlinear least-squares fitting of three parameters S_0, $S_{(TI = 0)}$, and T_1 was done for manually selected regions-of-interest with the Trust-Region Reflective Newton algorithm implemented in MATLAB. The quality of the fit was controlled by visual inspection and by calculating the mean errors and residuals.

Evaluation of the signal intensities in the T_1-weighted MR images were performed in ImageJ (http://rsb.info.nih.gov/ij) by defining a circular region of interest (ROI) inside one tube image and measuring the mean signal intensity and standard deviation in the included voxels. Further statistical analyses were performed in GraphPad Prism 5.03 (GraphPad Software, Inc., USA).

4.7 *In vivo* rat experiments

To test whether **[Gd.L¹]**, **[Gd.L²]** and **[Fluo.L¹]** were transported inside cells and could be visualized by MR and histological methods, we performed injections of all three compounds into the primary motor cortex of 8 albino rats (Sprague Dawley). Three of them (with

[Gd.L[1]]) were sacrificed after 24 h and the other three (one with **[Gd.L[1]]** and two with **[Gd.L[2]]**) were euthanized after 48 h. The remaining two (with **[Fluo.L[1]]**) were euthanized after 24 h.

4.7.1 Injections

All rats were anaesthetized with 2% isoflurane (Abbott) and placed in a stereotaxic frame (Kopf Instruments). After additional use of xylocain for local analgesia in the surgery area, a craniotomy was performed and a pulled fused silica capillary (ID 50μm; OD 150 μm; tip diameter 20-30 μm) was placed in the primary motor cortex at a depth of 1.2 mm below the surface. One compound per animal was then injected using a pressure cell containing the compound attached to the other end of the fused silica capillary. 100 nl of 4% tracer solution was injected at a flow rate of 3.3 nl/min. After injection, the capillary was left in place for 10 minutes before retracting it stepwise to avoid backflow of the injected solution.

In some cases we made iontophoretic injections, using borosilicate pipettes with tip diameters of 20-25 μm. In case of the injection shown in Fig. 6, injection time was 35 min (7s on, 7 s off) with a current of 4 μA. In case of the injection shown in Fig. 7, injection time was 70 min (7 s on, 7 s off) with a current of 10 μA.

At the end of the procedure, the animals received an intraperitoneal injection of analgesics and antibiotics [5mg/kg Baytril® (Bayer) and 2.5mg/kg Finadyne® (Essex)]. The animals to be left for 48 h received another injection of analgesics and antibiotics after 24 h.

4.7.2 *In vivo* MRI experiments

For the MRI experiments, the animals were anaesthetized with 1.5-2% isoflurane and placed in a home-made quadrature coil integrated within a stereotaxic animal holder. The head holder was adapted with movable bite and ear bars and positioned fixed on a magnet chair. This allowed precise positioning of the animal with respect to the coil and the magnet, avoiding movement artifacts. Body temperature, heart rate, CO_2 and SpO_2 were monitored throughout the scanning session. We typically scanned the animals before, immediately after and 24-48 h after the injection of CAs. One scan session consisted on 5 to 7 scans of 18 min each.

Experiments were carried out in a vertical 7T (300 MHz)/60-cm diameter bore magnet (Bruker BioSpin, Ettlingen). The saddle coil, which was designed to generate a homogeneous field over the whole rat brain, was used to transmit and receive. The MR system was controlled by a Bruker BioSpec console (ParaVision 3, 4 and 5 at different time periods) running under Linux operating system. We used a Modified Driven Equilibrium Fourier Transform (MDEFT) method with MDEFT-preparation (Lee et al., 1995) to obtain T_1-weighted anatomical images. The scan parameters were: TR = 22.2 ms, TE = 4.8 ms, FA = 20°, ID = 1000 ms and four segments. The geometric parameters of the 3D scans were: matrix 192×136×100, FOV = 48×34×25 mm and voxel size 0.25×0.25×0.25 mm.

The MRI images were analyzed with custom-developed Matlab functions (v7.5.0, MathWorks). An automated realignment procedure of SPM (statistical parametric mapping, www.fil.ion.ucl.ac.uk) was applied to co-register all scans. For statistical analysis the image intensity was normalized to reference signal intensity in the head muscles. Statistical maps were generated by implementing a Student's t-test (unpaired) at each voxel comparing brain images before and 24-48h after CAs injection. The significant voxels represent the pattern of T_1-weighted MRI signal enhancement induced by the neuronal transport of CAs. The arbitrary significance threshold was set to $P < 0.01$ (uncorrected for multiple comparisons) for individual voxels, and a minimum cluster size of 3 contiguous voxels constituting at least 3% of total number of voxels for a given region of interest (ROI). The same data were also tested for lower or higher p-values.

4.7.3 Perfusion

After the last MRI session, the animals received a lethal intraperitoneal injection of the barbiturate Pentobarbital sodium (Narcoren from Merial; 2.5 ml/kg body weight). After cessation of all reflexes, the chest of the animal was opened and 0.4 ml of Heparin-Sodium 25000 (ratiopharm) was injected into the heart in order to prevent coagulation. Then a cannula was inserted and the animal was perfused with iosotonic saline (using NaCl 0.9 E from Fresenius) for about 5 minutes and then with the fixative (commercially available 4% paraformaldehyde, phosphate buffered; Roti-Histofix 4% from Carl Roth).
The brain was removed from the skull and kept in the fixative over night. The next day the brain was transferred into 30% sucrose in demineralized water and kept there for at least 4 days until it had sunk. The brain was then sliced into serial sections with a cryotome at a thickness of 70 μm.

4.7.4 Histological procedure

The protocol for the biotin-avidin reaction largely followed that by Horikawa and Armstrong (Horikawa and Armstrong, 1988) with some modifications suggested by Dr. Michaela Schweizer (personal communication). In detail: the sections were collected in phosphate buffer (PB, 0.1 M; pH 7.3), rinsed again in PB and then transferred into 1% H_2O_2 in PB for 1 h, in order to block endogenous peroxidase activity. After rinsing 3 times in PB, the sections were kept for 90 min in Triton X-100 (2% in 0.1 M PB from Carl Roth). They were then incubated overnight in avidin-conjugated peroxidase (ABC Elite PK 6100 from Linaris, 1% in 0.1 M PB: i.e. adding 10 drops per 50 μl of each of the two solutions to 49 ml of buffer. Note that the ABC-mixture must stand for 30 min before use). On the next day, the sections were rinsed 2 x 10 min in PB (0.1 M) and then 2 x 10 min in Tris/HCl at pH 7.9 (using a 0.1 M solution of tris-(hydroxymethyl)-aminomethane and pH adjusted to 7.9 with HCl). The sections were then transferred into a solution of diamino benzidine (DAB) and H_2O_2 (DAB tablet were dissolved in demineralized water) for 30 - 45 min. After washing three times in Tris/HCl, the sections were transferred into 0.05 M PB and mounted on electrostatic slides (Superfrost Plus, Menzel, ThermoScientific), air-dried over night, dehydrated in ethanol (70%, 2 x 99%, 1 x 100% ethanol, 2 x terpineole and 2 x xylene), and covered in Eukitt or DePeX.

5. Acknowledgement

The authors thank Prof. Bernd Hamprecht, for the kind gift of the N18 mouse neuroblastoma cell line. The authors also thank Dr. Hellmut Merkle for providing the rf-coil for *in vivo* MRI imaging. This work was supported by the Max-Planck Society and the Hertie Foundation. S.C. acknowledges the support of the Human Frontiers Science Program Organization and the Ministry of Science and Innovation of Spain (BFU2009-09938) and the Consolider-Ingenio 2010 Program (CSD2007-0023). A.M. acknowledges the support of the EC for a Marie Curie IEF (PIEF-GA-2009-237253).

6. References

Aime, S., Botta, M., Parker, D., and Williams, J.A.G. (1996). Extent of hydration of octadentate lanthanide complexes incorporating phosphinate donors: Solution relaxometry and luminescence studies. Journal of the Chemical Society-Dalton Transactions, 17-23.

Baur, B., Suormala, T., and Baumgartner, E.R. (2002). Biocytin and biotin uptake into NB2a neuroblastoma and C6 astrocytoma cells. Brain Res *925*, 111-121.

Bickel, U., Yoshikawa, T., and Pardridge, W.M. (2001). Delivery of peptides and proteins through the blood-brain barrier. Adv Drug Deliv Rev *46*, 247-279.

Botta, M. (2000). Second coordination sphere water molecules and relaxivity of gadolinium(III) complexes: Implications for MRI contrast agents. European Journal of Inorganic Chemistry, 399-407.

Canals, S., Beyerlein, M., Keller, A.L., Murayama, Y., and Logothetis, N.K. (2008). Magnetic resonance imaging of cortical connectivity in vivo. Neuroimage *40*, 458-472.

Canals, S., Beyerlein, M., Merkle, H., and Logothetis, N.K. (2009). Functional MRI evidence for LTP-induced neural network reorganization. Curr Biol *19*, 398-403.

Cao, R., Gu, Z., Hsu, L., Patterson, G.D., and Armitage, B.A. (2003). Synthesis and characterization of thermoreversible biopolymer microgels based on hydrogen bonded nucleobase pairing. J Am Chem Soc *125*, 10250-10256.

Caravan, P., Ellison, J.J., McMurry, T.J., and Lauffer, R.B. (1999). Gadolinium(III) Chelates as MRI Contrast Agents: Structure, Dynamics, and Applications. Chem Rev *99*, 2293-2352.

Caswell, K.K., Wilson, J.N., Bunz, U.H., and Murphy, C.J. (2003). Preferential end-to-end assembly of gold nanorods by biotin-streptavidin connectors. J Am Chem Soc *125*, 13914-13915.

Chandra, S.V., Shukla, G.S., Srivastava, R.S., Singh, H., and Gupta, V.P. (1981). An exploratory study of manganese exposure to welders. Clin Toxicol *18*, 407-416.

Chklovskii, D.B., Mel, B.W., and Svoboda, K. (2004). Cortical rewiring and information storage. Nature *431*, 782-788.

Heller, A.J., Stanley, C., Shaia, W.T., Sismanis, A., Spencer, R.F., and Wolf, B. (2002). Localization of biotinidase in the brain: implications for its role in hearing loss in biotinidase deficiency. Hear Res *173*, 62-68.

Horikawa, K., and Armstrong, W.E. (1988). A versatile means of intracellular labeling: injection of biocytin and its detection with avidin conjugates. J Neurosci Methods *25*, 1-11.

Hymes, J., and Wolf, B. (1996). Biotinidase and its roles in biotin metabolism. Clin Chim Acta *255*, 1-11.

King, M.A., Louis, P.M., Hunter, B.E., and Walker, D.W. (1989). Biocytin: a versatile anterograde neuroanatomical tract-tracing alternative. Brain Res *497*, 361-367.

Kita, H., and Armstrong, W. (1991). A biotin-containing compound N-(2-aminoethyl)biotinamide for intracellular labeling and neuronal tracing studies: comparison with biocytin. J Neurosci Methods *37*, 141-150.

Kobbert, C., Apps, R., Bechmann, I., Lanciego, J.L., Mey, J., and Thanos, S. (2000). Current concepts in neuroanatomical tracing. Prog Neurobiol *62*, 327-351.

Koretsky, A.P., and Silva, A.C. (2004). Manganese-enhanced magnetic resonance imaging (MEMRI). NMR Biomed *17*, 527-531.

Lapper, S.R., and Bolam, J.P. (1991). The anterograde and retrograde transport of neurobiotin in the central nervous system of the rat: comparison with biocytin. J Neurosci Methods *39*, 163-174.

Lee, J.H., Garwood, M., Menon, R., Adriany, G., Andersen, P., Truwit, C.L., and Ugurbil, K. (1995). High contrast and fast three-dimensional magnetic resonance imaging at high fields. Magn Reson Med *34*, 308-312.

Leergaard, T.B., Bjaalie, J.G., Devor, A., Wald, L.L., and Dale, A.M. (2003). In vivo tracing of major rat brain pathways using manganese-enhanced magnetic resonance imaging and three-dimensional digital atlasing. Neuroimage *20*, 1591-1600.

Livramento, J.B., Weidensteiner, C., Prata, M.I., Allegrini, P.R., Geraldes, C.F., Helm, L., Kneuer, R., Merbach, A.E., Santos, A.C., Schmidt, P., *et al.* (2006). First in vivo MRI assessment of a self-assembled metallostar compound endowed with a remarkable high field relaxivity. Contrast Media Mol Imaging *1*, 30-39.

Marchisio, P.C., Weber, K., and Osborn, M. (1979). Identification of multiple microtubule initiating sites in mouse neuroblastoma cells. Eur J Cell Biol *20*, 45-50.

McMillan, D.E. (1999). A brief history of the neurobehavioral toxicity of manganese: some unanswered questions. Neurotoxicology *20*, 499-507.

Mishra, A., Dhingra, K., Schüz, A., Logothetis, N.K., and Canals, S. (2009). Improved Neuronal Tract Tracing with Stable Biocytin-Derived Neuroimaging Agents. ACS Chemical Neuroscience *1*, 129-138.

Mock, D.M., Lankford, G.L., Widness, J.A., Burmeister, L.F., Kahn, D., and Strauss, R.G. (1999). Measurement of circulating red cell volume using biotin-labeled red cells: validation against 51Cr-labeled red cells. Transfusion *39*, 149-155.

Murayama, Y., Weber, B., Saleem, K.S., Augath, M., and Logothetis, N.K. (2006). Tracing neural circuits in vivo with Mn-enhanced MRI. Magn Reson Imaging *24*, 349-358.

Pal, P.K., Samii, A., and Calne, D.B. (1999). Manganese neurotoxicity: a review of clinical features, imaging and pathology. Neurotoxicology *20*, 227-238.

Pautler, R.G., Silva, A.C., and Koretsky, A.P. (1998). In vivo neuronal tract tracing using manganese-enhanced magnetic resonance imaging. Magn Reson Med *40*, 740-748.

Pispa, J. (1965). Animal biotinidase. Ann Med Exp Biol Fenn *43*, Suppl 5:1-39.

Pope, S.J., Kenwright, A.M., Heath, S.L., and Faulkner, S. (2003). Synthesis and luminescence properties of a kinetically stable dinuclear ytterbium complex with differentiated binding sites. Chem Commun (Camb), 1550-1551.

Rivera, V.R., Merrill, G.A., White, J.A., and Poli, M.A. (2003). An enzymatic electrochemiluminescence assay for the lethal factor of anthrax. Anal Biochem *321*, 125-130.

Saleem, K.S., Pauls, J.M., Augath, M., Trinath, T., Prause, B.A., Hashikawa, T., and Logothetis, N.K. (2002). Magnetic resonance imaging of neuronal connections in the macaque monkey. Neuron *34*, 685-700.

Sloot, W.N., and Gramsbergen, J.B. (1994). Axonal transport of manganese and its relevance to selective neurotoxicity in the rat basal ganglia. Brain Res *657*, 124-132.

Suchy, S.F., McVoy, J.S., and Wolf, B. (1985). Neurologic symptoms of biotinidase deficiency: possible explanation. Neurology *35*, 1510-1511.

Tjalve, H., Mejare, C., and Borg-Neczak, K. (1995). Uptake and transport of manganese in primary and secondary olfactory neurones in pike. Pharmacol Toxicol *77*, 23-31.

Tsao, C.Y., and Kien, C.L. (2002). Complete biotinidase deficiency presenting as reversible progressive ataxia and sensorineural deafness. J Child Neurol *17*, 146.

Van der Linden, A., Verhoye, M., Van Meir, V., Tindemans, I., Eens, M., Absil, P., and Balthazart, J. (2002). In vivo manganese-enhanced magnetic resonance imaging reveals connections and functional properties of the songbird vocal control system. Neuroscience *112*, 467-474.

Watanabe, T., Frahm, J., and Michaelis, T. (2004). Functional mapping of neural pathways in rodent brain in vivo using manganese-enhanced three-dimensional magnetic resonance imaging. NMR Biomed *17*, 554-568.

Weizmann, Y., Patolsky, F., Katz, E., and Willner, I. (2003). Amplified DNA sensing and immunosensing by the rotation of functional magnetic particles. J Am Chem Soc *125*, 3452-3454.

Wilbur, D.S., Hamlin, D.K., Vessella, R.L., Stray, J.E., Buhler, K.R., Stayton, P.S., Klumb, L.A., Pathare, P.M., and Weerawarna, S.A. (1996). Antibody fragments in tumor pretargeting. Evaluation of biotinylated Fab' colocalization with recombinant streptavidin and avidin. Bioconjug Chem *7*, 689-702.

Wirsig-Wiechmann, C.R. (1994). Biocytin: a neuronal tracer compatible with rapid decalcification procedures. J Neurosci Methods *51*, 213-216.

Zaffanello, M., Zamboni, G., Fontana, E., Zoccante, L., and Tato, L. (2003). A case of partial biotinidase deficiency associated with autism. Child Neuropsychol *9*, 184-188.

10

The Use of 31-Phosphorus Magnetic Resonance Spectroscopy to Study Brain Cell Membrane Motion-Restricted Phospholipids

Basant K. Puri and Ian H. Treasaden
[1]*Imperial College London & West London Mental Health NHS Trust*
[2]*University of Limerick*
[1]*England, UK*
[2]*Ireland*

1. Introduction

Until relatively recently, the only way non-invasively to study brain cell membrane phospholipids in humans *in vivo* has been through the quantification of membrane phospholipid metabolism by means of ascertaining the levels of phosphomonoesters and phosphodiesters from 31-phosphorus neurospectroscopy scans. However, this only gives an indirect measure of the cell membrane phospholipid molecules. Ideally, one would want to study the brain cell membrane motion-restricted phospholipids directly, but it has previously proved almost impossible to obtain high-resolution magnetic resonance spectra of membrane phospholipids in living tissues owing to the large chemical-shift anisotropy of the 31-phosphorus confined to what is, in terms of nuclear magnetic resonance, the relatively rigid structure of the cell membrane, whether this be the external cell membrane or the membrane of an intracellular organelle.

2. 31-Phosphorus neurospectroscopy

Since structural imaging depends on the measurement of proton-based resonances, proton neurospectroscopy is readily achievable, in terms of hardware requirements, from magnetic resonance imaging scanners that are used for structural neuroimaging studies in humans. In contrast, the excitation of 31-phosphorus-containing relatively free moieties from the human brain and the measurement of the corresponding 31-phosphorus signals from relaxation of the 31-phosphorus nuclei require the use of a different coil tuned to the resonance frequency corresponding to the latter nuclei. The resonance frequency, ω, depends also on the strength of the static magnetic field, B_0, and is given by the Lamor equation:

$$\omega = \gamma B_0 \tag{1}$$

where γ refers to the gyromagnetic constant (or ratio) and is the ratio of the nuclear magnetic moment to the nuclear spin angular momentum. The gyromagnetic constant has a unique value for each nuclide possessing a nuclear magnetic moment, such as 31-phosphorus. For example, the value of the gyromagnetic constant for 31-phosphorus is 17.23 MHz T^{-1} while for the proton (1-hydrogen) it is 42.58 MHz T^{-1}. Hence, at a value of B_0 of 1.5 T, which is common for many magnetic resonance scanners in clinical use at the time of writing, whereas the value of the resonance frequency is 63.87 MHz for protons, it is just under 26 MHz for 31-phosphorus. A method our group have used to allow us to carry out 31-phosphorus neurospectroscopy studies without having to move each subject's head in relation to the magnetic resonance scanner, is to employ a birdcage quadrature head coil dual-tuned to proton (64 MHz) and 31-phosphorus (26 MHz); the proton tuned coil is required to enable T_1-weighted structural scans to be obtained, in order to allow subsequent spectral localization (Puri et al., 2008b).

Conventional 31-phosphorus neurospectroscopy allows us readily to discern seven narrow resonances from the adult human brain. In decreasing order of chemical shift, these are signals from phosphomonoesters, inorganic phosphate, phosphodiesters, phosphocreatine, gamma nucleotide triphosphate, alpha nucleotide triphosphate, and beta nucleotide triphosphate. The first and third narrow resonances, corresponding to phosphomonoesters and phosphodiesters, respectively, are considered further below.

2.1 Phosphomonoesters and phosphodiesters

The 31-phosphorus neurospectroscopy narrow resonances corresponding to phosphomonoesters and phosphodiesters are important in respect of membrane phospholipid metabolism for the following reasons.

The phosphomonoesters narrow resonance reflects membrane phospholipid anabolism. This is because it contains contributions from freely mobile phosphomonoesters, including phosphocholine, phosphoethanolamine, and even small contributions from inositol phosphate, glycerophosphate, phosphothreonine, and *L*-phosphoserine, and also contributions from less mobile phosphomonoester-containing molecules, such as certain phosphorylated proteins, and from certain proteins that are part of the neuronal cytoskeleton (Puri, 2006).

In contrast, the phosphodiesters narrow resonance reflects membrane phospholipid catabolism, since it contains contributions from freely mobile phosphodiesters, including glycerophosphocholine and glycerophosphoethanolamine. The phosphodiesters narrow resonance also contains contributions from less mobile phosphodiester-containing molecules, such as molecules involved in membrane structure (both cell membranes and intracellular organelle membranes) (Puri, 2006).

Traditionally, therefore, the ratio of phosphomonoesters to phosphodiesters has been used as an index of membrane phospholipid metabolism. We turn next to a consideration of the presence of a broad component in the 31-phosphorus neurospectroscopy spectrum, which enables brain cell membrane motion-restricted phospholipids to be assessed more directly than a consideration of just phosphomonoesters and phosphodiesters.

2.2 Broad component

In explaining the advantages of measuring the broad component in the 31-phosphorus neurospectroscopy signal, the reader may be struck by what is in retrospect a rather ironic fact that for many years this broad component has been treated as somewhat of a nuisance, with attempts being made to eliminate it altogether, as far as possible, from the final spectral analysis (Estilaei et al., 2001). For example, in previous neurospectroscopy research studies, our group have often used a fully automated approach to minimize the baseline roll in chemical shift imaging using a technique that employed knowledge-based data processing in the frequency domain, the broad component being regarded as an artefact that appeared as a result of the summation of several sinc functions; using prior knowledge, a mirror component corresponding to the 'artefact' was created and added to the delayed spectrum and this method compensated for noise and zero-order phase error when computing the roll artefact (Saeed and Menon, 1993).

The broad resonance which underlies the 31-phosphorus spectrum from the living mammalian brain is composed of signal directly from the cell membrane phospholipids (Hamilton et al., 2003a). Thus the quantification of this broad resonance from 31-phosphorus neurospectroscopy data provides a more direct measure of brain cell membrane motion-restricted phospholipids than does the evaluation of the ratio of phosphomonoesters, which index phospholipid anabolism, to phosphodiesters, which index phospholipid catabolism. The convolution difference resolution enhancement method may be used to obtain the broad component integral, from spectra obtained using an image-selected *in vivo* spectroscopy sequence (ISIS) (Estilaei et al., 2001, Roth and Kimber, 1982), whereby the broad component is the difference between the measured raw signal intensity, S, and S_{CD} given by:

$$S_{CD} = S(1 - fe^{-\pi L t}) \tag{2}$$

where f is the convolution-difference factor, representing the fraction of the broad component contributing to the acquired signal at a given echo time (TE), and L is an exponential filter; the broad component integral may then found by fitting the broad spectrum to multiple Gaussian lines, minimizing residuals, and summating over all Gaussian-line integrals. Estilaei and colleagues (2001) obtained transverse relaxation time (T_2)-magnetization decay curves by plotting the broad component area as a function of TE; having found that mono-exponential fitting did not adequately represent T_2-magnetization decay curves, they instead used the following bi-exponential fit:

$$S(t) = S_l e^{-A} + S_s e^{-B} \tag{3}$$

where $S(t)$ is the total magnetization at a given time t, S_l and S_s are the respective equilibrium magnetizations for the slow and fast decaying components, A is the quotient of the echo time and the spin-spin relaxation time for the long T_2 component, T_{2l}, and B is the quotient of the echo time and the spin-spin relaxation time for the short T_2 component, T_{2s}. Using the model of Radda's group in which T_{2l} is much greater than T_{2s} (Kilby et al., 1990), Estilaei and colleagues (2001) showed that the uncertainty in the determination of the long T_2 could be eliminated, and, with TE much less than T_{2l}, it followed that

$$\ln S(TE) = \ln (S_l + S_s) - S_s TE/(T_{2s} (S_l + S_s)) \tag{4}$$

and, with TE much greater than T_{2s}

$$\ln S(TE) \simeq \ln S_l - TE/T_{2l} \tag{5}$$

Linear regression was then used to carry out the corresponding fits.
Our group have tended to quantify the 31-phosphorus signals using prior knowledge in the temporal domain using the AMARES (advanced method for accurate, robust, and efficient spectral fitting) algorithm (Vanhamme et al., 1997) included in the Java-based MRUI (magnetic resonance user interface) software program, which allows time-domain analysis to be easily carried out (Naressi et al., 2001). Truncation of a specific early portion of the signal removes the broad component present in the 31-phosphorus spectra and allows initial analysis of the narrow components listed above using *a priori* knowledge in the AMARES algorithm (Hamilton et al., 2003a, Hamilton et al., 2003b). The broad hump can then be analyzed, using the above time-domain analysis, thereby allowing distinct separation of the narrow and broad components. The broad component is modelled as a Gaussian function and its area can be compared with the total peak area of the seven narrow resonances and then multiplied by 100 to give the percentage broad signal (Puri et al., 2008b).

2.3 Chronic alcohol consumption

It has been shown that ethanol increases the fluidity of spin-labelled membranes from normal mice, while membranes from mice that have been subjected to long-term ethanol treatment are relatively resistant to this fluidizing effect and have an altered phospholipid composition; this suggests that the membranes themselves had adapted to the alcohol, which constitutes a novel form of drug tolerance (Chin and Goldstein, 1977). This finding from this landmark 1977 study has been replicated using non- nuclear magnetic resonance techniques, including electron spin resonance and fluorescence polarization: chronic alcohol exposure in humans increases the rigidity of isolated brain membranes.
The related hypothesis that subjects who are heavy drinkers have stiffer brain cell membranes than have control subjects who are light drinkers, as reflected in a smaller broad signal component with a shorter T_2 of the broad signal from 31-phosphorus neurospectroscopy, was tested by Estilaei and colleagues (2001). They carried out localized 31-phosphorus neurospectroscopy at the level of the centrum ovale in 13 male alcohol-dependent heavy drinkers of average age 44 years (standard deviation 9 years) who had an average lifetime alcohol consumption of 239 (standard deviation 218) drinks per month, where one drink was taken to be an alcoholic beverage containing approximately 13 g ethanol, and who satisfied the Diagnostic and Statistical Manual of Mental Disorders, fourth edition (DSM-IV) criteria for lifetime dependence on alcohol (American Psychiatric Association, 1992). Seventeen male non-dependent light drinkers whose average lifetime alcohol consumption was 19 drinks (standard deviation 17 drinks) per month, and whose average age (37; standard deviation 10) years was similar to that of the first group, acted as the control group for this study. The broad component integral was found to be 13 per cent lower in the heavy drinkers compared with the light drinkers ($p = 0.000\ 5$), while no significant differences were found for any of the metabolite integrals. No significant main effect of a family history of alcohol use, assessed using a standard questionnaire, was found, and there was no significant family history-by-group interaction effect on the broad component integral. No significant correlations were found between, on the one hand, the broad component signal integral or its relaxation times, and, on the other hand, age, years of abuse, average monthly drinking or total lifetime consumption in either the heavy drinking group, or the control group or a combination of

both groups. A positive family history of alcohol abuse did not predict a smaller broad component integral or shorter relaxation times (Estilaei et al., 2001). In both the heavy drinkers and the control group, the T_2 distribution of the broad component consistently showed two resolvable components, with the fast relaxing component having the same T_2 in both groups while the slower relaxing component T_2 was 0.6 ms shorter in the heavy drinkers (Estilaei et al., 2001).

The authors concluded that 31-phosphorus neurospectroscopy 'provides a powerful and practical approach for measuring in vivo changes of the amount and fluidity of [phospholipids] in white matter regions of the human brain. Specifically, the smaller, broad component in [heavy drinkers] compared with [light drinkers] suggests altered white matter [phospholipids] associated with long-term chronic alcohol abuse...[and] may provide valuable information regarding possible biochemical mechanisms that [underlie] chronic alcohol-induced structural changes...' (Estilaei et al., 2001).

2.4 Hypoxia resulting from chronic obstructive pulmonary disease

The maintenance of cerebral metabolic homeostasis is required for the maintenance of consciousness and normal brain function, and this may be perturbed by a variety of insults, including hypoxia (Hamilton et al., 2003a). Taylor-Robinson's group at Hammersmith Hospital in London, U.K., had previously shown that abnormal cerebral bioenergetics can be detected readily using 31-phosphorus neurospectroscopy in a study of 10 patients with stable, but severe, chronic obstructive pulmonary disease and hypoxia; compared with controls, the patients with chronic obstructive pulmonary disease showed increased phosphomonoesters and inorganic phosphate signals but reduced phosphodiesters signals, thought to be caused by the utilization of anaerobic metabolism by the brains of hypoxic patients with this disease (Mathur et al., 1999). Since neonatal, animal and *in vitro* studies show an association between anaerobic glycolysis with a protective intracellular alkalosis, the same group attempted to identify such a compensatory intracellular alkalosis in eight hypoxic patients with chronic obstructive pulmonary disease, compared with eight age-matched control subjects, using 31-phosphorus neurospectroscopy (Hamilton et al., 2003a). As part of this study, the broad component was also quantified in the subjects.

Taylor-Robinson's group reported that the mean intracellular pH in patients with chronic obstructive pulmonary disease was similar to that in the control subjects, but decreased in the patients by a mean of 0.02 following the administration of supplemental oxygen, there being no such change in normal control subjects following oxygen administration. Of particular interest was their finding that the broad component increased in all the patients with chronic obstructive pulmonary disease following oxygen administration (Hamilton et al., 2003a). These findings point to altered phospholipid membrane fluidity in the brain being associated with the change in intracellular pH following oxygen administration. The change in the broad resonance was strongly and negatively correlated with the change in intracellular pH, and indeed *in vitro* studies have shown that membrane fluidity is sensitive to pH with, for example, the fusion process between synaptosomes, freshly isolated from rat brain cortex, and large unilamellar phosphatidylserine liposomes being shown to be pH dependent (an increase in both kinetics and extent occurring when the pH is lowered by 1.9 from 7.4) (Almeida et al., 1994).

Based on the above findings, including the results relating to the broad component from 31-phosphorus neurospectroscopy, the authors hypothesized that the transition from compensatory respiratory failure in patients with hypoxic chronic obstructive pulmonary disease to the clinical picture of confusion, disorientation and coma in patients with chronic obstructive pulmonary disease and with severe exacerbations may be associated with the failure of ion transport mechanisms, perturbation of membrane fluidity and the overwhelming of the compensatory intracellular alkalosis in neuronal and glial cells (Hamilton et al., 2003a).

2.5 Schizophrenia

A number of lines of evidence from biochemical studies have suggested that membrane phospholipid metabolism may be impaired in at least a subgroup of patients suffering from schizophrenia (Puri et al., 2008a). First, reduced levels of highly unsaturated (or polyunsaturated) fatty acids have been reported in erythrocyte membranes (Yao and van Kammen, 1994, Yao et al., 1994a, Yao et al., 1994b, Peet et al., 1995) in patients with schizophrenia. Second, increased levels of the phospholipase A_2 group of enzymes, which catalyze the removal of highly unsaturated (or polyunsaturated) fatty acids such as arachidonic acid and docosahexaenoic acid from the Sn2 position of membrane phospholipid molecules, have been found in both plasma (Gattaz, 1992, Gattaz et al., 1990, Gattaz et al., 1987, Tavares et al., 2003) and platelets (Gattaz et al., 1995) of patients with schizophrenia. Furthermore, the dermatological response to the niacin flush test, which indirectly indexes membrane phospholipid metabolism, has been found to be impaired in schizophrenia (Ward et al., 1998), including in its quantitative measurement form as the volumetric niacin response (Puri et al., 2002). These converging lines of evidence are consistent with the membrane phospholipid hypothesis of schizophrenia, associated with the late Professor David F. Horrobin, and also with Professor Iain Glen and Professor Krishna Vaddadi, which proposes a change in brain membrane phospholipids leading in turn to changes in the functioning of membrane-associated proteins and of cell signalling systems in schizophrenia (Horrobin, 1996, Horrobin, 1998, Horrobin et al., 1994).

Clearly, the above biochemical studies have not directly measured membrane phospholipids from the brains of patients suffering from schizophrenia. Similarly, as mentioned earlier, the quantification of the ratio of phosphomonoesters to phosphodiesters, gleaned from narrow resonances obtained from 31-phosphorus neurospectroscopy, also only provide an indirect measure of the ratio of brain cell membrane phospholipid anabolism to phospholipid catabolism. Therefore, there is a clear role for analyzing the broad component from 31-phosphorus neurospectroscopy in schizophrenia. Accordingly, our group were the first to do so.

In our initial study, we carried out the first analysis of the broad component resonance from the brain in forensic patients severely affected with schizophrenia and a comparison group of age- and gender-matched healthy normal control subjects, to assess directly whether, as expected under the membrane phospholipid hypothesis of schizophrenia, there was a change in cell membrane phospholipids in people suffering from schizophrenia who have a forensic history such as having perpetrated an act of serious violence while psychotic (Puri et al., 2008b). Fifteen male inpatients in a medium secure unit with a diagnosis of schizophrenia according to DSM-IV (American Psychiatric Association, 1992), and 12 male healthy control subjects underwent 31-phosphorus neurospectroscopy. Expert psychiatric opinion, accepted in court, was that all the patients had violently offended directly as a result of schizophrenia prior to admission to the unit, these offences consisting of homicide, attempted murder, or wounding with intent to cause grievous bodily harm. There was no history of alcohol dependency in these patients or in the control subjects. All the patients were suffering from severe positive symptoms of schizophrenia, mostly controlled by antipsychotic medication at the time of scanning. The average duration of illness since the index offence was 6.8 (standard error 0.4) years. Fourteen of the patients were being treated with typical antipsychotic medication, mainly in injectable depot form, while the remaining patient was being treated with clozapine. Spectra were obtained using an image-selected *in vivo* spectroscopy sequence with 64 signal averages localized on a 70 x 70 x 70 cubic millimetre voxel. Owing to the low abundance in the brain, and indeed the rest of the body, of 31-phosphorus compared with protons, the maximum size voxel was used to collect signal from the brain and thus maximize the signal-to-noise ratio. All spectral analyses were carried out by a single observer who was blinded to group allocation until after the spectral and statistical analyses were completed. It was found that the mean percentage broad component signal for the patients did not differ significantly from that for the control subjects and therefore it was not possible to reject the null hypothesis that there is no difference in the concentration of brain membrane-bound phospholipids in this group of forensic patients with schizophrenia compared with controls.

The above finding from analysis of the broad component in forensic patients with schizophrenia was a surprise to our group. An explanation based on the notion that the membrane phospholipid hypothesis applies not only to the outer cell membranes but also to the phospholipid membranes of intracellular organelles such as the nucleus and mitochondrion does not hold since the broad component resonance signal derives from both the outer cell membranes and the phospholipid membranes of these organelles (Puri et al., 2008b).

We carried out a review of the evidence relating to the membrane phospholipid hypothesis of schizophrenia (Puri et al., 2008b). There is strong evidence favouring this hypothesis. As alluded to above, much of this evidence is, as might be expected, primarily biochemical in nature. Plasma phospholipids that have been studied in schizophrenia have tended to show reduced levels of the *n*-6 (or omega-6) fatty acids linoleic acid and arachidonic acid and raised levels of *n*-3 (or omega-3) fatty acids (Horrobin et al., 1989). Interestingly, in a study of plasma phospholipids in patients with schizophrenia, patients with affective and paranoid disorders, and normal controls, from Japan, it was found that while the patients with schizophrenia had low linoleic acid levels (and a low ratio of linoleic acid to its metabolites), and while phospholipid fatty acid levels were in the normal range for the patients with paranoid or affective disorders, those patients with schizophrenia who showed reduced platelet sensitivity to the aggregation-inhibiting effects of prostaglandin E_1 had higher levels of oleic acid and lower levels of eicosapentaenoic acid (Kaiya et al., 1991). This possibility of a dichotomous nature to the fatty acid changes in plasma in schizophrenia also extends to erythrocyte membrane fatty acids.

Erythrocyte membrane fatty acid changes in schizophrenia have been found more consistently than plasma fatty acid changes (Puri et al., 2008b). They tend to point to reduced erythrocyte membrane levels of the long-chain polyunsaturated fatty acids arachidonic acid and docosahexaenoic acid, in the context of a biphasic distribution with one group of schizophrenia patients having essentially normal fatty acid levels, while the other has significantly low levels (Glen et al., 1994). It is of particular interest to note that when the schizophrenia patients were divided into those with predominantly negative symptoms, such as affective flattening, and predominantly positive syndromes, including positive symptoms such as auditory hallucinations and thought disorder, the low erythrocyte membrane levels of arachidonic acid and docosahexaenoic acid were largely confined to patients with a negative syndrome (Horrobin, 2003).

Clearly it was the case that the schizophrenia patients in the above broad component 31-phosphorus neurospectroscopy study would all fit into the category of a positive syndrome, given their history of seriously and violently offending while psychotic (Puri et al., 2008b) . Therefore, this may provide a possible explanation as to why the results of this study did not harmonize with the neurospectroscopy changes expected under the membrane phospholipid hypothesis of Horrobin, Glen and Vaddadi. It was therefore decided to carry to a further study of the broad component from 31-phosphorus neurospectroscopy scanning of patients with schizophrenia, but this time of a sample taken from patients who had not seriously or violently offended as a result of their illness and who suffered from predominantly negative symptoms.

For our new 31-phosphorus neurospectroscopy investigation, our group studied 16 psychiatric outpatients who had a diagnosis of schizophrenia according to DSM-IV (American Psychiatric Association, 1992), who had no history of dependency on psychoactive substances, and the same number of normal healthy controls, who had no previous history of psychiatric or neurological disorders. The two groups were matched with respect to age and gender. The patients suffered from mild to moderate negative symptoms of schizophrenia and had no history of having committed any violent or other offences as a result of their schizophrenic illness. The 31-phosphorus neurospectroscopy protocol was as mentioned above for the forensic schizophrenia study, with spectra being obtained from an image selected *in vivo* spectroscopy sequence with 64 signal averages localized on a 70 x 70 x 70 cubic millimetre voxel, with the signal-to-noise ratio again being improved by using this large voxel size (Puri et al., 2008a).

The broad component from each subject was quantified by an observer who at the time of this analysis was blinded to group status. Just as in our previous study mentioned above, analysis of these broad resonances in this new study showed no significant difference in the broad component between the group of patients with schizophrenia and the normal control group.

We considered that an explanation of these negative results might lie in the possibility that the membrane phospholipid hypothesis of schizophrenia could possibly be construed as predicting a change only in phospholipid metabolism in the cell membranes of the brain, rather than a change in the membrane-bound phospholipids themselves. To test this possibility, a further blinded analysis was carried out of the percentage phosphomonoesters (indexing phospholipid anabolism) and phosphodiesters (indexing phospholipid catabolism) levels in both groups. The mean (standard error) percentage phosphomonoesters level for the patients with schizophrenia was 11.4 (0.3) and did not differ significantly from that for the normal control subjects of 10.9 (0.5). Similarly, the mean (standard error) percentage phosphodiesters level for the schizophrenia patients was 44.4 (0.5), which did not differ significantly from that for the normal control subjects of 44.6 (0.9) (Puri et al., 2008a). In terms of ratios, the mean ratio of phosphomonoesters to phosphodiesters was 0.26 (standard error 0.01) in the case of the patients with schizophrenia and 0.25 (standard error 0.01) for the healthy controls (Puri et al., 2008a), and again these did not differ significantly. Therefore, on the basis of this second study, it was not possible to reject the null hypothesis that there was no difference in phospholipid metabolism in the brain in the schizophrenia patients compared with the age- and gender-matched control subjects.

Our two sets of 'negative' results in schizophrenia do not, of course, negate the value of quantifying the broad component gleaned from 31-phosphorus neurospectroscopy studies. Rather, they must give us cause to examine again the membrane phospholipid hypothesis of schizophrenia.

3. Conclusion

The above studies of chronic alcohol dependence, chronic obstructive pulmonary disease, forensic inpatients with schizophrenia who have seriously and violently offended while psychotic, and of outpatients with schizophrenia who are suffering from predominantly mild to moderate negative symptoms of schizophrenia, have demonstrated the feasibility of analyzing the broad component from 31-phosphorus neurospectroscopy studies in a wide range of patient groups. We have also shown the advantages over analysis of narrow resonances corresponding to levels of phosphomonoesters (indexing phospholipid anabolism) and phosphodiesters (indexing phospholipid catabolism) of the analysis of this broad component in order to quantify the level of motion-restricted membrane phospholipids in the brains of the individuals being studied.

The failure of our broad component analyses to yield results which harmonize with the rich biochemical literature that is consistent with the membrane phospholipid hypothesis of schizophrenia does insert a possible note of caution, however. It should be noted that, given the low signal-to-noise in 31-phosphorus magnetic resonance spectroscopy, the areas of the peaks obtained are inherently variable (Puri et al., 2008a). This is particularly true of the underlying broad component, which has a coefficient of variation double that of the other peaks visible in the spectrum (Hamilton et al., 2003b). One should take into account the possibility that this variability may be masking any changes in the broad component, leading to a reduction in the ability to monitor membrane phospholipids.

4. Acknowledgment

The authors wish to express their thanks to all the patients and healthy volunteers who took part in our 31-phosphorus neurospectroscopy studies. We also wish to thank our collaborators on these studies. We acknowledge with thanks the support that we received to conduct these studies from the British Medical Research Council (MRC) and from Marconi Medical Systems, Cleveland, Ohio.

5. References

Almeida, M. T., Ramalho-Santos, J., Oliveira, C. R. & de Lima, M. C. 1994. Parameters affecting fusion between liposomes and synaptosomes. Role of proteins, lipid peroxidation, pH and temperature. *J Membr Biol,* 142, 217-22.

American Psychiatric Association 1992. *Diagnostic and statistical manual of mental disorders : DSM-IV,* Washington, D.C., American Psychiatric Association.

Chin, J. H. & Goldstein, D. B. 1977. Drug tolerance in biomembranes: a spin label study of the effects of ethanol. *Science,* 196, 684-5.

Estilaei, M. R., Matson, G. B., Payne, G. S., Leach, M. O., Fein, G. & Meyerhoff, D. J. 2001. Effects of chronic alcohol consumption on the broad phospholipid signal in human brain: an in vivo 31P MRS study. *Alcohol Clin Exp Res,* 25, 89-97.

Gattaz, W. F. 1992. Phospholipase A2 in schizophrenia. *Biol Psychiatry,* 31, 214-6.

Gattaz, W. F., Hubner, C. V., Nevalainen, T. J., Thuren, T. & Kinnunen, P. K. 1990. Increased serum phospholipase A2 activity in schizophrenia: a replication study. *Biol Psychiatry,* 28, 495-501.

Gattaz, W. F., Kollisch, M., Thuren, T., Virtanen, J. A. & Kinnunen, P. K. 1987. Increased plasma phospholipase-A2 activity in schizophrenic patients: reduction after neuroleptic therapy. *Biol Psychiatry,* 22, 421-6.

Gattaz, W. F., Schmitt, A. & Maras, A. 1995. Increased platelet phospholipase A2 activity in schizophrenia. *Schizophr Res,* 16, 1-6.

Glen, A. I., Glen, E. M., Horrobin, D. F., Vaddadi, K. S., Spellman, M., Morse-Fisher, N., *et al.* 1994. A red cell membrane abnormality in a subgroup of schizophrenic patients: evidence for two diseases. *Schizophr Res,* 12, 53-61.

Hamilton, G., Mathur, R., Allsop, J. M., Forton, D. M., Dhanjal, N. S., Shaw, R. J., *et al.* 2003a. Changes in brain intracellular pH and membrane phospholipids on oxygen therapy in hypoxic patients with chronic obstructive pulmonary disease. *Metab Brain Dis,* 18, 95-109.

Hamilton, G., Patel, N., Forton, D. M., Hajnal, J. V. & Taylor-Robinson, S. D. 2003b. Prior knowledge for time domain quantification of in vivo brain or liver 31P MR spectra. *NMR Biomed,* 16, 168-76.

Horrobin, D. F. 1996. Schizophrenia as a membrane lipid disorder which is expressed throughout the body. *Prostaglandins Leukot Essent Fatty Acids,* 55, 3-7.

Horrobin, D. F. 1998. The membrane phospholipid hypothesis as a biochemical basis for the neurodevelopmental concept of schizophrenia. *Schizophr Res,* 30, 193-208.

Horrobin, D. F. 2003. Phospholipid and fatty acid biochemistry in schizophrenia. In: Peet, M., Glen, I. & Horrobin, D. F. (Eds.) *Phospholipid spectrum disorders in psychiatry and neurology,* 2nd ed. Carnforth, Marius Press.

Horrobin, D. F., Glen, A. I. & Vaddadi, K. 1994. The membrane hypothesis of schizophrenia. *Schizophr Res,* 13, 195-207.

Horrobin, D. F., Manku, M. S., Morse-Fisher, N., Vaddadi, K. S., Courtney, P., Glen, A. I., *et al.* 1989. Essential fatty acids in plasma phospholipids in schizophrenics. *Biol Psychiatry,* 25, 562-8.

Kaiya, H., Horrobin, D. F., Manku, M. S. & Fisher, N. M. 1991. Essential and other fatty acids in plasma in schizophrenics and normal individuals from Japan. *Biol Psychiatry,* 30, 357-62.

Kilby, P. M., Allis, J. L. & Radda, G. K. 1990. Spin-spin relaxation of the phosphodiester resonance in the 31P NMR spectrum of human brain. The determination of the concentrations of phosphodiester components. *FEBS Lett,* 272, 163-5.

Mathur, R., Cox, I. J., Oatridge, A., Shephard, D. T., Shaw, R. J. & Taylor-Robinson, S. D. 1999. Cerebral bioenergetics in stable chronic obstructive pulmonary disease. *Am J Respir Crit Care Med,* 160, 1994-9.

Naressi, A., Couturier, C., Devos, J. M., Janssen, M., Mangeat, C., de Beer, R., *et al.* 2001. Java-based graphical user interface for the MRUI quantitation package. *MAGMA,* 12, 141-52.

Peet, M., Laugharne, J., Rangarajan, N., Horrobin, D. & Reynolds, G. 1995. Depleted red cell membrane essential fatty acids in drug-treated schizophrenic patients. *J Psychiatr Res,* 29, 227-32.

Puri, B. K. 2006. Proton and 31-phosphorus neurospectroscopy in the study of membrane phospholipids and fatty acid intervention in schizophrenia, depression, chronic fatigue syndrome (myalgic encephalomyelitis) and dyslexia. *Int Rev Psychiatry,* 18, 145-7.

Puri, B. K., Counsell, S. J. & Hamilton, G. 2008a. Brain cell membrane motion-restricted phospholipids: A cerebral 31-phosphorus magnetic resonance spectroscopy study of patients with schizophrenia. *Prostaglandins Leukot Essent Fatty Acids,* 79, 233-35.

Puri, B. K., Counsell, S. J., Hamilton, G., Bustos, M. G. & Treasaden, I. H. 2008b. Brain cell membrane motion-restricted phospholipids in patients with schizophrenia who have seriously and dangerously violently offended. *Prog Neuropsychopharmacol Biol Psychiatry,* 32, 751-4.

Puri, B. K., Hirsch, S. R., Easton, T. & Richardson, A. J. 2002. A volumetric biochemical niacin flush-based index that noninvasively detects fatty acid deficiency in schizophrenia. *Prog Neuropsychopharmacol Biol Psychiatry,* 26, 49-52.

Roth, K. & Kimber, B. J. 1982. Determination of optimal parameters in the convolution difference resolution enhancement technique. *Org Mag Reson,* 18, 197-198.

Saeed, N. & Menon, D. K. 1993. A knowledge-based approach to minimize baseline roll in chemical shift imaging. *Magn Reson Med,* 29, 591-8.

Tavares, H., Yacubian, J., Talib, L. L., Barbosa, N. R. & Gattaz, W. F. 2003. Increased phospholipase A2 activity in schizophrenia with absent response to niacin. *Schizophr Res,* 61, 1-6.

Vanhamme, L., van den Boogaart, A. & Van Huffel, S. 1997. Improved method for accurate and efficient quantification of MRS data with use of prior knowledge. *J Magn Reson,* 129, 35-43.

Ward, P. E., Sutherland, J., Glen, E. M. & Glen, A. I. 1998. Niacin skin flush in schizophrenia: a preliminary report. *Schizophr Res,* 29, 269-74.

Yao, J. K. & van Kammen, D. P. 1994. Red blood cell membrane dynamics in schizophrenia. I. Membrane fluidity. *Schizophr Res,* 11, 209-16.

Yao, J. K., van Kammen, D. P. & Gurklis, J. 1994a. Red blood cell membrane dynamics in schizophrenia. III. Correlation of fatty acid abnormalities with clinical measures. *Schizophr Res,* 13, 227-32.

Yao, J. K., van Kammen, D. P. & Welker, J. A. 1994b. Red blood cell membrane dynamics in schizophrenia. II. Fatty acid composition. *Schizophr Res,* 13, 217-26.

11

Pediatric Cranial Ultrasound: Techniques, Variants and Pitfalls

Kristin Fickenscher[1,2], Zachary Bailey[3],
Megan Saettele[1,4], Amy Dahl[1,2] and Lisa Lowe[1,2]
[1]*Department of Radiology, University of Missouri-Kansas City, Kansas City, MO,*
[2]*Department of Radiology, Children's Mercy Hospital and Clinics, Kansas City, MO,*
[3]*Kansas City University of Medicine and Biosciences, Kansas City, MO,*
[4]*Department of Radiology, Saint Luke's Hospital, Kansas City, MO,*
USA

1. Introduction

Recent advances in sonographic technology have made ultrasound an increasingly accurate and adequate means to detect cranial morphology and intracranial pathology in infants. When modern equipment is combined with thorough imaging technique, ultrasound delivers similar results to MRI in terms of sensitivity and ability to direct initial management (Daneman et. al, 2006; Epelman et. al., 2010). Furthermore, ultrasound offers certain advantages over other imaging modalities such as MRI and CT. Cranial sonography is less expensive, spares the patient from radiation, does not require sedation, and its portability allows for bedside evaluation in gravely ill infants who cannot be transported to radiology for imaging.

The goal of this chapter is to provide an updated approach to modern cranial ultrasound in order to improve diagnostic accuracy and increase recognition of normal anatomical structures, anatomical variants, pathologic processes, and imaging pitfalls that may simulate disease. The discussion will begin with an overview of the approach and interpretation of gray-scale imaging. The chapter will continue with a review of Doppler imaging, the use of additional fontanels, and linear imaging. The chapter will conclude by reviewing pitfalls and normal variants which may simulate pathology.

2. Ultrasound techniques and interpretation

2.1 Gray-scale

The cranial ultrasound examination is performed with a linear-array transducer. Six-eight coronal plane images are taken through the anterior fontanel, beginning in the frontal lobes anterior to the frontal horns and progressing posteriorly to the occipital lobes past the trigones of the lateral ventricles. (**Figure 1**) The first coronal image acquired at the level of the frontal lobes allows the observer to examine the frontal lobes, orbital cones, and the hyperechoic falx cerebri located within the interhemispheric fissure (Slovis et. al., 1981). The second coronal image is taken through the frontal horns of the lateral ventricles, which allows multiple structures to be imaged at once. The frontal horns and cavum septum pellucidum appear as anechoic, CSF-filled spaces. The corpus callosum is a linear, hypoechoic structure crossing the hemispheres that is contained within echogenic superior and inferior borders. Finally, the globus pallidus, putamen, caudate nucleus, and thalamus of each side can be visualized in their respective locations with their characteristic gray matter appearance (Seigel, 2002). The third image is obtained at the level of the foramen of Monro and further illustrates many of the structures mentioned above. The third ventricle can be visualized as an anechoic structure beneath the septum pellucidum. Brainstem structures such as the pons and medulla can also be seen (Seigel, 2002). Moving posteriorly, the fourth image is taken at the level of the cerebral peduncles and shows hyperechoic choroid plexus along the floor of the lateral ventricles and the roof of the third ventricle. The tentorium cerebelli and fourth ventricle are also demonstrated (Seigel, 2002). The quadrigeminal plate cistern serves as a marker for the fifth image, which enables the viewer to see both temporal horns of the lateral ventricles as well as cerebellar structures including the hemispheres and vermis. Below the vermis, the cisterna magna is visible. Occasionally, the mammillary bodies can be discerned on this image (Seigel, 2002). The sixth image is taken through the lateral ventral trigones and shows their innate hyperechoic choroid plexus (Seigel, 2002). The perventricular white matter halo is also seen and should be less echogenic than the choroid plexus (Grant et. al., 1981; Seigel, 2002). The final image is obtained through the cerebral convexities and displays the interhemispheric fissure and occipital lobes (Seigel, 2002).

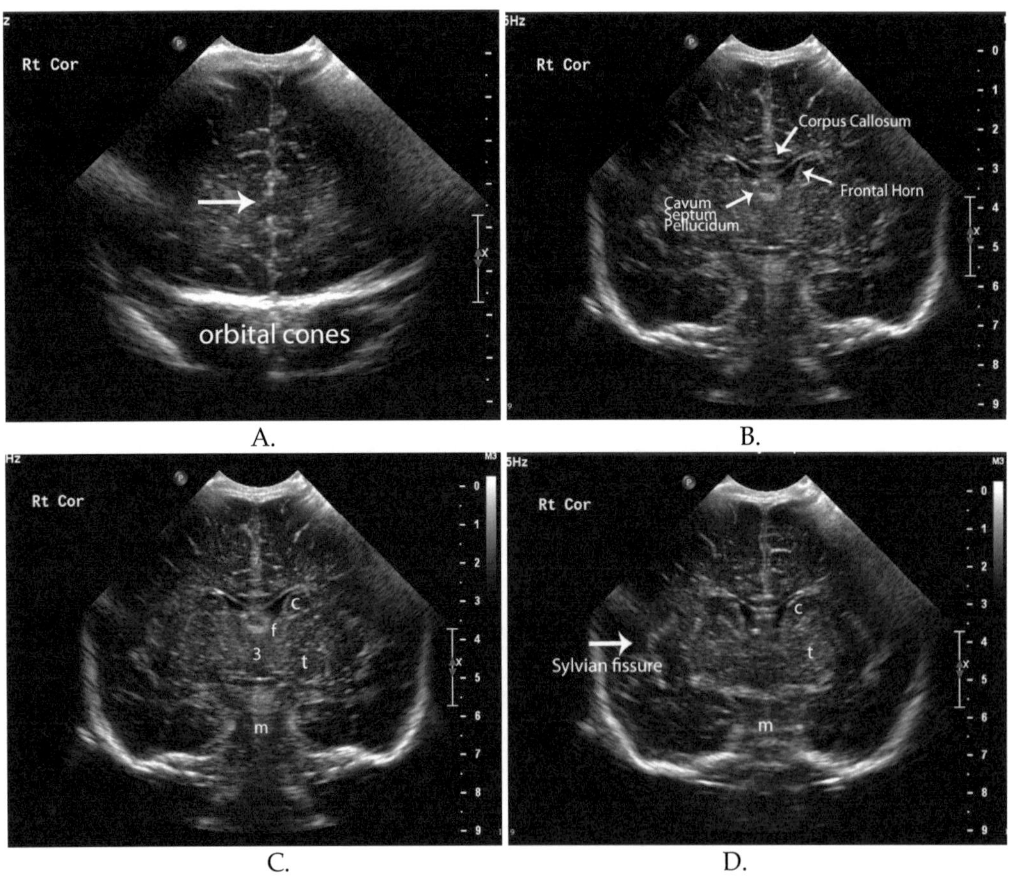

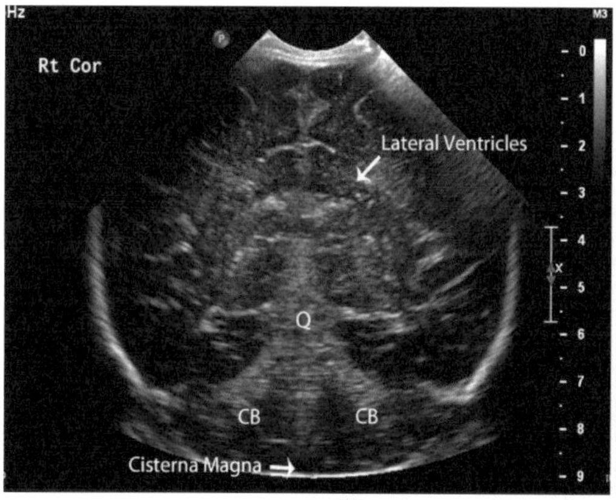

E.

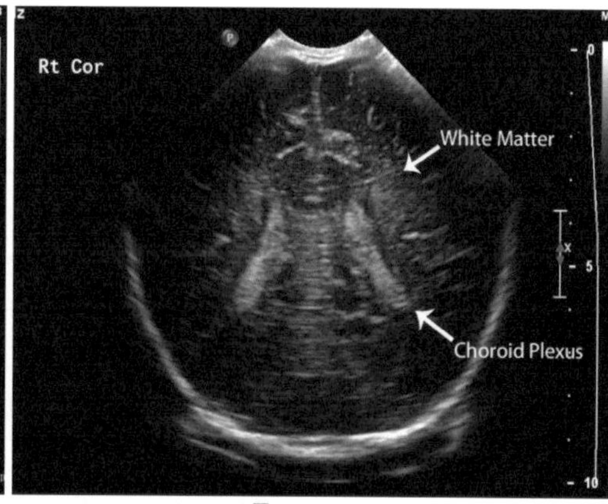

F.

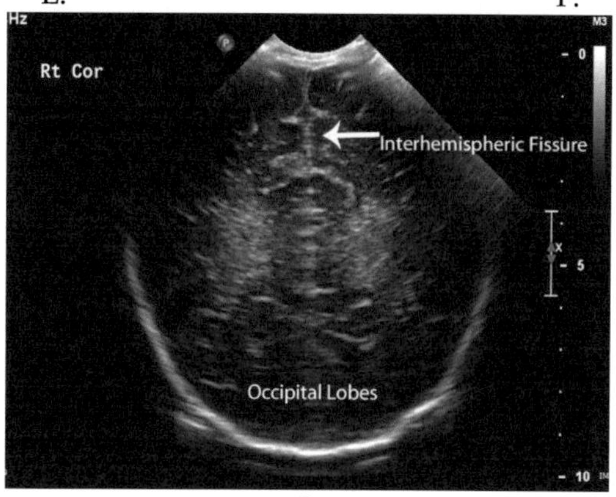

G.

Fig. 1. (a-g). Coronal images of a normal neonatal brain. C (caudate) t (thalamus) f (Foramen of Monro) m (midbrain) 3 (third ventricle) Q (quadrigeminal plate cistern) CB (cerebellar hemispheres)

Next, the transducer is turned 90 degrees on the anterior fontanel, and five more images are acquired in the sagittal and parasagittal planes. (**Figure 2**) The first image is a midline sagittal view which includes the corpus callosum and cerebellar vermis. Additional parasagittal views are obtained laterally on either side, allowing for the inspection of the lateral horns and choroid plexus (Epelman et. al., 2010; Seigel 2002; Rumack et. al. 2005). The first midline sagittal image displays a number of important structures. The C-shaped corpus callosum appears as a hypoechoic structure bound by echogenic superior and inferior borders (Seigel, 2002). The cingulate gyrus is seen above the corpus callosum, while the septum cavum pellucidum is seen below. The third and fourth ventricles along with the cisterna magna appear anechoic at their respective positions (Seigel, 2002). The white matter containing pons and cerebellar vermis are also seen (Grant et. al., 1981 Seigel, 2002). Additional views are obtained in the parasagittal plane by cutting through the lateral ventricles. The intraventricular echogenic choroid plexus is well evaluated in this plane. The temporal lobe and caudothalamic groove, which separates the caudate nucleus from the thalamus, are also visualized. Progressing laterally, parasagittal images are obtained through the temporal horns of the lateral ventricles further demonstrating the hyperechoic choroid plexus (Seigel, 2002). A final view can be made on either side through the lateral thalamus.

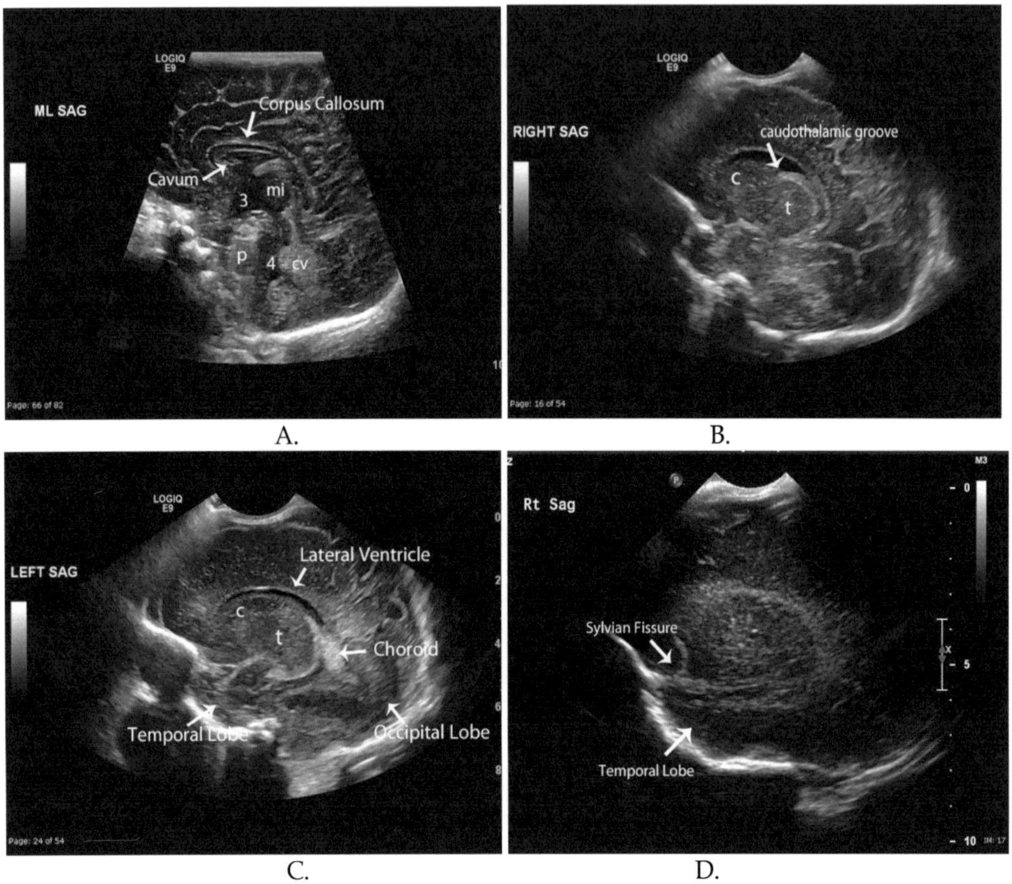

Fig. 2. (a-d). Sagittal images of a normal neonatal brain. 3 (third ventricle) mi (mass intermedia) p (belly of the pons) 4 (fourth ventricle) cv (cerebellar vermis) c (caudate nucleus) t (thalamus)

Interpretation of cranial gray-scale imaging relies not only on neuro-anatomical knowledge but also on recognition of the normal echogenic patterns of cranial structures. The following concepts are important to keep in mind when examining cranial sonographic images. Gray matter is normally hypoechoic while white matter is hyperechoic. Therefore, an anomaly is indicated when the appearance of the two is switched (North & Lowe, 2009). Secondly, though the normal brain is always symmetric, symmetry is not always normal. A prime example is seen in bilaterally symmetric hyperechoic thalami which may signal thalamic edema, ischemia, or infarct (Huang & Castillo, 2008; North & Lowe, 2009). Thirdly, it is important to visualize the pia mater, cortical gray matter, and white matter to detect focal hemorrhages and infarcts (Grant et. al. 1981). From superficial to deep, a hyperechoic, hypoechoic, hyperechoic pattern should be seen in these layers, respectively (**Figure 3**) (Slovis & Kuhns, 1981). Finally, periventricular white matter should look homogenous with an echogenicity less than or equal to the neighboring choroid plexus (North & Lowe, 2009; Seigel, 2002). A change from this appearance including asymmetry, heterogeneity, or hyperechogenicity greater than that of adjacent choroid could be indicative of periventricular leukomalacia (**Figure 4**).

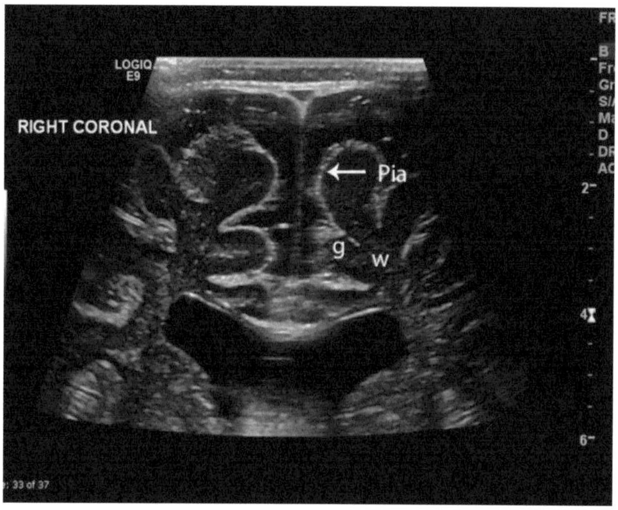

Fig. 3. High resolution linear image of the cerebral cortex. Note the hyperechoic pia matter, hypoechoic gray matter, and hyperechoic white matter. This image displays normal gray-white matter differentiation in a term neonate.

2.2 Doppler imaging

The next step in pediatric cranial sonography is Doppler screening of the vasculature (North & Lowe, 2009). First, the Circle of Willis is investigated with color Doppler imaging using either the anterior or temporal fontanels. Spectral tracings of the internal cerebral arteries are obtained and used to calculate the peak systolic velocity (PSV), end diastolic velocity (EDV), and resistive index (RI). Color Doppler images are then performed in the sagittal plane to evaluate the sagittal sinus and vein of Galen. Power Doppler imaging can be utilized to detect signs of ischemia which may present as areas of hyper- or hypovascularity (Epelman et. al., 2010).

Doppler imaging, whether color, spectral, or power, can be achieved in either the anterior or temporal fontanels according to ease or vessels to be examined (**Figure 5a &b**) (Lowe & Bulas, 2005). While either fontanel enables the inspection of the circle of Willis, use of the anterior fontanel better displays the internal cerebral arteries (**Figure 5c**) (Rumack et. al. 2005; Seigel, 2002). Color Doppler imaging is used to screen the vasculature for patency and resistance to flow. Arteries are usually evaluated in the coronal plane, while venous structures are best imaged in sagittal. Indices, including the resistive index (RI), systolic, and diastolic velocities, typically of the middle or internal cerebral arteries are obtained from spectral tracings. The RI is calculated from the peak systolic velocity and end diastolic velocity by the following formula:

$$RI= (PSV-EDV)/PSV$$

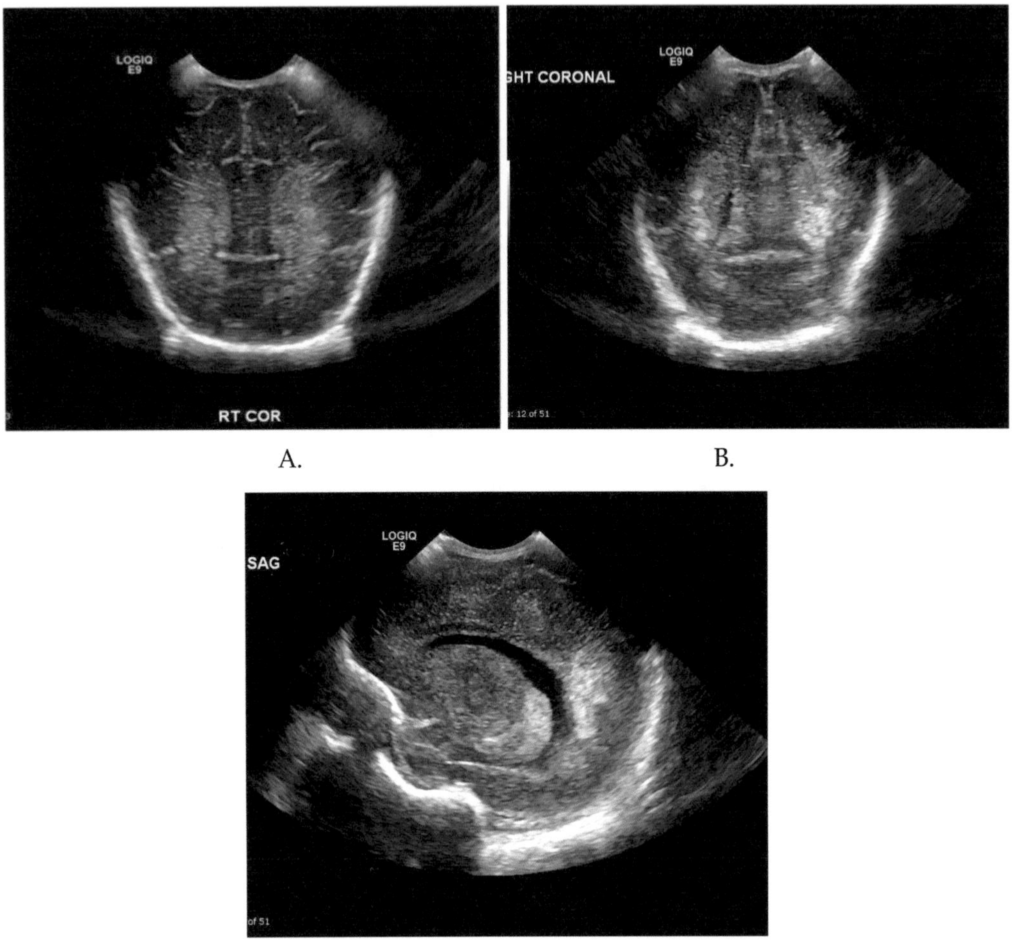

C.

Fig. 4. (a) Normal echogenicity in the periventricular white matter is symmetric and homogenous. It is less echogenic than the neighboring choroid. (b and c) Periventricular leukomalacia is asymmetric, heterogeneous, and more echogenic than the adjacent choroid plexus.

The RI may be impacted by flow velocity, blood volume, congenital cardiac anomalies, and peripheral vascular resistance (Bulas & Vezina, 1999; Soetaert et. al., 2009). The RI tends to decline with age as diastolic flow increases with the progression from fetal to newborn circulation. Premature infants exhibit a normal RI of .62-.92 that typically drops to .43-.58 by the time the child is older than 2 years (Allison et. al., 2000; Lowe & Bulas, 2005). Therefore, a value ranging from .6-.9 is used to estimate a normal RI in premature and full-term infants. Lower values may indicate acute hypoxia or ischemia, which may trigger increased diastolic flow through cerebral vasodilation. Higher values may suggest cerebral swelling where intracranial pressures rise higher than systemic pressures leading to decreased diastolic flow (North & Lowe, 2009).

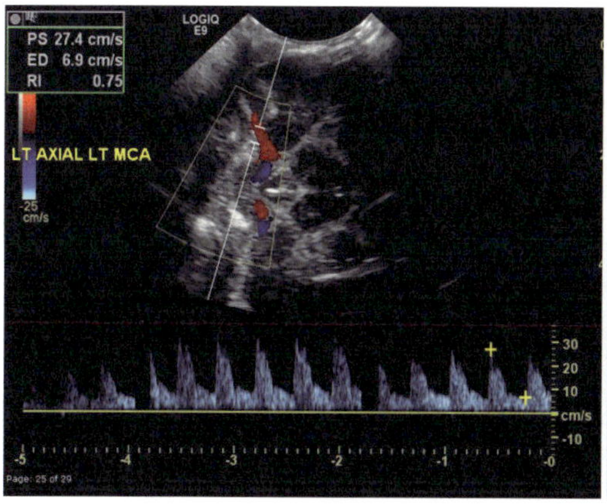

A.

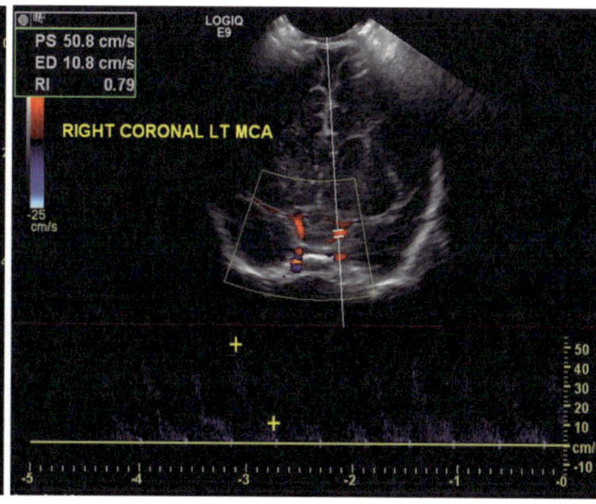

B.

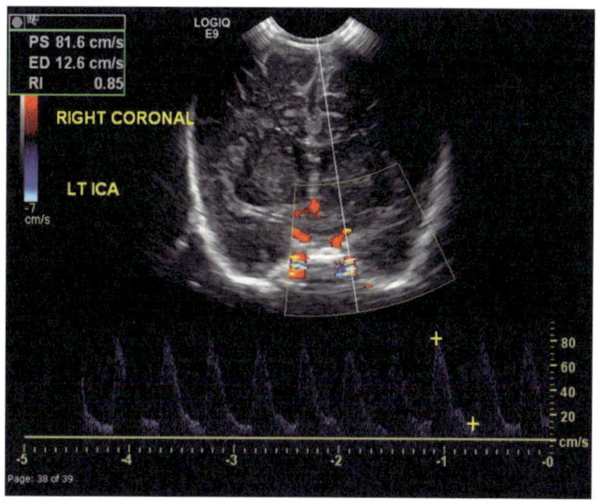

C.

Fig. 5. (a) Axial and (b) coronal Doppler images and spectral waveforms of the normal Circle of Willis. Axial images were obtained through the temporal fontanel. Coronal images were obtained through the anterior fontanel. (c) Coronal Doppler images and spectral waveforms of a normal ICA obtained through the anterior fontanel.

As mentioned above, the RI is not always reliable. This is especially true in children with extra cardiac shunts or congenital cardiac malformations with left to right intracardiac shunt, particularly a patent ductus arteriosis (Lipman et. al., 1982). In addition, vessel velocity fluctuations are common leading to the need to acquire multiple measurements.

2.3 Additional fontanels and linear imaging

A state of the art approach to head sonography requires utilization of additional fontanels and high-resolution linear imaging. The mastoid fontanels enable inspection of the cerebellar hemispheres and aid in detection of posterior fossa hemorrhages and congenital anomalies (**Figure 6**) (Di Salvo, 2001). Mastoid fontanels are also used to evaluate the size and appearance of the fourth ventricle and cisterna magna. Due to improved posterior fossa hemorrhage discovery, these views are now part of the standard of care for hindbrain

imaging (Seigel, 2002). The transverse sinuses can be examined through posterior fontanels or foramen magnum. Color Doppler can aid in evaluating vascular flow and patency (Brennan et. al., 2005; Epelman et. al, 2010; Lowe & Bulas, 2005, Sudakoff et. al., 1993).
Linear imaging should be used to assess the subarachnoid space and superficial cortex via the anterior fontanel (**Figure 7**) (Epelman et. al., 2010). Supplementary fontanels may be explored to gain accessory views.

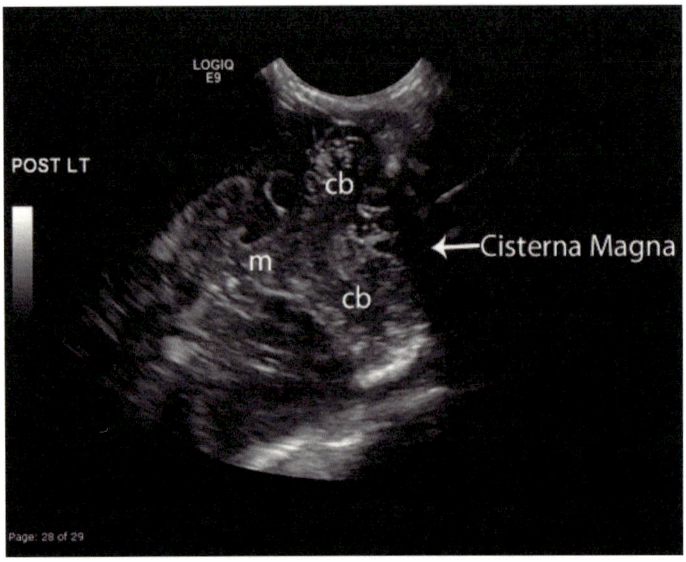

Fig. 6. Normal posterior fossa image obtained using the mastoid fontanel.
cb (cerebellar hemispheres) m (midbrain)

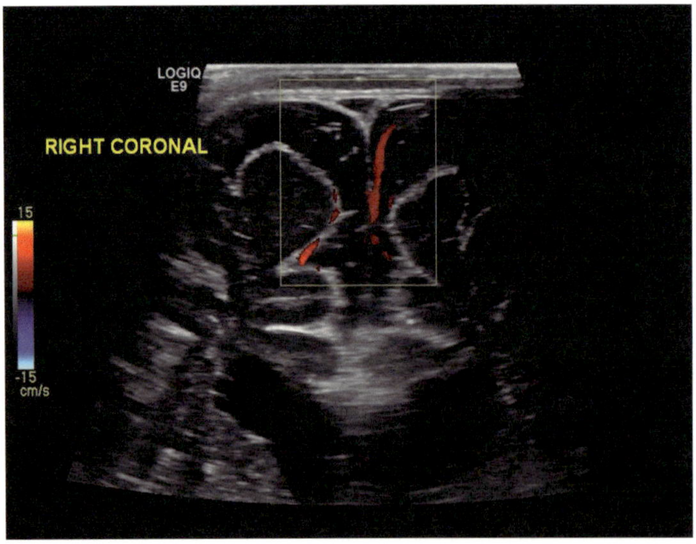

Fig. 7. High resolution linear image demonstrating prominent extra axial CSF spaces. Doppler interrogation demonstrates a vessel crossing the space, confirming subarachnoid fluid rather than subdural.

3. Pitfalls and normal variants

3.1 Immature sulcation in premature infants

The infant brain becomes increasingly sulcated during development. Cerebral cortices in neonates born prior to the 24th week gestational age contain only Sylvian fissures in an otherwise smooth cerebral cortex making lissencephaly in this age group an avoidable diagnosis (**Figure 8**). At 24 weeks gestational age, the parietooccipital fissure is seen. This is followed by the appearance of the cingulate sulci at 28 weeks gestational age with additional branching occurring into full term (North & Lowe, 2009; Rumack et. al., 2005).

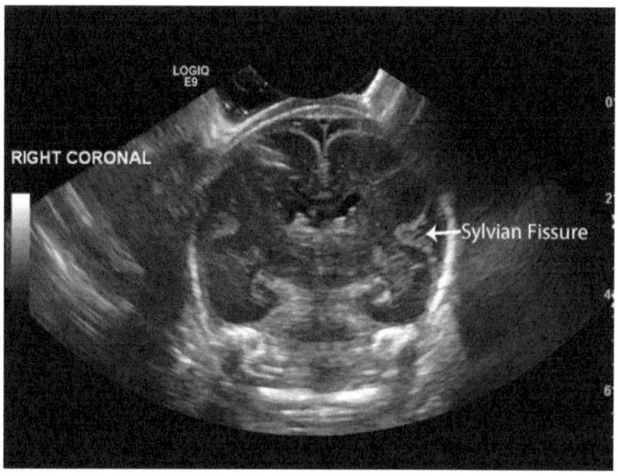

Fig. 8. Coronal image of a 24 week gestation preterm infant. Note the lack of cerebral sulci. Only the Sylvian Fissures are clearly visible.

3.2 Persistent fetal fluid-filled spaces

Healthy infants commonly exhibit persistent fetal fluid-filled spaces. Typical findings consist of cavum septum pellucidum (CSP), cavum vergae, and cavum veli interpositi. Usually, these spaces start to close around the 6th month of gestational age, and most (85%) are completely closed by 3-6 months of chronological age, although some may remain present into adulthood (Epelman, 2006; Faruggia & Babcock, 1981; Needleman et. al., 2007; Osborn, 1991). The CSP is a midline fluid-filled space located anteriorly and between the frontal horns of the lateral ventricles (**Figure 9**). It is formed from failed septal laminae fusion (Epelman, 2006). If the space extends posterior to the fornices, it is termed cavum vergae. (Bronshtein & Weiner, 1992; Epelman et. al., 2006). A cavum veli interpositi is located even further posteriorly as a separate fluid-filled space found in the pineal region. Due to the location of the cavum veli interpositi. It must be distinguished from other commonly occurring manifestations in this region, specifically, congenital pineal cysts and vein of Galen malformations (Chen et. al., 1998; Epelman et. al., 2006).

3.3 Mega cisterna magna

A mega cisterna magna is defined as a cisterna magna that measures greater than 8mm in either sagittal or axial planes. It is present in approximately 1% of infant brains and is a benign finding of no clinical significance. It is, therefore, key not to mistake a mega cisterna magna for other malformations that can occur in the posterior fossa (Bernard et. al., 2001; Epelman et.al., 2006; Nelson et. al., 2004). Unlike arachnoid cysts, a mega cisterna magna will not exhibit mass effect on adjacent structures. It can also be differentiated from Dandy-

Walker malformations by visualization of the cerebellar vermis (Epelman et.al., 2006; Nelson et. al., 2004).

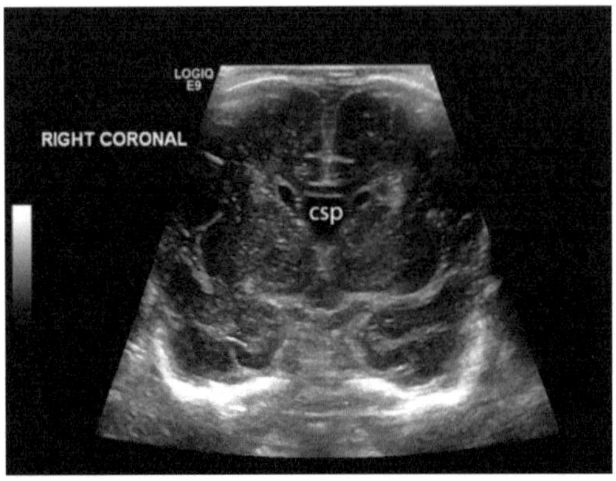

Fig. 9. Coronal image of a term neonate demonstrating a midline fluid-filled space between the frontal horns of the lateral ventricles consistent with a cavum septum pellucidum (csp).

3.4 Asymmetric ventricular size

20-40% of infants may exhibit asymmetrical ventricular size (Middleton et. al., 2009; Seigel, 2002; Winchester et. al., 1986). This can appear as a discrepancy between the frontal and occipital horn size termed colpocephaly or as variations in sizes of the left and right ventricles. The former may co-occur with agenesis of the corpus callosum or Chiari II malformations. (Achiron et. al., 1997; Horbar et. al., 1983; Seigel, 2002). The latter is a common finding in which the less dependent ventricle is the largest. The left ventricle is most commonly the bigger of the two with sizes varying depending on patient position (Enriquez et. al., 2003; Koeda et. al., 1988; Seigel, 2002).

3.5 Choroid plexus variants

The choroid plexus is located at the roof of the third ventricle and travels through the foramen of Monro into the lateral ventricles (North & Lowe, 2009; Seigel, 2002). It does not extend into the frontal or occipital horns, so hyperechoic material in these areas should suggest pathology. Choroid appearing substance anterior to the caudothalamic groove is likely a germinal matrix hemorrhage, while interventricular hemorrhage may be indicated by hyperechoic material in the dependent portions of the occipital horns (Grant et. al., 1983; Seigel, 2002). Choroid plexus morphology, however, is variable and should not be confused with hemorrhage. This is especially true in the glomus of the lateral ventricles and ventricular atria where lobular and bulbous choroid is commonly seen (**Figure 10**). The occipital horns may also display bulbous and drumstick-shaped choroid variations, particularly in conjunction with Chiari II malformations (Di Salvo, 2001; Seigel, 2002).

In addition, choroid cysts are commonly identified (**Figure 11**). When seen in isolation and measuring less than 1cm, they are considered a benign finding (DeRoo et. al., 1988; Epelman et. al., 2006; Ostlere et. al., 1990; van Baalen & Versmold, 2004). When choroid cysts are found to be multiple, bilateral, or greater than 1 cm in size, this may suggest a chromosomal abnormality (Gupta et. al., 1995; Seigel, 2002).

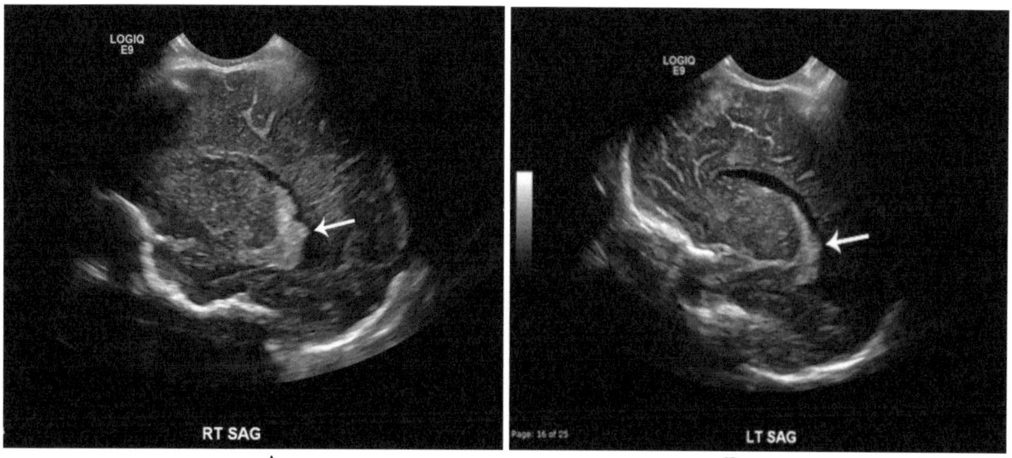

A. B.

Fig. 10. Sagittal images of the (a) right and (b) left lateral ventricles demonstrating asymmetry in the choroid plexus (arrows) with the right being larger and more lobulated than the left. Both are normal.

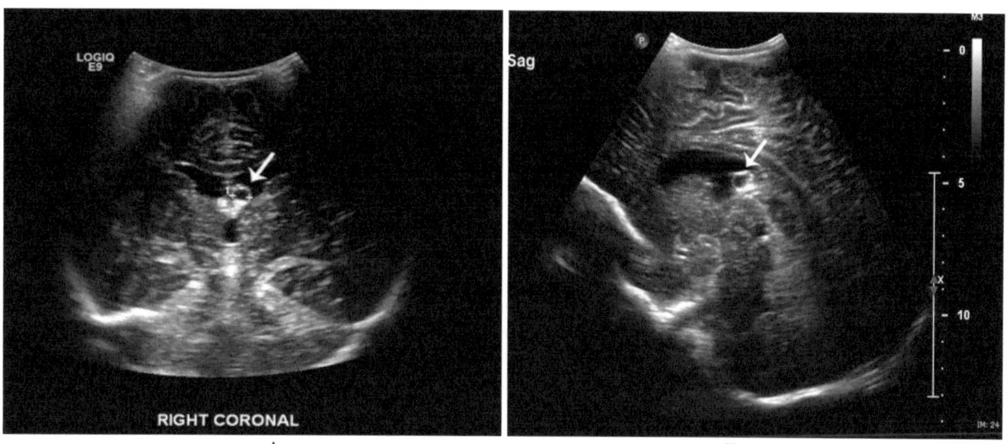

A. B.

Fig. 11. Coronal (a) and Sagittal (b) images demonstrate and anechoic, cystic structure (arrows) arising from the anterior choroid consistent with a choroid plexus cyst.

3.6 Periventricular cystic lesions

Connatal cysts, subependymal cysts, germinolytic cysts, and white matter cysts can all appear in the periventricular area (Epelman et. al., 2006; North & Lowe, 2009). Connatal cysts are always found in immediate proximity with the frontal horns where they are found in multiples and exhibit a string of pearls appearance (**Figure 12**). They are a normal variant believed to be caused by deficient coaptation of the ventricles (Chang et. al., 2006; Enriquez et. al., 2003; Epelman et. al, 2006; Pal et. al., 2001; Rosenfeld et. al., 1997). These cysts are often discovered shortly after birth and usually undergo spontaneous regression (Chang et. al., 2006; Rosenfeld et. al., 1997). Subependymal cysts and germinolytic cysts both occur at the caudothalamic groove. Subependymal cysts are the sequlae of germinal matrix hemorrhages and geminolytic cysts are commonly seen in metabolic disorders. Despite the differing pathophysiology, the imaging characteristics are identical and the two cysts cannot be distinguished from one another. (Epelman et. al., 2006; Herini et. al., 2003). Lastly, hypoxia and ischemic injury in preterm infants can lead to white matter cysts located near the lateral ventricles in cases of cystic periventricular leukomalacia (**Figure 13**) (Epelman et. al., 2006; North & Lowe, 2009).

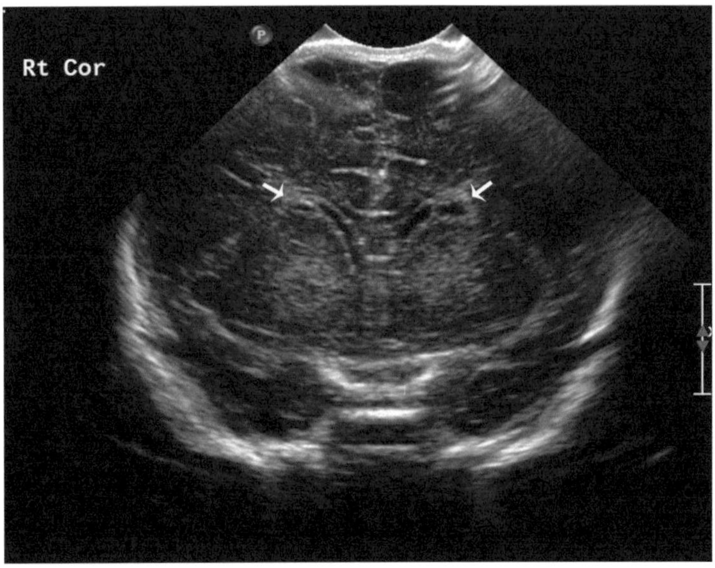

Fig. 12. Cystic lesions in the bilateral frontal periventricular white matter (arrows) consistent with connatal cysts. Connatal cysts are considered to be a normal variant.

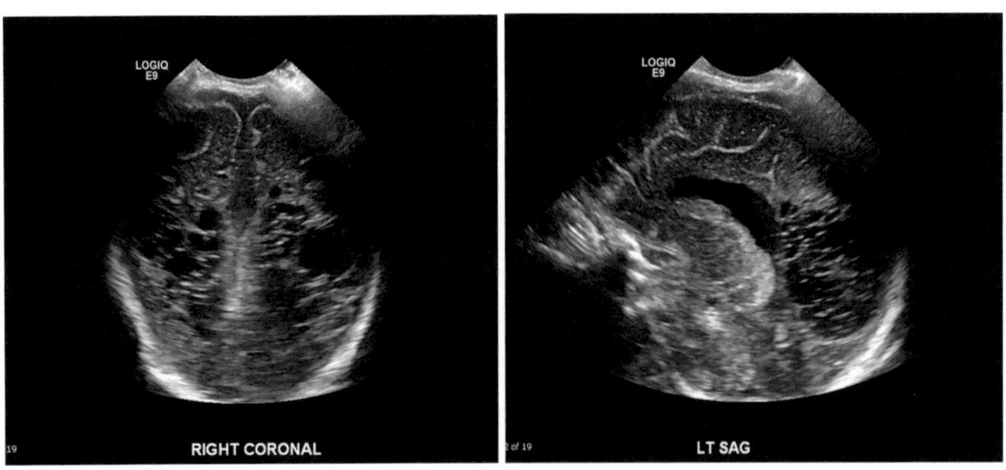

A. B.

Fig. 13. (a) Coronal and (b) Sagittal images demonstrating multiple cystic lesions in the posterior periventricular white matter consistent with cystic periventricular leukomalacia.

3.7 Periventricular halos

Periventricular halos are hyperechoic white matter pseudolesions found adjacent to ventricles (**Figure 14**). They are discovered more often in preterm than term infants and are caused by anisotropic effect. These artifacts tend to disappear on tangential imaging and should have less echogenicity than neighboring choroid plexus (Enriquez et. al., 2003; Seigel, 2002). Linear imaging may serve a complimentary role in evaluation, helping distinguish between normal and abnormal processes. Pathological findings such as periventricular hemorrhage, leukmalacia, or other abnormalities, are seen in two planes (DiPietro et. al., 1986; Schafer et. al., 2009).

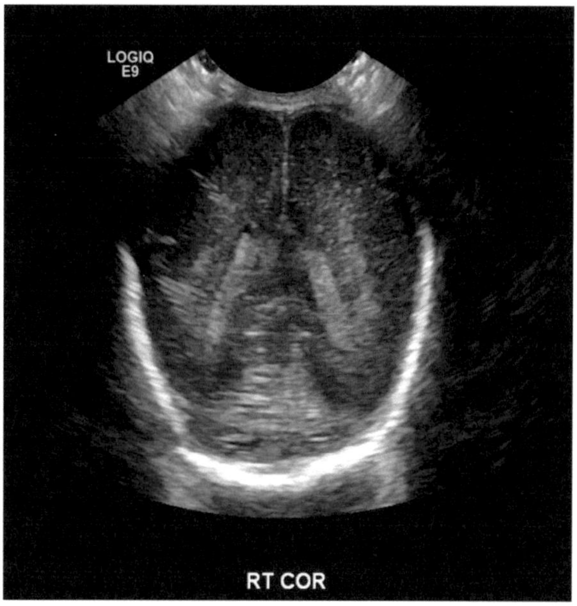

Fig. 14. Coronal image in a premature infant (note the lack of sulci) demonstrating hyperechoic psedudolesions in the periventricular white matter consistent with normal "periventricular halo". This should not be confused with the more echogenic, less homogeneous findings of periventricular luekomalacia.

3.8 Lenticulostriate vasculopathy

Lenticulostriate vasculopathy appears as linear, branching or punctate increased echogenicity within the thalami (**Figure 15**). It can be unilateral or bilateral (Cabanas et. al., 1994; Coley et. al., 2000; Makhoul et. al., 2003). It is associated with congenital infections (TORCH infections), metabolic syndromes (peroxisomal biogenesis disorders), severe congenital heart disease, and chromosomal anomalies (Patau's syndrome) which are all believed to cause lenticulostriate artery wall thickening (Cabanas et. al. 1994; Leijser et. al., 2007; Makhoul et. al., 2003; Te Pas et. al., 2005; Teele et. al., 1988). Sometimes, however, no specific cause can be ascertained making lenticulostriate vasculopathy a non-specific finding on sonography(Cabanas et. al., 1994; Coley et. al., 2000; Makhoul et. al., 2003).

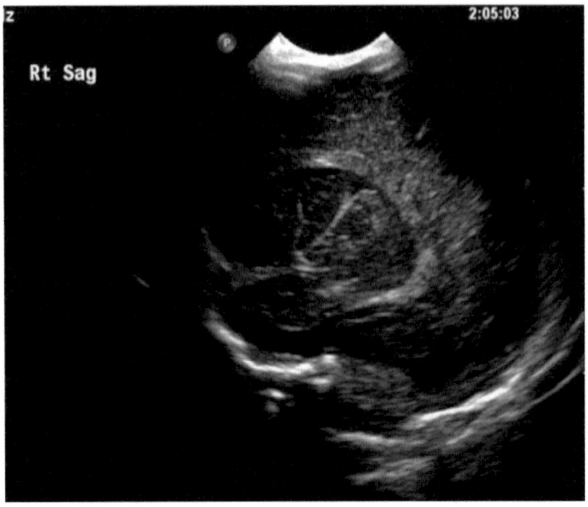

Fig. 15. Sagittal image of the right lateral ventricle and thalamus demonstrating echogenic linear and branching vessels in the thalamus consistent with lenticulostriate vasculopthy.

4. Conclusion

Technical advances in ultrasound examination have made this a highly sensitive means to detect and guide treatment for pediatric cranial pathologies. When performing a head ultrasound, it is important to use modern modalities to full advantage. Doppler and linear sonography as well as the use of additional fontanels play a key role in the evaluation of the pediatric brain. Further knowledge of normal anatomy, normal variants, and imaging pitfalls increases diagnostic accuracy and helps to limit misdiagnoses.

5. References

Achiron R, Yagel S, Rotstein Z, Inbar O, Mashiach S, Lipitz S. Cerebral lateral ventricular asymmetry: is this a normal ultrasonographic finding in the fetal brain? *Obstet Gynecol* 1997; 89:233–237

Allison JW, Faddis LA, Kinder DL, Roberson PK, Glasier CM, Seibert JJ. Intracranial resistive index (RI) values in normal term infants during the first day of life. *Pediatr Radiol* 2000; 30:618–620

Bernard JP, Moscoso G, Renier D, Ville Y. Cystic malformations of the posterior fossa. *Prenat Diagn* 2001; 21:1064-1069

Brennan KC, Lowe LH, Yeaney GA. Pediatric central nervous system posttransplant lymphoproliferative disorder. *AJNR* 2005; 26:1695–1697

Bronshtein M, Weiner Z. Prenatal diagnosis of dilated cava septi pellucidi et vergae: associated anomalies, differential diagnosis, and pregnancy outcome. *Obstet Gynecol* 1992; 80:838–842

Bulas DI, Vezina GL. Preterm anoxic injury: radiologic evaluation. *Radiol Clin North Am* 1999; 37:1147–1161

Cabanas F, Pellicer A, Morales C, Garcia-Alix A, Stiris TA, Quero J. New pattern of hyperechogenicity in thalamus and basal ganglia studied by color Doppler flow imaging. *Pediatr Neurol* 1994; 10:109–116

Chang CL, Chiu NC, Ho CS, Li ST. Frontal horn cysts in normal neonates. *Brain Dev* 2006; 28: 426–430

Chen CY, Chen FH, Lee CC, Lee KW, Hsiao HS. Sonographic characteristics of the cavum velum interpositum. *AJNR* 1998; 19:1631-1635

Coley BD, Rusin JA, Boue DR. Importance of hypoxic/ischemic conditions in the development of cerebral lenticulostriate vasculopathy. *PediatrRadiol* 2000; 30:846-855

Daneman A, Epelman M, Blaser S, Jarrin JR. Imaging of the brain in full-term neonates: does sonography still play a role? *Pediatr Radiol* 2006; 36:636-646

DeRoo TR, Harris RD, Sargent SK, Denholm TA, Crow HC. Fetal choroid plexus cysts: prevalence, clinical significance, and sonographic appearance. *AJR* 1988; 151:1179-1181

DiPietro MA, Brody BA, Teele RL. Peritrigonal echogenic "blush" on cranial sonography: pathologic correlates. *AJR* 1986; 146:1067-1072

Di Salvo DN. A new view of the neonatal brain: clinical utility of supplemental neurologic US imaging windows. *RadioGraphics* 2001; 21:943-955

Enriquez G, Correa F, Lucaya J, Piqueras J, Aso C, Ortega A. Potential pitfalls in cranial sonography. *Pediatr Radiol* 2003; 33:110-117

Epelman M. The whirlpool sign. *Radiology* 2006; 240:910-911

Epelman M, Daneman A, Blaser SI, et al. Differential diagnosis of intracranial cystic lesions at head US: correlation with CT and MR imaging. *RadioGraphics* 2006; 26:173-196

Epelman M, Daneman A, Kellenberger CJ, et al. Neonatal encephalopathy: a prospective comparison of head US and MRI. *Pediatr Radiol* 2010; 40:1640-1650

Farruggia S, Babcock DS. The cavum septi pellucidi: its appearance and incidence with cranial ultrasonography in infancy. *Radiology* 1981; 139: 147-150

Grant EG, Schellinger D, Borts FT, et al. Realtime sonography of the neonatal and infant head. *AJR* 1981; 136:265-270

Grant EG, Schellinger D, Richardson JD, Coffey ML, Smirniotopoulous JG. Echogenic periventricular halo: normal sonographic finding or neonatal cerebral hemorrhage. *AJR* 1983; 140:793-796

Gupta JK, Cave M, Lilford RJ, et al. Clinical significance of fetal choroid plexus cysts. *Lancet* 1995; 346:724-729

Herini E, Tsuneishi S, Takada S, Sunarini, Nakamura H. Clinical features of infants with subependymal germinolysis and choroid plexus cysts. *Pediatr Int* 2003; 45:692-696

Horbar JD, Leahy KA, Lucey JF. Ultrasound identification of lateral ventricular asymmetry in the human neonate. *J Clin Ultrasound* 1983; 11:67-69

Huang BY, Castillo M. Hypoxic-ischemic brain injury: imaging findings from birth to adulthood. *RadioGraphics* 2008; 28:417-439; quiz, 617

Koeda T, Ando Y, Takashima S, Takeshita K, Maeda K. Changes in the lateral ventricle with the head position: ultrasonographic observation. *Neuroradiology* 1988; 30:315-318

Leijser LM, de Vries LS, Rutherford MA, et al. Cranial ultrasound in metabolic disorders presenting in the neonatal period: characteristic features and comparison with MR imaging. *AJNR* 2007; 28:1223-1231

Lipman B, Serwer GA, Brazy JE. Abnormal cerebral hemodynamics in preterm infants with patent ductus arteriosus. *Pediatrics* 1982; 69:778-781

Lowe LH, Bulas DI. Transcranial Doppler imaging in children: sickle cell screening and beyond. *Pediatr Radiol* 2005; 35:54–65

Makhoul IR, Eisenstein I, Sujov P, et al. Neonatal lenticulostriate vasculopathy: further characterisation. *Arch Dis Child Fetal Neonatal Ed* 2003; 88:F410–F414

Middleton WD, Kurtz AB, Hertzbert BS. *Ultrasound: the requisites*. St. Louis, MO: Mosby-Year Book, 2009:377

Needelman H, Schroeder B, Sweeney M, Schmidt J, Bodensteiner JB, Schaefer GB. Postterm closure of the cavum septi pellucidi and developmental outcome in premature infants. *J Child Neurol* 2007; 22:314–316

Nelson MD Jr, Maher K, Gilles FH. A different approach to cysts of the posterior fossa. *Pediatr Radiol* 2004; 34:720–732

North K, Lowe L. Modern head ultrasound: normal anatomy, variants, and pitfalls that may simulate disease. *Ultrasound Clin* 2009; 4:497–512

Osborn A. *Handbook of neuroradiology*. St. Louis, MO: Mosby-Year Book, 1991

Ostlere SJ, Irving HC, Lilford RJ. Fetal choroid plexus cysts: a report of 100 cases. *Radiology* 1990; 175:753–755

Pal BR, Preston PR, Morgan ME, Rushton DI, Durbin GM. Frontal horn thin walled cysts in preterm neonates are benign. *Arch Dis Child Fetal Neonatal Ed* 2001; 85:F187–F193

Rosenfeld DL, Schonfeld SM, Underberg-Davis S. Coarctation of the lateral ventricles: an alternative explanation for subependymal pseudocysts. *Pediatr Radiol* 1997; 27:895–897

Rumack C, Wilson S, Charboneau J. *Diagnostic ultrasound*. St. Louis, MO: Mosby, 2005

Schafer RJ, Lacadie C, Vohr B, et al. Alterations in functional connectivity for language in prematurelyborn adolescents. *Brain* 2009; 132:661–670

Seigel M, ed. *Pediatric sonography*, 3rd ed. Philadelphia, PA: Lippincott Williams & Wilkins, 2002

Slovis TL, Kuhns LR. Real-time sonography of the brain through the anterior fontanel. *AJR* 1981; 136:277–286

Soetaert AM, Lowe LH, Formen C. Pediatric cranial Doppler sonography in children: non-sickle cell applications. *Curr Probl Diagn Radiol* 2009; 38:218–227

Sudakoff GS, Montazemi M, Rifkin MD. The foramen magnum: the underutilized acoustic window to the posterior fossa. *J Ultrasound Med* 1993; 12:205–210

Te Pas AB, van Wezel-Meijler G, Bokenkamp-Gramann R, Walther FJ. Preoperative cranial ultrasound findings in infants with major congenital heart disease. *Acta Paediatr* 2005; 94:1597–1603

Teele RL, Hernanz-Schulman M, Sotrel A. Echogenic vasculature in the basal ganglia of neonates:a sonographic sign of vasculopathy. *Radiology* 1988; 169:423–427

van Baalen A, Versmold H. Choroid plexus cyst: comparison of new ultrasound technique with old histological finding. *Arch Dis Child* 2004; 89:426

Winchester P, Brill PW, Cooper R, Krauss AN, Peterson HD. Prevalence of "compressed" and asymmetric lateral ventricles in healthy full-term neonates: sonographic study. *AJR* 1986; 146

12

Impact of White Matter Damage After Stroke

Robert Lindenberg[1,2] and Rüdiger J. Seitz[3,4]
[1]*Department of Neurology, Beth Israel Deaconess Medical Center and Harvard Medical School, Boston, Massachusetts,*
[2]*Department of Neurology, Charité – Universitaetsmedizin Berlin, Berlin,*
[3]*Department of Neurology, University Hospital Düsseldorf and Biomedical Research Centre, Heinrich-Heine-University Düsseldorf*
[4]*Florey Neuroscience Institutes, Melbourne, Victoria,*
[1]*USA*
[2,3]*Germany*
[4]*Australia*

1. Introduction

Ischemic stroke is one of the leading causes of persistent disability in Western countries (Bejot *et al.*, 2007). It results from cessation of blood supply due to an occlusion of a cerebral artery. Many patients benefit from thrombolysis with the approved drug recombinant tissue plasminogen activator (rtPA). Nevertheless, the clinical effect of intravenously administered rtPA is variable (Hallevi *et al.*, 2009; Wahlgren *et al.*, 2008) which is of particular importance for middle cerebral artery (MCA) stroke: It has been demonstrated that early artery recanalisation yields unevenly distributed, circumscribed infarct lesions within the MCA territory with a great potential for functional recovery; in contrast, failed recanalisation results in large infarcts with a limited potential for functional recovery (Figure 1). Accordingly, an important factor contributing to recovery from stroke is the early restoration of cerebral blood flow. Spontaneous recovery is known to continue for the subsequent weeks to months (Cramer, 2008). Furthermore, recovery can be facilitated by dedicated rehabilitative training with greater effects in greater dosing of training (Kwakkel, 2006) even years after the stroke (Stinear *et al.*, 2007).

Animal studies (Dancause *et al.*, 2005) as well as imaging and electrophysiological studies in humans (Butefisch *et al.*, 2006) have suggested that recovery is brought about by cerebral plasticity. Cerebral plasticity pertains to *functional* changes such as synaptic efficiency as well as *structural* changes such as synaptic sprouting (Dancause *et al.*, 2005; Nudo *et al.*, 1996). Even in the adult brain, a loss of hand motor function due to small cortical lesions within the sensorimotor cortex can be completely restored (Binkofski and Seitz, 2004). However, there are limits to plasticity. For example, severe damage to major pathways such as the pyramidal tract (PT) can be compensated for to some extent, but full functional recovery is often not possible (Lang and Schieber, 2004).

To date, neuroimaging studies of brain infarcts have mostly examined grey matter alterations. Recent advances in diffusion tensor imaging (DTI) and lesion-symptom mapping techniques provided novel ways to investigate the white matter in the context of recovery from stroke (Johansen-Berg *et al.*, 2010). The crucial role of the white matter for functional outcome can be illustrated by the observation that small cortical infarcts, e.g. in the precentral gyrus, typically allow for profound recovery from stroke, whereas infarcts of similar volume in the peri-ventricular white matter or the internal capsule may induce a severe and persistent hemiparesis (Kretschmann, 1988; Wenzelburger *et al.*, 2005). Focusing on DTI and lesion mapping, we will discuss recent studies that established white matter damage as an important factor for functional outcome in the acute stroke phase. Furthermore, alterations of fibre tracts will be presented as a critical determinant of functional recovery due to cerebral plasticity in the subacute and chronic phases after stroke.

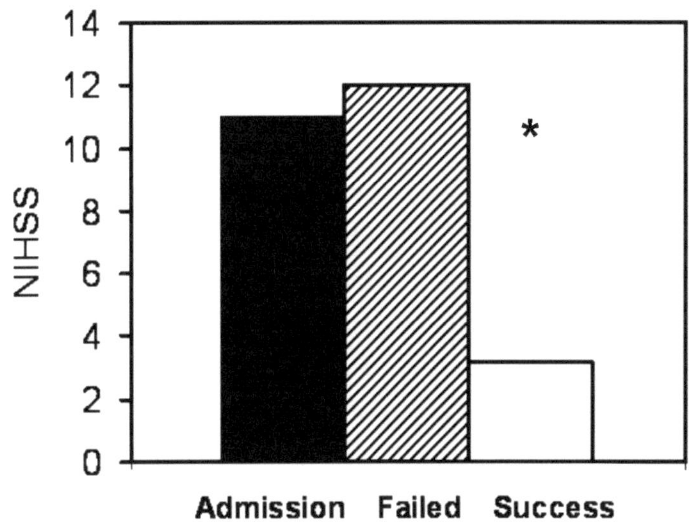

Fig. 1. Neurological deficit as assessed with the NIHSS in 108 MCA stroke patients. Successful thrombolysis with early MCA recanalization resulted in a significant neurological improvement (*: $p<0.0001$). Adapted from (Seitz *et al.*, 2009).

2. Lesion mapping in the acute phase after stroke

Different modalities of magnetic resonance imaging (MRI) are widely used to visualise brain lesions. In acute stroke, perfusion-weighted imaging (PWI) and diffusion-weighted imaging (DWI) can identify the area of acute ischemia. After reperfusion, PWI deficits can be resolved (Davis *et al.*, 2008; Seitz *et al.*, 2005), and also DWI alterations are partly reversible (Kranz and Eastwood, 2009). By use of lesion mapping it has been found that the hemispheric white matter is preferentially affected in patients with major MCA stroke as compared to patients with lesion regression (Stoeckel *et al.*, 2007). Similarly, patients with a lacking response to rtPA and no recanalization of the MCA, showed larger brain lesions with greater hemispheric white matter damage than those with successful thrombolysis (Seitz *et al.*, 2009). The large infarct lesions in patients non-responsive to thrombolysis occurred adjacent to the insular cortex and basal ganglia in the internal capsule and periventricular white matter and were predicted by the maximal perfusion deficit in the acute phase of stroke. These infarcts corresponded to the type II.2 MCA infarcts as described recently (Seitz and Donnan, 2010). Note the close topographic correspondence of the mean area of the most severe perfusion deficit, the DWI abnormalities, and the lesion overlap in the periventricular white matter found in the patients with severe MCA stroke (Figure 2). Since the structural alterations project onto the corona radiate, the corresponding damage of well-defined fibre bundles—such as corticospinal motor tracts—can be assessed specifically by electrophysiology and MRI techniques such as DTI in order to correlate imaging measures with parameters of functional outcome.

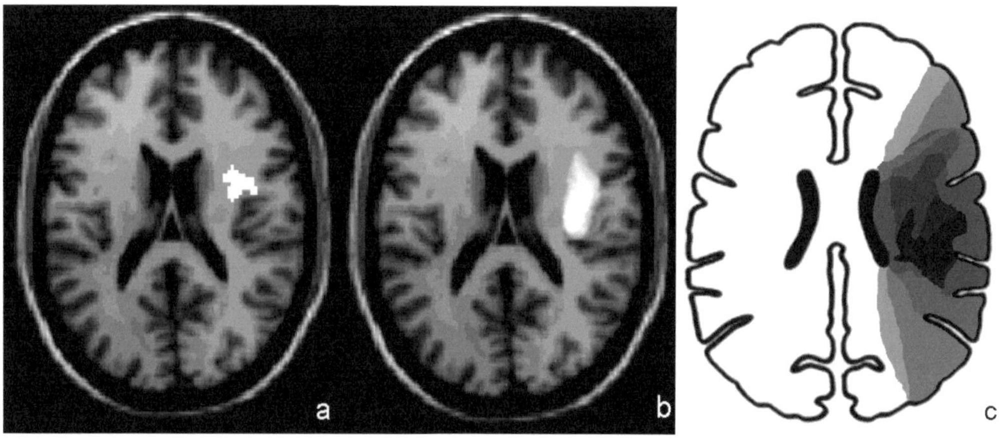

Fig. 2. Lesion pattern in severe MCA stroke. a) Area of the maximal PWI deficit in severely as compared to slightly affected patients. b) Area of common DWI-changes before acute stroke therapy (n=64). c) Overlap of the residual infarct lesions in hemispheric white matter (n=13). Adapted from (Seitz *et al.*, 2009; Stoeckel *et al.*, 2007).

3. Diffusion tensor imaging: Methodological considerations

DTI allows for inferences of the microstructural status of regions of interest in the white matter or reconstructed tracts (Beaulieu, 2009). DTI is a DWI technique that uses the measurement of Brownian motion of water molecules in different directions to reconstruct three-dimensional images of diffusivity (Jones, 2008). Whereas molecules can diffuse relatively freely in water, structural boundaries such as cell membranes or myelin sheaths cause restrictions and yield anisotropic diffusion (Beaulieu, 2002). The degree of diffusion anisotropy can then be used to characterise neural tissue and reveal potential pathological processes (Beaulieu, 2002; Jones, 2008). As an example, Figure 3 shows images of fibre distributions according to the main directions of diffusivity in each voxel of the image. Here, the colour-coding allows for the detection of diffusion abnormalities. Main diffusion directions of single voxels also provide the basis for deterministic tractography, which reconstructs trajectories through a combination of adjacent voxels with similar main directions. Probabilistic tractography, in contrast, propagates numerous pathways through the tensor field so that each voxel can be coded with a number that reflects its likelihood of being connected with a given seed region from which the tracking is started (see (Jones, 2008) for a review).

With both the deterministic and probabilistic approaches, major fibre bundles can be reliably reconstructed (Mori and Zhang, 2006; Wakana *et al.*, 2004). Furthermore, tractography not only allows for the visualisation of tract alterations after lesions, but can be used to quantify those alterations (Johansen-Berg and Behrens, 2006). Furthermore, fractional anisotropy (FA) has been used to describe microstructural abnormalities of white matter. FA indicates the coherence of aligned fibres and is calculated from directional diffusivities (axial and radial). Based on animal experiments, axial diffusivity is thought to primarily reflect axonal integrity whereas radial diffusivity has been suggested to relate to myelin degradation (Acosta-Cabronero *et al.*, 2009; Naismith *et al.*, 2009; Sidaros *et al.*, 2008; Song *et al.*, 2003; Sun *et al.*, 2008). However, the model of a specific relationship of directional diffusivities with discrete pathological processes such as axonal damage or demyelination is controversial, especially in regions of complex fibre architecture (Wheeler-Kingshott and Cercignani, 2009). Interpretations of these parameters with respect to "fibre integrity" should therefore be made with caution.

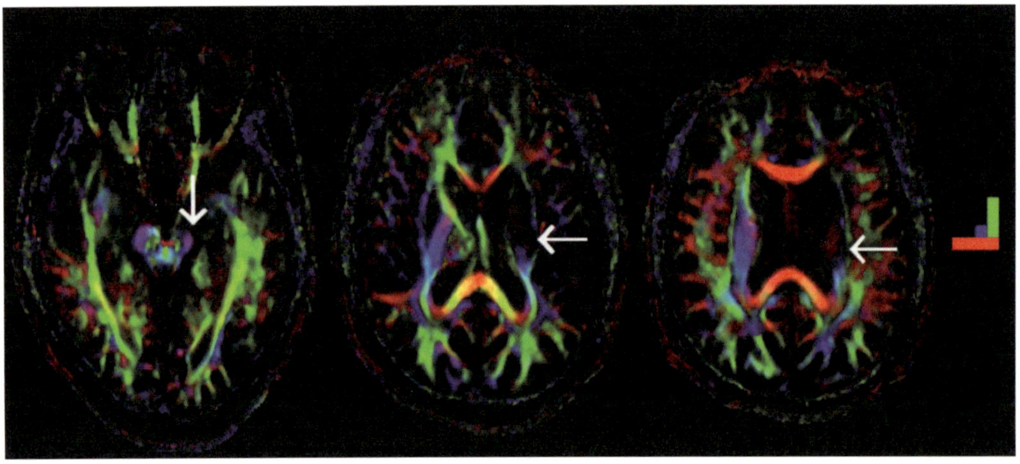

Fig. 3. DTI image of a patient with persistent hemiplegia in a striatocapsular infarct. Arrows point to severe diffusion alteration of corticospinal fibres descending in the posterior limb of the internal capsule and the cerebral pedunculus. The colour bar indicates the spatial orientation of fibres; blue: predominantly inferior – superior orientation, green: predominantly anterior – posterior orientation, red: predominantly left – right orientation.

4. Assessing the impact of white matter damage on motor function using DTI

Although the concept of disconnection syndromes is well established and helps explaining functional deficits after lesions (Geschwind, 1965a; Geschwind, 1965b), the involvement of the white matter in stroke has not received much attention until recently (e.g., (Catani and ffytche, 2005). White matter damage has been found to be particularly prominent in large cerebral infarcts with hemispatial neglect, apraxia and severe hemiparesis (Karnath *et al.*, 2009; Pazzaglia *et al.*, 2008; Seitz *et al.*, 2009; Stoeckel *et al.*, 2007). However, it is not merely the size of the infarct but preferentially its location that determines the functional outcome after stroke (Binkofski *et al.*, 1996; Chen *et al.*, 2000; Zhu *et al.*, 2010).

The importance of corticospinal fibres for recovery of motor function after stroke has been demonstrated with different imaging modalities as well as electrophysiological measures (Binkofski *et al.*, 1996; Fries *et al.*, 1991; Schaechter *et al.*, 2008; Stinear *et al.*, 2007). Based on animal studies, it has been suggested that so-called alternate motor fibres (aMF) can compensate for motor impairment after severe damage to the PT (Lang and Schieber, 2004). In monkeys and cats, the cortico-reticulo-spinal and cortico-rubro-spinal tracts may mediate motor functions in case of PT lesions (Canedo, 1997), whereas these tracts have been described as functionally redundant in healthy animals (Kennedy, 1990). In more detail, it has been observed that damage to the PT and the rubro-spinal tract of monkeys yielded therapy-refractory impairment of the contralateral upper extremity, but monkeys with lesions to the PT that spared the rubro-spinal tract were able to recover considerably (Lawrence & Kuypers, 1968a; Lawrence & Kuypers, 1968b). Furthermore, changes in the synaptic organization of rubro-spinal neurons in response to PT lesions have been reported in monkeys (Belhaj-Saïf & Cheney, 2000).

The first neuroimaging study that translated these findings into motor recovery after human stroke combined structural MRI and electrophysiology to demonstrate that, despite severe degeneration of the PT, motor evoked potentials (MEP) could still be elicited from the ipsilesional motor cortex in patients who had recovered from stroke (Fries *et al.*, 1991). Similarly, patients with hemiparesis due to focal PT lesions were still able to execute individuated finger movements contralateral to the lesion, but with reduced selectivity (Lang and Schieber, 2004). These studies in humans illustrate the role of aMF after stroke similar to that observed in non-human primates.

Using diffusivity parameters and tractography, researchers can examine fibre degeneration at different stages of motor recovery after stroke (Kang *et al.*, 2000; Lindberg *et al.*, 2007; Thomalla *et al.*, 2004; Werring *et al.*, 2000). In the chronic stage, structural damage to the PT could be related to measures of functional impairment (Schaechter *et al.*, 2009; Stinear *et al.*, 2007). Besides the PT, DTI has been applied to reconstruct aMF using deterministic fibre tracking algorithms and, thereby, to explore their role for motor recovery after stroke (Lindenberg *et al.*, 2010). Consistent with previous animal and human studies mentioned above, the differential affection of PT and aMF yielded a three-tier classification system suggesting that (1) when both PT and aMF could be reconstructed, patients showed only mild impairment, (2) when damage occurred to the PT but aMF remained relatively preserved, patients were only moderately impaired, and (3) when pronounced damage to both the PT and aMF was visible, patients was most severely impaired (Figure 4). In addition, DTI-based tractography allows to topographically relate lesions to corticospinal fibres and provides insights into their somatotopic organisation (Konishi *et al.*, 2005; Kunimatsu *et al.*, 2003; Lee *et al.*, 2005; Nelles *et al.*, 2008; Newton *et al.*, 2006; Yamada *et al.*, 2004). Furthermore, the calculation of the overlap between lesion and tracts can explain some of the variance in motor outcome after stroke (Zhu *et al.*, 2010).

5. Predicting functional potential for motor recovery using DTI

One of the most important clinical questions after stroke is a patient's potential for recovery from stroke-induced deficits. Small cortical infarcts in the precentral gyrus typically allow for a profound recovery from hemiparesis. In contrast, infarcts of similar volume in the periventricular hemispheric white matter or the posterior limb of the internal capsule may induce a severe persistent hemiparesis (Kretschmann, 1988). Electrophysiological studies suggest that the functional integrity of ipsilesional motor circuits as well as interhemispheric interactions play a major role in motor recovery from hemiparesis after stroke (Perez and Cohen, 2009). Although transcranial magnetic stimulation (TMS) has been shown to strongly correlate with motor impairment in the acute and subacute phase after stroke, its predictive value appears unclear in the chronic stage (Talelli *et al.*, 2006). However, a combination of TMS and DTI-derived parameters of corticospinal tracts proved to be useful in estimating a patient's potential for recovery when undergoing motor rehabilitation even years after the stroke (Stinear *et al.*, 2007). Similarly, DTI in the acute stroke phase helped predicting outcome at three months (Jang *et al.*, 2008).

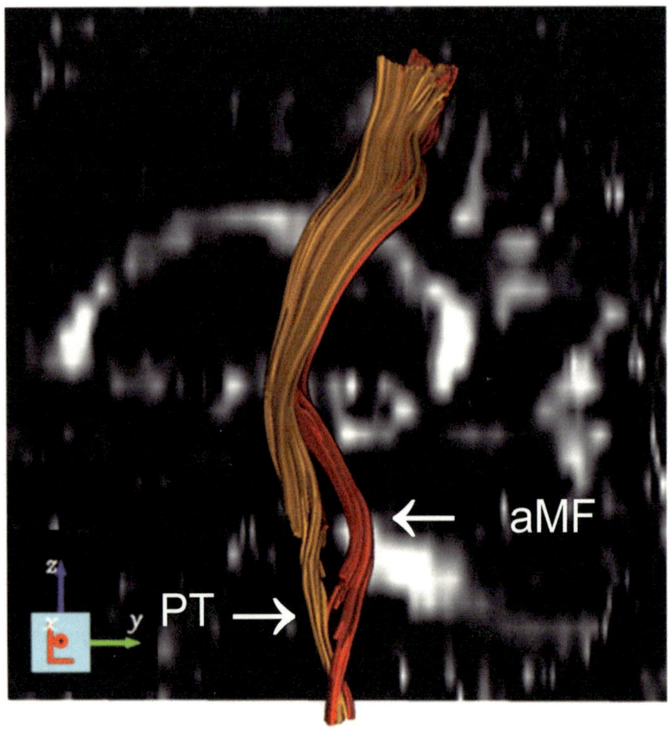

Fig. 4. The course of the pyramidal tract (PT) and alternate motor fibres (aMF) from the white matter underlying the precentral gyrus to the brainstem in a healthy subject.

In order to define predictors of therapeutic response to novel rehabilitation techniques such as non-invasive brain stimulation, it may be useful to examine transcallosal motor fibres as well. Using transcranial direct current stimulation (tDCS) or repetitive TMS, it has been demonstrated that both the up-regulation of intact portions of the ipsilesional and down-regulation of contralesional motor cortices facilitates motor recovery after stroke (Schlaug *et al.*, 2008). Together with evidence from electrophysiological investigations (Perez and Cohen, 2009) and functional MRI (Carter *et al.*, 2009; Grefkes *et al.*, 2008), there is ample evidence for the importance of inter-hemispheric interactions in functional recovery from a stroke. To complement these findings, a study in healthy subjects revealed an association of function and microstructure of transcallosal motor connections (Wahl *et al.*, 2007). In chronic stroke patients, DTI-derived measures of transcallosal motor fibres as well as ipsilesional corticospinal tracts (PT and aMF) could be used to explain the therapeutic response to rehabilitation: the more the diffusivity profiles resembled those observed in healthy subjects, the greater a patient's potential for functional recovery (Lindenberg *et al.*, 2011). Thus, diffusivity profiles of motor tracts, particularly, in combination with electrophysiological measures can serve as predictors of a patient's potential for spontaneous recovery as well as in response to different types of neurorehabilitation techniques.

6. Impact of white matter damage for functional deficits beyond hemiparesis

Brain infarcts with white matter involvement lead to disconnection of areas in perilesional tissue, but also remote locations. This has been shown using positron emission tomography of cerebral blood flow and metabolism as well as with MRI (Feeney and Baron, 1986). Lesion analysis by use of statistical parametric mapping revealed that cortical infarcts result in remote changes in the ipsilesional thalamus, while striatocapsular infarcts induce changes in the contralesional cerebellum (Seitz *et al.*, 1994). Consequently, functional changes occur in regions spatially distant from the area of infarction, an event which has been termed diaschisis. In the chronic phase after stroke, scar formation and fibre degeneration have been shown to result in brain atrophy (Kraemer *et al.*, 2004). Many patients retain functional impairments which can be documented by dedicated investigations including neuropsychology, electrophysiology and DTI. A clinical example is ataxic hemiplegia resulting from infarct lesions around the internal capsule with cortico-cerebellar disconnection (Classen *et al.*, 1995). Similarly, callosal infarcts can induce a lasting decoupling of both hands (Seitz *et al.*, 2004). Infarcts in the frontal parasagittal white matter can produce a deficit of visual face processing probably due to disruption of fronto-occipitotemporal projections (Schafer *et al.*, 2007). Lesion studies in neglect have demonstrated subcortical white matter involvement in the peri-insular area and the internal capsule (Karnath *et al.*, 2004). In Gerstmann's syndrome it has been shown recently that the different parietal cortical subareas which process finger naming, colour naming, right-left orientation, and calculation can all be impaired by a single subcortical white matter lesion affecting the point of convergence of their subcortical projections (Rusconi et al. 2009). These data are of considerable interest given the impact of white matter abnormalities for cognitive decline and the development of dementia after stroke (Dufouil *et al.*, 2009). Taken together, many clinically well-established syndromes are likely to result from cortico-cortical and cortico-subcortical disconnections.

7. Fibre tract changes in white matter and cerebral plasticity

As observed in lesion experiments, intensive rehabilitation allowed animals with damage of corticospinal tracts to recover considerably (Maier *et al.*, 2008). In these animals, collateral fibres increased their innervation density and extended toward the ventral and dorsal horn in response to forced limb use. In contrast, animals that were impeded in their usage of the affected limbs remained impaired and did not show such plastic changes. This highlights the importance of examining white matter structures to determine the extent of potential recovery. In monkeys it has been found that damage of white matter adjacent to lesions in the visual cortex determined the extent of remote and transneural degeneration in the dorsal geniculate and retina (Cowey *et al.*, 1999). Preliminary results in humans undergoing intonation-based speech therapy for chronic aphasia suggest plastic changes in the contralesional arcuate fasciculus associated with improvement in speech production (Schlaug *et al.*, 2009). In healthy subjects, it has already been demonstrated that DTI allows for the detection of white matter changes in response to training, as indicated by an increase in FA after training (Scholz *et al.*, 2009). Taken together, homologous contralesional regions or partially preserved perilesional areas and their associated fibre tracts seem to exhibit plastic reorganisation upon dedicated training. However, more work in experimental animals is needed to come to a better understanding which microstructural and physicochemical changes underlie the signal changes assessed with DTI in men. In the future, DTI may serve as a surrogate marker of cerebral plasticity and help evaluating a patient's response to rehabilitation.

8. Conclusions

White matter changes after stroke are important determinants for presentation and severity of the neurological deficits as well as for prospects of recovery or secondary cognitive decline. Notably, DTI appears to be a valuable tool for predicting the individual patient's perspective for recovery in order to tailor an optimized rehabilitation regime.

9. References

Acosta-Cabronero J, Williams GB, Pengas G, Nestor PJ. Absolute diffusivities define the landscape of white matter degeneration in Alzheimer's disease. Brain 2009: Epub ahead of print.

Beaulieu C. The basis of anisotropic water diffusion in the nervous system - a technical review. NMR Biomed 2002; 15: 435-55.

Beaulieu C. The biological basis of diffusion anisotropy. In: Johansen-Berg H, Behrens TE, editors. Diffusion MRI: From quantitative measurement to in vivo neuroanatomy. London: Academic Press; 2009. p. 105-26.

Bejot Y, Benatru I, Rouaud O, Fromont A, Besancenot JP, Moreau T, et al. Epidemiology of stroke in Europe: geographic and environmental differences. J Neurol Sci 2007; 262: 85-8.

Binkofski F, Seitz RJ. Modulation of the BOLD-response in early recovery from sensorimotor stroke. Neurology 2004; 63: 1223-9.

Binkofski F, Seitz RJ, Arnold S, Classen J, Benecke R, Freund HJ. Thalamic metabolism and corticospinal tract integrity determine motor recovery in stroke. Ann Neurol 1996; 39: 460-70.

Butefisch CM, Kleiser R, Seitz RJ. Post-lesional cerebral reorganisation: evidence from functional neuroimaging and transcranial magnetic stimulation. J Physiol Paris 2006; 99: 437-54.

Canedo A. Primary motor cortex influences on the descending and ascending systems. Prog Neurobiol 1997; 51: 287-335.

Carter AR, Astafiev SV, Lang CE, Connor LT, Rengachary J, Strube MJ, et al. Resting inter-hemispheric fMRI connectivity predicts performance after stroke. Ann Neurol 2009; 67: 365-75.

Catani M, ffytche DH. The rises and falls of disconnection syndromes. Brain 2005; 128: 2224-39.

Chen CL, Tang FT, Chen HC, Chung CY, Wong MK. Brain lesion size and location: effects on motor recovery and functional outcome in stroke patients. Arch Phys Med Rehabil 2000; 81: 447-52.

Classen J, Kunesch E, Binkofski F, Hilperath F, Schlaug G, Seitz RJ, et al. Subcortical origin of visuomotor apraxia. Brain 1995; 118 (Pt 6): 1365-74.

Cowey A, Stoerig P, Williams C. Variance in transneuronal retrograde ganglion cell degeneration in monkeys after removal of striate cortex: effects of size of the cortical lesion. Vision Res 1999; 39: 3642-52.

Cramer SC. Repairing the human brain after stroke: I. Mechanisms of spontaneous recovery. Ann Neurol 2008; 63: 272-87.

Dancause N, Barbay S, Frost SB, Plautz EJ, Chen D, Zoubina EV, et al. Extensive cortical rewiring after brain injury. J Neurosci 2005; 25: 10167-79.

Davis SM, Donnan GA, Parsons MW, Levi C, Butcher KS, Peeters A, et al. Effects of alteplase beyond 3 h after stroke in the Echoplanar Imaging Thrombolytic Evaluation Trial (EPITHET): a placebo-controlled randomised trial. Lancet Neurol 2008; 7: 299-309.

Dufouil C, Godin O, Chalmers J, Coskun O, MacMahon S, Tzourio-Mazoyer N, et al. Severe cerebral white matter hyperintensities predict severe cognitive decline in patients with cerebrovascular disease history. Stroke 2009; 40: 2219-21.

Feeney DM, Baron JC. Diaschisis. Stroke 1986; 17: 817-30.

Fries W, Danek A, Witt TN. Motor responses after transcranial electrical stimulation of cerebral hemispheres with a degenerated pyramidal tract. Ann Neurol 1991; 29: 646-50.

Geschwind N. Disconnexion syndromes in animals and man. I. Brain 1965a; 88: 237-94.

Geschwind N. Disconnexion syndromes in animals and man. II. Brain 1965b; 88: 585-644.

Grefkes C, Nowak DA, Eickhoff SB, Dafotakis M, Kust J, Karbe H, et al. Cortical connectivity after subcortical stroke assessed with functional magnetic resonance imaging. Ann Neurol 2008; 63: 236-46.

Hallevi H, Albright KC, Martin-Schild SB, Barreto AD, Morales MM, Bornstein N, et al. Recovery after ischemic stroke: criteria for good outcome by level of disability at day 7. Cerebrovasc Dis 2009; 28: 341-8.

Jang SH, Bai D, Son SM, Lee J, Kim DS, Sakong J, et al. Motor outcome prediction using diffusion tensor tractography in pontine infarct. Ann Neurol 2008; 64: 460-5.

Johansen-Berg H, Behrens TE. Just pretty pictures? What diffusion tractography can add in clinical neuroscience. Curr Opin Neurol 2006; 19: 379-85.

Johansen-Berg H, Scholz J, Stagg CJ. Relevance of structural brain connectivity to learning and recovery from stroke. Front Syst Neurosci 2010; 4: 146.

Jones DK. Studying connections in the living human brain with diffusion MRI. Cortex 2008; 44: 936-52.

Kang DW, Chu K, Yoon BW, Song IC, Chang KH, Roh JK. Diffusion-weighted imaging in Wallerian degeneration. J Neurol Sci 2000; 178: 167-9.

Karnath HO, Fruhmann Berger M, Kuker W, Rorden C. The anatomy of spatial neglect based on voxelwise statistical analysis: a study of 140 patients. Cereb Cortex 2004; 14: 1164-72.

Karnath HO, Rorden C, Ticini LF. Damage to white matter fiber tracts in acute spatial neglect. Cereb Cortex 2009; 19: 2331-7.

Konishi J, Yamada K, Kizu O, Ito H, Sugimura K, Yoshikawa K, et al. MR tractography for the evaluation of functional recovery from lenticulostriate infarcts. Neurology 2005; 64: 108-13.

Kraemer M, Schormann T, Hagemann G, Qi B, Witte OW, Seitz RJ. Delayed shrinkage of the brain after ischemic stroke: preliminary observations with voxel-guided morphometry. J Neuroimaging 2004; 14: 265-72.

Kranz PG, Eastwood JD. Does diffusion-weighted imaging represent the ischemic core? An evidence-based systematic review. AJNR Am J Neuroradiol 2009; 30: 1206-12.

Kretschmann HJ. Localisation of the corticospinal fibres in the internal capsule in man. J Anat 1988; 160: 219-25.

Kunimatsu A, Aoki S, Masutani Y, Abe O, Mori H, Ohtomo K. Three-dimensional white matter tractography by diffusion tensor imaging in ischaemic stroke involving the corticospinal tract. Neuroradiology 2003; 45: 532-5.

Kwakkel G. Impact of intensity of practice after stroke: issues for consideration. Disabil Rehabil 2006; 28: 823-30.

Lang CE, Schieber MH. Reduced muscle selectivity during individuated finger movements in humans after damage to the motor cortex or corticospinal tract. J Neurophysiol 2004; 91: 1722-33.

Lee JS, Han MK, Kim SH, Kwon OK, Kim JH. Fiber tracking by diffusion tensor imaging in corticospinal tract stroke: Topographical correlation with clinical symptoms. Neuroimage 2005; 26: 771-6.

Lindberg PG, Skejo PH, Rounis E, Nagy Z, Schmitz C, Wernegren H, et al. Wallerian degeneration of the corticofugal tracts in chronic stroke: a pilot study relating diffusion tensor imaging, transcranial magnetic stimulation, and hand function. Neurorehabil Neural Repair 2007; 21: 551-60.

Lindenberg R, Renga V, Zhu LL, Betzler F, Alsop D, Schlaug G. Structural integrity of corticospinal motor fibers predicts motor impairment in chronic stroke. Neurology 2010; 74: 280-7.

Lindenberg R, Zhu LL, Rüber T, Schlaug G. Predicting functional motor potential in chronic stroke patients using diffusion tensor imaging. Hum Brain Mapp 2011; epub ahead of print.

Maier IC, Baumann K, Thallmair M, Weinmann O, Scholl J, Schwab ME. Constraint-induced movement therapy in the adult rat after unilateral corticospinal tract injury. J Neurosci 2008; 28: 9386-403.

Mori S, Zhang J. Principles of diffusion tensor imaging and its applications to basic neuroscience research. Neuron 2006; 51: 527-39.

Naismith RT, Xu J, Tutlam NT, Snyder A, Benzinger T, Shimony J, et al. Disability in optic neuritis correlates with diffusion tensor-derived directional diffusivities. Neurology 2009; 72: 589-94.

Nelles M, Gieseke J, Flacke S, Lachenmayer L, Schild HH, Urbach H. Diffusion tensor pyramidal tractography in patients with anterior choroidal artery infarcts. AJNR Am J Neuroradiol 2008; 29: 488-93.

Newton JM, Ward NS, Parker GJ, Deichmann R, Alexander DC, Friston KJ, et al. Non-invasive mapping of corticofugal fibres from multiple motor areas--relevance to stroke recovery. Brain 2006; 129: 1844-58.

Nudo RJ, Wise BM, SiFuentes F, Milliken GW. Neural substrates for the effects of rehabilitative training on motor recovery after ischemic infarct. Science 1996; 272: 1791-4.

Pazzaglia M, Smania N, Corato E, Aglioti SM. Neural underpinnings of gesture discrimination in patients with limb apraxia. J Neurosci 2008; 28: 3030-41.

Perez MA, Cohen LG. Interhemispheric inhibition between primary motor cortices: what have we learned? J Physiol 2009; 587: 725-6.

Rusconi E, Pinel P, Eger E, LeBihan D, Thirion B, Dehaene S, et al. A disconnection account of Gerstmann syndrome: functional neuroanatomy evidence. Ann Neurol 2009; 66: 654-62.

Schaechter JD, Fricker ZP, Perdue KL, Helmer KG, Vangel MG, Greve DN, et al. Microstructural status of ipsilesional and contralesional corticospinal tract correlates with motor skill in chronic stroke patients. Hum Brain Mapp 2009; 30: 3461-74.

Schaechter JD, Perdue KL, Wang R. Structural damage to the corticospinal tract correlates with bilateral sensorimotor cortex reorganization in stroke patients. Neuroimage 2008; 39: 1370-82.

Schafer R, Popp K, Jorgens S, Lindenberg R, Franz M, Seitz RJ. Alexithymia-like disorder in right anterior cingulate infarction. Neurocase 2007; 13: 201-8.

Schlaug G, Marchina S, Norton A. Evidence for plasticity in white-matter tracts of patients with chronic Broca's aphasia undergoing intense intonation-based speech therapy. Ann N Y Acad Sci 2009; 1169: 385-94.

Schlaug G, Renga V, Nair D. Transcranial direct current stimulation in stroke recovery. Arch Neurol 2008; 65: 1571-6.

Scholz J, Klein MC, Behrens TE, Johansen-Berg H. Training induces changes in white-matter architecture. Nat Neurosci 2009; 12: 1370-1.

Seitz RJ, Donnan GA. Role of neuroimaging in promoting long-term recovery from ischemic stroke. J Magn Reson Imaging 2010; 32: 756-72.

Seitz RJ, Kleiser R, Butefisch CM, Jorgens S, Neuhaus O, Hartung HP, et al. Bimanual recoupling by visual cueing in callosal disconnection. Neurocase 2004; 10: 316-25.

Seitz RJ, Meisel S, Weller P, Junghans U, Wittsack HJ, Siebler M. Initial ischemic event: perfusion-weighted MR imaging and apparent diffusion coefficient for stroke evolution. Radiology 2005; 237: 1020-8.

Seitz RJ, Schlaug G, Kleinschmidt A, Knorr U, Nebeling B, Wirrwar A, et al. Remote depressions of cerebral metabolism in hemiparetic stroke: Topography and relation to motor and somatosensory functions. Hum Brain Mapp 1994; 1: 81-100.

Seitz RJ, Sondermann V, Wittsack HJ, Siebler M. Lesion patterns in successful and failed thrombolysis in middle cerebral artery stroke. Neuroradiology 2009; 51: 865-71.

Sidaros A, Engberg AW, Sidaros K, Liptrot MG, Herning M, Petersen P, et al. Diffusion tensor imaging during recovery from severe traumatic brain injury and relation to clinical outcome: a longitudinal study. Brain 2008; 131: 559-72.

Song SK, Sun SW, Ju WK, Lin SJ, Cross AH, Neufeld AH. Diffusion tensor imaging detects and differentiates axon and myelin degeneration in mouse optic nerve after retinal ischemia. Neuroimage 2003; 20: 1714-22.

Stinear CM, Barber PA, Smale PR, Coxon JP, Fleming MK, Byblow WD. Functional potential in chronic stroke patients depends on corticospinal tract integrity. Brain 2007; 130: 170-80.

Stoeckel MC, Wittsack HJ, Meisel S, Seitz RJ. Pattern of cortex and white matter involvement in severe middle cerebral artery ischemia. J Neuroimaging 2007; 17: 131-40.

Sun SW, Liang HF, Cross AH, Song SK. Evolving Wallerian degeneration after transient retinal ischemia in mice characterized by diffusion tensor imaging. Neuroimage 2008; 40: 1-10.

Talelli P, Greenwood RJ, Rothwell JC. Arm function after stroke: neurophysiological correlates and recovery mechanisms assessed by transcranial magnetic stimulation. Clin Neurophysiol 2006; 117: 1641-59.

Thomalla G, Glauche V, Koch MA, Beaulieu C, Weiller C, Rother J. Diffusion tensor imaging detects early Wallerian degeneration of the pyramidal tract after ischemic stroke. Neuroimage 2004; 22: 1767-74.

Wahl M, Lauterbach-Soon B, Hattingen E, Jung P, Singer O, Volz S, et al. Human motor corpus callosum: topography, somatotopy, and link between microstructure and function. J Neurosci 2007; 27: 12132-8.

Wahlgren N, Ahmed N, Eriksson N, Aichner F, Bluhmki E, Davalos A, et al. Multivariable analysis of outcome predictors and adjustment of main outcome results to baseline data profile in randomized controlled trials: Safe Implementation of Thrombolysis in Stroke-MOnitoring STudy (SITS-MOST). Stroke 2008; 39: 3316-22.

Wakana S, Jiang H, Nagae-Poetscher LM, van Zijl PCM, Mori S. Fiber Tract-based Atlas of Human White Matter Anatomy. Radiology 2004; 230: 77-87.

Wenzelburger R, Kopper F, Frenzel A, Stolze H, Klebe S, Brossmann A, et al. Hand coordination following capsular stroke. Brain 2005; 128: 64-74.

Werring DJ, Toosy AT, Clark CA, Parker GJ, Barker GJ, Miller DH, et al. Diffusion tensor imaging can detect and quantify corticospinal tract degeneration after stroke. J Neurol Neurosurg Psychiatry 2000; 69: 269-72.

Wheeler-Kingshott CA, Cercignani M. About "axial" and "radial" diffusivities. Magn Reson Med 2009; 61: 1255-60.

Yamada K, Ito H, Nakamura H, Kizu O, Akada W, Kubota T, et al. Stroke patients' evolving symptoms assessed by tractography. J Magn Reson Imaging 2004; 20: 923-9.

Zhu LL, Lindenberg R, Alexander MP, Schlaug G. Lesion load of the corticospinal tract predicts motor impairment in chronic stroke. Stroke 2010; 41: 910-5.

13

Tissue Fate Prediction from Regional Imaging Features in Acute Ischemic Stroke

Fabien Scalzo, Xiao Hu and David Liebeskind
University of California, Los Angeles (UCLA)
USA

1. Introduction

Stroke is a leading cause of death and a major cause of long term disabilities worldwide. According to the World Health Organization (WHO), a total of 15 million people suffer from a stroke each year comprising 5 million with a fatal outcome and another 5 million with permanent disabilities. While prevention research identifies factors and specific drugs that may lower the risk of a future stroke, the treatment of ischemic stroke patients aims at maximizing the recovery of brain tissue at risk. It is typically done by arterial recanalization of the vessel where the clot is located. Identification of salvageable brain tissue is essential during the clinical decision-making process. As a general rule for the decision to intervene, the expected benefits of the intervention should outweigh its potential risks and costs. To identify viable brain tissue, time is considered as a determining factor in the treatment of stroke patients. A perfect illustration of this timing issue is the thrombolytic therapy which uses specific drugs to break-up or dissolve the blood clot. As shown in a recent study (Hacke et al, 2008), thrombolysis applied with recombinant tissue plasminogen activator (rt-PA) is effective for acute ischemic stroke patients when administered intra-venously within a specific time window (3 hours, or 4 hours 30 min for patients meeting additional criteria). However, this time frame is arbitrary and might be too restrictive for some patients (Schaefer et al., 2007). For example, some patients could have benefited from this therapy but, instead, have been unnecessarily excluded. Beyond this ongoing debate about the length of the time window, there is a recognized need for accurate strategies to quantify the extent of viable tissue for victims of ischemic strokes and therefore to be able to identify the patients who could benefit from such a therapy.

Estimating the dynamic of infarct growth in ischemic stroke is extremely complex and its mechanisms are still poorly understood. Various factors such as quality of collateral perfusion, energy delivery, and age of the patient are known to have a significant impact on the outcome. However, their interactions over time is not clearly established and has not been quantified. The most commonly used techniques currently available to predict tissue outcome are based on imaging. It is widely accepted that the combination of diffusion (DWI) and perfusion-weighted (PWI) magnetic resonance imaging (MRI) provide useful information to identify the tissue at risk at an early stage. Several groups (Chen et al., 2008; Fisher & Ginsberg, 2004; Kidwell et al., 2004; Schlaug et al., 1999) have studied the mismatch between DWI and PWI to determine the penumbral tissue. However, DWI-PWI mismatch approaches have limitations: increased diffusion signals may be reversible (although a recent study (Chemmanam et al., 2010) has concluded that it does not seem to be a common phenomenon), and the determination of the threshold of critical perfusion by PWI has been controversial (Heiss & Sobesky, 2005). DWI-PWI technique is based on the static thresholding of images and additional analysis is necessary to predict the final infarct size.

More recently, considerable attention has been given to the development of automatic, quantitative predictive models that can estimate the likely evolution of the endangered tissue. These approaches that have been proposed in the literature differ on the types of images, and the prediction techniques they employ. Initially, automatic prediction models have been trained on a voxel-by-voxel basis by integrating multimodal perfusion information from cases with known follow-up tissue fate. WU *et al* (Wu et al., 2001; 2007) proposed in one of their studies a framework based on a generalized linear model (GLM) and evaluated 14 ischemic stroke patients. Results showed that combining parameters computed from DWI and PWI offers higher specificity and sensitivity than models trained on DWI, or PWI alone. ROSE *et al* (Rose et al., 2001) used Gaussian models trained on multiple parameters (DWI, CBF, CBV, mean transit time (MTT)) to predict tissue outcome on 19 ischemic stroke patients. Other studies based on logistic regression (Yoo et al., 2010), on ISODATA clustering (Shen et al., 2005) applied to ADC and CBF have also led to similar conclusions; the combination of various parameters improves the prediction accuracy. In addition to the DWI-PWI mismatch, several studies (Olivot, Mlynash, Zaharchuk, Straka, Bammer, Schwartz, Lansberg, Moseley & Albers, 2009; Olivot, Mlynash, Thijs, Purushotham, Kemp, Lansberg, Wechsler, Gold, Bammer, Marks & Albers, 2009) have demonstrated that time-to-maximum (Tmax) of the residue function is a reliable parameter to detect penumbra in acute stroke because it implicitly captures a complex combination of delay and dispersion. It has been shown to predict actual CBF more accurately than mean transit time (MTT) (Olivot, Mlynash, Zaharchuk, Straka, Bammer, Schwartz, Lansberg, Moseley & Albers, 2009).

The regional information contained in the surrounding voxels of the location to be predicted has been shown in recent works to improve the accuracy of the predictive model in comparison with a single-voxel-based method. Although some regional information may implicitly be included by single-voxel-based methods via the convolution of the image with a smoothing filter, it is usually not taken into account by the models. Promising approaches have attempted to take into account the regional distribution explicitly by exploiting spatial correlation between voxels (Nguyen et al., 2008), using a prior map of spatial frequency-of-infarct (Shen & Duong, 2008), and Neural Networks (Huang et al., 2010). All these studies have demonstrated signs of improvement in comparison with single-voxel-based approaches.

Drawing from these findings, this chapter introduces a predictive model of tissue fate that captures the relationship between spatial patterns observed in perfusion images after onset and tissue outcome. This work presents a comparative analysis of the predictive power of different flow parameters extracted from Perfusion Weighted Images (PWI) during the acute phase of the stroke. Specifically, Cerebral Blood Volume (CBV), Cerebral Blood Flow (CBF), Mean Transit Time (MTT), Tmax, Time-To-Peak (TTP), and Peak are extracted and evaluated in this study. The predictive model is formalized as a nonlinear regression problem. It combines the tissue information available at onset in terms of Fluid Attenuated Inversion Recovery (FLAIR) images with parameters extracted from PWI to predict the tissue outcome four days after intervention. FLAIR images are used in this study to identify lesions from previous strokes and, to a lesser extent, early lesions in the acute phase. They are also used to assess the survival outcome of the brain tissue four days after intervention. While FLAIR is the gold standard in neurology to depict irreversible lesions, PWI parameters represent flow-related features that may be useful for the prediction of tissue outcome.

The novelty of the proposed work is to study the impact of a regional model on each of these perfusion maps (CBV, CBF, MTT, Tmax, Peak, TTP). The regional distribution among neighboring voxels is represented by *cuboids* (*i.e.* rectangular volumes) (Fig 1(a)). By varying the size of these cuboids, we expect to determine what is the optimal size for each map that leads to the most accurate tissue fate prediction. Such an approach can be seen as a 3D generalization of subwindows-based stochastic methods (Maree et al., 2005) that have been successfully used on a wide variety of image classification problems.

During learning, the cuboids are sampled at similar locations in FLAIR and one of the perfusion images, and each pair of cuboids is combined into a single vector and used as input to the predictive model. The output is the tissue fate, in terms of FLAIR voxel intensity, measured 4-days after an arterial recanalization intervention. A Kernel Spectral Regression (SR-KDA) (Cai et al., 2007) model is used to represent the relation that exists between PWI parameters combined with FLAIR images at onset and the tissue fate.

2. Image-based prediction of tissue outcome

2.1 Patients, and MRI data acquisition

MRI data was collected from patients identified with symptoms of ischemic stroke and admitted at the University of California-Los Angeles Medical Center. The use of these data was approved by the local institutional review board (IRB). Inclusion criteria for this study included: (1) presenting symptoms suggestive of acute stroke, (2) last known well time within six hours, (3) MRI (including PWI) of the brain performed before recanalization therapy and approximately four days later, (4) final diagnosis of ischemic stroke. A total of 25 patients (mean age, 56 ± 21 years; age range, 27 to 89; 15 women; average NIHSS of 14 ± 6.3) satisfied the above criteria and underwent MRI using a 1.5 Tesla echo planar MR imaging scanner (Siemens Medical Systems). The PWI scanning was performed with a timed contrast-bolus passage technique (0.1 mg/kg contrast administered intravenously at a rate of 5 cm3/s) and with the following parameters on average: repetition time (TR), 2000 ms; echo time (TE), 60 ms. The FLAIR sequence was acquired with the following parameters: repetition time (TR), 7000 ms; echo time (TE), 105 ms; inversion time (TI), 2000 ms. All the images were resized using bilinear interpolation to match a resolution of $1 \times 1 \times 5$ mm per voxel.

The median time from symptom onset to baseline MRI was 4h38 (IQR 1h43, 5h39), and to followup MRI was 4 days 13h30 (IQR 3 days 15h08, 4 days 22h17). Median time from onset to intervention was 6h20. The degree of success of the intervention in terms of recanalization and reperfusion, as well as the quality of collaterals have a significant impact on the tissue fate. These factors are not taken into account in our predictive model because it relies only on onset images.

2.2 Prediction framework

The prediction framework proposed in this chapter relies on a regression model that is learned in a supervised fashion from a set of training images with known outcome. Once the model has been trained, it can be used to predict the tissue fate, in terms of followup FLAIR intensity, on new cases. The following subsections describe a series of preprocessing steps (Figure 1(b)) prior to the predictive modeling.

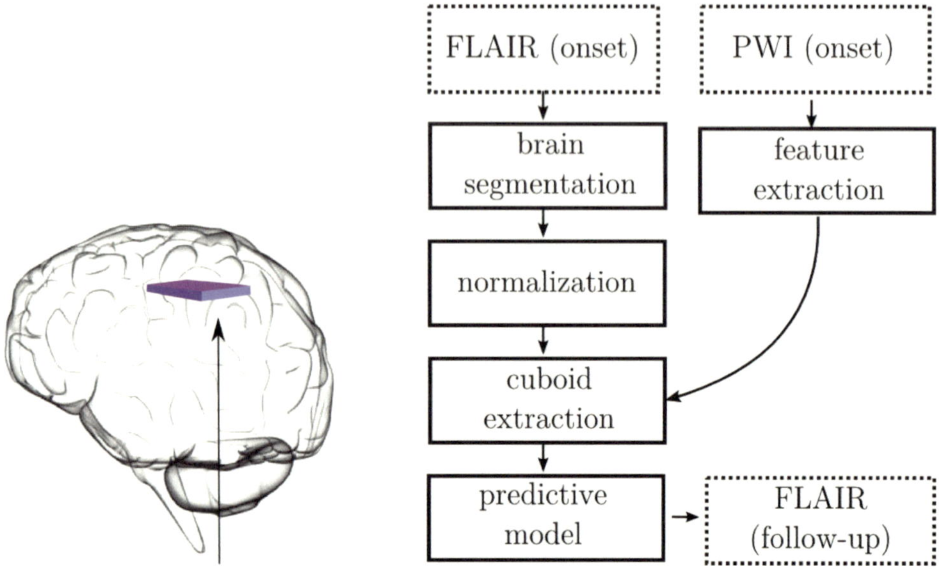

(a) Cuboid (b) Prediction Framework

Fig. 1. (a) Illustration of a cuboid extracted from the brain volume. (b) During prediction, the skull is first stripped from the FLAIR image and the result is normalized. A parameter map is extracted from PWI images and registered to FLAIR images. Cuboids are sampled at the same locations from both images and used as input to the regression model to predict the tissue outcome.

2.2.1 Automatic brain volume segmentation

Before learning, the framework requires FLAIR images acquired immediately after onset and at followup to be co-registered. The skull and non-brain tissue could interfere with the registration process and therefore have been stripped.

To perform this brain extraction step, we use the FSL Brain Extraction Tool (BET) (Smith., 2002) that is integrated into a pipeline software developed by the Laboratory of Neuro Imaging (LONI) at UCLA (`http://www.loni.ucla.edu/`). BET estimates an intensity threshold to discriminate between brain/non-brain voxels. Then, it determines the center of gravity of the head, defines a sphere based on the center of gravity of the volume, and finally deforms it toward the brain surface.

2.2.2 FLAIR image normalization

Because FLAIR images were acquired with different settings and originated from different patients, their intensity value was not directly comparable. To allow for inter-patient comparisons, FLAIR images were normalized with respect to the average intensities within the contralateral white matter. The normal-appearing white matter was delineated manually by an experienced researcher for both onset and follow-up brain volumes.

2.2.3 Perfusion imaging features

Imaging features are extracted from PWI images with a software developed at UCLA, the Stroke Cerebral Analysis (SCAN) package. The tissue contrast agent concentration $C(t)$ is expressed as a convolution of the arterial input function (AIF) identified from the contralateral middle cerebral artery (MCA) and the residue function $R(t)$ (Calamante et al., 2010)

$$C(t) = CBF \times (AIF(t) \otimes R(t)), \tag{1}$$

where CBF is the cerebral blood flow. The residue function is obtained by deconvolution, and the time to its maximum value is used to specify Tmax. Therefore, Tmax is the arrival delay between the AIF and C(t).

After applying a gamma variate fit on a pixel-by-pixel basis, cerebral blood volume (CBV) is estimated in each voxel by computing the area under the fitted gadolinium concentration time curve, measured in the corresponding image pixel at every time point after bolus arrival:

$$CBV = \sum_{t=0}^{N_c} C(t). \tag{2}$$

The mean transit time (MTT) is computed as the normalized first moment of the fitted curve, up to the peak of the curve. The time to peak contrast concentration (TTP) is another perfusion-related parameter that corresponds to the time it takes for signal intensity to reach its minimum in each pixel. The value of this minimum is used to define another feature called Peak.

Finally, CBV and MTT are used to calculate the cerebral blood flow (CBF) through the tissue voxel, according to the central volume theorem:

$$CBF = \frac{CBV}{MTT}. \tag{3}$$

2.2.4 Image registration

Registration of FLAIR and PWI images is necessary because the outcome of an extracted cuboid, measured as a voxel value in the followup image, has to correspond to the same anatomical location in the different volumes. Co-registration was performed for each patient independently. Because the intensity of FLAIR images may present large variations between onset and followup due to changes in the tissue perfusion caused by the stroke, several attempts to use automatic image registration methods failed to accurately align the volumes. Instead, our framework utilized five landmark points placed manually at specific anatomical locations (center, plus four main cardinal directions) on the slice of the brain that had the largest ventricular area. An affine projection was applied to project the followup FLAIR and acute Tmax on the original FLAIR volume.

2.2.5 Ground truth

During evaluation, we pose the prediction task as a two-class classification problem, where the voxel of the groundtruth is set to 1 if it is infarcted and 0 if it is not. The groundtruth is obtained by manual outline of infarcts on FLAIR images by an expert in neurology from UCLA who was asked to precisely delineate infarcts, comparing the infarcted hemisphere with the contralateral hemisphere. Outlining was performed with the help of the commercially available medical imaging software 3D DOCTOR developed by ABLE SOFTWARE CORP (`http://www.ablesw.com/`). No manual outlining is made on the predicted images.

2.2.6 Cuboid sampling

For training, we exploit a set of FLAIR images F at onset, their corresponding co-registered PWI feature map M, and followup FLAIR images F'.

The dataset $\{X, Y\}$ used to train and to evaluate the predictive model is created by extracting cuboids of fixed size $w \times l \times d$ among onset images with their corresponding outcome. Each cuboid $c \in \mathbb{R}^s$ is described by its raw voxel values, yielding an input vector of $s = w \times l \times d$ numerical attributes. Our method extracts a large number of cuboids at random positions from training images. In practice, given a sampled location $\{i, j, k\}$, we extract a cuboid c_F in the acute FLAIR image at $F(i, j, k)$ and a corresponding cuboid c_M in the perfusion map at $M(i, j, k)$. To improve the generalization power of the predictive model, the cuboids c_M, c_F are normalized with respect to the direction θ of the image gradient in the XY plane using an image rotation, performed with bilinear interpolation. Normalized patches $c_{M'}, c_{F'}$ thus become invariant to orientation changes in the XY plane. Orientation normalization is particularly useful when considering the case where cuboids are located at the same distance from a circular infarction but at different directions. If no rotational normalization is performed, all the cuboids have a different appearance and the model has to be trained for all the directions around the infarct and requires more training examples.

$$c_{M'} = \text{imrotate}(c_M, -\theta_M) \qquad \theta_M = \tan^{-1} \frac{L^{\sigma}_{y,M}(x, y, z)}{L^{\sigma}_{x,M}(x, y, z)} \tag{4}$$

$$c_{F'} = \text{imrotate}(c_F, -\theta_F) \qquad \theta_F = \tan^{-1} \frac{L^{\sigma}_{y,F}(x, y, z)}{L^{\sigma}_{x,F}(x, y, z)} \tag{5}$$

where $L^{\sigma}_{x,F}, L^{\sigma}_{x,F}, L^{\sigma}_{x,M}, L^{\sigma}_{y,M}$ are the Gaussian derivatives in X and Y directions, computed from the acute FLAIR image F and perfusion map M,

$$L^{\sigma}_{x,M} = \frac{\partial}{\partial x} \mathcal{G}_{\sigma} \otimes M \qquad L^{\sigma}_{y,M} = \frac{\partial}{\partial y} \mathcal{G}_{\sigma} \otimes M \tag{6}$$

$$L^{\sigma}_{x,F} = \frac{\partial}{\partial x} \mathcal{G}_{\sigma} \otimes F \qquad L^{\sigma}_{y,F} = \frac{\partial}{\partial y} \mathcal{G}_{\sigma} \otimes F \tag{7}$$

where $\mathcal{G}_{\sigma}$ is a 2D isotropic Gaussian filter with standard deviation $\sigma = 3$ in our experiments. The two cuboids are merged into a single, multi-modal cuboid $x = \{c_{F'}, c_{M'}\}$ that corresponds to the concatenation of the cuboids extracted at the same location in the different volumes. Each multi-modal cuboid x is then labeled with the intensity y of the central voxel in the corresponding follow-up FLAIR image $y = F'(i, j, k)$. The dataset consists of the set of multi-modal cuboids $x \in X$ and their corresponding outputs $y \in Y$ that represent the followup FLAIR intensities.

2.3 Regression-based predictive model

Our predictive model takes the form a regression model $y = f(x)$ that maps the tissue outcome $y \in Y$, described in terms of the voxel intensity in the followup FLAIR image, as a function of the multi-modal cuboid $x \in X$ extracted at the same location. Defining outputs y in a continuous space, in contrast with a binary one, allow us to easily change the sensitivity and specificity of the framework, by varying the threshold on the predictions. A greyscale (or color) output image is also more adapted than a binary image to visualize complex patterns.

In the context of pattern recognition, the literature of regression analysis has been particularly proficient in the last couple of years with the emergence of robust, nonlinear methods. In this study, the comparative analysis will be based on a Kernel Spectral Regression (SR-KDA) analysis (Cai et al., 2007) that we successfully used in our preliminary study (Scalzo et al., 2010), and other regression-based pattern recognition applications Scalzo et al. (2009; 2010).

2.3.1 Kernel spectral regression

Kernel Spectral Regression (SR-KDA) (Cai et al., 2007) is a recently proposed method to solve Kernel Discriminant Analysis (KDA) problems efficiently. Specifically, it poses the discriminant analysis as a regularized regression problem that exploits a graph representation. SR-KDA utilizes a kernel projection of the data (also called "kernel trick" in the literature). Input data samples X are projected onto a high-dimensional space via a Gaussian kernel K,

$$K(i,j) = \exp -\|x_i - x_j\|^2/2\sigma^2 \tag{8}$$

where σ is the user-specified standard deviation of the kernel.
In addition, from the set of n input data samples X, a $n \times n$ symmetric affinity matrix W is generated with W_{ij} having a positive constant value if $x_i, x_j \in X$ are from the same class (i.e. $y_i \in Y$ is equal to $y_j \in Y$), and zero otherwise. From matrix K and W, SR-KDA uses the Gram-Schmidt method to obtain eigenvectors ϕ,

$$W\phi = \lambda\phi \tag{9}$$

and estimates the mapping α efficiently using a Cholesky decomposition,

$$\alpha^{\mathrm{T}}(K + \delta I) = \phi \tag{10}$$

where I is the identity matrix, $\delta > 0$ the regularization parameter, and ϕ are the eigenvectors of W. When a new multi-modal cuboid, x_{new}, is extracted from the image of a new patient, the FLAIR intensity at followup, $\hat{y}_{\text{new}}$, is computed using

$$k(i) = \exp -\|x_i - x_{\text{new}}\|^2/2\sigma^2, i = 1 \ldots n \tag{11}$$

$$\hat{y}_{\text{new}} = \hat{\alpha}^{\mathrm{T}}(k + \delta I) \tag{12}$$

where k is the vector resulting from the kernel projection of x_{new} into the kernel space using training data X.

2.4 Experimental setup

This section describes how the predictive power in terms of tissue fate of the different perfusion images will be evaluated on our dataset of ischemic stroke patients. The proposed experiments are designed to answer the following questions: *Do the neighboring voxels significantly improve the prediction of the tissue outcome at a specific voxel in the different maps? If so, what is the optimal size of this neighborhood in ischemic strokes? Does it differ depending on the type of image?* Specifically, these questions will be addressed by evaluating the tissue fate prediction accuracy of the Kernel Spectral Regression (SR-KDA) (Section 2.3.1) method on our dataset (Section 2.1). The problem is posed as a classification task where the output Y (*i.e.* followup FLAIR image) was manually binarized to create the ground truth (Section 2.2.5).
A specific model will be trained for each of the six types of perfusion parameter; CBV, CBF, MTT, Tmax, TTP, Peak. The training of a specific regression model is made from a set of training samples that, in the ideal case, should be uniformly distributed throughout the data space. However, this is not the case for most of the stroke patients where the brain volume

contains a larger number of noninfarcted voxels. A recent study (Jonsdottir et al., 2009) has shown that an unequal number of infarcted and noninfarcted voxels can negatively impact the overall performance of the system. Following the methods of the study, we perform a random sampling on the input cuboids so that an equal number of infarcted and noninfarcted cuboids are present in the training set. The number of training samples for each slice was set to a maximum of 85 cuboids of class 0 and 85 cuboids of class 1. In theory, this could create a large dataset of $170 \times nbSlice \times nbCases$ training samples. In practice, however, we reduce the size of the dataset during the extraction process such that the number of extracted cuboids for a slice is equal to the minimum number of occurrence of either class (0 or 1). For example, if only 10 voxels are infarcted (class 1) on the followup of one slice, only 10 cuboids will be extracted for class 1 as well as 10 other cuboids for class 0. This procedure has the advantage of speeding up the cuboid extraction process and generates less than 10,000 training samples equally distributed between the two classes.

2.4.1 Cuboid size

For each PWI parameter map, we evaluate the accuracy of the SR-KDA regression method to predict tissue fate for different sizes of cuboids. A predictive model is evaluated for each cuboid size using a leave-one-patient-out crossvalidation so that the data from the patient evaluated is excluded from the training set at each iteration. In this experiment, cuboids are symmetric; w, l have the same length (Section 2.2.6). The tested sizes [1] spanned from 1×1 to 23×23. During the leave-one-out crossvalidation, the Area Under the Curve (AUC) is computed from the ROC curve for each patient. The average AUC and standard deviation across patients are calculated and constitute our measure of performance. The parameters of SR-KDA σ, δ were optimized at each iteration of the leave-one-out procedure by running another leave-one-out cross-validation on the data excluding the patient to be tested.

2.4.2 Global ROC curves

Global ROC curves are also generated for each PWI parameter map. For fair comparison, the cuboid size of each image was the one that led to the best accuracy in the experiment presented in the previous paragraph and reported in Figure 2. To generate the global ROC curve, predictions $\hat{Y}_i$ are first computed for each specific patient i during the crossvalidation. Then, all the prediction vectors $\{\hat{Y}_1, \hat{Y}_2, \ldots, \hat{Y}_n\}$ are concatenated into a single vector $\hat{Y}_{total}$, and the global ROC curve is computed from the data of all patients $\hat{Y}_{total}$.

2.4.3 McNemar's significance test

Although differences in average AUCs can be used to rank the predictive power of the different PWI parameter maps and to observe the improvements of the regional model versus a single-voxel-based approach, differences are not necessarily statistically significant. We propose to use a McNemar's test (Siegel & Castellan, 1988) to verify if the difference between between regional and single-voxel-based models are statistically significant for each PWI map. McNemar's test, which is based on a Fisher-test with one degree of freedom, is a useful tool in determining if two methods have comparable error rates. Given the null hypothesis that the two methods A and B have the same error rate, and the following contingence table (Table 1),

[1] The low sagittal resolution (≥ 7 mm per voxel) of PWI images did not allow us to test the z-size of the cuboid which was set to 1 slice.

McNemar's test can be written as a Fisher-test,

$$\chi^2 = \frac{(|b-c|-1)^2}{b+c}. \tag{13}$$

	Correct (B)	Error (B)	Total
Correct (A)	a	b	a+b
Error (A)	c	d	c+d
	a+c	b+d	n

Table 1. Classification contingence table between two methods (A, B).

McNemar's test is applied to investigate if the main hypothesis of this paper is supported by a statistical significance test. We verify that the improvement in performance obtained by the regional cuboids versus a single voxel is significant. To do so, the McNemar's test is performed between the models obtained using SR-KDA with their optimal cuboid size and with a single voxel 1×1. We perform the experiment for each PWI parameter map with the following optimal cuboids size (identified in the previous experiment): Tmax, 15×15; MTT, 15×15; CBV, 9×9; CBF, 11×11; TTP, 13×13; Peak, 11×11.

3. Results

3.1 Cuboid size

AUC after a leave-one-patient-out crossvalidation for an increased cuboid size is reported in Figure 2 for each PWI parameter map. The AUC can be interpreted as the probability of correct classification for a randomly selected pair of positive and negative samples. Usually, any AUC result above .9 is considered as excellent.

Baseline average accuracy for Tmax parameter reaches 0.83 ± 0.01 with cuboid size 1×1 and increases to 0.90 ± 0.05 at a size of 15×15. MTT parameter reaches 0.76 ± 0.02 and increases to 0.87 ± 0.06 at a size of 15×15. CBV parameter reaches 0.67 ± 0.03 and increases to 0.74 ± 0.10 at a size of 9×9. CBF parameter reaches 0.71 ± 0.02 and increases to 0.81 ± 0.08 at a size of 11×11. TTP parameter reaches 0.84 ± 0.02 and increases to 0.91 ± 0.04 at a size of 13×13. Peak parameter reaches 0.74 ± 0.02 and increases to 0.82 ± 0.08 at a size of 11×11.

These results suggest that Tmax and TTP parameters are the most accurate single maps to predict the tissue outcome. Interestingly, the optimal size of the cuboids vary across the different modalities, however all of them outperform their respective single-voxel-based model. These results demonstrate that a regional approach, which takes into account neighboring voxels may improve the prediction accuracy regardless of the modality used.

Global ROC curves that illustrate the results in terms of true positive and false positive rates are depicted in Figure 3. The ROC are produced for each parameter map, comparing the results between a baseline cuboid size of 1×1 and the optimal size.

The similarity between the prediction and the actual outcome of the brain tissue for each parameter can be visualized in Figure 4 on arbitrary slices. The columns respectively correspond (from left to right, top to bottom) to follow-up FLAIR, prediction from Tmax, TTP, MTT, the manually outlined ground truth of followup FLAIR, and prediction from CBV, CBF, and Peak. The prediction are produced from the SR-KDA model trained using a leave-one-out crossvalidation with optimal cuboid size for each modality.

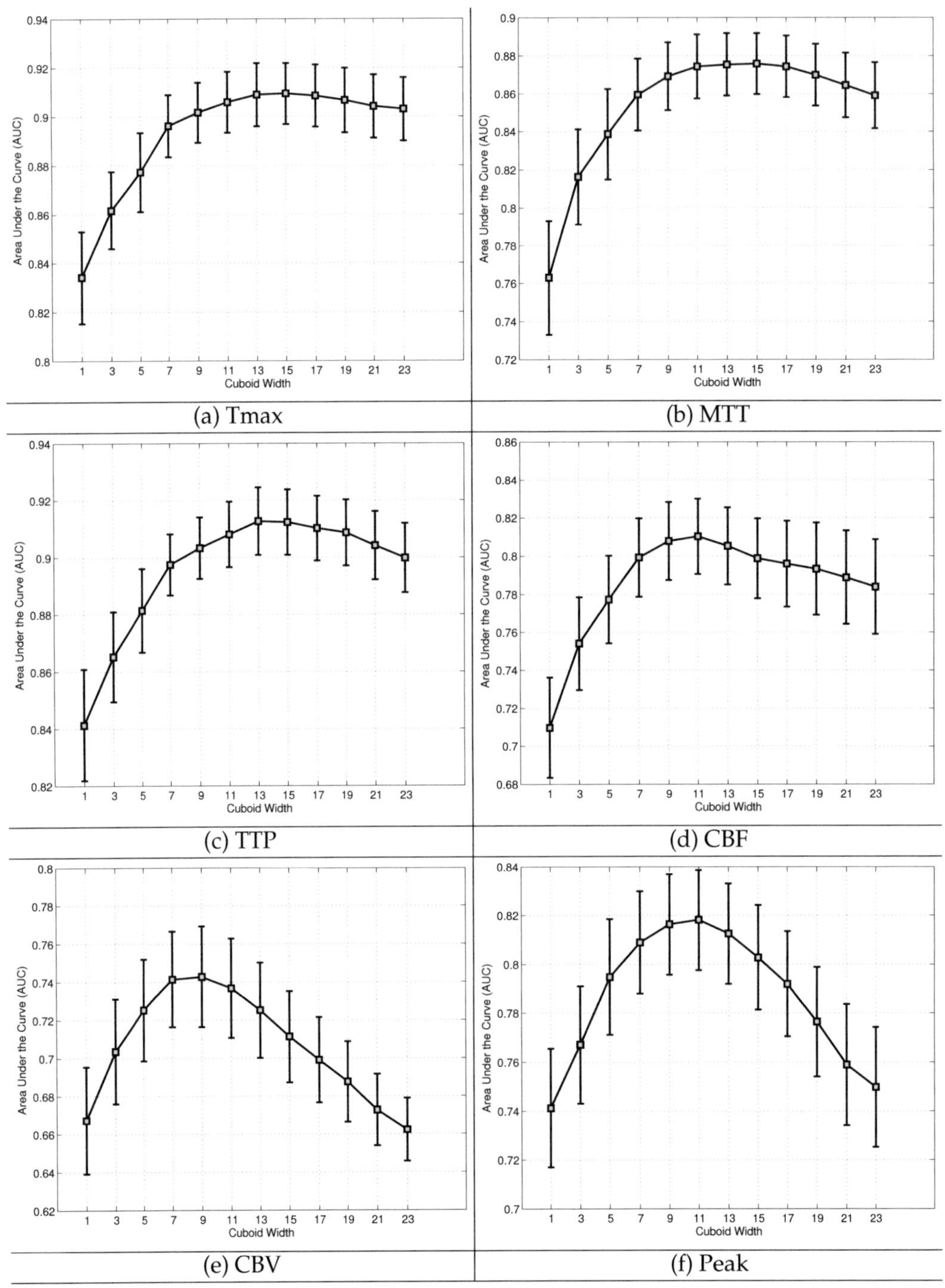

(a) Tmax
(b) MTT
(c) TTP
(d) CBF
(e) CBV
(f) Peak

Fig. 2. Effect of the cuboid size on the average Area Under the Curve (AUC) for SR-KDA regression models using a leave-one-out crossvalidation strategy.

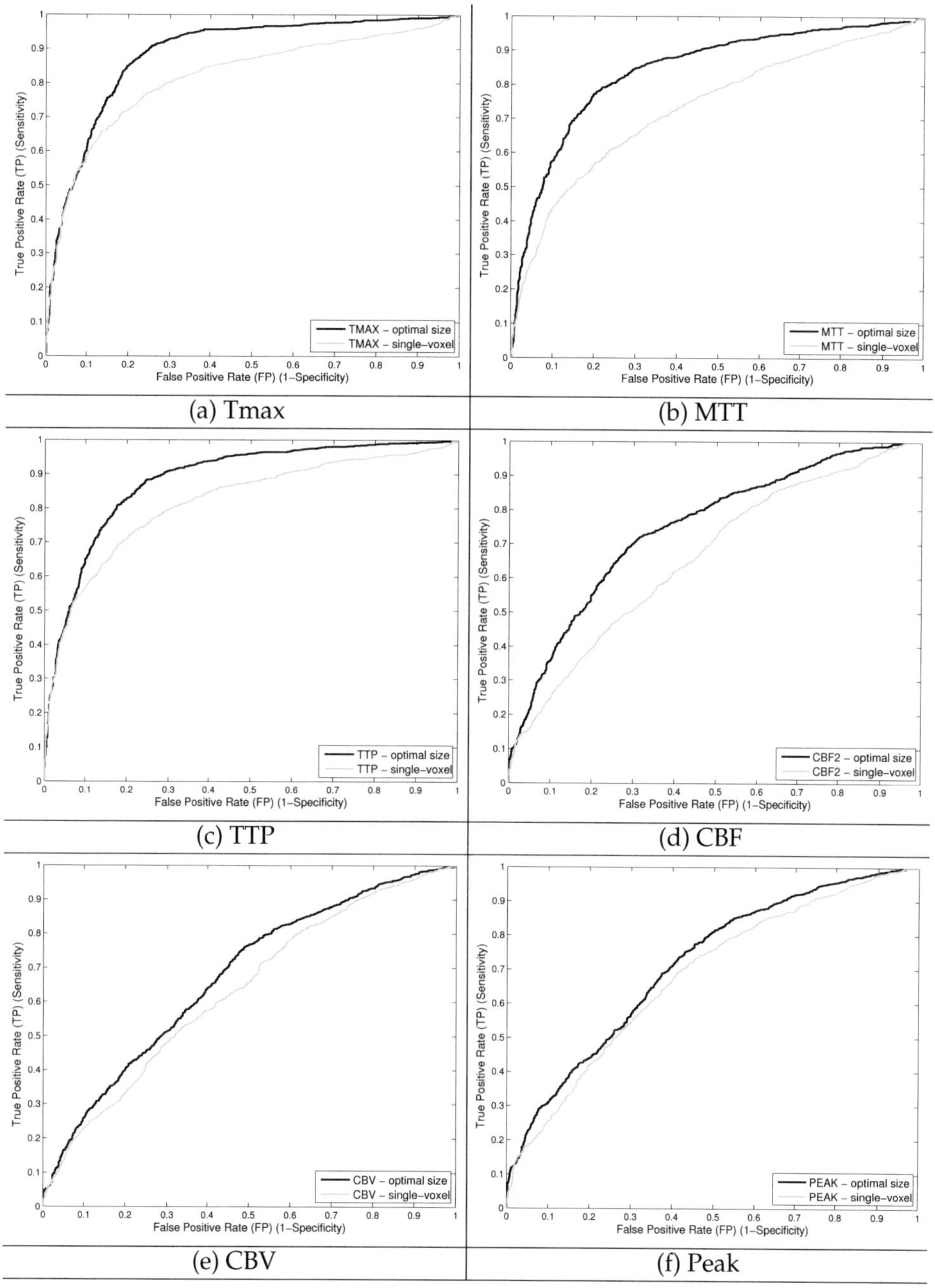

Fig. 3. For each parameter, ROC curves (dark line) are generated using the cuboid size that led to the best average AUC for each method as reported in Fig 2, and compared to single-voxel-based models (gray line). The difference between the dark and gray lines is proportional to the improvement obtained by a regional model versus single-voxel-based model.

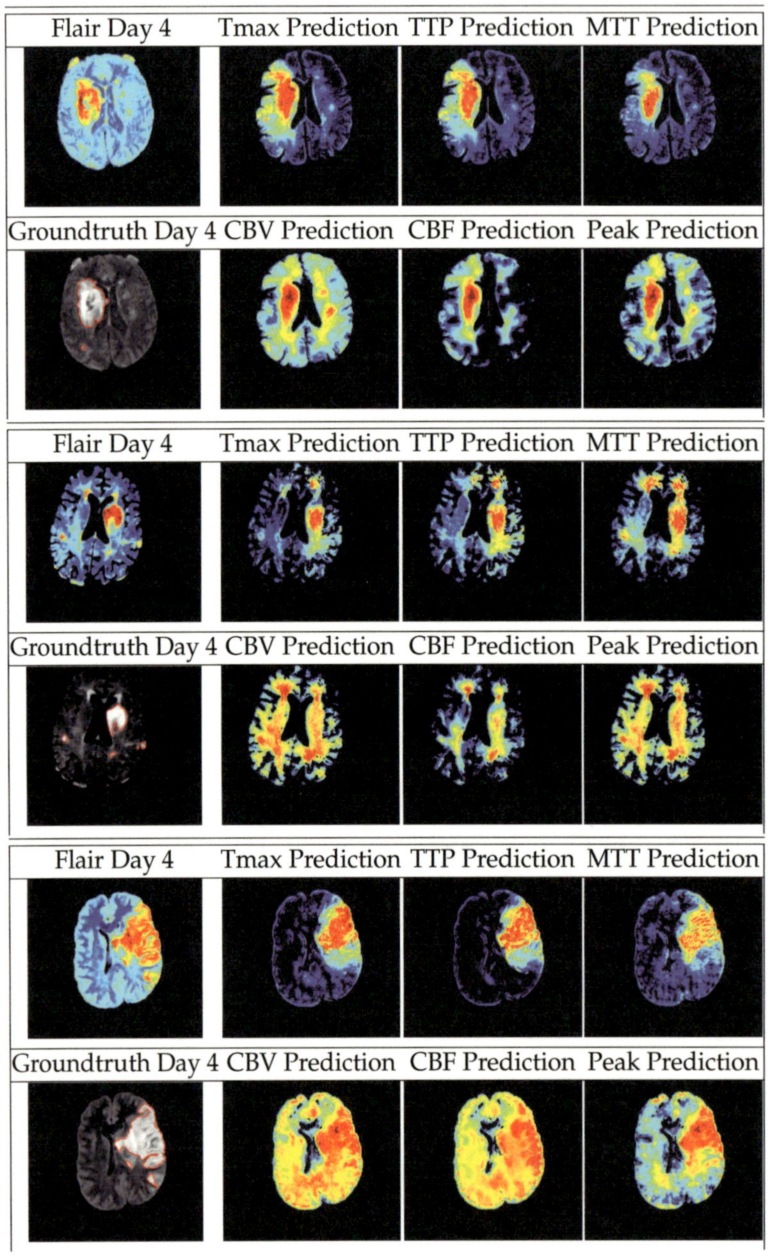

Fig. 4. Prediction results for three patients. FLAIR at followup, and predictions from onset Tmax, TTP, MTT, perfusion map are illustrated on the first row. Predictions are compared to the ground truth manually outlined in followup FLAIR at day 4 on the second row, followed by CBV, CBF, and Peak predictions.

3.2 McNemar's test

Significance results of the McNemar's test are summarized in Table 2. With a 95% confidence interval and one degree of freedom, two models are considered significantly different if the value χ^2 is above 3.8414. McNemar's values between a baseline model of size 1×1 versus an optimal regional model are 25.56, 116.8, 54.04, 5.81, 23.313.12, for Tmax, MTT, TTP, CBF, CBV, Peak, respectively. Because they are way over 3.8414, regional models for Tmax, MTT, CBF, CBV (and CBF to some extent) can be considered to improve the prediction accuracy significantly. However, Peak was just below the threshold and therefore the impact of the regional model on this feature map cannot be considered significant on our dataset.

Test	McNemar value
Tmax 15x15 vs Tmax 1x1	25.56
MTT 15x15 vs MTT 1x1	116.8
TTP 13x13 vs TTP 1x1	54.04
CBF 11x11 vs CBF 1x1	5.81
CBV 9x9 vs CBV 1x1	23.31
Peak 11x11 vs Peak 1x1	3.12

Table 2. Results of McNemar's test to measure the significance of using single-voxel-based versus regional models using the optimal cuboid size for each PWI parameter map.

3.3 Computational performance

The predictive model was implemented in Matlab and executed on a Dell Optiplex 760 desktop computer equipped with an Intel Core2 Duo CPU cadenced at 3.33GHz. The training of the predictive model, excluding image normalization, volume registration, and ground truth selection took less than ten minutes for 10×10 cuboids, while the prediction on an entire volume took less than two minutes. Note that the speed depends on the size of the cuboids, larger cuboids require more memory and computational time.

4. Discussion

The prediction of brain tissue fate in ischemic stroke, and therefore the identification of salvageable tissue, is a challenging problem that holds useful information for the clinician during the decision making process. Ultimately, automatic tissue fate predictive models could help us understand the underlying mechanisms of infarct growth. These mechanisms are complex, as they depend on a wide variety of factors such as: quality of blood perfusion to the area, quality of colaterals, energy delivery, age and medical history of the patient, etc. Integrating all these elements within a unified predictive model is the long-term goal of our research.

In this chapter, we have proposed a comparative analysis about the predictive power of PWI parameter maps. A generic framework based on a nonlinear regression method was introduced to predict the likely outcome of brain tissue in ischemic stroke patients. Although the models were trained on a rather small dataset (25 patients), our experimental results have demonstrated that significant improvement can be obtained by a regional model in comparison with a single-voxel-based approach. Several feature maps achieve an average

AUC of over .8 using optimal cuboid sizes. These good performances may be explained by the three following reasons:

- Regional: The use of optimized cuboids significantly improves a single-voxel-based approach. A possible explanation of this improvement is that cuboids implicitly represent the regional distribution of intensity and correlation among voxels and are more robust to noise.
- Nonlinear: The predictive model is based on Kernel Spectral Regression (SR-KDA) that has demonstrated excellent performances in a wide variety of applications. For the current application, a possible explanation for this difference is that the relation between the cuboids extracted at onset from PWI parameters and the followup FLAIR intensity is not a linear one, and it is, therefore, better captured by a nonlinear model such as SR-KDA.
- Randomness: Because machine learning techniques are often limited in the number of training samples they can handle in a reasonable time, efficiently exploiting the millions of cuboids available in the training set is a complex task. To obtain a representative training set, we randomly sample cuboids across images so that a similar number of cuboids is sampled for each outcome (infarcted or not). This is similar in spirit to what has been shown in a previous study (Jonsdottir et al., 2009).

In principle, even after normalization, FLAIR images are not necessarily comparable between patients. However, in practice, the "leave-one-patient-out" approach excludes all the data of the patient to be evaluated from the training set, and therefore, solely relies on the other patients to make predictions. Results obtained in terms of average AUC show that after normalization, infarcted and non-infarcted tissue can, with a reasonable confidence, be predicted across patients.
The proposed study is not only useful to identify the optimal size of the regional model for a given perfusion map, but may also serve as a starting point to help us understand the limitations of current perfusion maps and to identify in which cases other factors may improve the predictions. While a correct prediction tells us that the relation between different PWI parameters and the outcome of the tissue can be captured by the model, a prediction error may originate from several technical errors (co-registration of images, normalization, classifier, data sampling, perfusion map) or come from physiological reasons (quality of collaterals, degree of success of arterial recanalization intervention). For example, in the case of an arterial occlusion, the infarct core might not grow after an unsuccessful intervention (failed opening of the vessel) due to good collateral blood supply to the territory. There is, therefore, a margin for improvement by taking into account additional physiological parameters (*e.g.* collateral flow) and a larger dataset.

5. Acknowledgments

This work was supported by the National Institutes of Health [K23-NS054084 and P50-NS044378 to D.S.L.] and [R01-NS066008 to X.H.].

6. References

Cai, D., He, X. & Han, J. (2007). Spectral Regression for Efficient Regularized Subspace Learning, *ICCV*.

Calamante, F., Christensen, S., Desmond, P. M., Ostergaard, L., Davis, S. M. & Connelly, A. (2010). The physiological significance of the time-to-maximum (Tmax) parameter in perfusion MRI, *Stroke* 41: 1169–1174.

Chemmanam, T., Campbell, B. C., Christensen, S., Nagakane, Y., Desmond, P. M., Bladin, C. F., Parsons, M. W., Levi, C. R., Barber, P. A., Donnan, G. A. & Davis, S. M. (2010). Ischemic diffusion lesion reversal is uncommon and rarely alters perfusion-diffusion mismatch, *Neurology* 75: 1040–1047.

Chen, F., Liu, Q., Wang, H., Suzuki, Y., Nagai, N., Yu, J., Marchal, G. & Ni, Y. (2008). Comparing two methods for assessment of perfusion-diffusion mismatch in a rodent model of ischaemic stroke: a pilot study, *Br J Radiol* 81: 192–198.

Fisher, M. & Ginsberg, M. (2004). Current concepts of the ischemic penumbra: introduction, *Stroke* 35: 2657–2658.

Hacke et al, W. (2008). Thrombolysis with alteplase 3 to 4.5 hours after acute ischemic stroke, *N. Engl. J. Med.* 359(13): 1317–1329.

Heiss, W. & Sobesky, J. (2005). Can the penumbra be detected: MR versus PET imaging, *J Cereb Blood Flow Metab* 25: S702.

Huang, S., Shen, Q. & Duong, T. Q. (2010). Artificial neural network prediction of ischemic tissue fate in acute stroke imaging, *J Cereb Blood Flow Metab* .

Jonsdottir, K., Ostergaard, L. & Mouridsen, K. (2009). Predicting Tissue Outcome From Acute Stroke Magnetic Resonance Imaging: Improving Model Performance by Optimal Sampling of Training Data, *Stroke* 40: 3006–3011.

Kidwell, C. S., Alger, J. R. & Saver, J. L. (2004). Evolving Paradigms in Neuroimaging of the Ischemic Penumbra, *Stroke* 35: 2662–2665.

Maree, R., Geurts, P., Piater, J. & Wehenkel, L. (2005). Random subwindows for robust image classification, *CVPR*, Vol. 1, pp. 34–40.

Nguyen, V., Pien, H., Menenzes, N., Lopez, C., Melinosky, C., Wu, O., Sorensen, A., Cooperman, G., Ay, H., Koroshetz, W., Liu, Y., Nuutinen, J., Aronen, H. & Karonen, J. (2008). Stroke Tissue Outcome Prediction Using A Spatially-Correlated Model, *PPIC*.

Olivot, J. M., Mlynash, M., Zaharchuk, G., Straka, M., Bammer, R., Schwartz, N., Lansberg, M. G., Moseley, M. E. & Albers, G. W. (2009). Perfusion MRI (Tmax and MTT) correlation with xenon CT cerebral blood flow in stroke patients, *Neurology* 72: 1140–1145.

Olivot, J., Mlynash, M., Thijs, V., Purushotham, A., Kemp, S., Lansberg, M., Wechsler, L., Gold, G., Bammer, R., Marks, M. & Albers, G. (2009). Geography, structure, and evolution of diffusion and perfusion lesions in Diffusion and perfusion imaging Evaluation For Understanding Stroke Evolution (DEFUSE), *Stroke* 40(10): 3245–3251.

Rose, S., Chalk, J., Griffin, M., Janke, A., Chen, F., McLachan, G., Peel, D., Zelaya, F., Markus, H., Jones, D., Simmons, A., O'Sullivan, M., Jarosz, J., Strugnell, W., Doddrell, D. & Semple, J. (2001). MRI based diffusion and perfusion predictive model to estimate stroke evolution, *Magnetic Resonance Imaging* 19(8): 1043–1053.

Scalzo, F., Hao, Q., Alger, J., Hu, X. & Liebeskind, D. (2010). Tissue Fate Prediction in Acute Ischemic Stroke Using Cuboid Models, *LNCS* 6454: 292–301.

Scalzo, F., Xu, P., Asgari, S., Bergsneider, M. & Hu, X. (2009). Regression analysis for peak designation in pulsatile pressure signals, *Med Biol Eng Comput* 47: 967–977.

Scalzo, F., Xu, P., Asgari, S., Kim, S., Bergsneider, M. & Hu, X. (2010). Robust Peak Recognition in Intracranial Pressure Signals, *Biomed Eng Online* 9: 61.

Schaefer, P., Barak, E., Kamalian, S., Romero, J., Koroshetz, W., Gonzalez, R. & Lev, M. (2007). Visual estimation of mri core/penumbra mismatch, versus quantitative measurement, unnecessarily excludes patients from thrombolytic clinical trials, *Stroke* 38: 453–607.

Schlaug, G., Benfield, A., Baird, A. E., Siewert, B., Lovblad, K. O., Parker, R. A., Edelman, R. R. & Warach, S. (1999). The ischemic penumbra: operationally defined by diffusion and perfusion MRI, *Neurology* 53: 1528–1537.

Shen, Q. & Duong, T. (2008). Quantitative Prediction of Ischemic Stroke Tissue Fate, *NMR Biomedicine* 21: 839–848.

Shen, Q., Ren, H., Fisher, M. & Duong, T. (2005). Statistical prediction of tissue fate in acute ischemic brain injury, *J Cereb Blood Flow Metab* 25: 1336–1345.

Siegel, S. & Castellan, N. (1988). *Nonparametric statistics for the behavioral sciences*, second edn, McGraw–Hill, Inc.

Smith., S. (2002). Fast robust automated brain extraction, *Human Brain Mapping* 17(3): 143–155.

Wu, O., Koroshetz, W., Ostergaard, L., Buonanno, F., Copen, W., Gonzalez, R., Rordorf, G., Rosen, B., Schwamm, L., Weisskoff, R. & Sorensen, A. (2001). Predicting tissue outcome in acute human cerebral ischemia using combined diffusion- and perfusion-weighted MR imaging, *Stroke* 32(4): 933–42.

Wu, O., Sumii, T., Asahi, M., Sasamata, M., Ostergaard, L., Rosen, B., Lo, E. & Dijkhuizen, R. (2007). Infarct prediction and treatment assessment with MRI-based algorithms in experimental stroke models, *Journal of Cerebral Blood Flow and Metabolism* 27: 196–204.

Yoo, A. J., Barak, E. R., Copen, W. A., Kamalian, S., Gharai, L. R., Pervez, M. A., Schwamm, L. H., Gonzalez, R. G. & Schaefer, P. W. (2010). Combining acute diffusion-weighted imaging and mean transmit time lesion volumes with NIHSSS improves the prediction of acute stroke outcome, *Stroke* 41: 1728–1735.

14

MRI Assessment of Post-Ischemic Neuroinflammation in Stroke: Experimental and Clinical Studies

Fabien Chauveau, Marilena Marinescu, Cho Tae-Hee,
Marlène Wiart, Yves Berthezène and Norbert Nighoghossian
University of Lyon, Lyon 1, CNRS UMR5220, INSERM U1044, INSA-Lyon, CREATIS
France

1. Introduction

Stroke is a major healthcare issue in both industrialized and developing countries (Yach et al., 2004): it is the third leading cause of death, after myocardial infarction and cancer, the second leading cause of dementia, and the leading cause of permanent disability in Western countries (Pendlebury et al., 2009; Rothwell et al., 2011). Ischemic stroke accounts for up to 85% of total stroke events (Feigin et al., 2003). Cerebral ischemia is caused by blood-clot obstruction of a cerebral artery. Occlusion of a brain vessel leads to a critical reduction in cerebral perfusion and, within minutes, to ischemic infarction. The resulting lesion comprises a central infarct core of irreversibly damaged brain tissue and a surrounding area of hypoperfused but still viable brain tissue (the ischemic penumbra), which can potentially be salvaged by rapid restoration of the blood flow. Intravenous thrombolysis with tissue plasminogen activator (tPA) within 4.5 hours of symptom onset can improve the clinical outcome (NINDS, 1995; Hacke et al., 2008). Endovascular strategies (e.g. thrombectomy) can enhance reperfusion rates in large artery occlusions, but remain to be validated in randomized clinical trials. Although approved by North American and European authorities, only a small proportion of patients receive acute revascularization therapies, mainly because of late diagnosis and limited access to specialized stroke units.
Neuroprotective drugs aim at salvaging the ischemic brain by targeting multiple pathophysiological processes: prolonging the time window for reperfusion therapies, limiting reperfusion injury and the risk of hemorrhage, minimizing the deleterious effects of inflammation. Compounds regulating the inflammatory response are being evaluated by the pharmaceutical industry (Barone & Parsons, 2000). Indeed, stroke triggers a marked inflammatory reaction, involving several types of immune cells, including those of the mononuclear phagocyte system. There has been a longstanding controversy about the respective role of these cells, whether they are infiltrating blood-borne macrophages or resident microglia. On one hand, there is evidence that inflammation can contribute to secondary ischemic injury and worsening of neurological status (Iadecola & Alexander, 2001). On the other hand, inflammation under certain circumstances could promote functional recovery, by supporting neurogenesis and plasticity (Ekdahl et al., 2009). Therefore, targeted intervention to control specific aspects of post-ischemic neuro-

inflammation is a promising strategy in human stroke, with a potentially wide therapeutic window. A thorough understanding of these processes is required in order to develop safe and effective anti-inflammatory therapies for stroke patients.

Microglial cells are the main brain-resident population of the mononuclear phagocyte system. Microglial activation is considered a hallmark of central nervous system (CNS) inflammation. Activated microglial cells become immunohistochemically indistinguishable from infiltrating myeloid cells (monocytes/macrophages) (Raivich et al., 1999). In particular, activated cells of the monocytic lineage, whether resident microglia or blood-borne macrophages, overexpress an outer mitochondrial membrane protein formerly known as the peripheral benzodiazepine receptor (PBR), now renamed "translocator protein (18kDa)" (TSPO 18kDa) (Papadopoulos et al., 2006). Nearly 30 years ago, radiolabeling of the prototypic PBR/TSPO ligand PK11195 with carbon-11 enabled in vivo imaging of microglial activation using Positron Emission Tomography (PET scan) (Camsonne et al., 1984), and paved the road for neuroinflammation imaging. However, [^{11}C]PK11195 has shown limitations that until now slowed clinical application of neuroinflammation imaging by PET (Venneti et al., 2006). Although the field is still very active, as seen from the plethora of radioligands for PBR/TSPO that have been radiolabeled these last few years (Chauveau et al., 2008), large-scale clinical PET studies are difficult to set up in the context of emergency stroke management.

In contrast, magnetic resonance imaging (MRI) is being increasingly used in the diagnosis and management of acute ischemic stroke patients. Abnormalities observed on diffusion-weighted imaging (DWI) allow early identification of severely ischemic brain regions that typically evolve into infarction (i.e. the ischemic core). Perfusion-weighted imaging (PWI) provides information about the hemodynamic status of the cerebral tissue. PWI lesions are frequently larger than the corresponding DWI lesions during the first hours of stroke evolution. Subsequent infarct enlargement has been described in the region of DWI/PWI mismatch, supporting the hypothesis that this area represents the ischemic penumbra. Combined DWI and PWI imaging at the acute stage of stroke might thus help to identify patients with salvageable tissue, who may benefit from thrombolytic therapy. These MRI techniques are increasingly used for the evaluation of neuroprotectants, as PWI/DWI mismatch is considered a valuable estimate of penumbra in both animal models (Chauveau et al., 2011) and patients (Donnan et al., 2009). Given its pivotal role in the management of stroke patients, an additional MRI-based technique to image inflammation is thus particularly compelling. MRI has an unparalleled ability to image brain structure and function in both humans and small animals.

This chapter focuses on the MRI techniques that have been developed so far to image inflammation in stroke.

2. In vivo imaging of phagocytic cells using endogenous mechanisms

Magnetic Resonance Imaging of inflammation was first attempted in stroke models by taking advantage of endogenous contrast mechanisms. Schroeter et al. (Schroeter et al., 2001) thus used high resolution multimodal MRI to investigate inflammatory and glial response following focal cerebral ischemia. Images were acquired in rats, with transient occlusion of the middle cerebral artery 3, 7 and 14 days after stroke onset, and compared to immunostaining of phagocytic cells and astrocytes. This MRI approach, however, failed to visually discriminate inflammatory regions from healthy tissue, and highlighted the need to develop new MRI techniques for specific detection of inflammatory cells. Two subsequent studies (Justicia et al., 2008; Weber et al., 2005) demonstrated the potential of 3D T2*-weighted sequences for detecting regions with phagocytic activity, due to cell accumulation of endogenous iron, which induces strong susceptibility artifacts. However, both studies were performed at late stages of stroke (starting 10 weeks post-injury), in a time-window that was less than optimal for therapeutic intervention.

3. In vivo labeling of phagocytic cells

Cellular imaging of inflammation using MRI coupled with the injection of iron oxide nanoparticles has recently emerged as a promising non-invasive technique for pre-clinical and clinical studies of several inflammatory diseases. Two distinct classes of iron oxide nanoparticles are currently used in MRI, depending on hydrodynamic particle size: superparamagnetic iron oxide (SPIO) particles, with a mean particle diameter of more than 50 nm, and ultrasmall superparamagnetic iron oxide (USPIO) particles with a smaller hydrodynamic diameter (Corot et al., 2006). When injected intravenously, both types of nanoparticles are phagocytosed by macrophages, whether within the blood-pool (circulating monocytes) or locally at the inflammation site (tissue macrophages/activated microglia). Macrophages can thus be labeled and monitored in vivo with exogenous magnetic contrast agents. Importantly, this technique can be applied in patients, as several (U)SPIOs are already being used in humans.

3.1 Pre-clinical studies

To date, few teams have monitored phagocytic cell trafficking after focal cerebral ischemia on MRI coupled with (U)SPIO injection. Investigations were mostly conducted in rats, using differing protocols (various stroke models, rat strains, contrast agents, magnetic field strengths and imaging protocols), which render inter-study comparisons difficult. Of note, an early study (Doerfler et al., 2000) showed no impact of USPIO injection on clinical scores and lesion size in a model of permanent focal cerebral ischemia in rats; the dose, however, was ten times as low as in the following studies, the aim being to use USPIO as a marker of perfusion, not inflammation.

Table 1 synthesizes the studies published so far, using a permanent model of focal cerebral ischemia (pMCAO). Administration of iron oxide nanoparticles was performed at different times after ischemia. T2/T2*-weighted imaging was used in all studies to detect MR signal changes following (U)SPIO injection, typically showing decreasing signal intensity. The most relevant protocol in terms of T2/T2* effects involved injection at day 5 post-injury with a dose of 300 μmol Fe/kg, and follow-up at day 6, whether with USPIO (Ferumoxtran-10) or with SPIO (Ferucarbotran) (Engberink et al., 2008; Kleinschnitz et al., 2003; Saleh et al., 2004b; Schroeter et al., 2004). This 24-hour interval between injection and imaging is necessary in order for the iron oxide particles to wash out from the vascular compartment (the half-life of Ferumoxtran 10 in plasma is 5 hours in rat). T2/T2* hypointense signals were usually observed at day 6 in the perilesional area (Saleh et al., 2004b; Schroeter et al., 2004). At later time-points, these hyposignals were detected in the lesion core (Kleinschnitz et al., 2003). The hypothesis of passive diffusion of iron oxide nanoparticles through a disrupted blood brain barrier (BBB) was rejected, because post-gadolinium and post-(U)SPIO MR signal changes did not superimpose, suggesting an active mechanism of brain entry, via (U)SPIO-laden infiltrating macrophages (Engberink et al., 2008; Kleinschnitz et al., 2003).

Animal model		Contrast Agent			MRI			Ref.
Species	Stroke model	Name	Dose (µmol/kg)	Injection time	Imaging times	Field strength	Sequences	
Rat	EC	Ferumo-xtran-10	100	T0+5h	D0, D1, D2, D4, D7	4.7T	T2 map	(Rausch et al., 2001)
Rat	PT	Ferucar-botran	200	MRI-24h	D1-9, D11, D12, D14	1.5T	T2, 3D CISS, Gd-T1	(Kleinsch nitz et al., 2003)
Rat	PT	Ferumo-xtran-10	300	MRI-24h	D6	7T	3D T2*	(Schroeter et al., 2004)
Rat	PT	Ferumo-xtran-10	300	MRI-24h	D6	7T	T2*, 3D T2*	(Saleh et al., 2004b)
Rat	PT	Ferucar-botran	300	T0, T0+2h, T0+24h	D1, D2, D5, D7, D14	1.5T	T2, 3D CISS	(Kleinsch nitz et al., 2005)
Rat	PT	Ferumo-xtran-10	300	MRI-24h	D6, D8, D11	4.7T	T2 map, T2, Gd-T1	(Engberink et al., 2008)
Mouse	EC	Ferumo-xtran-10	2000	T0+5h,	D0, D1,D2, D3	7T	T2, T1, Gd-T1	(Wiart et al., 2007)
Mouse	EC	Ferumo-xtran-10	2000	T0+5h,	D0, D1	7T	T2, T1, Gd-T1	(Desestret et al., 2009)

Table 1. Literature review of USPIO-enhanced MRI in the permanent middle cerebral artery occlusion (pMCAO) model. EC- Electrocoagulation; PT- Photothrombosis; T0 = Occlusion time; T0+5h = 5h after occlusion; MRI-24h = 24h before MRI; Gd-T1: T1-weighted MRI with gadolinium chelate injection (to assess BBB integrity).

Despite the number of post-ischemia time points investigated (between D0 and D14), few animals were followed longitudinally, because most were usually sacrificed after MRI for comparison with immunohistochemistry. Post-mortem analysis typically comprised immunostaining of phagocytic cells (ED1) and Prussian Blue (PB) staining to detect iron. Spatial co-location between macrophages, iron and MR hypointense signals was well documented at the periphery of the lesion in a photothrombosis model at D6 (Saleh et al., 2004b). Double immunostaining on the same histological slices confirmed internalization of iron inside macrophages in this set-up (Kleinschnitz et al., 2003). Co-location was also suggested in an electrocoagulation model (Rausch et al., 2001). It should be noted, however, that in all cases ED1 immunostaining exceeded iron staining, suggesting that only part of the inflammatory response was revealed by (U)SPIO-enhanced MRI.

We sought to investigate the feasibility of macrophage imaging in mice using MRI. USPIOs were injected into mice 5h after pMCAO (Wiart et al., 2007). The timing of injection and imaging (from D0 to D3) was early compared to previous studies, because we aimed at assessing the early, potentially pathological role of macrophages, anticipating future studies of anti-inflammatory drugs at the acute stage. Hypointense MR signals were detected in the perilesional area at 48h and 72h post-injury, in accordance with published data obtained in rats with a similar protocol (Rausch et al., 2001). More surprisingly, USPIO-enhanced MRI kinetic analysis disclosed a hypointense MR signal in the contralateral hemisphere: this hyposignal spread along to the corpus callosum (ipsilateral to contralateral) from D0 to D3. Imaging data correlated with histochemical analysis at 48h and 72h post-injury, showing macrophage activation remote from the lesion, and macrophage ingestion of USPIO (Figure 1). Remote inflammatory response to brain injury was previously reported in animal models of focal cerebral ischemia using invasive techniques (Dubois et al., 1988; Schroeter et al., 1999) and in stroke patients using PET-scan (Gerhard et al., 2005; Pappata et al., 2000), but to our knowledge the present study provided the first evidence obtained in living animals.

Whereas the accumulation of (U)SPIOs in cells is well explained by phagocytosis activity of macrophages, their route of transport to brain macrophages is not yet well described. Three hypotheses have been put forward to explain the MR signal changes observed after (U)SPIO injection: (i) intravascular trapping of iron particles (Bendszus et al., 2007; Kleinschnitz et al., 2005); (ii) (U)SPIO uptake by phagocytes, on the assumption that (U)SPIOs are primarily taken up by circulating phagocytes (Kleinschnitz et al., 2003); and (iii) interstitial iron particle diffusion into damaged tissue after nonspecific leakage through a disrupted blood-brain barrier (Engberink et al., 2008). To assess the early brain distribution of iron particles, MRI signal changes after intravenous USPIO injection were then compared with the histological iron and macrophage distribution from 6h to 24h, using the same experimental set-up as before (Desestret et al., 2009). In this electrocoagulation model of stroke, USPIO-related MR signal changes were indisputably paralleled by phagocyte-associated iron deposits detected on histology after 24h post-ischemia, but the pattern of results suggested that early USPIO-related MR signal changes were mainly caused by passive diffusion of free USPIOs after BBB leakage or by intravascular trapping, rather than by peripheral phagocyte infiltration. Indeed, at early time-points after USPIO injection, BBB disruption matches the spatiotemporal pattern of MR signal change. These results were in accordance with a previous study investigating both early and delayed time-points after SPIO injection in a photothrombosis model in rats (Kleinschnitz et al., 2005). Intravascular trapping was found to be the main mechanism of particle entry into peripheral areas and lesion core. These findings highlight the fact that several mechanisms of (U)SPIO entry into the brain may co-exist, so that MR data interpretation should take account of the experimental set-up used (post-ischemia time-points, model characteristics, and nature of the contrast agent used).

Table 2 synthesizes the studies published so far, to our knowledge, using a transient model of focal cerebral ischemia (tMCAO). Transient ischemia was in all cases performed using the suture model, which allows mechanical reperfusion by withdrawing the suture from the artery. This model is thought to be more representative of the clinical situation than permanent ischemia models. Results of these studies are contradictory and all the more difficult to interpret since protocols differed on many points (in particular in terms of the type of iron oxide nanoparticles used, and timing of injection). The first study (Rausch et al., 2002) presented the most unexpected results, with the observation of a transient T1 hyperintense signal inside the lesion, without corresponding T2 hypointense signal, although the study was performed at high field (4.7T). Furthermore, while macrophages (ED1) were detected in the lesion from day 1 to day 7, Prussian Blue immunostaining was positive only at day 7, i.e. 5 days after the onset of the hyperintense signal. The authors

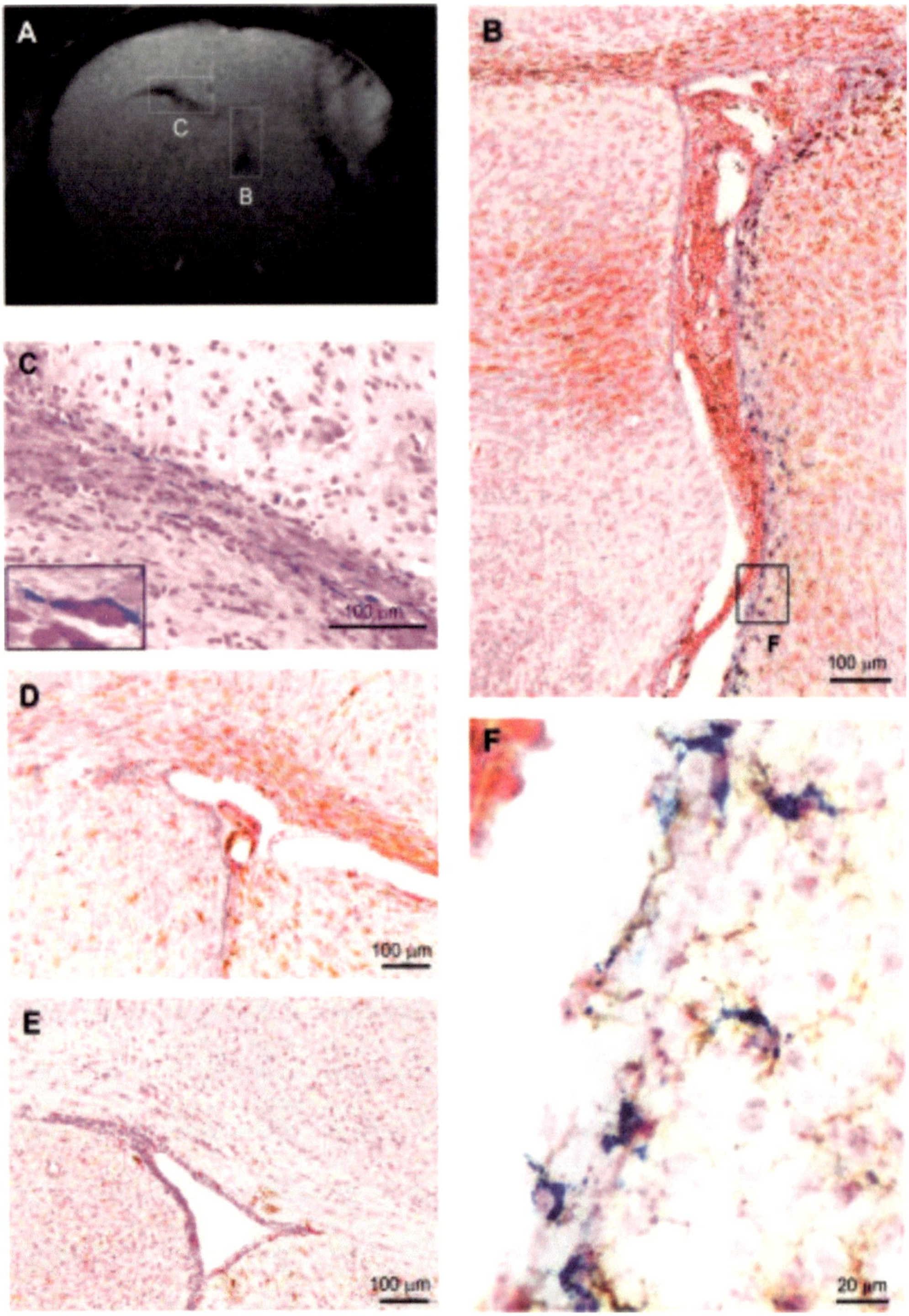

Fig. 1. Correlation of gradient echo (GRE) MR signals with immunohistology (Bregma 0mm according to Franklin and Paxinos's atlas). A- GRE MRI 72h post-pMCAO and i.v. injection

of USPIO. Note the hyposignal around the lesion, the contralateral corpus callosum and the ipsilateral peri-ventricular area. B- Double staining with Prussian Blue and F4/80 of the right (ipsilateral) ventricle. Iron-stained microglia/macrophages are clearly visible along the lateral wall, in correlation with the hyposignal observed in GRE images (A). C- Prussian Blue staining for iron in the contralateral corpus callosum of the corresponding slice. Positive staining was observed around cell nuclei, which suggests cytoplasm uptake (insert). D- F4/80 immunostaining for mouse microglia/macrophages in the contralateral corpus callosum. Note the F4/80+ brown cells, in spatial agreement with iron+ cells (B) and MRI hypointense signal (A). E- F4/80 immunostaining of a non-operated control mouse in the left corpus callosum, with no positive staining. F- Double staining with Prussian Blue and F4/80: magnification of B. Microglia/macrophages, as identified by their brown color and typical ramified shape, were also blue-stained, suggesting USPIO intra-cellularity. From (Wiart et al., 2007).

proposed the following explanations: (i) that USPIOs might be leaked by the infiltrating macrophages before being re-ingested by secondarily recruited macrophages, and (ii) that Prussian Blue might become sensitive to iron oxide nanoparticles only after degradation of their dextran coating, an enzymatic process that could take several days. The second study (Kim et al., 2008) presented results more in line with those obtained in the permanent model, with an hypointense signal appearing relatively late (day 3-4) after stroke onset. Macrophages (ED1) and focal iron deposition were detected in the lesion at these time-points, in agreement with T2/T2* hypointense areas. However, these results obtained with SPIO injection failed to be reproduced with USPIO in a recent study : Farr and colleagues did not observed T1,T2, nor T2* signal changes, despite a three-dose assay and extensive ED-1-positive macrophage accumulation at the sub-acute stage (Farr et al., 2011). In line with this negative results, the single study performed with a mouse model of transient ischemia reported no detectable MRI changes in the first 72h following stroke onset (Denes et al., 2007). It should be noted, however, that the dose used in that study was particularly low (160 µmol/kg) and perhaps not optimal for MRI detection. Besides, this study confirmed the predominance of microglial response, demonstrated by a panoply of immunohistological markers, at acute and subacute stages, compared to monocytic infiltration (Denes et al., 2007).

Henning and colleagues (Henning et al., 2009) used an original strategy of "in vivo pre-labeling". The methodology is based (i) on the fact that iron oxide nanoparticles injected intravenously target, amongst other phagocytic cells, those from bone marrow (Denes et al., 2007; Simon et al., 2005); and (ii) on the hypothesis of resident macrophage turnover from bone-marrow progenitor cells (Priller et al., 2001). SPIO injection was performed 7 days before tMCAO, in order to pre-label bone marrow-derived macrophages. A T2/T2* hypointense signal was observed in the lesion periphery with a peak at D4 post-reperfusion in pre-loaded rats, and remained constant until D7 in the perilesional area. Conversely, post-loaded animals (which received the same SPIO injection 5 minutes after occlusion) showed no significant signal changes. Another interesting result of the study concerned the nature of the subpopulation of labeled macrophages, which were confined to three distinct locations: the perivascular regions, the meninges and the choroid plexus. In these areas, Prussian blue co-located with differentiated macrophages staining (ED2 marker) rather than with the non-specific staining of macrophages (ED1 marker) and activated microglia staining (IBA). In line with previous studies, Prussian Blue staining was found in only a small proportion of cells. Although the exact mechanisms of cell labeling by SPIOs and migration of these labeled cells into the central nervous system were not elucidated in this study, the proposed approach is elegant in the sense that it solves the question of passive diffusion of SPIOs (since they are washed out from the plasma before stroke onset). Other independent studies are nevertheless mandatory to confirm these results.

Animal model		**Contrast Agent**			**MRI**			**Ref.**
Species	**Extent (min)**	**Name**	**Dose (μmol/kg)**	**Injection time**	**Imaging times**	**Field strength**	**Sequences**	
Rat	30	Ferumo xtran-10	300	T0+5h	D0, D1, D2, D3, D4, D7	4.7T	T2, T1	(Rausch et al., 2002)
Mouse	30/60	Ferumo xtran-10	160	MRI-2h	D0, D1, D2, D3	7T	T2, Gd-T1	(Denes et al., 2007)
Rat	60	Ferucar botran	200	MRI-24h	D1-6, D8, D10, D14	3T	T2, 3D T2*, Gd-T1	(Kim et al., 2008)
Rat	30	Ferumo xide	286	T0-7days	D1-4, D7	7T	T2 map, 3D T2*	(Henning et al., 2009)
Rat	60	Ferumo xtran-10	300 / 600 / 1000	T0+3days T0+6days	D3-4, D6-7	4.7T	T2, T2*, T1	(Farr et al., 2011)

Table 2. Literature review of USPIO-enhanced MRI in the transient middle cerebral artery occlusion (tMCAO) model. All transient models were performed with the intraluminal thread model. T0 = Reperfusion time; T0+5h = 5h after reperfusion; MRI-24h = 24h before MRI; Gd-T1: T1-weighted MRI with gadolinium chelate injection (to assess BBB integrity); PB- Prussian Blue

3.2 Clinical studies

The first clinical study was published in 2004 by Saleh et al. (Saleh et al., 2004a). USPIOs (Ferumoxtran-10) were injected in 10 stroke patients at the end of the first week after symptom onset (6 to 9 days). MRI was performed at 1.5T before injection, then between 24h and 36h and again between 48h and 72h post-injection. Parenchymal enhancement was observed on T1-weighted imaging in most cases (8 out of 10). However, T2/T2* effects were not systematically observed and seemed to be associated with vessels. As in experimental studies, there was a mismatch between regions showing BBB disruption (as assessed by post-gadolinium T1 enhancement) and regions showing USPIO enhancement. The authors suggested that USPIO enhancement was due to the infiltration of magnetically-labeled macrophages. We conducted a similar study, in which USPIOs were injected at D6 after stroke onset and MRI was performed 72h post-injection (Nighoghossian et al., 2007). In the 10 included patients, USPIO response was heterogeneous and not related to subacute lesion volume. As in the study by Saleh et al. (Saleh et al., 2004a), T1 enhancement was observed in most cases (9 out of 10), while T2/T2* effects were not systematically observed (5 patients out of 10) (Figure 2). No obvious relationship was observed between regions with BBB disruption and those showing USPIO-induced signal changes: for example, 3 patients without BBB disruption showed enhancement following USPIO administration, whereas one patient with severe BBB disruption showed no USPIO-induced signal change.

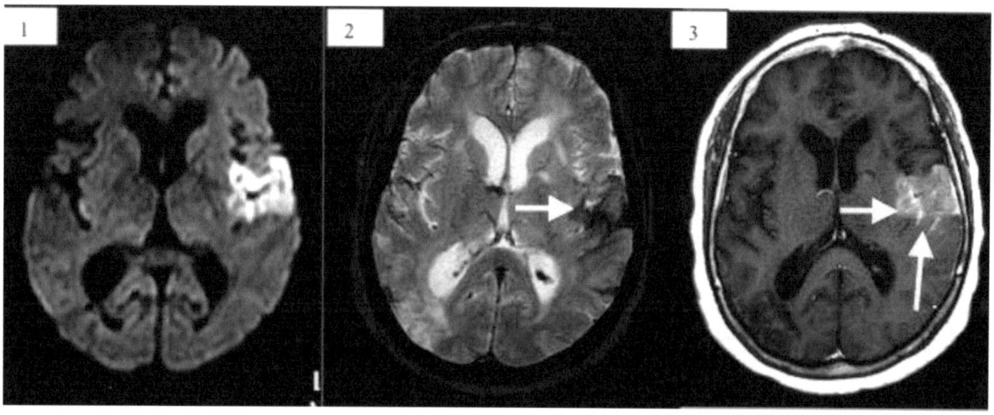

Fig. 2. A 55–year-old woman, with a past history of transient confusional state 2 months before admission, which was likely related to a right posterior middle cerebral artery (MCA) stroke, was admitted for acute left MCA stroke with nonfluent aphasia and severe right hemiplegia. From left to right: (1) Day 6 diffusion-weighted imaging (DWI) without contrast; (2) Day 9 T2*-weighted imaging; and (3) Day 9 T1-weighted imaging 72 hours after USPIO infusion. Right, old posterior superficial MCA ischemic infarction and recent left superficial MCA stroke with a large USPIO enhancement (arrow) compared with DWI lesion volume. From (Nighoghossian et al., 2007).

In their second study, Saleh et al. (Saleh et al., 2007) investigated an earlier time window: USPIOs were injected 2 to 3 days following symptom onset and MRI was performed at different post-injection time points (24h-36h, 48h-72h, 10-11 days). Only 3 of the 9 patients included in the analysis showed signal change on post-injection MRI. None of these patients showed T1 enhancement following gadolinium chelate administration. As in the previous study, signal changes consisted in enhancement on T1-weighted images, with an increase in enhancement between the first two post-injection examinations, and a decrease between the last two. A subsequent study involving the same earlier time-window (2 days after stroke onset with MRI performed 48h after) confirmed these findings (Cho et al., 2007). T1 enhancement was observed inside the lesion in only 1 of the 5 included patients. In this patient, post-gadolinium enhancement was more extensive than post-USPIO enhancement. The heterogeneity of USPIO-labeling was thought to reflect inter-individual variability of post-ischemic inflammation (Saleh et al., 2007). Accordingly, MRI may be of use in selecting patients for targeted anti-inflammatory therapies.

Interpretation of clinical data is mainly based on experimental studies. Since (U)SPIOs have been found in macrophages following ischemic stroke, signal changes observed in patients are thought to reflect the phagocytic response. There are, however, several obstacles for direct translation from small animals to humans. Firstly, the animal model may not properly represent the clinical situation, so that the route of (U)SPIO transport to brain macrophages might not be the same. Secondly, there are some differences in the time-windows investigated: in the perspective of therapy, it is more attractive to treat in the very first days or even hours after symptom onset; experimental and clinical protocols performed during the early stage failed to produce consistent signal changes. Thirdly, the dose used in humans (2.6 mg iron/kg body weight) is far less than in animals. Finally, the interpretation of MR signal changes may differ according to the field strength at which they were acquired. Animal experiments are usually performed at very high field compared to clinical studies, which obviously influences relaxation properties. The latter two elements (high dose/high field in pre-clinical studies and small dose/low field in clinical studies) could partly explain why T1 effects were mostly observed in clinical studies, whereas T2/T2* effects were always observed in experimental studies. Besides, though compartmentalization of USPIO inside cells is thought to induce magnetic susceptibility gradients leading to T2* effects, it seems that SPIO-labeled macrophages could produce T1 effects at 1.5T (Daldrup-Link et al., 2003). This shows the importance of performing quantitative studies in order to characterize the effects of compartmentalization and concentration on MR signal, at different field strengths for each contrast agent (Brisset et al., 2010a). In the future, the development of MR sequences specifically dedicated to detection and quantification of (U)SPIO-labeled macrophages, such as positive contrast techniques (Brisset et al., 2010b; Mani et al., 2008), may help data interpretation and analysis of longitudinal studies.

4. Ex vivo labeling of phagocytic cells

MRI techniques using intravenously injected SPIO/USPIO fail to distinguish between non-specific diffusion of free particles and magnetically labeled phagocytes. Thus, signal changes might be wrongly attributed to inflammatory processes. This limitation could be overcome in part by magnetically labeling macrophages before their injection (ex vivo labeling). To date, the majority of studies using ex vivo labeling in stroke models addressed cellular therapy, using subventricular zone progenitor cells (Athiraman et al., 2009; Cicchetti et al., 2007; Jiang et al., 2005; Zhang et al., 2003), embryonic neural stem cells (Hoehn et al., 2002; Modo et al., 2004) mesenchymal stem cells (Lee et al., 2009; Walczak et al., 2008), spleen-derived mononuclear cells (Stroh et al., 2006) or adipose-derived stem cells (Rice et al., 2007). To our knowledge, only one study was published using ex vivo labeling of macrophages in a rat stroke model (Engberink et al., 2008): 4 rats were intravenously injected with 5 million SPIO-labeled monocytes after induction of cerebral ischemia by photothrombosis. MRI was performed at 4.7T pre- and 24h, 72h and 120h post-injection. Although visual examination of T2*-weighted images and Prussian Blue staining were not conclusive, quantitative analysis (percentage of hypointense voxels compared to baseline) showed significant differences in MR signal changes compared to control animals (non-injected or injected with free USPIOs). According to the authors, the differences observed between groups are suggestive of an active monocytic infiltration into the lesion. One limitation of this method is that injected monocytes may not reflect the actual behavior of endogenous monocytes.

5. Conclusion

Despite abundant evidence for an inflammatory response after stroke, anti-inflammatory treatments have so far failed in clinical trials (Savitz & Fisher, 2007). In this context, non-invasive detection of inflammatory cells after brain ischemia could be helpful (i) to select patients who may benefit from anti-inflammatory treatment; (ii) to identify the optimal therapeutic time window; (iii) to develop therapies targeting specific pathophysiological processes. MRI coupled with (U)SPIO, a contrast agent taken up by macrophages ex vivo and in vivo, appears to be a promising tool for this purpose. Current limitations of this approach include the difficulty in identifying non-specific signal changes. Additional studies on long-term monitoring of (U)SPIO-related signal changes are required. This will be of crucial importance for clinical trials aiming to assess immunomodulatory drugs. Multiple factors are likely to account for post-treatment modifications of MR signal: modulation of inflammation, changes in the iron microenvironment and biotransformation. Well-designed pre-clinical studies including dedicated quantitative MR sequences are still warranted before application of the technique in larger patient cohorts.

6. References

NINDS. (1995). Tissue plasminogen activator for acute ischemic stroke. *N Engl J Med,* Vol.333, No.24, (n.d.), pp. 1581-1587, ISSN 0028-4793 (Print)

Athiraman, H., Jiang, Q., Ding, G. L., Zhang, L., Zhang, Z. G., Wang, L., Arbab, A. S., Li, Q., Panda, S., Ledbetter, K., Rad, A. M., & Chopp, M. (2009). Investigation of relationships between transverse relaxation rate, diffusion coefficient, and labeled cell concentration in ischemic rat brain using MRI. *Magn Reson Med,* Vol.61, No.3, (n.d.), pp. 587-594, ISSN 1522-2594 (Electronic)

Barone, F. C., & Parsons, A. A. (2000). Therapeutic potential of anti-inflammatory drugs in focal stroke. *Expert Opin Investig Drugs,* Vol.9, No.10, (n.d.), pp. 2281-2306, ISSN 1354-3784 (Print)

Bendszus, M., Kleinschnitz, C., & Stoll, G. (2007). Iron-enhanced MRI in ischemic stroke: intravascular trapping versus cellular inflammation. *Stroke,* Vol.38, No.5, (n.d.), pp. e12; author reply e13, ISSN 1524-4628 (Electronic)

Brisset, J. C., Desestret, V., Marcellino, S., Devillard, E., Chauveau, F., Lagarde, F., Nataf, S., Nighoghossian, N., Berthezene, Y., & Wiart, M. (2010a). Quantitative effects of cell internalization of two types of ultrasmall superparamagnetic iron oxide nanoparticles at 4.7 T and 7 T. *Eur Radiol,* Vol.20, No.2, (n.d.), pp. 275-285, ISSN 1432-1084 (Electronic) 0938-7994 (Linking)

Brisset, J. C., Sigovan, M., Chauveau, F., Riou, A., Devillard, E., Desestret, V., Touret, M., Nataf, S., Honnorat, J., Canet-Soulas, E., Nighoghossian, N., Berthezene, Y., & Wiart, M. (2010b). Quantification of Iron-Labeled Cells with Positive Contrast in Mouse Brains. *Mol Imaging Biol,* (n.d.), pp., ISSN 1860-2002 (Electronic) 1536-1632 (Linking)

Camsonne, R., Crouzel, C., Comar, D., Maziere, M., Prenant, C., Sastre, J., Moulin, M. A., & Syrota, A. (1984). Synthesis of N-(C-11) Methyl, N-(Methyl-1 Propyl), (Chloro-2 Phenyl)-1 Isoquinoleine Carboxamide-3 (PK11195) - a New Ligand for Peripheral Benzodiazepine Receptors. *Journal of Labelled Compounds & Radiopharmaceuticals,* Vol.21, No.10, (n.d.), pp. 985-991

Chauveau, F., Boutin, H., Van Camp, N., Dolle, F., & Tavitian, B. (2008). Nuclear imaging of neuroinflammation: a comprehensive review of [11C]PK11195 challengers. *Eur J Nucl Med Mol Imaging,* Vol.35, No.12, (n.d.), pp. 2304-2319, ISSN 1619-7089 (Electronic)

Chauveau, F., Cho, T. H., Perez, M., Guichardant, M., Riou, A., Aguettaz, P., Picq, M., Lagarde, M., Berthezene, Y., Nighoghossian, N., & Wiart, M. (2011). Brain-Targeting Form of Docosahexaenoic Acid for Experimental Stroke Treatment: MRI

Evaluation and Anti-Oxidant Impact. *Curr Neurovasc Res,* (n.d.), pp., ISSN 1875-5739 (Electronic) 1567-2026 (Linking)

Cho, T. H., Nighoghossian, N., Wiart, M., Desestret, V., Cakmak, S., Berthezene, Y., Derex, L., Louis-Tisserand, G., Honnorat, J., Froment, J. C., & Hermier, M. (2007). USPIO-enhanced MRI of neuroinflammation at the sub-acute stage of ischemic stroke: preliminary data. *Cerebrovasc Dis,* Vol.24, No.6, (n.d.), pp. 544-546, ISSN 1421-9786 (Electronic)

Cicchetti, F., Gross, R. E., Bulte, J. W., Owen, M., Chen, I., Saint-Pierre, M., Wang, X., Yu, M., & Brownell, A. L. (2007). Dual-modality in vivo monitoring of subventricular zone stem cell migration and metabolism. *Contrast Media Mol Imaging,* Vol.2, No.3, (n.d.), pp. 130-138, ISSN 1555-4317 (Electronic)

Corot, C., Robert, P., Idee, J. M., & Port, M. (2006). Recent advances in iron oxide nanocrystal technology for medical imaging. *Adv Drug Deliv Rev,* Vol.58, No.14, (n.d.), pp. 1471-1504, ISSN 0169-409X (Print)

Daldrup-Link, H. E., Rudelius, M., Oostendorp, R. A., Settles, M., Piontek, G., Metz, S., Rosenbrock, H., Keller, U., Heinzmann, U., Rummeny, E. J., Schlegel, J., & Link, T. M. (2003). Targeting of hematopoietic progenitor cells with MR contrast agents. *Radiology,* Vol.228, No.3, (n.d.), pp. 760-767, ISSN 0033-8419 (Print)

Denes, A., Vidyasagar, R., Feng, J., Narvainen, J., McColl, B. W., Kauppinen, R. A., & Allan, S. M. (2007). Proliferating resident microglia after focal cerebral ischaemia in mice. *J Cereb Blood Flow Metab,* Vol.27, No.12, (n.d.), pp. 1941-1953, ISSN 0271-678X (Print)

Desestret, V., Brisset, J. C., Moucharrafie, S., Devillard, E., Nataf, S., Honnorat, J., Nighoghossian, N., Berthezene, Y., & Wiart, M. (2009). Early-stage investigations of ultrasmall superparamagnetic iron oxide-induced signal change after permanent middle cerebral artery occlusion in mice. *Stroke,* Vol.40, No.5, (n.d.), pp. 1834-1841, ISSN 1524-4628 (Electronic)

Doerfler, A., Engelhorn, T., Heiland, S., Knauth, M., Wanke, I., & Forsting, M. (2000). MR contrast agents in acute experimental cerebral ischemia: potential adverse impacts on neurologic outcome and infarction size. *J Magn Reson Imaging,* Vol.11, No.4, (n.d.), pp. 418-424, ISSN 1053-1807 (Print)

Donnan, G. A., Baron, J. C., Ma, H., & Davis, S. M. (2009). Penumbral selection of patients for trials of acute stroke therapy. *Lancet Neurol,* Vol.8, No.3, (n.d.), pp. 261-269, ISSN 1474-4422 (Print) 1474-4422 (Linking)

Dubois, A., Benavides, J., Peny, B., Duverger, D., Fage, D., Gotti, B., MacKenzie, E. T., & Scatton, B. (1988). Imaging of primary and remote ischaemic and excitotoxic brain lesions. An autoradiographic study of peripheral type benzodiazepine binding sites in the rat and cat. *Brain Res,* Vol.445, No.1, (n.d.), pp. 77-90, ISSN 0006-8993 (Print) 0006-8993 (Linking)

Ekdahl, C. T., Kokaia, Z., & Lindvall, O. (2009). Brain inflammation and adult neurogenesis: the dual role of microglia. *Neuroscience,* Vol.158, No.3, (n.d.), pp. 1021-1029, ISSN 0306-4522 (Print) 0306-4522 (Linking)

Engberink, R. D., Blezer, E. L., Hoff, E. I., van der Pol, S. M., van der Toorn, A., Dijkhuizen, R. M., & de Vries, H. E. (2008). MRI of monocyte infiltration in an animal model of neuroinflammation using SPIO-labeled monocytes or free USPIO. *J Cereb Blood Flow Metab,* Vol.28, No.4, (n.d.), pp. 841-851, ISSN 0271-678X (Print)

Farr, T. D., Seehafer, J. U., Nelles, M., & Hoehn, M. (2011). Challenges towards MR imaging of the peripheral inflammatory response in the subacute and chronic stages of transient focal ischemia. *NMR Biomed,* Vol.24, No.1, (n.d.), pp. 35-45, ISSN 1099-1492 (Electronic) 0952-3480 (Linking)

Feigin, V. L., Lawes, C. M., Bennett, D. A., & Anderson, C. S. (2003). Stroke epidemiology: a review of population-based studies of incidence, prevalence, and case-fatality in the late 20th century. *Lancet Neurol,* Vol.2, No.1, (n.d.), pp. 43-53, ISSN 1474-4422 (Print) 1474-4422 (Linking)

Gerhard, A., Schwarz, J., Myers, R., Wise, R., & Banati, R. B. (2005). Evolution of microglial activation in patients after ischemic stroke: a [11C](R)-PK11195 PET study. *Neuroimage,* Vol.24, No.2, (n.d.), pp. 591-595, ISSN 1053-8119 (Print) 1053-8119 (Linking)

Hacke, W., Kaste, M., Bluhmki, E., Brozman, M., Davalos, A., Guidetti, D., Larrue, V., Lees, K. R., Medeghri, Z., Machnig, T., Schneider, D., von Kummer, R., Wahlgren, N., & Toni, D. (2008). Thrombolysis with alteplase 3 to 4.5 hours after acute ischemic stroke. *N Engl J Med,* Vol.359, No.13, (n.d.), pp. 1317-1329, ISSN 1533-4406 (Electronic) 0028-4793 (Linking)

Henning, E. C., Ruetzler, C. A., Gaudinski, M. R., Hu, T. C., Latour, L. L., Hallenbeck, J. M., & Warach, S. (2009). Feridex preloading permits tracking of CNS-resident macrophages after transient middle cerebral artery occlusion. *J Cereb Blood Flow Metab,* (n.d.), pp., ISSN 1559-7016 (Electronic)

Hoehn, M., Kustermann, E., Blunk, J., Wiedermann, D., Trapp, T., Wecker, S., Focking, M., Arnold, H., Hescheler, J., Fleischmann, B. K., Schwindt, W., & Buhrle, C. (2002). Monitoring of implanted stem cell migration in vivo: a highly resolved in vivo magnetic resonance imaging investigation of experimental stroke in rat. *Proc Natl Acad Sci U S A,* Vol.99, No.25, (n.d.), pp. 16267-16272, ISSN 0027-8424 (Print) 0027-8424 (Linking)

Iadecola, C., & Alexander, M. (2001). Cerebral ischemia and inflammation. *Curr Opin Neurol,* Vol.14, No.1, (n.d.), pp. 89-94, ISSN 1350-7540 (Print)

Jiang, Q., Zhang, Z. G., Ding, G. L., Zhang, L., Ewing, J. R., Wang, L., Zhang, R., Li, L., Lu, M., Meng, H., Arbab, A. S., Hu, J., Li, Q. J., Pourabdollah Nejad, D. S., Athiraman, H., & Chopp, M. (2005). Investigation of neural progenitor cell induced angiogenesis after embolic stroke in rat using MRI. *Neuroimage,* Vol.28, No.3, (n.d.), pp. 698-707, ISSN 1053-8119 (Print) 1053-8119 (Linking)

Justicia, C., Ramos-Cabrer, P., & Hoehn, M. (2008). MRI detection of secondary damage after stroke: chronic iron accumulation in the thalamus of the rat brain. *Stroke,* Vol.39, No.5, (n.d.), pp. 1541-1547, ISSN 1524-4628 (Electronic)

Kim, J., Kim, D. I., Lee, S. K., Kim, D. J., Lee, J. E., & Ahn, S. K. (2008). Imaging of the inflammatory response in reperfusion injury after transient cerebral ischemia in rats: correlation of superparamagnetic iron oxide-enhanced magnetic resonance imaging with histopathology. *Acta Radiol,* Vol.49, No.5, (n.d.), pp. 580-588, ISSN 1600-0455 (Electronic)

Kleinschnitz, C., Bendszus, M., Frank, M., Solymosi, L., Toyka, K. V., & Stoll, G. (2003). In vivo monitoring of macrophage infiltration in experimental ischemic brain lesions by magnetic resonance imaging. *J Cereb Blood Flow Metab,* Vol.23, No.11, (n.d.), pp. 1356-1361, ISSN 0271-678X (Print) 0271-678X (Linking)

Kleinschnitz, C., Schutz, A., Nolte, I., Horn, T., Frank, M., Solymosi, L., Stoll, G., & Bendszus, M. (2005). In vivo detection of developing vessel occlusion in photothrombotic ischemic brain lesions in the rat by iron particle enhanced MRI. *J Cereb Blood Flow Metab,* Vol.25, No.11, (n.d.), pp. 1548-1555, ISSN 0271-678X (Print) 0271-678X (Linking)

Lee, E. S., Chan, J., Shuter, B., Tan, L. G., Chong, M. S., Ramachandra, D. L., Dawe, G. S., Ding, J., Teoh, S. H., Beuf, O., Briguet, A., Chiu Tam, K., Choolani, M., & Wang, S. C. (2009). Microgel Iron Oxide Nanoparticles for Tracking Human Fetal Mesenchymal Stem Cells Through Magnetic Resonance Imaging. *Stem Cells,* Vol.27, No.8, (n.d.), pp. 1921-1931, ISSN 1549-4918 (Electronic)

Mani, V., Adler, E., Briley-Saebo, K. C., Bystrup, A., Fuster, V., Keller, G., & Fayad, Z. A. (2008). Serial in vivo positive contrast MRI of iron oxide-labeled embryonic stem cell-derived cardiac precursor cells in a mouse model of myocardial infarction. *Magn Reson Med,* Vol.60, No.1, (n.d.), pp. 73-81, ISSN 0740-3194 (Print)

Modo, M., Mellodew, K., Cash, D., Fraser, S. E., Meade, T. J., Price, J., & Williams, S. C. (2004). Mapping transplanted stem cell migration after a stroke: a serial, in vivo magnetic resonance imaging study. *Neuroimage,* Vol.21, No.1, (n.d.), pp. 311-317, ISSN 1053-8119 (Print) 1053-8119 (Linking)

Nighoghossian, N., Wiart, M., Cakmak, S., Berthezene, Y., Derex, L., Cho, T. H., Nemoz, C., Chapuis, F., Tisserand, G. L., Pialat, J. B., Trouillas, P., Froment, J. C., & Hermier, M. (2007). Inflammatory response after ischemic stroke: a USPIO-enhanced MRI study in patients. *Stroke,* Vol.38, No.2, (n.d.), pp. 303-307, ISSN 1524-4628 (Electronic) 0039-2499 (Linking)

Papadopoulos, V., Baraldi, M., Guilarte, T. R., Knudsen, T. B., Lacapere, J. J., Lindemann, P., Norenberg, M. D., Nutt, D., Weizman, A., Zhang, M. R., & Gavish, M. (2006). Translocator protein (18kDa): new nomenclature for the peripheral-type benzodiazepine receptor based on its structure and molecular function. *Trends Pharmacol Sci,* Vol.27, No.8, (n.d.), pp. 402-409, ISSN 0165-6147 (Print) 0165-6147 (Linking)

Pappata, S., Levasseur, M., Gunn, R. N., Myers, R., Crouzel, C., Syrota, A., Jones, T., Kreutzberg, G. W., & Banati, R. B. (2000). Thalamic microglial activation in ischemic stroke detected in vivo by PET and [11C]PK1195. *Neurology,* Vol.55, No.7, (n.d.), pp. 1052-1054, ISSN 0028-3878 (Print) 0028-3878 (Linking)

Pendlebury, S. T., & Rothwell, P. M. (2009). Prevalence, incidence, and factors associated with pre-stroke and post-stroke dementia: a systematic review and meta-analysis. *Lancet Neurol,* Vol.8, No.11, (n.d.), pp. 1006-1018, ISSN 1474-4465 (Electronic) 1474-4422 (Linking)

Priller, J., Flugel, A., Wehner, T., Boentert, M., Haas, C. A., Prinz, M., Fernandez-Klett, F., Prass, K., Bechmann, I., de Boer, B. A., Frotscher, M., Kreutzberg, G. W., Persons, D. A., & Dirnagl, U. (2001). Targeting gene-modified hematopoietic cells to the central nervous system: use of green fluorescent protein uncovers microglial engraftment. *Nat Med,* Vol.7, No.12, (n.d.), pp. 1356-1361, ISSN 1078-8956 (Print)

Raivich, G., Bohatschek, M., Kloss, C. U., Werner, A., Jones, L. L., & Kreutzberg, G. W. (1999). Neuroglial activation repertoire in the injured brain: graded response, molecular mechanisms and cues to physiological function. *Brain Res Brain Res Rev,* Vol.30, No.1, (n.d.), pp. 77-105

Rausch, M., Baumann, D., Neubacher, U., & Rudin, M. (2002). In-vivo visualization of phagocytotic cells in rat brains after transient ischemia by USPIO. *NMR Biomed,* Vol.15, No.4, (n.d.), pp. 278-283, ISSN 0952-3480 (Print) 0952-3480 (Linking)

Rausch, M., Sauter, A., Frohlich, J., Neubacher, U., Radu, E. W., & Rudin, M. (2001). Dynamic patterns of USPIO enhancement can be observed in macrophages after ischemic brain damage. *Magn Reson Med,* Vol.46, No.5, (n.d.), pp. 1018-1022, ISSN 0740-3194 (Print) 0740-3194 (Linking)

Rice, H. E., Hsu, E. W., Sheng, H., Evenson, D. A., Freemerman, A. J., Safford, K. M., Provenzale, J. M., Warner, D. S., & Johnson, G. A. (2007). Superparamagnetic iron oxide labeling and transplantation of adipose-derived stem cells in middle cerebral artery occlusion-injured mice. *AJR Am J Roentgenol,* Vol.188, No.4, (n.d.), pp. 1101-1108, ISSN 1546-3141 (Electronic)

Rothwell, P. M., Algra, A., & Amarenco, P. (2011). Medical treatment in acute and long-term secondary prevention after transient ischaemic attack and ischaemic stroke. *Lancet,* Vol.377, No.9778, (n.d.), pp. 1681-1692, ISSN 1474-547X (Electronic) 0140-6736 (Linking)

Saleh, A., Schroeter, M., Jonkmanns, C., Hartung, H. P., Modder, U., & Jander, S. (2004a). In vivo MRI of brain inflammation in human ischaemic stroke. *Brain,* Vol.127, No.Pt 7, (n.d.), pp. 1670-1677, ISSN 0006-8950 (Print) 0006-8950 (Linking)

Saleh, A., Schroeter, M., Ringelstein, A., Hartung, H. P., Siebler, M., Modder, U., & Jander, S. (2007). Iron oxide particle-enhanced MRI suggests variability of brain inflammation at early stages after ischemic stroke. *Stroke,* Vol.38, No.10, (n.d.), pp. 2733-2737, ISSN 1524-4628 (Electronic)

Saleh, A., Wiedermann, D., Schroeter, M., Jonkmanns, C., Jander, S., & Hoehn, M. (2004b). Central nervous system inflammatory response after cerebral infarction as detected by magnetic resonance imaging. *NMR Biomed,* Vol.17, No.4, (n.d.), pp. 163-169, ISSN 0952-3480 (Print)

Savitz, S. I., & Fisher, M. (2007). Future of neuroprotection for acute stroke: in the aftermath of the SAINT trials. *Ann Neurol,* Vol.61, No.5, (n.d.), pp. 396-402, ISSN 0364-5134 (Print)

Schroeter, M., Franke, C., Stoll, G., & Hoehn, M. (2001). Dynamic changes of magnetic resonance imaging abnormalities in relation to inflammation and glial responses after photothrombotic cerebral infarction in the rat brain. *Acta Neuropathol,* Vol.101, No.2, (n.d.), pp. 114-122, ISSN 0001-6322 (Print)

Schroeter, M., Jander, S., Witte, O. W., & Stoll, G. (1999). Heterogeneity of the microglial response in photochemically induced focal ischemia of the rat cerebral cortex. *Neuroscience,* Vol.89, No.4, (n.d.), pp. 1367-1377, ISSN 0306-4522 (Print) 0306-4522 (Linking)

Schroeter, M., Saleh, A., Wiedermann, D., Hoehn, M., & Jander, S. (2004). Histochemical detection of ultrasmall superparamagnetic iron oxide (USPIO) contrast medium uptake in experimental brain ischemia. *Magn Reson Med,* Vol.52, No.2, (n.d.), pp. 403-406, ISSN 0740-3194 (Print)

Simon, G. H., Raatschen, H. J., Wendland, M. F., von Vopelius-Feldt, J., Fu, Y., Chen, M. H., & Daldrup-Link, H. E. (2005). Ultrasmall superparamagnetic iron-oxide-enhanced MR imaging of normal bone marrow in rodents: original research original research. *Acad Radiol,* Vol.12, No.9, (n.d.), pp. 1190-1197, ISSN 1076-6332 (Print)

Stroh, A., Zimmer, C., Werner, N., Gertz, K., Weir, K., Kronenberg, G., Steinbrink, J., Mueller, S., Sieland, K., Dirnagl, U., Nickenig, G., & Endres, M. (2006). Tracking of systemically administered mononuclear cells in the ischemic brain by high-field magnetic resonance imaging. *Neuroimage,* Vol.33, No.3, (n.d.), pp. 886-897, ISSN 1053-8119 (Print) 1053-8119 (Linking)

Venneti, S., Lopresti, B. J., & Wiley, C. A. (2006). The peripheral benzodiazepine receptor (Translocator protein 18kDa) in microglia: from pathology to imaging. *Prog Neurobiol,* Vol.80, No.6, (n.d.), pp. 308-322, ISSN 0301-0082 (Print) 0301-0082 (Linking)

Walczak, P., Zhang, J., Gilad, A. A., Kedziorek, D. A., Ruiz-Cabello, J., Young, R. G., Pittenger, M. F., van Zijl, P. C., Huang, J., & Bulte, J. W. (2008). Dual-Modality Monitoring of Targeted Intraarterial Delivery of Mesenchymal Stem Cells After Transient Ischemia. *Stroke,* Vol.39, No.5, (n.d.), pp. 1569-1574, ISSN 1524-4628 (Electronic) 0039-2499 (Linking)

Weber, R., Wegener, S., Ramos-Cabrer, P., Wiedermann, D., & Hoehn, M. (2005). MRI detection of macrophage activity after experimental stroke in rats: new indicators for late appearance of vascular degradation? *Magn Reson Med,* Vol.54, No.1, (n.d.), pp. 59-66, ISSN 0740-3194 (Print)

Wiart, M., Davoust, N., Pialat, J. B., Desestret, V., Moucharaffie, S., Cho, T. H., Mutin, M., Langlois, J. B., Beuf, O., Honnorat, J., Nighoghossian, N., & Berthezene, Y. (2007). MRI monitoring of neuroinflammation in mouse focal ischemia. *Stroke,* Vol.38, No.1, (n.d.), pp. 131-137, ISSN 1524-4628 (Electronic) 0039-2499 (Linking)

Yach, D., Hawkes, C., Gould, C. L., & Hofman, K. J. (2004). The global burden of chronic diseases: overcoming impediments to prevention and control. *JAMA,* Vol.291, No.21, (n.d.), pp. 2616-2622, ISSN 1538-3598 (Electronic)

Zhang, Z. G., Jiang, Q., Zhang, R., Zhang, L., Wang, L., Arniego, P., Ho, K. L., & Chopp, M. (2003). Magnetic resonance imaging and neurosphere therapy of stroke in rat. *Ann Neurol,* Vol.53, No.2, (n.d.), pp. 259-263, ISSN 0364-5134 (Print) 0364-5134 (Linking)

15

Intracerebral Hemorrhage: Influence of Topography of Bleeding on Clinical Spectrum and Early Outcome

Adrià Arboix[1] and Elisenda Grivé[2]
[1]*Cerebrovascular Division, Department of Neurology, Hospital Universitari del Sagrat Cor, Universitat de Barcelona, Barcelona,*
[2]*Servei de Neuroradiologia, CRC, Hospital Universitari del Sagrat Cor, Barcelona, Spain*

1. Introduction

Approximately 10-20% of strokes are due to intracerebral hemorrhage (ICH) [1]. Hospital admissions for ICH have increased by 18% in the past 10 years. ICH is a medical emergency. Rapid diagnosis and attentive management of patients with ICH is crucial because hematoma expansion and early deterioration is common in the first few hours after ICH onset. The clinical spectrum and outcome of a patient with ICH is directly related to the site of bleeding. The prognosis and treatment of ICH often depends on the areas affected by the hemorrhage [3-5]. Particular locations, such as the cerebral lobes, right putamen and cerebellum are relatively accesible to surgical drainage, whereas other areas, such as the thalamus and the brainstem are inaccesible [6].

It is very difficult to determine whether the presenting neurological symptoms are due to cerebral ischemia or ICH based on the clinical characteristics alone. Vomiting, elevated systolic blood pressure (SBP) (>220 mmHg), severe headache, coma or decreased level of consciousness, and progression of neurological deficit over minutes or hours are suggestive of ICH, although none of these features are specific and, therefore, neuroimaging examination is mandatory. Neuroimaging data, particularly computed tomography (CT) is needed to rule out stroke mimics, to confirm the clinical diagnosis, and to distinguish ischemia from ICH [4,5].

The influence of the site of bleeding on the clinical spectrum and outcome in patients with ICH is still a poorly defined aspect of the disease. Factors associated with outcome in ICH have been evaluated in many studies but the findings are of limited utility because they have tipically considered broad groups of patients with different etiologies or have otherwise employed univariate rather than factorial techniques for the analysis of data. Moreover, prognostic variables related to morbidity and mortality are of great importance but remain difficult to establish clearly because of methodological problems, including sample selection bias, timing of initial assessment, criteria for measuring outcome, and the role of other confounding factors. Although community-based studies and prospective stroke registries have provided data on the identification of prognostic factors in ICH patients, there is a scarcity of information on the differences across the clinical spectrum and outcome of hemorrhagic stroke according to the site of bleeding [5-8].

The aim of this chapter is to determine the influence of topography of hemorrhage on the clinical spectrum, in-hospital mortality, and early outcome in ICH patients according to data collected from a review of the literature and the authors' experience based on a large hospital-based stroke registry (Sagrat Cor Hospital of Barcelona Stroke Registry) in Barcelona, Spain.

In relation to the site of bleeding, seven topographies were analyzed. These included the thalamus, internal capsule and basal ganglia, cerebral lobes, cerebellum, brainstem, multiple topographic involvement (when more then one of these areas was affected), and primary intraventricular hematoma. Secondary intraventricular blood expansion (evidence of intraventricular blood on CT and/or magnetic resonance imaging [MRI] scans) for each topography was also assessed.

In relation to localization of the hemorrhage in the Sagrat Cor Hospital of Barcelona Stroke Registry (Table 1), lobar ICH was the most frequent (33.2%) followed by hemorrhages in the

Anatomic localization	No. patients (%)
Lobar	76 (33.2)
Frontal	8
Parietal	23
Temporal	14
Occipital	13
Frontoparietal	3
Temporoparietal	6
Temporo-occipital	6
Parieto-occipital	2
Frontoparietotemporal	1
Thalamus	31 (13.5)
Cerebellum	15 (6.6)
Brainstem	15 (6.6)
Mesencephalon	2
Pons	6
Medulla oblongata	1
Pons and mesencephalon	6
Internal capsule	7 (3.0)
Basal ganglia	24 (10.5)
Internal capsule and basal ganglia	18 (7.9)
Multiple topographic involvement	34 (14.8)
Thalamus, internal capsule/basal ganglia	18
Lobar, internal capsule/basal ganglia	10
Lobar, internal capsule/basal ganglia, thalamus	5
Brainstem, basal ganglia	1
Primary intraventricular hemorrhage	9 (3.9)

Table 1. Site of bleeding in 229 patients with hemorrhagic stroke in the Sagrat Cor Hospital of Barcelona Stroke Registry

thalamus (13.5%), basal ganglia (10.5%), internal capsule and basal ganglia (7.9%), cerebellum (6.6%), and brainstem (6.6%). Multiple topographic involvement was found in 14.8% of the patients and primary intraventricular hemorrhage in 3.9%. In these series of 229 consecutive cases, the main cause of ICH was hypertension in 124 patients, arteriovenous malformations in 11, hematologic disorders in 9, and other causes in 12. In 73 patients, the cause of bleeding was not identified [5].

MRI and CT with angiographic studies (where relevant), MR angiography (MRA), MR venography or CT angiography (CTA), are reasonably sensitive at identifying secondary causes of hemorrhage, including arteriovenous malformations, aneurysms, cavernous malformations, tumors, moyamoya, vasculitis and dural venous thrombosis. Digital subtraction angiography (DSA) may be considered if clinical suspicion is high but noninvasive studies do not show a clear cause particularly in young, normotensive and surgical candidates. DSA remains the gold standard for the evaluation of vascular anomalies and allows endovascular treatment, however the use of non-invasive MRA or CTA may help to exclude unnecessary invasive DSA [6].

Risk factors and clinical variables associated with different topographic locations are shown in Tables 2 and 3. Sensory deficit was significantly associated with thalamic ICH; lacunar syndrome and hypertension with internal capsule/basal ganglia ICH; seizures and non-sudden stroke onset with lobar ICH; ataxia with hemorrhage in the cerebellum; cranial nerve palsy with brainstem ICH; and limb weakness, diabetes, and altered consciousness with multiple topographic involvement. On the other hand, hypertension and sensory deficit were inversely associated with lobar and cerebellar ICH, respectively.

The in-hospital mortality rate was 30.6% (n = 70). Causes of death included cerebral herniation in 44 patients, pneumonia in 8, sepsis in 8, sudden death in 3, myocardial infarction in 1, pulmonary thromboembolism in 1, and unknown cause in 5.

Mortality at 3 months was 34% in a review of 586 patients with ICH from 30 centers. In other studies it was 31% at 7 days, 59% at 1 year, 82% at 10 years and more than 90% at 16 years [5].

According to the different sites of bleeding, in-hospital mortality rates were 16.3% in internal capsule/basal ganglia ICH, 20% in cerebellar ICH, 25% in lobar ICH, 25.8% in thalamic ICH, 40% in brainstem ICH, 44.4% in primary intraventricular hemorrhage, and 64.7% in multiple topographic involvement. Intraventricular extension of the hemorrhage was associated with a significantly higher in-hospital mortality rate in all ICH topographies except for lobar hemorrhage (presence of intraventricular hemorrhage *vs.* absence 41.1 *vs.* 0%, in thalamic ICH; 50 *vs.* 9.8%, in internal capsule/basal ganglia ICH; 66.7 *vs.* 8.3%, in cerebellar ICH; 100 *vs.* 25%, in brainstem ICH; and 87.5 *vs.* 44.4%, in multiple topographic involvement). Survivors were significantly younger than patients who died (mean age 69.07 [12.75] *vs.* 73.94 [10.32] years), for whom the overall mean survival time was 15 (23) days [5].

2. Internal capsule/basal ganglia

The commonest location of hypertensive ICH is the lateral basal-ganglionic-capsular region (classical deep subcortical intracerebral hemorrhages) [9,10]. Patients with small hematomas in this topography have a good outcome. Small hematomas of subcortical topography in the internal capsule, but also in the basal ganglia and more infrequently in the pons, may cause a lacunar syndrome [11]. In a clinical series hypertension and lacunar syndrome were significantly associated with internal capsule/basal ganglia ICH (Table 4). The selection of

Variable	Thalamus (n=31) *vs* remaining ICH	Internal capsule basal ganglia (n= 49) *vs.* remaining ICH	Lobar (n=76) *vs.* remaining ICH	Cerebellum (n=15) vs. remaining ICH	Brainstem (n=15) *vs.* remaining ICH	Multiple sites (n=34) *vs.* remaining ICH	Intrave-ntricular (n=9) *vs.* Remaining ICH
Hypertension		77.6 *vs.* 55.5%*	42.1 *vs.* 69.9†				
Diabetes						35.3 *vs.* 11.8†	
Heart valve disease							22.2 *vs.* 0.5‡
Atrial dysrhythmia							44.4 *vs.* 9.5*
Previous cerebral hemorrhage			6.0 *vs.* 1.3§				
Anticoagulant treatment							22.2 *vs.* 0.5§
Suddent onset			57.9 *vs.* 73.8§				
Non-sudden onset			38.1 *vs.* 23.5§				
Dizziness				60.0 *vs.* 5.6‡			
Seizures		4.1 *vs.* 5.0§	11.8 *vs.* 1.3§				
Nausea, vomiting				66.7 *vs.* 20.6†			
Altered consciousness						76.5 *vs.* 40.5‡	
Limb weakness				40.0 *vs.* 79.9†		97.1 *vs.* 73.8¶	
Sensory deficit	72.4 *vs.* 46.4*			6.7 *vs.* 53.7†		73.5 *vs.* 46.1**	
Ataxia		0 *vs.* 11.1§		86.7 *vs.* 3.7‡			
Cranial nerve palsy			0 vs. 13.1††		66.7 *vs.* 4.7†		
Lacunar syndrome		18.4 vs. 4.4‡‡					

Data expressed as percentages; **P* < 0.2; †*P* < 0.01; ‡*P* < 0.001; §*P* < 0.3; ¶*P* < 0.07; ***P* < 0.08; ††*P* < 0.05; ‡‡*P* < 0.06.

Table 2. Frequency of vascular risk factors and clinical features according to site of bleeding in 229 patients with intracerebral hemorrhage (ICH) in the Sagrat Cor Hospital of Barcelona Stroke Registry

Bleeding topography	β	SE (β)	Odds ratio (95% CI)
Thalamus			
Sensory deficit	1.1729	0.4365	3.23 (1.37 to 7.60)
Internal capsule/basal ganglia			
Lacunar syndrome	1.3373	0.5346	3.81 (1.33 to 10.86)
Hypertension	0.8065	0.3855	2.24 (1.05 to 4.77)
Lobar			
Seizures	2.4178	0.8278	11.22 (2.21 to 56.84)
Non-sudden stroke onset	0.8045	0.3344	2.24 (1.16 to 4.31)
Hypertension	–1.0669	0.3091	0.34 (0.19 to 0.63)
Cerebellum			
Ataxia	5.7560	1.1653	316.09 (32.2 to 3102.63)
Sensory deficit	–4.0215	1.5093	0.02 (0.009 to 0.35)
Brainstem			
Cranial nerve palsy	3.7108	0.6393	40.89 (11.67 to 143.15)
Sensory deficit	–4.0215	1.5093	0.02 (0.009 to 0.35)
Multiple topography			
Limb weakness	2.3628	1.0662	10.62 (1.31 to 85.84)
Diabetes mellitus	1.5992	0.5099	4.95 (1.82 to 13.44)
Altered consciousness	1.3950	0.4631	4.03 (1.63 to 10.0)

Table 3. Predictive value of different risk factors and clinical variables on the site of bleeding in the Sagrat Cor Hospital of Barcelona Stroke Registry

hypertension may be explained because blood supply of the putamen is derived predominantly from penetrating branches of the middle cerebral artery, which are the arterioles most frequently affected by hypertension [9,12]. This finding is consistent with other studies showing that the lateral ganglionic region is the most common topography of deep hypertensive ICH, and that a great proportion of hematomas found in the putaminal region are hypertensive [3,12] (Figures 1 and 2).

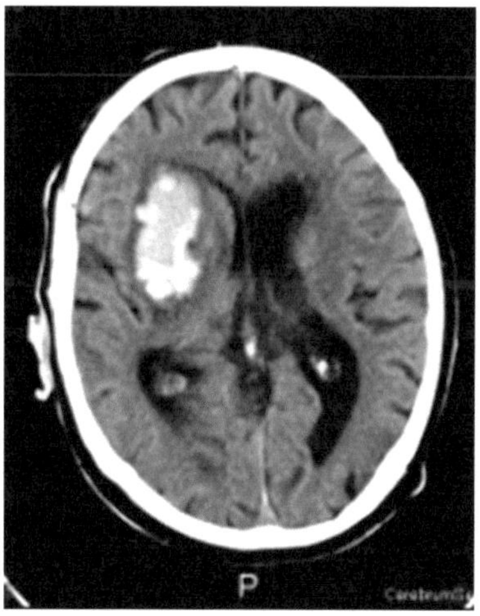

Fig. 1. Axial CT shows acute hypertensive putaminal hematoma with early peripheral edema.

Hemorrhage in the caudate nucleus accounts for approximately 7% of ICH. The symptoms and signs in caudate hemorrhage closely mimic SAH but the CT appearance of blood in the caudate and lateral ventricles is distinctive. Larger hemorrhages are more likely to rupture into the ventricle and have a much higher mortality than do small putaminal hematomas [4,12].

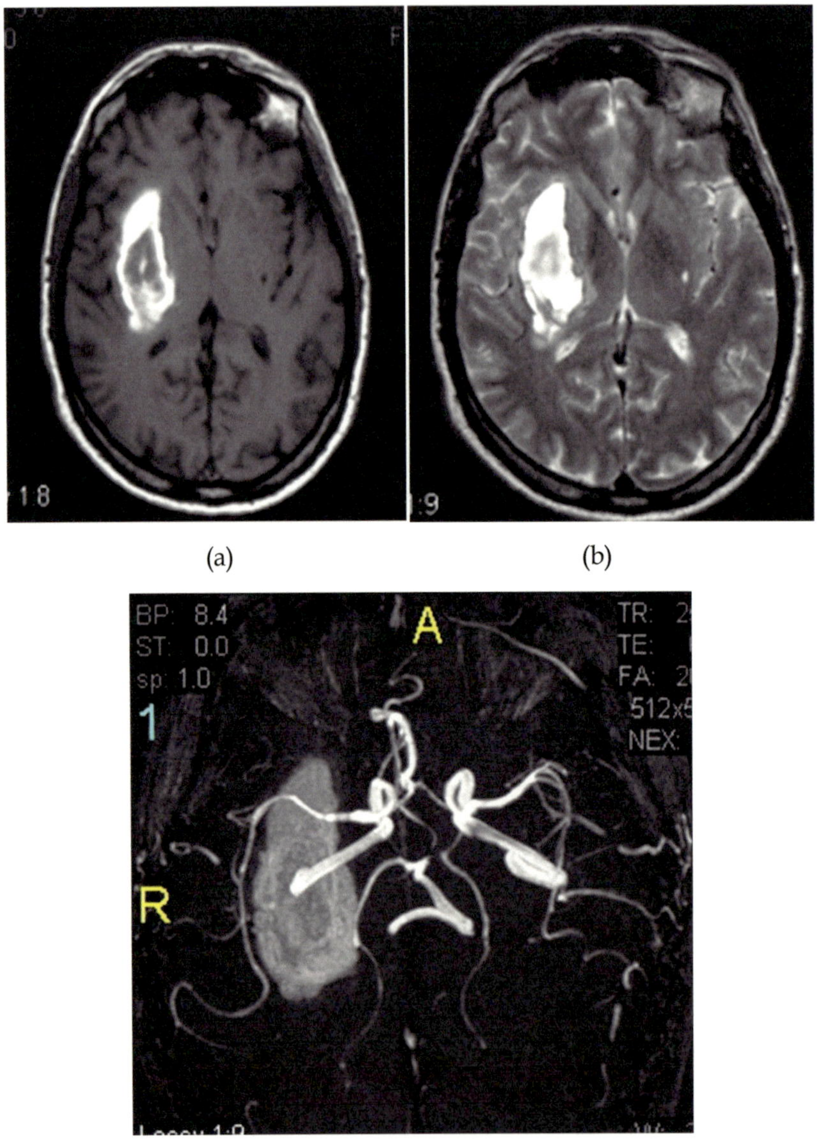

(a) (b)

(c)

Fig. 2. Subacute intraparenchymatous hematoma in the right basal ganglia/external capsule. A) Axial T1WI MR showing peripheral hyperintensity and central isointensity related to different ICH temporal staging. Signal changes first occur peripherally and progress centrally; B) Axial T2WI MR; C) Axial MRA (3D TOF) MIP image shows no vascular malformation.

Variable	Lobar hemorrhage	Deep subcortical hemorrhage	*P* value
Demographic data			
Male sex	44 (45.4)	59 (64.1)	0.007
Age, years, mean (SD)	70.3 (14.3)	71.8 (10.9)	0.414
Vascular risk factors			
Hypertension	41 (42.3)	64 (69.6)	0.001
Diabetes mellitus	10 (10.3)	13 (14.1)	0.281
Ischemic heart disease	6 (6.2)	6 (6.5)	0.579
Atrial fibrillation	10 (10.3)	11 (12)	0.448
Valvular heart disease	5 (5.2)	1 (1.1)	0.118
Congestive heart failure	3 (3.1)	2 (2.2)	0.525
Previous transient ischemic attack	7 (7.2)	3 (3.3)	0.188
Previous cerebral infarction	8 (8.2)	9 (9.8)	0.454
Previous intracerebral hemorrhage	8 (8.2)	1 (1.1)	0.021
Chronic obstructive pulmonary disease	6 (6.2)	5 (5.4)	0.537
Chronic renal disease		2 (2.2)	0.236
Chronic liver disease	8 (8.2)	2 (2.2)	0.060
Obesity	1 (1)	7 (7.6)	0.027
Alcohol consumption (> 80 g/day)	3 (3.1)	6 (6.5)	0.444
Smoking (> 20 cigarettes/day)	11 (11.3)	8 (8.7)	0.360
Hyperlipidemia	9 (9.3)	13 (14.1)	0.208
Anticoagulant treatment	4 (4.1)	2 (2.2)	0.367
Peripheral vascular disease	2 (2.1)	6 (6.5)	0.123
Clinical features			
Suden onset (min)	59 (60.8)	65 (70.7)	0.102
Acute onset (hours)	28 (28.9)	20 (21.7)	0.169
Headache	45 (46.4)	27 (29.3)	0.012
Seizures	11 (11.3)	2 (2.2)	0.012
Nausea, vomiting	18 (18.6)	17 (18.5)	0.569
Decreased consciousness	44 (45.4)	31 (37.5)	0.068
Motor deficit	66 (68)	77 (83.7)	0.009
Sensory deficit	36 (37.1)	55 (59.8)	0.001
Homonymous hemianopsia	31 (32)	19 (20.7)	0.055
Aplasia, dysarthria	35 (36.1)	32 (34.8)	0.486
Ataxia	3 (3.1)	3 (3.3)	0.633
Absence of neurological deficit at discharge	6 (6.2)	5 (5.4)	0.537
In-hospital mortality	26 (26.8)	18 (19.6)	0.158
Respiratory complications	7 (7.2)	10 (10.9)	0.267
Urinary complications	13 (13.4)	15 (16.3)	0.361
Infectious complications	15 (15.5)	24 (26.1)	0.052
Length of hospital stay, median (IQR)	17 (18)	20 (16)	0.383

Table 4. Comparison between 97 patients with lobar hemorrhage and 92 patients with deep subcortical bleeding

3. Thalamic hemorrhage

Thalamic hematomas (Figures 3 and 4) is a subgroup of hemorrhagic stroke that accounted for 1.4% of all cases of stroke and 13% of intracerebral hemorrhages, a percentage in the range between 6% and 25.6% in the series of other authors [3,7,13].

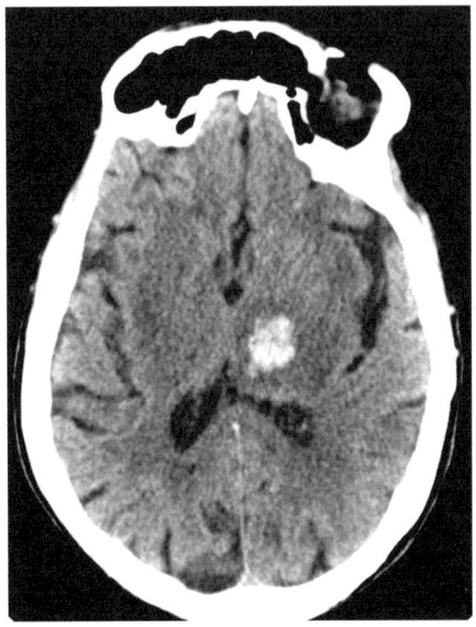

Fig. 3. Axial CT reveals an acute anterior left thalamic hematoma.

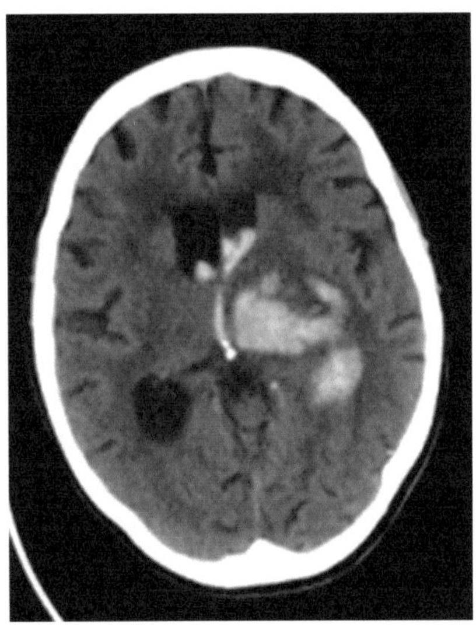

Fig. 4. Axial CT shows a large thalamic hematoma with intraventricular rupture.

Sensory deficit was significantly associated with thalamic ICH [4,5]. It has been shown that 74.2% of patients with hemorrhage in the thalamus showed sensory deficit, which coincide in part with early observations emphasizing that the predominance of sensory deficit over motor is one cardinal feature of thalamic ICH [4]. Sometimes the contralateral limbs are ataxic or have choreic movements. The commonest oculomotor abnormalities include paralysis of upward gaze, often with one or both eyes resting downward, and hyperconvergence of one or both eyes. These ocular abnormalities are due to direct extension of the hematoma to the diencephalic-mesencephalic junction or to compression of the quadrigeminal plate region.

The topography of thalamic lesion [14] was anterior in 6% of cases (behavioral abnormalities predominate), posteromedial in 24% (abnormalities of consciousness, papillary function and vertical gaze predominate), posterolateral in 48% (sensorimotor signs predominate), dorsal in 2% (slights sensorimotor signs usually transients and aphasia and behavioral are common) and affected all thalamic vascular territories in 20%. Intraventricular involvement was present in 42.6% of patients.

Thalamic hemorrhage is a severe clinical condition with in-hospital mortality rate of 19%, and symptom-free at discharge from the hospital documented in only 2.1% [15]. The mortality rate of thalamic hemorrhage ranges between 17% and 52% in the experience of different authors [14,16]. On the other hand, the mortality rate of thalamic hemorrhage is generally lower than that of brainstem hemorrhages or cerebral hemorrhages of multiple topographies, which show a very high in-hospital mortality rate usually greater than 40% [5]. The mortality rate in patients with thalamic hemorrhage, however, is higher than that of patient with capsular stroke [5,17]. Altered consciousness, intraventricular hemorrhage and age have been shown to be independent predictors of in-hospital mortality in patients with thalamic hematoma [15,17]. In summary, approximately one of each 10 patients with acute intracerebral hemorrhage had a thalamic hematoma. Patients with thalamic hemorrhage show a differential clinical profile than patients with internal capsule-basal ganglia ICH. Altered consciousness, intraventricular involvement and advanced age have been found to be independent predictors of in-hospital mortality.

4. Lobar hemorrhage

The frequency of lobar hemorrhage varies between 24% to 49% in the different clinical series reported in the literature [1,5,18]. In our experience, lobar bleeding was the most common ICH (33% of cases) [18]. The symptoms and signs in lobar hemorrhages are similar to cerebral infarctions. Seizures, non-sudden stroke onset, and hypertension were independent clinical factors related to the site of bleeding. Seizures occurred more frequently in lobar ICH than in the remaining ICH. Other studies have shown that seizures are more frequent in hemorrhagic than in ischemic stroke as well as more frequent in lobar than in deep hematomas mainly in the parietal and temporal lobes [19,20]. On the other hand, it has been generally considered that bleeding in ICH lasts only a few minutes. However, recent data show that substantial early hemorrhage growth in patients with ICH is common [21]. Explanation of the gradual onset of symptoms found in 38% of our patients with lobar ICH, suggests that the period of hematoma enlargement can extend for a number of hours from onset as a result of active bleeding, a phenomenon that is frequently but not always associated with clinical deterioration [4]. Lobar ICH was less commonly associated with hypertension than any of the remaining topographies. For this reason, non-hypertensive mechanisms of ICH including cerebral amyloid angiopathy (Figure 5), vascular malformations, sympathomimetic drugs, and bleeding disorders all have a tendency to cause predominantly subcortical lobar ICH with a lower frequency of deep hemispheric and brainstem hemorrhages [6,19].

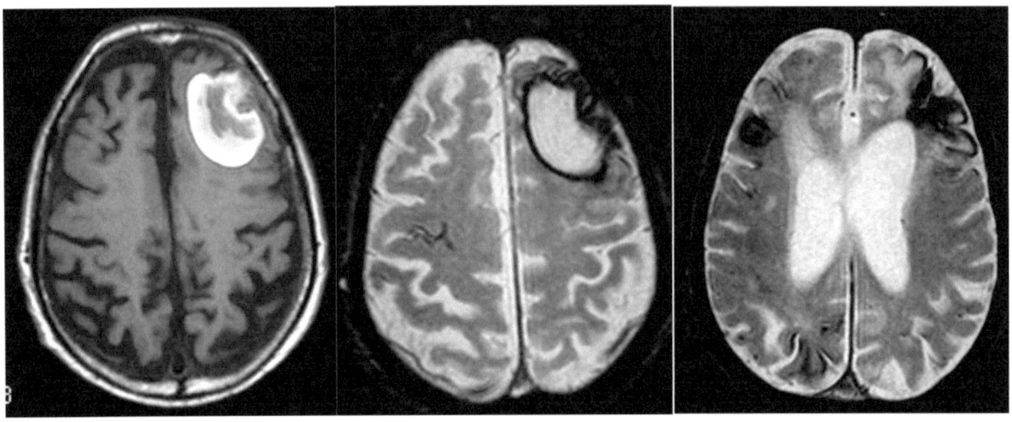

Fig. 5. Lobar hemorrhage related to cerebral amyloid angiopathy. A) Axial T1WI MR shows subacute lobar hematoma in the left frontal lobe; in B) and C) axial T2*GRE MR, apart from the subacute lobar hematoma, superficial hemosiderosis, scattered microbleeds and a chronic right frontal cortical hematoma are shown.

In the comparative analysis between lobar hemorrhages and deep subcortical hemorrhages (Table 4), lobar hemorrhages were more common in women, in patients with previous ICH as well in those presenting with headache and seizures. In contrast, deep subcortical hemorrhages occurred more frequently in obese patients and were associated with motor and sensory deficits.

Lobar ICH is a severe disease, with in-hospital mortality (26.8%) and absence of neurological deficit at the time of hospital discharge being observed occasionally (6.2%). Lobar ICH may be considered a more benign condition as compared with brainstem hemorrhages or mutiple topographic location [5,10] in which in-hospital mortality may be as high as 40%, but is more severe than capsular hemorrhages, which may even present as a lacunar syndrome, mainly pure motor hemiparesis or sensorimotor syndrome [11].

The lower frequency of hypertension in lobar ICH (42.3% *vs.* 69.6% in subcortical ICH) is a relevant clinical aspect that coincides with datas reported in the literature [6], because high blood pressure has the lowest frequency as compared with other topographies of bleeding. However, other causes different from hypertension, such as arteriovenous malformations (8.5%), blood dyscrasias (5.5%) or anticoagulant iatrogenia (3%) are more common in lobar ICH. Because of the higher incidence of vascular malformations and other bleeding lesions in patients with lobar hematomas angiography is often indicated [6]. For patients presenting with lobar clots > 30 mL and with 1 cm of the surface, evacuation of supratentorial ICH by standard craniotomy might be considered [6].

In our experience of the Sagrat Cor of Barcelona Stroke Registry, chronic obstructive pulmonary disease (COPD), altered consciousness, previous cerebral infarction, chronic liver disease, female sex, seizures and headache were clinical variables independently associated with in-hospital mortality in the logistic regression analyses.

5. Cerebellar hemorrhage

This subgroup of hemorrhagic stroke account for 0.73% of total stroke and 6.9% of ICH, a percentage similar to 5–10% reported in the literature [4,9].

Establishing the diagnosis of cerebellar hemorrhage is important because of the potentially serious outcome if not treated and the contrasting good prognosis after surgical treatment. Cerebellar hemorrhage usually originates in the region of the dentate nucleus, arising from distal branches of the superior cerebellar artery and the posterior inferior cerebellar artery (Figure 6). Characteristic presenting symptoms of cerebellar ICH include headache, vertigo, vomiting, and inability to stand and walk. Ataxia is an independent clinical factor associated with cerebellar ICH. In our experience, ataxia was found in 87% of patients and this finding agrees with the high frequency of cerebellar signs including gait ataxia, truncal ataxia, and ipsilateral limb ataxia reported by others [4,9].

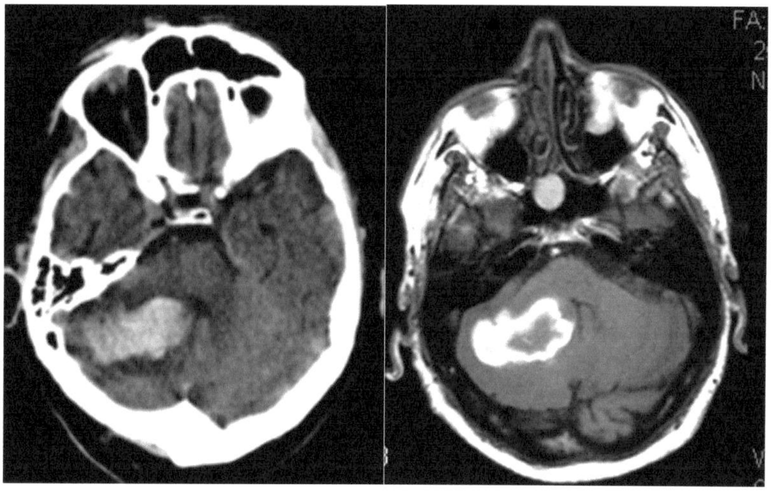

(a) (b)

Fig. 6. Right cerebellar hematoma in the region of the dentate nucleus. A) Axial CT shows acute hematoma with halo of surrounding edema; B) axial T1WI MR discloses the same hematoma in early subacute stage. Mass effect partially effaces the 4th ventricle.

Cerebellar hemorrhages are severe, with a high in-hospital mortality (21.4%) and functional deficit at hospital discharge in practically all patients. The in-hospital mortality of 21.4% observed in our patients [5] is lower than 39–47% observed in other studies [22-24] and similar to death rates (13% and 25%) reported by other authors [25,26].

Patients with larger cerebellar hematomas ussually develop brainstem compression [25,28]. If the hematoma affects the caudal cerebellum, the medulla is the portion of the brainstem compressed and for this reason vasomotor disturbances and respiratory arrest may develop. Ocassionally, patients with cerebellar hemorrhage present with symptoms and signs of hydrocephalus. In deteriorating patients with accesible lesions, surgery should not be delayed. Patients with cerebellar hemorrhage who are deteriorating neurologically or who have brainstem compression and/or hydrocephalus from ventricular obstruction should undergo surgical removal of the hemorrhage as soon as possible [6].

6. Pontine and brainstem hematomas

Hematomas affecting the pons and the brainstem are one of the topographies associated with a more severe clinical outcome [4]. Primary brainstem hemorrhages are located most often in the pons. Midbrain and medullary hemorrhages are rare. Pontine hematomas (Figure 7) constitute a subgroup of hemorrhagic stroke that accounts for 0.36% of the total number of strokes and 3.4% of ICH, which is similar to 3–6% reported in most studies [4,8,9].

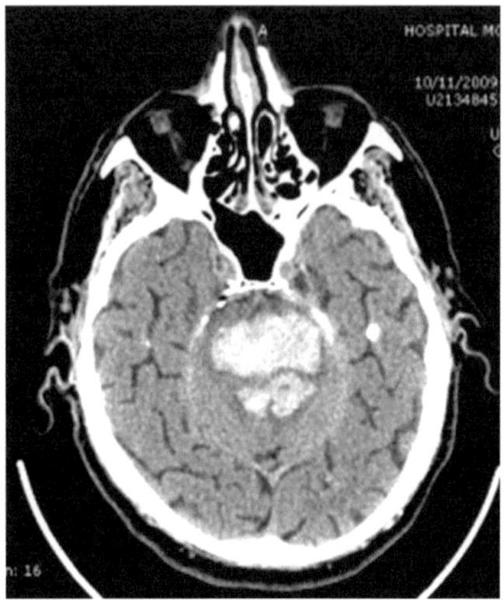

Fig. 7. Axial CT demonstrates a large pontine hemorrhage.

Early cranial nerve dysfunction was the independent clinical factor associated with brainstem ICH. Cranial nerve palsy found in 66.7% of our patients may be explained by involvement of the brainstem tegmentum by the hematoma either primarily or indirectly causing nuclear palsies and conjugate gaze abnormalities [4].

Pontine hematomas are severe, with a high mortality rate (50%). A small percentage of patients are symptom-free at the time of hospital discharge (7.1%) [5]. The 50% in-hospital mortality rate observed in our study [5] is lower than 55–60% reported by others [29,30] but higher than 31–47.5% of other series [31,32].

It should be noted that a pure motor hemiparesis, clinically indistinguishable from a lacunar infarction is an infrequent presenting form of pontine hematoma [11,33]. In this cases, there are two unilateral pontine hematomas localized in the basis pontis or at the union of basis pontis and tegmentum.

7. Multiple topographic involvement

In multiple topographic involvement with large-size hematomas (Figure 8), limb weakness, diabetes, and altered consciousness were independent clinical factors selected in the multivariate analysis. In relation to limb weakness (found in 97% of the cases), persistent hemiplegia is caused by involvement of the pyramidal tract fibers. It is well known that severity of hemiplegia is related to survival [4,9]. The state of alertness of the patient is a clinical feature that correlates with prognosis in ICH and, in general, in acute stroke patients. In the Lausanne Stroke Registry [35], 50% of ICH patients had some reduction in the level of consciousness, which is similar to 45.9% of our series. However, in patients with hemorrhage of multiple topographies, altered consciousness was found in 76.5% of cases. Reduced alertness in ICH is due to either a generalized increase in intracranial pressure, or to compromise of both hemispheres, or to the reticular activating system bilaterally in the brainstem tegmentum [4].

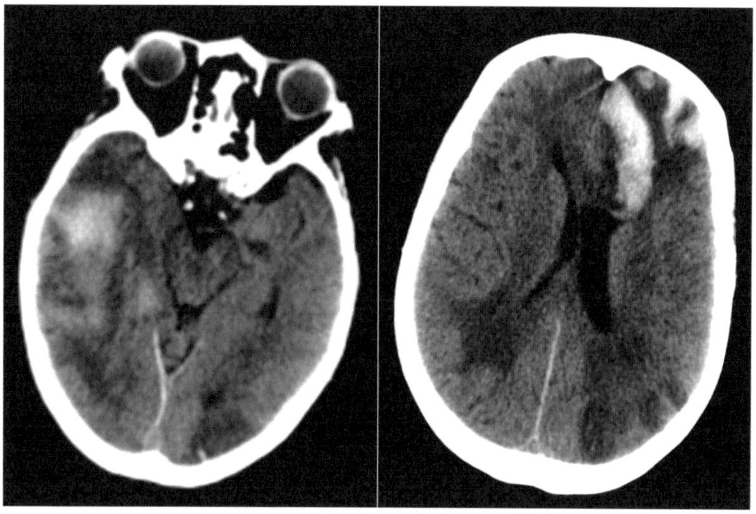

(a) (b)

Fig. 8. A) and B) Multiple parenchymal hematoma in cerebral amyloid angiopathy

In patients with ICH, diabetes was more frequently associated with multiple parenchymal hematoma (35.3%) [35]. Little is known about the influence of diabetes on the volume of damaged brain tissue in ICH patients. Diabetes is known to produce deleterious effects on the microvasculature that may result in increased bleeding risk. The ICH of multiple topography in patients with diabetes might be related to the specific angiopathy induced by diabetes in small vessels. The vasculopathy of perforating cerebral arteries, the walls of which are weakened by lipid and hyaline material (lipohyalinosis and fibrinoid necrosis), microaneurysms and/or microangiopathy may be a real risk for hematoma of multiple topography in diabetic patients [35]. These changes in cerebral vessels would perhaps make diabetics more prone to develop hemorrhages of large size than nondiabetics. More information, however, is needed on the cerebrovascular pathology whereby diabetes affects large and small blood vessels.

8. Primary intraventricular hemorrhage

Data regarding the frequency of primary intraventricular hemorrhage in the different hospital-based stroke registries are scarce. In our experience, primary intraventricular hemorrhage (Figure 9) is a rare subgroup of haemorrhagic stroke that accounted for 0.31% of all cases of stroke and 3.3% of intracerebral hemorrhages [5]. The clinical syndrome closely mimics subarachnoid hemorrhage, with sudden headache, stiff neck, vomiting and lethargy [36]. In childhood ventricular bleeding usually arises from small subependymal arteriovenous malformations. In adults, most intraventricular hemorrhages are due to ventricular spread of primary hypertensive bleeds into periventricular structures. Primary intraventricular hemorrhage is a severe clinical condition with an in-hospital mortality rate, in the present study, of 41.7%, and only one patient (8.3%) was symptom-free at discharge [5]. In other series, the mortality rate ranged between 33.3% and 43% [36-38].

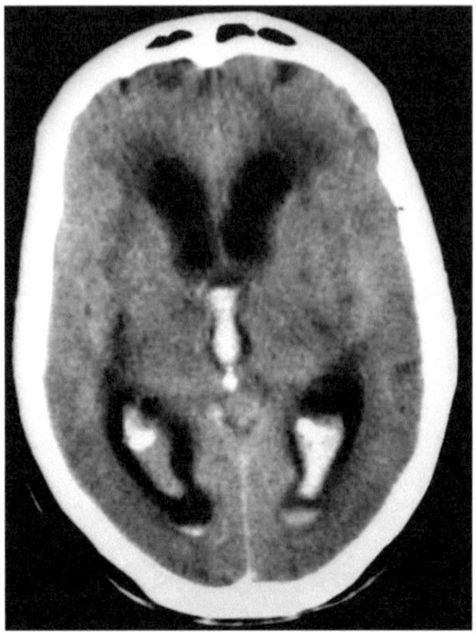

Fig. 9. Axial CT showing hemorrhage within the 3rd and both lateral ventricles with small layering fluid-fluid levels.

In conclusion, different topographies of ICH have an influence on the clinical spectrum and early outcome of patients with hemorrhagic stroke. Sensory deficit is frequently associated with ICH in the thalamus, lacunar syndrome and hypertension with internal capsule/basal ganglia ICH, seizures and non-sudden stroke onset with lobar ICH, ataxia with hemorrhage in the cerebellum, cranial nerve palsy with brainstem ICH, and limb weakness, diabetes, and altered consciousness with multiple topographic involvement. In-hospital mortality rates are also different according to the site of bleeding, varying from 16% in patients with internal capsule/basal ganglia hematomas, 20% in those with cerebellar hemorrhage and 25% for lobar and thalamic hematomas. Brainstem, primary intraventricular hemorrhage, and multiple topographic involvement are very severe conditions, with in-hospital mortality rates ranging between 40% to 65%.The morbidity and mortality associated with ICH remain high despite recent advances in our understanding of the clinical course of ICH. Rapid recognition and diagnosis of ICH as well as identification of early prognostic indicators are essential for planning the level of care and avoiding acute rapid progression during the first hours. Aggressive treatment of hypertension is essential in the primary and secondary prevention of ICH.

9. Acknowledgements

We thank M. Balcells, MD, for valuable participation in the study and Marta Pulido, MD, for editing the manuscript and editorial assistance. This study was supported in part by a grant from the Fondo de Investigación Sanitaria (FIS PI081514). Instituto de Salud Carlos III, Madrid, Spain.

10. References

[1] Rosenow F, Hojer CH, Meyer-Lohmann CH, Hilgers RD, Mühlhofer H, Kleindienst A, et al. Spontaneous intracerebral hemorrhage. Prognostic factors in 896 cases. Acta Neurol Scand 1997;96:174–182.

[2] Lisk DR, Pasteur W, Rhoades H, Putnam RD, Grotta JC. Early presentation of hemispheric intracerebral hemorrhage: prediction of outcome and guidelines for treatment allocation. Neurology 1994;44:133–139.
[3] Juvela S. Risk factors for impaired outcome after spontaneous intracerebral hemorrhage. Arch Neurol 1995;52:1193–1200.
[4] Kase CS, Mohr JP, Caplan LR. Intracerebral hemorrhage. In: Mohr JP, Choi DW, Grotta JC, Weir B, Wolf PhA, eds. Stroke. Pathophysiology, diagnosis, and management. Churchill Livingstone, Philadelphia, 2004, pp 327-376.
[5] Arboix A, Comes E, García-Eroles L, Massons J, Oliveres M, Balcells M, et al. Site of bleeding and early outcome in primary intracerebral hemorrhage. Acta Neurol Scand 2002;105:282–288.
[6] Morgenstern LB, Hemphill JC 3rd, Anderson C, Becker K, Broderick JP, Connolly ES Jr, et al. Guidelines for the Management of Spontaneous Intracerebral Hemorrhage. A Guidelines for Healthcare Professionals from the American Heart Association/American Stroke Association. Stroke 2010;4:2108–2129.
[7] Tatu L, Moulin Th, Mohamad RE, Vuillier F, Rumbach L, Czorny A. Primary intracerebral hemorrhages in the Besançon Stroke Registry. Initial clinical and CT findings, early course and 30-day outcome in 350 patients. Eur Neurol 2000;43:209–214.
[8] Qureshi A, Mendelow AD, Hanley DF. Intracerebral haemorrhage. Lancet 2009;373:1632–1644.
[9] Kase CS. Subcortical hemorrhages. In: Donnan G, Norrving B, Bamford J, Bogousslavsky J, eds. Subcortical stroke (2 edition). Oxford Medical Publications, Great Britain, 2002, pp 347–377.
[10] Arboix A, Martínez-Rebollar M, Oliveres M, García-Eroles L, Massons J, Targa C. Acute isolated capsular stroke: a clinical study of 148 cases. Clin Neurol Neurosurg 2005;107:88–94.
[11] Arboix A, García-Eroles L, Massons J, Oliveres M, Balcells M. Hemorrhagic pure motor stroke. Eur J Neurol 2007;14:219–223.
[12] Miyai I, Suzuki T, Kang J, Volpe BT. Functional outcome in patients with hemorrhagic stroke in putamen and thalamus compared with those with stroke restricted to the putamen or thalamus. Stroke 2000;31:1365–1369.
[13] Kumral E, Kocaer T, Ertubey NO, Kumral K. Thalamic hemorrhage. A prospective study of 100 patients. Stroke 1995;26:964–970.
[14] Chung CS, Caplan LR, Han W, Pessin MS, Lee KH, Kim JM. Thalamic hemorrhage. Brain 1996;119:1973–1886.
[15] Arboix A, Rodríguez-Aguilar R, Oliveres M, Comes E, García-Eroles L, Massons J. Thalamic haemorrhage vs internal capsule-basal ganglia haemorrhage: clinical profile and predictors of in-hospital mortality. BMC Neurol 2007;7:32, doi: 10.1186/1471-2377-7-32.
[16] Mori S, Sadoshima S, Ibayashi S, Fujishima M. Impact of thalamic hematoma on six-month mortality and motor and cognitive outcome. Stroke 1995;26:620–626.
[17] Shah SA, Kalita J, Misra UK, et al. Prognostic predictors of thalamic hemorrhage. J Clin Neurosci 2005;12:559–561.
[18] Arboix A, Manzano C, García-Eroles L, Massons J, Oliveres M, Parra O, et al. Determinants of early outcome in spontaneous lobar cerebral hemorrhage. Acta Neurol Scand 2006;114:187–192.

[19] Hårdemark HG, Wesslén N, Persson L. Influence of clinical factors, CT findings and early management on outcome in supratentorial intracerebral hemorrhage. Cerebrovasc Dis 1999;9:10–21.

[20] Broderick J, Brott Th, Tomsick Th, Leach A. Lobar hemorrhage in the elderly. The undiminishing importance of hypertension. Stroke 1993;24:49–51.

[21] Brott T, Broderick J, Kothari R, Barsan W, Tomsick T, Sauerbeck L, et al. Early hemorrhage growth in patients with intracerebral hemorrhage. Stroke 1997;28:1-5.

[22] Van der Hoop RG, Vermeulen M , van Gijn J. Cerebellar hemorrhage: diagnosis and treatment. Surg Neurol 1988;29:6–10.

[23] Melamed N, Satya-Murti S.Cerebellar hemorrhage. A review and reappraisal of benign cases. Arch Neurol 1984;41:425–428.

[24] Dunne JW, Chakera T, Kermode. Cerebellar hemorrhage. Diagnosis and treatment: a study of 75 consecutive cases. Q J Med 1987;64:739–754.

[25] González-García J, Gelabert-González M, García-Allut A, Fernández-Villa JM, López-García E, García-Pravos A. Hematomas de cerebelo: un ictus con tratamiento quirúrgico. Rev Neurol 2000;31:1119–1126.

[26] Toyoda K, Okada Y, Ibayashi S, Inoue T, Yasumori K, Fukui D, et al. Antithrombotic therapy and predilection for cerebellar hemorrhage. Cerebrovasc Dis 2007;23:109–116.

[27] Turgut M, Özcan OE, Ertürk Ö, Saribas O, Erbengi A. Spontaneous cerebellar strokes. Clinical observations in 60 patients. Angiology 1996;47:841–848.

[28] Arboix A, Rennie M. Clinical study of 28 patients with cerebellar hemorrhage. Med Clin (Barc) 2009;132:665–668.

[29] Wijdicks EFM, Louis ES. Clinical profiles predictive of outcome in pontine hemorrhage. Neurology 1997;49:1342–1346.

[30] Chung CS, Park CH. Primary pontine hemorrhage: a new CT classification. Neurology 1992;42:830–834.

[31] Wessels T, Möller-Hartmann W, Noth J, Klötzsch C. CT findings and clinical features as markers for patient outcome in primary pontine hemorrhage. Am J Neuroradiol 2004;25:257–260.

[32] Murata Y, Yamaguchi S, Kajikawa H, Yamamura K, Sumioka S, Nakamura S. Relationship between the clinical manifestations, computed tomographic findings and the outcome in 80 patients with primary pontine hemorrhage. J Neurol Sci 1999;167:107–111

[33] Arboix A. Clinical study of 14 patients with pontine hemorrhage. Med Clin (Barc) 2008;130:339–341.

[34] Bogousslavski J, Van Melle J, Regli F. The Lausanne Stroke Registry: analysis of 1.000 consecutive patients with first stroke. Stroke 1988;19:1083–1092.

[35] Arboix A, Massons J, Garcia-Eroles L, Oliveres M, Targa C. Diabetes is an independent risk factor for in-hospital mortality from acute spontaneous intracerebral hemorrhage. Diabetes Care 2000;23:1527–1532.

[36] Angelopoulos M, Gupta SR, Hia AB. Primary intraventricular hemorrhage in adults: clinical features, risk factors, and outcome. Surg Neurol 1995;44:433-436.

[37] Passero S, Ulivelli M, Reale F. Primary intraventricular haemorrhage in adults. Acta Neurol Scand 2002;105:115–119.

[38] Verma A, Maheshwari MC, Bhargava S. Spontaneous intraventricular haemorrhage. J Neurol 1987;234:233–236.

16

Genetic Risk Factors of Imaging Measures Associated with Late-Onset Alzheimer's Disease

Christiane Reitz[1,2,3]
[1]*Taub Institute for Research on Alzheimer's Disease and the Aging Brain College of Physicians and Surgeons, Columbia University, New York, NY*
[2]*Department of Neurology, College of Physicians and Surgeons Columbia University, New York, NY*
[3]*Gertrude H. Sergievsky Center, College of Physicians and Surgeons Columbia University, New York, NY*
USA

1. Introduction

Late-onset Alzheimer's disease (LOAD) is the most common cause of dementia and the fifth leading cause of death in Americans older than 65 years.[1] Although other major causes of death have decreased, deaths due to LOAD have been rising dramatically over the past two decades, between 2000 and 2006 they increased by 46.1%.[1] Clinically, LOAD is characterized by progressive cognitive decline in particular in the memory domain. Neuropathologically it is characterized by the aggregation and deposition of misfolded proteins, in particular aggregated β-amyloid (Aβ) peptide in the form of extracellular senile (or neuritic) "plaques," and hyperphosphorlylated tau (τ) protein in the form of intracellular neurofibrillary "tangles" (NFTs). These changes are often accompanied by microvascular damage, vascular amyloid deposits, inflammation, microgliosis, and loss of neurons and synapses.

Although twin studies suggest that 37% to 78% of the variance in the age-at-onset of LOAD can be attributed to additive genetic effects,[2] few genes have been identified and validated, and these genes likely explain less than 50% of the genetic contribution to LOAD. This is the upper bound of explained heritability in other complex diseases for which—unlike LOAD—significant association has been demonstrated for several common loci of large effect (i.e., ORs > 2 to > 3), such as age-related macular degeneration. Thus, a substantial proportion of the heritability for LOAD remains unexplained by the currently known susceptibility genes. A likely explanation for the difficulty in gene identification is that LOAD is a multifactorial complex disorder with both genetic and environmental components, and that multiple genes with small effects are likely to contribute.

Several neuroimaging measures correlate with LOAD risk and progression, in particular the volumes of the hippocampus, parahippocampus and entorhinal cortex, and the cerebral grey matter. Also these measures appear to have a substantial genetic contribution reflected by heritability estimates ranging from 40% to 80%.[3-5] Advances in brain imaging and high throughput genotyping enable new approaches to study the influence of genetic variation on brain structure and function. As a result, imaging genetics has become an emergent transdisciplinary research field, where genetic variation is evaluated using imaging measures as quantitative traits (QTs) or continuous phenotypes. Imaging genetics studies have advantages over traditional case-control designs. An important consideration is that QT association studies have increased statistical power and thus decreased sample size requirements. Additionally, imaging phenotypes may be closer to the underlying biological etiology of AD, making it easier to identify underlying genes. Together with studies of the genetics of brain structure and function among normal individuals which have been extended to the entire human lifespan from childhood through extreme old age,6-8 the data of such studies provide an invaluable backdrop for understanding the genetic influences on neuroanatomy and neurophysiology and are powerful tools for understanding the genetics of neurodegenerative diseases associated with changes in these brain structures such as LOAD. In this chapter, we summarize the current evidence relating genetic variation with LOAD and review the usefulness of imaging endophenotypes in identification of genes increasing susceptibility to LOAD.

2. Imaging endophenotypes in LOAD

Structural MRI. On structural magnetic resonance imaging (LOAD) is characterized by atrophy of the medial temporal lobe, foremostly the hippocampus and the amygdala (Figure 1),[9] which may further involve the posterior cortex,[1] occipital lobes, precuneus and posterior cingulate.[10] Atrophy in the hippocampus and entorhinal cortex is associated with a decline in memory function, progression of memory impairment and an increased risk of LOAD.[11] However, these structural changes on MRI are not specific to LOAD and not sufficient to establish a definitive diagnosis of LOAD, as similar atrophy is observed in other neurodegenerative disorders and normal aging. In addition, while nonspecific white matter changes appear frequently in healthy elderly individuals, such changes are also common in elderly people with cognitive decline, stroke or MCI. Nevertheless, several studies have suggested that certain structural MRI biomarkers possess some degree of discriminative diagnostic power. For example, evidence exists that in LOAD, the corpus callosum (particularly the anterior area) exhibits atrophy. This change helps to distinguish LOAD from frontotemporal dementia, in which the posterior area of the corpus callosum shows greater atrophy than the anterior area of this brain structure.[12] There is also evidence that among patients with amnestic MCI, those who convert to LOAD show greater atrophy in the hippocampus and the inferior and middle temporal gyri than those who do not convert to LOAD.[13]

Functional MRI. Functional MRI (fMRI) can visualize neuronal activity either during rest or in association with a task that activates specific brain regions. The most common method is blood oxygen level-dependent (BOLD) fMRI, which measures alterations in blood flow on the basis of changes in deoxyhemoglobin. As the deoxyhemoglobin concentration depends on neuronal activity, BOLD reflects brain activity. This technique is widely used in research and in the diagnosis of various brain disorders because of its high sensitivity and easy implementation.

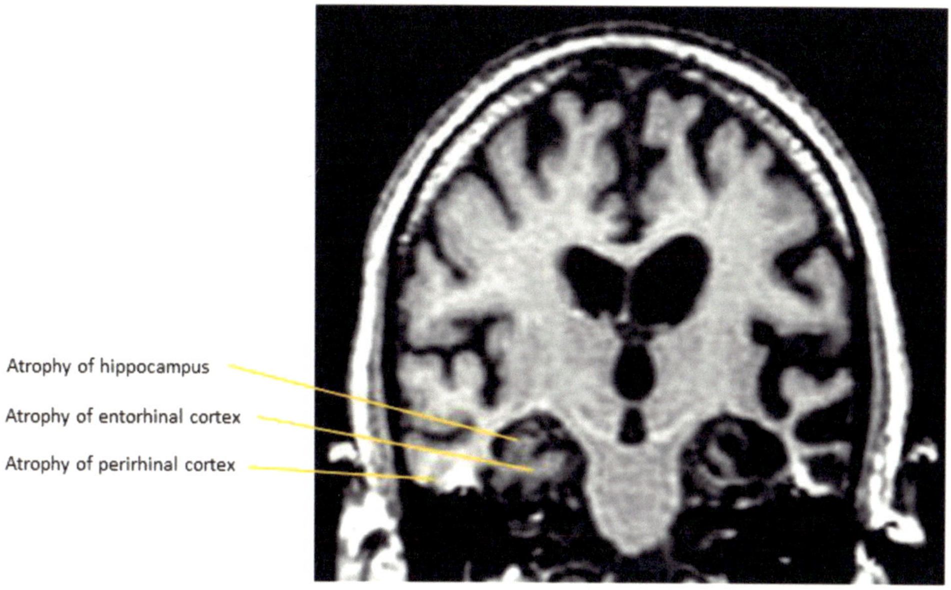

Fig. 1. LOAD Endophenotypes on MRI

BOLD signals depend on several anatomical, physiological and imaging parameters, and can be interpreted qualitatively or semiquantitatively. As a result, interindividual and intraindividual variability limits the use of such signals in the differential diagnosis of dementia- causing disorders. Nevertheless, fMRI can facilitate the characterization of functional abnormalities in specific diseases. People with LOAD exhibit reduced brain activity in parietal and hippocampal regions in comparison with healthy controls when undergoing memory encoding tasks.[14-16] In addition, some studies have found different neuronal activity patterns in healthy controls and patients with MCI. Recent advances in fMRI have allowed intrinsic functional networks in the human brain to be defined. The study of cognitive–behavioral function in the early stages of neurodegenerative disorders may allow the identification of the neuroanatomical networks affected by these diseases, and may assist in the differential diagnosis of the various disorders that underlie dementia.

PET and single-photon emission CT. PET and single-photon emission CT (SPECT) have been widely explored as diagnostic tools for dementia, and both techniques have shown good diagnostic and prognostic capabilities. PET studies have mostly used the tracer 2-[18F]-fluoro-2-deoxy-d-glucose (18F-FDG), which provides a measure of cerebral glucose metabolism and, hence, indirectly demonstrates synaptic activity. In the early stages of LOAD, 18F-FDG-PET reveals a characteristic pattern of symmetric hypometabolism in the posterior cingulate and parietotemporal regions that spreads to the prefrontal cortices (Figure 2a). These changes are distinct from the changes in cerebral glucose metabolism that are seen in healthy controls and cases of other forms of dementia, and the extent of hypometabolism inversely correlates with the degree of cognitive impairment.[17] 18F-FDG-PET has a high sensitivity (94%) but a low specificity (73–78%) for the diagnosis of dementia.[18] SPECT, which involves studying regional blood flow with Tc-hexamethylpropyleneamine oxime, has a similar specificity to 18F-FDG-PET for this condition.[19] A number of low-molecular-weight tracers have been developed for PET to assess Aβ deposits in vivo. The most frequently used tracer is Pittsburgh compound B (PIB). Compared with healthy controls, patients with LOAD show increased 11C-PIB retention in cortical regions targeted by Aβ deposits (Figure 2b).[20] Deposition of this peptide seems to reach a plateau by the early stages of LOAD. In MCI, PIB binding is bimodal, with ≈ 50% of patients showing an increase in 11C-PIB binding, resembling the 11C-PIB retention that is seen in LOAD, while the other ≈ 50% of patients exhibit low levels of 11C-PIB binding that are similar to the levels seen in controls.[21] In MRI studies, 11C-PIB binding correlated positively with atrophy in the amygdala and hippocampus but not other cortical areas, suggesting that various brain areas have different susceptibilities to Aβ deposit-mediated toxicity, or that amyloid deposition is nonessential for neurodegeneration.[21] New PET tracers for amyloid deposits, such as 18F-FDDNP, are being developed. In studies comparing 11C-PIB and 18F-FDDNP, these tracers showed differences in regional binding and in the cognitive domains with which they seem to be associated, suggesting that these tracers measure related but different characteristics of LOAD.[22]

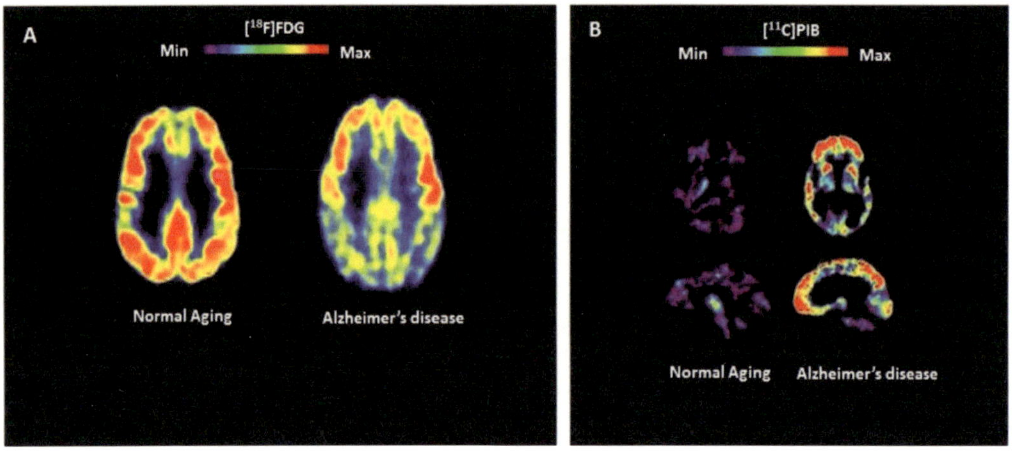

Fig. 2. A) FDG PET patterns characteristic of metabolic activity in cognitively normal individuals and patients with LOAD. Red: high FDG uptake, Blue: low FDG uptake. Compared to persons aging normally, persons with LOAD show decreased bilateral glucose metabolism particularly in the temporal and parietal regions. B) PIB PET images characteristic of elderly individuals without cognitive impairment and patients with LOAD. Red: high PiB retention, Purple: low PiB retention. The image of the LOAD case shows red and yellow areas indicating high concentrations of PiB in the brain thereby suggesting high amounts of amyloid deposits.

3. Genetic influences on brain morphological endophenotypes

Elucidating the extent to which genetic and environmental factors influence normal brain structure is of great importance for understanding age-related normal and pathological changes in brain and cognition. Twin studies, which estimate heritability based on data from monozygotic (MZ) and dizygotic (DZ) twin pairs, provide the optimal genetic method for clarifying this issue because they allow decomposing the variance of any variable into genetic, shared environmental influences, and unique individual-specific environmental influences.

As MZ twin pairs are genetically identical (with rare exceptions due to somatic mutations) while DZ twin pairs share on average 50% of their segregating genes, variation of a certain measure is considered heritable if MZ twin pairs resemble each other for this measure more closely than DZ twin pairs. An influence of shared environmental factors is suspected when correlations in DZ twin pairs are >50% of the MZ twin pair correlation.[23] Unique environmental factors determine the extent to which MZ twins do not resemble each other. Extended twin-studies include additional relatives thereby increasing the statistical power to detect the influences of environmental influences shared by members from the same family.

Heritability of Brain Volumes and Structures. To date, more than 30 twin studies on brain imaging measures have been performed that aim to define the genetic contribution to brain structures (reviewed by Krasuski et al. and Karas et al[9, 10]). Overall, these studies demonstrated substantial heritability of these endophenotypes, particularly for larger structures.

Twin studies using magnetic resonance imaging (MRI), found high heritability estimates of global brain measures including intracranial volume (>72%),[3, 9, 11, 24-26] total brain volume (66–97%),[3, 11, 24, 27-30] lobar tissue (in particular the temporal and parietal cortices),[25, 30, 31] total gray matter volume[3, 11, 24] and total white matter volume.[3, 11, 24] Brain areas that in contrast seem to be under stronger environmental control include the gyral patterning of the cortex,[27, 32] the volume of the lateral ventricles,[12, 24, 26, 29, 33] and the volume of the hippocampus.[11, 12, 24, 29, 34, 35] It is important to point out that some of these studies did not correct for total cranial volume or height when measuring brain volumes. Although it is likely that the ratio of brain volume/total cranial volume is comparable among monozygotic twins, it remains possible that this lack of correction has led in some studies to spurious results.

More recent studies have predominantly examined possible genetic effects on specific brain areas using voxel-based morphometry[36] and cortical thickness measures. Overall, these studies confirmed in particular the high heritabilities for the frontal, parietal and temporal cortices. In a study by Thompson et al., that constructed detailed three-dimensional maps based on a genetic continuum of similarity in grey matter in groups of unrelated subjects as well as DZ and MZ twins, genetic factors influenced in particular anatomical regions that include frontal and language-related cortices (ie., sensorimotor, middle frontal, anterior temporal and Wernicke's cortices; $r2(MZ) > 0.8$, $p < 0.05$).[5] In a study by Holshoff Pol et al.[37] which examined both gray and white matter density in a large sample of 54 monozygotic and 58 dizygotic twin pairs and 34 of their siblings, genetic factors significantly influenced white matter density of the superior occipitofrontal fascicle, corpus callosum, optic radiation, and corticospinal tract, as well as grey matter density of the medial frontal, superior frontal, superior temporal, occipital, postcentral, posterior cingulate, and parahippocampal cortices (heritability>0.69).[37] In a study by Wright et al., voxel-based morphometry revealed moderate heritabilities (42-66%) for temporal/parietal neocortical areas and paralimbic structures.[29] In a study by Rijsdijk et al.,[38] heritability estimates were only significant for left posterior cingulate and right dorsal anterior cingulate gray matter concentrations (46% and 37%, respectively). In a recent study that derived both surface-based and voxel-based representations of brain structure,[39] both heritability estimates for thickness and surface area were highest for the temporal and parietal lobes. In addition, this

study suggested that grey matter volume is more closely related to surface area than cortical thickness suggesting that surface area and cortical thickness measurements should be considered separately and preferred over gray matter volumes for imaging genetic studies.
Only one study has measured the heritability estimates for changes in brain volumes over time. In this study which used structural MRI, the genetic contributions to variability in intracranial volume, corpus callosum, and lateral ventricles in healthy elderly were high (88-92%)[26] but did not change after 4 years follow-up.40

4. Genetic epidemiology of LOAD

Genetically, AD is categorized into two forms: (1) familial cases with Mendelian inheritance of predominantly early-onset (<60 years, early-onset familial AD [EOFAD]), and (2) "sporadic" cases with less apparent or no familial aggregation and later age of onset (≥60 years, late-onset AD [LOAD]). It is important to note that this traditional dichotomization is overly simplistic as there are cases of early-onset AD without evidence for Mendelian transmission while, conversely, LOAD is frequently observed with a strong familial clustering, sometimes resembling a Mendelian pattern.
In contrast to early-onset Alzheimer's disease which is caused by autosomal dominant mutations in the *APP* (amyloid precursor protein), *PSEN1* (presenilin 1) and *PSEN2* (presenilin 2) genes, the genetics of LOAD is more complex. The genes involved in LOAD increase disease risk and are not inherited in a Mendelian fashion. First-degree relatives of patients with LOAD have twice the expected lifetime risk of this disease of people who do not have a LOAD-affected first-degree relative.[41] In addition, LOAD occurs more frequently in monozygotic than in dizygotic co-twins,42 suggesting a substantial genetic contribution to this disorder. In the largest twin study of dementia, involving 11,884 participants in the Swedish registry who were aged >65 years, 395 twin pairs were identified in which either one or both twins had LOAD.42 This study demonstrated a heritability of 58-79% for LOAD, depending on the model that was used in the data analysis.
Apolipoprotein E. APOE is the only established susceptibility gene for LOAD and maps to chromosome 19 in a cluster with the genes encoding translocase of outer mitochondrial membrane 40 (TOMM40), apolipoprotein C1 and apolipoprotein C2. APOE is a lipid-binding protein that is expressed in humans as one of three common isoforms, which are encoded by three different alleles, namely APOE ε2, APOE ε3 and APOE ε4. The presence of a single APOE ε4 allele is associated with a 2-3-fold increase in the risk of LOAD, while the presence of two copies of this allele is associated with a fivefold increase in the risk of this disease.
Each inherited APOE ε4 allele lowers the age of LOAD onset by 6–7 years. Furthermore, the presence of this allele is associated with memory impairment, MCI, and progression from MCI to dementia.[38] APOE ε4 has been suggested to account for as much as 20–30% of LOAD risk.
Despite the studies linking APOE ε4 with LOAD, the presence of this allele is neither necessary nor sufficient for disease: among participants in the Framingham study,[39] 55% of those who were homozygous for APOEε4, 27% of those with one copy of this allele and 9% of those without an APOE ε4 allele developed LOAD by 85 years of age. Segregation analyses conducted in families of patients with LOAD support the presence of at least four to six additional major LOAD risk genes.43 **Additional genetic risk variants**. After APOE,

the best-validated gene LOAD risk is the sortilin-related receptor 1 (SORL1) gene, which is located on chromosome 11q23. SorL1 belongs to a group of five type I transmembrane receptors (the others being sortilin, SorCS1, SorCS2 and SorCS3) that are highly expressed in the CNS and are characterized by a luminal, extracellular vacuolar protein sorting 10 domain. From family-based and population-based studies that, together, included over 6,000 individuals from four ethnic groups, Rogaeva et al. identified two haplotypes in the 3′ and 5′ regions of *SORL1* that are associated with LOAD risk.44 In addition, these researchers demonstrated that SorL1 promotes the translocation and retention of APP in subcellular compartments that exhibit low secretase activity, thereby reducing the extent of proteolytic breakdown into both amyloidogenic and nonamyloidogenic products.44 As a consequence, underexpression of SORL1 leads to overexpression of Aβ and an increased risk of LOAD. Several subsequent studies replicated these initial genetic association findings, and the results were further validated by a collaborative, unbiased metaanalysis of all published genetic data sets that included a total of 12,464 LOAD cases and 17,929 controls.45 In the past year, several studies demonstrated that, in addition, genetic variation in the *SORL1* homolog *SORCS1* influences LOAD risk, cognitive performance, APP processing and Aβ1–40 and Aβ1–42 levels through an effect on γ-secretase processing of APP,46, 47 further emphazising the role of sortilin-related proteins in LOAD etiology.

Genome-wide association studies[48-50] for LOAD using large numbers of cases and controls have revealed modest effect sizes for several genes on LOAD risk, with odds ratios in the range of 1.1–1.5, although most of these studies have only confirmed the association of APOE with this disease. One such study showed that variants of *TOMM40*—which is proximally located to and in linkage disequilibrium with *APOE*—were associated with LOAD risk, but whether these genetic associations are independent of the *APOE* locus remains unclear.

Together, two genome-wide association studies identified variants in the clusterin gene (*CLU*),[16,] 51 the phosphatidylinositol- binding clathrin assembly protein gene (*PICALM*)16 and complement receptor type 1 gene (*CR1*)51 as being associated with LOAD and several subsequent studies replicated these findings, but functional data confirming the roles in LOAD of the proteins encoded by these genes are still lacking. Clusterin is a lipoprotein that is expressed in mammalian tissues and is incorporated into amyloid plaques. This protein binds to soluble Aβ in CSF, forming complexes that can penetrate the BBB. Clusterin levels are positively correlated with the number of *APOE ε4* alleles, suggesting a compensatory induction of *CLU* in the brains of LOAD patients with the *APOE ε4* allele, who show low brain levels of APOE. *CR1* encodes a protein that is likely to contribute to Aβ clearance from the brain, while PICALM protein is involved in clathrin-mediated endocytosis, allowing intracellular trafficking of proteins and lipids such as nutrients, growth factors and neurotransmitters. PICALM protein also has a role in the trafficking of vesicle-associated membrane protein 2, a soluble *N*-ethylmaleimide-sensitive factor attachment protein receptor that is involved in the fusion of synaptic vesicles to the presynaptic membrane in neurotransmitter release. A third large genome-wide association study confirmed the associations of *PICALM* and *CLU* with LOAD and reported two additional loci as being associated with LOAD52: rs744373, which is near the bridging integrator 1 gene *(BIN1)* on chromosome 2q14.3, and rs597668, which is located on chromosome 19q13.3. BIN1 is a member of the BAR (BIN–amphiphysin–Rvs) adaptor family, which has been implicated in caspase-independent apoptosis and membrane dynamics, including vesicle fusion and trafficking, neuronal membrane organization, and clathrin-mediated synaptic vesicle formation. Of note, the latter process is disrupted by Aβ. Changes in *BIN1* expression have also been shown in aging mice and in transgenic mouse models of LOAD. The locus rs597668 is not in linkage disequilibrium with *APOE*, suggesting that the effect of this locus on LOAD risk is independent. Six genes are found in this region, of which at least two (genes encoding biogenesis of lysosomal organelles complex 1 subunit 3 and microtubule associated protein–microtubule affinity-regulating kinase 4) are implicated in molecular pathways linked to LOAD or other brain disorders.

It is important to note, that the results of the published genome-wide association studies are informative, but that the genetic associations need functional validation. Indeed, such studies alone cannot prove causality or assess the biological significance of an observed genetic association. Genomewide association studies represent a method of screening the genome, but are limited in their ability to detect true associations.

5. Genetic variation and neuroimaging measures in LOAD

As described above, multiple neuroimaging measures that correlate with LOAD risk and progression appear to have genetic underpinnings, with heritability estimates ranging from 40% to 80%. Recent studies that aimed to determine whether the discovered genetic risk factors for LOAD also influence these neuroimaging traits suggest that several of these candidate genes also influence specific LOAD imaging endophenotypes. Most studies chose hippocampal volume as the quantitative phenotype because of its sensitivity to the changes of early LOAD, and by far the best studied gene is APOE. In line with the strong and consistent results for APOE when using LOAD as the phenotype, most T-1 weighted MRI studies reported an association of APOE e4 with accelerated LOAD-related volume loss in the hippocampal region.[53-56] This is supported by several studies exploring the effect of the APOE e4 allele on glucose metabolism using FDG-PET,[57-60] or amyloid deposition using ([^{11}C] PiB-PET. [61-63]

Few studies have examined the association between other genes and LOAD imaging measures, and most of these were GWAS studies. In a GWAS of 381 participants of the Alzheimer's Disease Neuroimaging Initiative (ADNI) cohort, 21 chromosomal areas were associated with hippocampal atrophy.[64] These candidate regions included the APOE, EFNA5, CAND1, MAGI2, ARSB, and PRUNE2 genes, which are involved in the regulation of protein degradation, apoptosis, neuronal loss and neurodevelopment. In the same study, APOE and TOMM40 were confirmed when LOAD was used as the phenotype of interest.64 Additional studies by the same group, that included a larger set of imaging phenotypes and used T1-weighted MRI, 65 voxel-based morphometry/FreeSurfer methods 66or 3D mapping of temporal lobe volume differences using tensor-based morphometry,67 confirmed SNPs in APOE and TOMM40 as strongly associated with multiple brain regions (including hippocampal volume, entorhinal cortex volume, amygdala volume, cortical thickness measures, grey-matter density) and revealed other SNPs in or close to candidate genes that have been repeatedly associated with LOAD as described above (PICALM, SORL1, SORCS1, APP, CR1, BIN1). In addition these studies reported novel SNPs in proximity to the EPHA4, TP63, NXPH1, GRIN2B, NEDD9, DAPK1, IL1B, MYH13, TNK1, ACE, PRNP, PCK1 and GAPDHS genes. Several of these genes are biologically plausible. NXPH1 codes for neurexophilin-1, a protein implicated in synaptogenesis, that forms a tight complex with alpha neurexins, a group of proteins that promote adhesion between dendrites and axons. This adhesion is a key factor in synaptic integrity, the loss of which is a hallmark of AD. GRIN2B encodes the N-methyl-D-aspartate glutamate receptor NR2B subunit, which is a target for memantine therapy to decrease excitotoxic damage. ACE has been shown to cleave amyloid beta *in vitro* and is in addition involved in blood pressure regulation. Both high and low blood pressure have been associated with LOAD.

There have been few studies exploring the effects of specific candidate genes (other than APOE) on brain imaging phenotypes. Ho et al.[68] investigated the relationship between an obesity-associated candidate gene (FTO) and regional brain volume differences in 206 ADNI control participants. Systematic brain volume deficits were detected in cognitively normal obesity-associated risk allele carriers, as well as in subjects with increased body mass index indicating that this obesity susceptibility gene is associated with detectable deficits in brain structure, which may indirectly influence future risk for neurodegenerative disease. In 129 hypertensive individuals from a family-based cohort sampled from a Dutch genetically isolated population,69 four SNPs located at the 3'-end of SORL1 (rs1699102, rs3824968, rs2282649, rs1010159) were associated with frequency of microbleeds which is potentially related to amyloid angiopathy. In the MIRAGE Study70 several SORL1 SNPs that have been reported to be associated with LOAD, were associated with hippocampal atrophy, cerebrovascular disease, and white matter hyperintensities. In a candidate gene study that used (FDG-PET) measurements as a quantitative pre-symptomatic endophenotype in 158 cognitively normal late-middle-aged APOEε4 homozygotes, heterozygotes, and non-carriers,71 the GAB2 protective haplotype was associated with higher regional-to-whole brain FDG uptake in APOEε4 carriers.

6. Discussion

The work reviewed above indicates that there are various brain imaging measures that are useful endophenotypes associated with genetic liability for LOAD. The strongest evidence of heritability, linkage and/or association in studies of normal brain aging have been found for the medial frontal cortex, Heschl's gyrus and postcentral gyrus, Broca's area, anterior cingulate, gray matter of the parahippocampal gyrus and white matter of the superior occipitofrontal fasciculus. The high heritability for these endophenotypes seems to be present throughout life and seems to be functionally relevant. In contrast, the heritability of volume of the hippocampus, which is central to the formation of new memories and memory consolidation, the process for converting short-term memory into stored or long-term memory,[72] seems to be modest. Support for an environmental component of hippocampus volume comes from a twin study of Ammon's horn sclerosis73 in which only the twin of MZ pairs who had experienced prolonged, childhood febrile seizures developed sclerosis. This discordance in hippocampal response to trauma suggests susceptibility of this structure to environmental events. Mammalian studies reporting neurogenesis of the hippocampal dentate gyrus in adult animals even into senescence74, 75 suggest that the relatively stable size of the hippocampus throughout adulthood76, 77 may reflect a lifelong relative maintenance of volume 78, 79 through mechanisms such as neurogenesis and synaptogenesis with rich environmental stimulation75 even when genetically compromised.[80, 81] This speculation must, however, be tempered by the relatively small number of new neurons generated in confined regions of the hippocampus[82] and the lack of evidence that volume necessarily reflects cell number. In any case, if neurogenesis could be adequately and functionally amplified, it may carry new promise for conditions affecting the hippocampus such as LOAD.

The GWAS and candidate gene studies, however, which explored the impact of genetic variation on imaging endophenotypes of LOAD, do support an impact of genetic factors. In particular studies exploring the effect of APOE genotype on morphological changes consistently suggest a modulation of volume/structure dependent on level of genetic risk. Thus, taken together these studies of the genetics of brain structure and function among normal individuals suggest that variation in brain structure and function can be expected and that pathological states represent the extremes of this variation. They further indicate that the morphological characteristics of several brain structures represent both differential vulnerability to environmental influences and phenotypical expressions of different sets of genes, which may operate on morphology at different times throughout development and aging. As a consequence, these data provide a valuable background for understanding the genetics of neurodegenerative diseases associated with changes in brain structures including LOAD. They suggest that using these quantitative imaging traits may provide an informative phenotype and may increase statistical power.

Although encouraging, this also raises some additional questions and challenges. First, are the genes mediating each endophenotype involved in abnormal brain aging and cognition at least partially distinct from each other? This is a key assumption of the endophenotype approach, yet empirical proof of this remains to be determined. A substantial degree of overlap appears likely for a number of the known genes associated with early- and late-onset AD, at least including the APP, PSEN1, PSEN2, APOE, SORL1 and SORCS1, given that these genes are involved in either the production or processing of the β-amyloid peptide. Nevertheless, each gene has a unique role in this cascade and it thus seems likely these loci will differ in their magnitudes of influence across the brain systems affected in this disorder. How do these genes (along with others that remain to be identified) coalesce in influencing liability to overt expression of LOAD? Are their effects additive or interactive? The answers to these questions depend on large-scale studies of genetically at-risk samples with and without environmental exposures and the use of sophisticated statistical modeling algorithms that can powerfully probe the resulting datasets for evidence of gene-gene and gene-environment interactions. Finally, are these endophenotypes and associated genes unique to cognitive impairment in LOAD, or are they shared by other diseases such as Dementia with Lewy Bodies, Parkinson's disease or depression? Lewy body inclusions and Lewy neurites, the key pathological hallmarks of dementia with Lewy Bodies and Parkinson's disease, are a frequent coexistent pathologic change observed in autopsy-confirmed LOAD.

The questions posed above raise considerable challenges for investigators attempting to unravel the genetic complexity of LOAD. Nevertheless, we have entered a new era in which conjoint advances in molecular genetics and dissection of the dementing phenotype are enabling rapid progress with multiple gene discoveries. These discoveries validate the dissection of this disorder into its more discretely determined subcomponents in order to elucidate the mechanisms underlying cognitive impairment in the elderly.

Author	Subjects	Age in years, mean (range)	Brain region	Heritability in % (95% CI)
Reveley et al.[33] (1984)	18 MZ, 18 DZ	NA	LV	82-85% (NA)
Bartley et al.[27] (1997)	10 MZ, 9 DZ	MZ: 31 (19-54), DZ: 33 (18-29)	TB	94% (NA)
Carmelli et al.[25] (1998)	74 MZ, 71 DZ	68-79 years	IC	91% (NA)
Pennington et al.[28] (2000)	Reading disability: 25 MZ, 23 DZ; Non-Reading disability: 9 MZ, 9 DZ	Reading disability: MZ: 17.1, DZ: 16.8; Non-reading disability: MZ: 19.4, DZ: 18.7	TB Neocortex	97% (NA) 56% (NA)
Pfefferbaum et al.[26] (2000)	45 MZ, 40 DZ	MZ: 72.2, DZ: 71.4, range: 68-78	Subcortex IC CC LV	70% (NA) 81% (72-90) 79% (69-89) 79% (55-100)
Posthuma et al.[3] (2000)	See Baaré et al (2001)	See Baaré et al (2001)	CB	88% (81-92)
Sullivan et al.[34] (2001)	45 MZ, 40 DZ	MZ: 72.2, DZ: 71.4, range: 68-78	HIP	40% (NA)
Thompson et al.[5] (2001)	10 MZ, 10 DZ	48.2 ±3.4	Middle frontal sensimotor and anterior temporal cortices, Broca`s and Wernicke`s region (cortical thickness)	90-95% (NA)
Baaré et al.[24] (2001)	54 MZ, 58 DZ, 34 sibs 15 MZ, 18 DZ	MZM: 31.2, MZF: 34.1, DZM: 30.3, DZF: 30.6, OS: 30.3, sibs: 29.0; range: 19-69 75.7 ± years	IC TB GM WM LV Size CC Microstructure CC (DTI)	88% (82-92) 90% (85-93) 82% (73-88) 87% (80-91) C: 59% (47-69), E: 41% (31-53) 5:1 (NA) 3:1 (NA)
Geschwind et al.[30] (2002)	72 MZ, 67 DZ	MZ: 72.3, DZ: 71.8	Cerebral hemispheres	65% (NA)
Eckert et al.[32] (2002)	27 MZ, 12 DZ	MZ: 6.9-16.4, DZ: 6.1-15.0	Planum temporale asymmetry	NA (NA)

Author	Subjects	Age in years, mean (range)	Brain region	Heritability in % (95% CI)
Wright et al.[29] (2002)	10 MZ, 10 DZ	MZ: 31 (19-54), DZ: 23 (18-29)	TB LV CB Ventrolateral FR, cingulate, anterior/superior/transverse temp, retrosplenium	66% (17-100) C: 48% (0-97), E: 50% (32-84) 63%, E: 22% (NA) 58-73% (NA)
White et al.[83] (2002)	12 MZ, 12 control pairs	MZ: 24.5±7.2, controls: 24.4 ±7.2	TB, GM, WM, CB CAU, PUT, THAL, cortical depth	r>0.90 r>0.75
Scamvougeras et al.[84] (2003)	14 MZ, 12 DZ	MZ: 16-41, DZ: 18-32	CC	94% (NA)
Pfefferbaum et al.[40] (2004)	34 MZ, 37 DZ	4-year longitudinal follow-up T1: 68-80 years, T2: 72-84 years	CC (T1) CC (T2) LV (T1) LV (T2)	89% (NA) 92% (NA) 92% (NA) 88% (NA)
Wallace et al.[31] (2006)	90 MZ, 37 DZ	MZ: 11.9, DZ: 10.9, range: 5-19	TB GM WM FR, TEMP, PAR CB LV	89% (67-92) 82% (50-87) 85% (56-90) 77-88% (50-90) 49% (13-83) 31% (0-67), C: 24% (0-58), E: 45% (33-60)
Hulshoff Pol et al.[37] (2006)	See Baaré et al (2001)	See Baaré et al (2001)	WM (SOF, CC, CST) GM, MFL, SFL, STL, CING, PARAHIP, AMYG, OCC	69-82% (NA) 55-85% (NA)

AMYG, amygdala; CAU, caudate; CB, cerebellum; CC, corpus callosum; CI, confidence interval; CING, cingulate; CST, corticospinal tract; DTI, diffusion tensor imaging; DZ, dizygotic; DZF, dizygotic female; DZM, dizygotic male; FR, frontal lobe; GM, gray matter; HIP, hippocampus; IC, intracranial volume; LH, left handed; LV, lateral ventricles; MFL, medial frontal lobe; MZ, monozygotic; MZF, monozygotic female; MZM, monozygotic male; NA, not available; OCC, occipital lobe; occ-front-temp, occipito-fronto temporal; PAR, parietal lobe; PARAHIP, parahippocampal gyrus; PUT, putamen; SOF, superior orbitofrontal; TB, total brain; TEMP, temporal lobe; THAL, thalamus; SFL, superior frontal lobe; STL, superior temporal lobe; WM, white matter.

Table 1. Studies on heritability of human brain volumes

It is important to note that - despite their utility in the context of etiological research on LOAD - endophenotypes have not proven to have great utility in the clinical distinction of dementing disorders. As described above, the different forms of dementia show substantial clinical and pathological overlap, and likely do not reflect completely separate underlying pathologies or genetic causes but rather a continuous spectrum of disease. Therefore, although they more realistically reflect variation in the underlying causes of illness, the use of endophenotypic assessments in diagnostic or treatment contexts is difficult.
In conclusion, given that the pathways from genotypes to end-stage phenotypes are circuitous at best, discernment of endophenotypes more proximal to the effects of genetic variation can improve statistical power and thereby be a powerful tool in the identification of genes linked to complex disorders. They can help understand how environmental and genetic factors interact to influence disease susceptibility and expression, and can help identify targets for the development of new treatment and prevention strategies.

7. Acknowledgements

This work was supported by grants from the National Institute of Health and the National Institute on Aging: R37-AG15473, P01-AG07232, The Blanchett Hooker Rockefeller Foundation, The Charles S. Robertson Gift from the Banbury Fund, and The Merrill Lynch Foundation. Dr. Reitz was further supported by a Paul B. Beeson Career Development Award (K23AG034550).

8. References

[1] Teipel SJ, Schapiro MB, Alexander GE, Krasuski JS, Horwitz B, Hoehne C, Moller HJ, Rapoport SI, Hampel H. Relation of corpus callosum and hippocampal size to age in nondemented adults with down's syndrome. *The American journal of psychiatry*. 2003;160:1870-1878

[2] Meyer JM, Breitner JC. Multiple threshold model for the onset of alzheimer's disease in the nas-nrc twin panel. *American journal of medical genetics*. 1998;81:92-97

[3] Posthuma D, de Geus EJ, Neale MC, Hulshoff Pol HE, Baare WEC, Kahn RS, Boomsma D. Multivariate genetic analysis of brain structure in an extended twin design. *Behavior genetics*. 2000;30:311-319

[4] Thompson P, Cannon TD, Toga AW. Mapping genetic influences on human brain structure. *Annals of medicine*. 2002;34:523-536

[5] Thompson PM, Cannon TD, Narr KL, van Erp T, Poutanen VP, Huttunen M, Lonnqvist J, Standertskjold-Nordenstam CG, Kaprio J, Khaledy M, Dail R, Zoumalan CI, Toga AW. Genetic influences on brain structure. *Nature neuroscience*. 2001;4:1253-1258

[6] Gogtay N, Giedd JN, Lusk L, Hayashi KM, Greenstein D, Vaituzis AC, Nugent TF, 3rd, Herman DH, Clasen LS, Toga AW, Rapoport JL, Thompson PM. Dynamic mapping of human cortical development during childhood through early adulthood. *Proceedings of the National Academy of Sciences of the United States of America*. 2004;101:8174-8179

[7] Sowell ER, Peterson BS, Thompson PM, Welcome SE, Henkenius AL, Toga AW. Mapping cortical change across the human life span. *Nature neuroscience*. 2003;6:309-315

[8] Thompson PM, Hayashi KM, Dutton RA, Chiang MC, Leow AD, Sowell ER, De Zubicaray G, Becker JT, Lopez OL, Aizenstein HJ, Toga AW. Tracking alzheimer's disease. *Ann N Y Acad Sci*. 2007;1097:183-214

[9] Krasuski JS, Alexander GE, Horwitz B, Daly EM, Murphy DG, Rapoport SI, Schapiro MB. Volumes of medial temporal lobe structures in patients with alzheimer's disease and mild cognitive impairment (and in healthy controls). *Biological psychiatry*. 1998;43:60-68

[10] Karas G, Scheltens P, Rombouts S, van Schijndel R, Klein M, Jones B, van der Flier W, Vrenken H, Barkhof F. Precuneus atrophy in early-onset alzheimer's disease: A morphometric structural mri study. *Neuroradiology*. 2007;49:967-976

[11] Mungas D, Harvey D, Reed BR, Jagust WJ, DeCarli C, Beckett L, Mack WJ, Kramer JH, Weiner MW, Schuff N, Chui HC. Longitudinal volumetric mri change and rate of cognitive decline. *Neurology*. 2005;65:565-571

[12] Likeman M, Anderson VM, Stevens JM, Waldman AD, Godbolt AK, Frost C, Rossor MN, Fox NC. Visual assessment of atrophy on magnetic resonance imaging in the diagnosis of pathologically confirmed young-onset dementias. *Archives of neurology*. 2005;62:1410-1415

[13] Chetelat G, Landeau B, Eustache F, Mezenge F, Viader F, de la Sayette V, Desgranges B, Baron JC. Using voxel-based morphometry to map the structural changes associated with rapid conversion in mci: A longitudinal mri study. *NeuroImage*. 2005;27:934-946

[14] Wolk DA, Dickerson BC. Fractionating verbal episodic memory in alzheimer's disease. *NeuroImage*. 2011;54:1530-1539

[15] Rombouts SA, Barkhof F, Veltman DJ, Machielsen WC, Witter MP, Bierlaagh MA, Lazeron RH, Valk J, Scheltens P. Functional mr imaging in alzheimer's disease during memory encoding. *AJNR Am J Neuroradiol*. 2000;21:1869-1875

[16] Bokde AL, Karmann M, Born C, Teipel SJ, Omerovic M, Ewers M, Frodl T, Meisenzahl E, Reiser M, Moller HJ, Hampel H. Altered brain activation during a verbal working memory task in subjects with amnestic mild cognitive impairment. *J Alzheimers Dis*. 2010;21:103-118

[17] Small GW, Bookheimer SY, Thompson PM, Cole GM, Huang SC, Kepe V, Barrio JR. Current and future uses of neuroimaging for cognitively impaired patients. *Lancet neurology*. 2008;7:161-172

[18] Silverman DH, Small GW, Chang CY, Lu CS, Kung De Aburto MA, Chen W, Czernin J, Rapoport SI, Pietrini P, Alexander GE, Schapiro MB, Jagust WJ, Hoffman JM, Welsh-Bohmer KA, Alavi A, Clark CM, Salmon E, de Leon MJ, Mielke R, Cummings JL, Kowell AP, Gambhir SS, Hoh CK, Phelps ME. Positron emission tomography in evaluation of dementia: Regional brain metabolism and long-term outcome. *JAMA*. 2001;286:2120-2127

[19] O'Brien JT. Role of imaging techniques in the diagnosis of dementia. *Br J Radiol*. 2007;80 Spec No 2:S71-77

[20] Klunk WE, Engler H, Nordberg A, Wang Y, Blomqvist G, Holt DP, Bergstrom M, Savitcheva I, Huang GF, Estrada S, Ausen B, Debnath ML, Barletta J, Price JC, Sandell J, Lopresti BJ, Wall A, Koivisto P, Antoni G, Mathis CA, Langstrom B. Imaging brain amyloid in alzheimer's disease with pittsburgh compound-b. *Ann Neurol*. 2004;55:306-319

[21] Frisoni GB, Lorenzi M, Caroli A, Kemppainen N, Nagren K, Rinne JO. In vivo mapping of amyloid toxicity in alzheimer disease. *Neurology*. 2009;72:1504-1511

[22] Tolboom N, van der Flier WM, Yaqub M, Koene T, Boellaard R, Windhorst AD, Scheltens P, Lammertsma AA, van Berckel BN. Differential association of [11c]pib and [18f]fddnp binding with cognitive impairment. *Neurology*. 2009;73:2079-2085

[23] Boomsma D, Busjahn A, Peltonen L. Classical twin studies and beyond. *Nature reviews*. 2002;3:872-882

[24] Baare WF, Hulshoff Pol HE, Boomsma DI, Posthuma D, de Geus EJ, Schnack HG, van Haren NE, van Oel CJ, Kahn RS. Quantitative genetic modeling of variation in human brain morphology. *Cereb Cortex*. 2001;11:816-824

[25] Carmelli D, DeCarli C, Swan GE, Jack LM, Reed T, Wolf PA, Miller BL. Evidence for genetic variance in white matter hyperintensity volume in normal elderly male twins. *Stroke; a journal of cerebral circulation*. 1998;29:1177-1181

[26] Pfefferbaum A, Sullivan EV, Swan GE, Carmelli D. Brain structure in men remains highly heritable in the seventh and eighth decades of life. *Neurobiology of aging*. 2000;21:63-74

[27] Bartley AJ, Jones DW, Weinberger DR. Genetic variability of human brain size and cortical gyral patterns. *Brain*. 1997;120 (Pt 2):257-269

[28] Pennington BF, Filipek PA, Lefly D, Chhabildas N, Kennedy DN, Simon JH, Filley CM, Galaburda A, DeFries JC. A twin mri study of size variations in human brain. *Journal of cognitive neuroscience*. 2000;12:223-232

[29] Wright IC, Sham P, Murray RM, Weinberger DR, Bullmore ET. Genetic contributions to regional variability in human brain structure: Methods and preliminary results. *NeuroImage*. 2002;17:256-271

[30] Geschwind DH, Miller BL, DeCarli C, Carmelli D. Heritability of lobar brain volumes in twins supports genetic models of cerebral laterality and handedness. *Proceedings of the National Academy of Sciences of the United States of America*. 2002;99:3176-3181

[31] Wallace GL, Eric Schmitt J, Lenroot R, Viding E, Ordaz S, Rosenthal MA, Molloy EA, Clasen LS, Kendler KS, Neale MC, Giedd JN. A pediatric twin study of brain morphometry. *Journal of child psychology and psychiatry, and allied disciplines*. 2006;47:987-993

[32] Eckert MA, Leonard CM, Molloy EA, Blumenthal J, Zijdenbos A, Giedd JN. The epigenesis of planum temporale asymmetry in twins. *Cereb Cortex*. 2002;12:749-755

[33] Reveley AM, Reveley MA, Chitkara B, Clifford C. The genetic basis of cerebral ventricular volume. *Psychiatry research*. 1984;13:261-266

[34] Sullivan EV, Pfefferbaum A, Swan GE, Carmelli D. Heritability of hippocampal size in elderly twin men: Equivalent influence from genes and environment. *Hippocampus*. 2001;11:754-762

[35] Chetelat G, Fouquet M, Kalpouzos G, Denghien I, De la Sayette V, Viader F, Mezenge F, Landeau B, Baron JC, Eustache F, Desgranges B. Three-dimensional surface mapping of hippocampal atrophy progression from mci to ad and over normal aging as assessed using voxel-based morphometry. *Neuropsychologia*. 2008;46:1721-1731

[36] Ashburner J, Friston KJ. Why voxel-based morphometry should be used. *NeuroImage*. 2001;14:1238-1243

[37] Hulshoff Pol HE, Schnack HG, Posthuma D, Mandl RC, Baare WF, van Oel C, van Haren NE, Collins DL, Evans AC, Amunts K, Burgel U, Zilles K, de Geus E, Boomsma DI, Kahn RS. Genetic contributions to human brain morphology and intelligence. *J Neurosci*. 2006;26:10235-10242

[38] Farlow MR, He Y, Tekin S, Xu J, Lane R, Charles HC. Impact of apoe in mild cognitive impairment. *Neurology*. 2004;63:1898-1901

[39] Myers RH, Schaefer EJ, Wilson PW, D'Agostino R, Ordovas JM, Espino A, Au R, White RF, Knoefel JE, Cobb JL, McNulty KA, Beiser A, Wolf PA. Apolipoprotein e epsilon4 association with dementia in a population-based study: The framingham study. *Neurology*. 1996;46:673-677

[40] Pfefferbaum A, Sullivan EV, Carmelli D. Morphological changes in aging brain structures are differentially affected by time-linked environmental influences despite strong genetic stability. *Neurobiology of aging*. 2004;25:175-183

[41] Green RC, Cupples LA, Go R, Benke KS, Edeki T, Griffith PA, Williams M, Hipps Y, Graff-Radford N, Bachman D, Farrer LA. Risk of dementia among white and african american relatives of patients with alzheimer disease. *JAMA*. 2002;287:329-336

[42] Gatz M, Reynolds CA, Fratiglioni L, Johansson B, Mortimer JA, Berg S, Fiske A, Pedersen NL. Role of genes and environments for explaining alzheimer disease. *Archives of general psychiatry*. 2006;63:168-174

[43] Daw EW, Payami H, Nemens EJ, Nochlin D, Bird TD, Schellenberg GD, Wijsman EM. The number of trait loci in late-onset alzheimer disease. *American journal of human genetics*. 2000;66:196-204

[44] Rogaeva E, Meng Y, Lee JH, Gu Y, Kawarai T, Zou F, Katayama T, Baldwin CT, Cheng R, Hasegawa H, Chen F, Shibata N, Lunetta KL, Pardossi-Piquard R, Bohm C, Wakutani Y, Cupples LA, Cuenco KT, Green RC, Pinessi L, Rainero I, Sorbi S, Bruni A, Duara R, Friedland RP, Inzelberg R, Hampe W, Bujo H, Song YQ, Andersen OM, Willnow TE, Graff-Radford N, Petersen RC, Dickson D, Der SD, Fraser PE, Schmitt-Ulms G, Younkin S, Mayeux R, Farrer LA, St George-Hyslop P. The neuronal sortilin-related receptor sorl1 is genetically associated with alzheimer disease. *Nature genetics*. 2007;39:168-177

[45] Reitz C, Cheng R, Rogaeva E, Lee JH, Tokuhiro S, Zou F, Bettens K, Sleegers K, Tan EK, Kimura R, Shibata N, Arai H, Kamboh MI, Prince JA, Maier W, Riemenschneider M, Owen M, Harold D, Hollingworth P, Cellini E, Sorbi S, Nacmias B, Takeda M, Pericak-Vance MA, Haines JL, Younkin S, Williams J, van Broeckhoven C, Farrer LA, St George-Hyslop PH, Mayeux R. Meta-analysis of the association between variants in sorl1 and alzheimer disease. *Archives of neurology*. 2011;68:99-106

[46] Reitz C, Lee J, Clark L, Rogers R, Rogaeva E, St George-Hyslop P, Mayeux R. Impact of genetic variation in sorcs1 on memory retention. *Neurobiology of aging*. 2011;In press

[47] Reitz C, Tokuhiro S, Clark L, Conrad C, Vonsattel JP, Hazrati L-N, Palotas A, Lantigua R, Medrano M, Jimenez-Velazquez I, Vardarajan B, Simkin I, Haines JL, Pericak-Vance MA, Farrer L, Lee J, Rogaeva E, St George-Hyslop P, Mayeux R. Sorcs1 alters amyloid precursor protein processing and variants may increase alzheimer's disease risk. *Ann Neurol*. 2011;In press

[48] Beecham GW, Martin ER, Li YJ, Slifer MA, Gilbert JR, Haines JL, Pericak-Vance MA. Genome-wide association study implicates a chromosome 12 risk locus for late-onset alzheimer disease. *American journal of human genetics.* 2009;84:35-43

[49] Bertram L, McQueen MB, Mullin K, Blacker D, Tanzi RE. Systematic meta-analyses of alzheimer disease genetic association studies: The alzgene database. *Nature genetics.* 2007;39:17-23

[50] Carrasquillo MM, Zou F, Pankratz VS, Wilcox SL, Ma L, Walker LP, Younkin SG, Younkin CS, Younkin LH, Bisceglio GD, Ertekin-Taner N, Crook JE, Dickson DW, Petersen RC, Graff-Radford NR. Genetic variation in pcdh11x is associated with susceptibility to late-onset alzheimer's disease. *Nature genetics.* 2009;41:192-198

[51] Lambert JC, Heath S, Even G, Campion D, Sleegers K, Hiltunen M, Combarros O, Zelenika D, Bullido MJ, Tavernier B, Letenneur L, Bettens K, Berr C, Pasquier F, Fievet N, Barberger-Gateau P, Engelborghs S, De Deyn P, Mateo I, Franck A, Helisalmi S, Porcellini E, Hanon O, de Pancorbo MM, Lendon C, Dufouil C, Jaillard C, Leveillard T, Alvarez V, Bosco P, Mancuso M, Panza F, Nacmias B, Bossu P, Piccardi P, Annoni G, Seripa D, Galimberti D, Hannequin D, Licastro F, Soininen H, Ritchie K, Blanche H, Dartigues JF, Tzourio C, Gut I, Van Broeckhoven C, Alperovitch A, Lathrop M, Amouyel P. Genome-wide association study identifies variants at clu and cr1 associated with alzheimer's disease. *Nature genetics.* 2009;41:1094-1099

[52] Seshadri S, Fitzpatrick AL, Ikram MA, DeStefano AL, Gudnason V, Boada M, Bis JC, Smith AV, Carassquillo MM, Lambert JC, Harold D, Schrijvers EM, Ramirez-Lorca R, Debette S, Longstreth WT, Jr., Janssens AC, Pankratz VS, Dartigues JF, Hollingworth P, Aspelund T, Hernandez I, Beiser A, Kuller LH, Koudstaal PJ, Dickson DW, Tzourio C, Abraham R, Antunez C, Du Y, Rotter JI, Aulchenko YS, Harris TB, Petersen RC, Berr C, Owen MJ, Lopez-Arrieta J, Varadarajan BN, Becker JT, Rivadeneira F, Nalls MA, Graff-Radford NR, Campion D, Auerbach S, Rice K, Hofman A, Jonsson PV, Schmidt H, Lathrop M, Mosley TH, Au R, Psaty BM, Uitterlinden AG, Farrer LA, Lumley T, Ruiz A, Williams J, Amouyel P, Younkin SG, Wolf PA, Launer LJ, Lopez OL, van Duijn CM, Breteler MM. Genome-wide analysis of genetic loci associated with alzheimer disease. *JAMA.* 2010;303:1832-1840

[53] Bigler ED, Tate DF, Miller MJ, Rice SA, Hessel CD, Earl HD, Tschanz JT, Plassman B, Welsh-Bohmer KA. Dementia, asymmetry of temporal lobe structures, and apolipoprotein e genotype: Relationships to cerebral atrophy and neuropsychological impairment. *J Int Neuropsychol Soc.* 2002;8:925-933

[54] Burggren AC, Zeineh MM, Ekstrom AD, Braskie MN, Thompson PM, Small GW, Bookheimer SY. Reduced cortical thickness in hippocampal subregions among cognitively normal apolipoprotein e e4 carriers. *NeuroImage.* 2008;41:1177-1183

[55] Morra JH, Tu Z, Apostolova LG, Green AE, Avedissian C, Madsen SK, Parikshak N, Toga AW, Jack CR, Jr., Schuff N, Weiner MW, Thompson PM. Automated mapping of hippocampal atrophy in 1-year repeat mri data from 490 subjects with alzheimer's disease, mild cognitive impairment, and elderly controls. *NeuroImage.* 2009;45:S3-15

[56] Chen K, Reiman EM, Alexander GE, Caselli RJ, Gerkin R, Bandy D, Domb A, Osborne D, Fox N, Crum WR, Saunders AM, Hardy J. Correlations between apolipoprotein

e epsilon4 gene dose and whole brain atrophy rates. *The American journal of psychiatry*. 2007;164:916-921

[57] Valla J, Yaari R, Wolf AB, Kusne Y, Beach TG, Roher AE, Corneveaux JJ, Huentelman MJ, Caselli RJ, Reiman EM. Reduced posterior cingulate mitochondrial activity in expired young adult carriers of the apoe epsilon4 allele, the major late-onset alzheimer's susceptibility gene. *J Alzheimers Dis*. 2010;22:307-313

[58] Mosconi L, Perani D, Sorbi S, Herholz K, Nacmias B, Holthoff V, Salmon E, Baron JC, De Cristofaro MT, Padovani A, Borroni B, Franceschi M, Bracco L, Pupi A. Mci conversion to dementia and the apoe genotype: A prediction study with fdg-pet. *Neurology*. 2004;63:2332-2340

[59] Scarmeas N, Anderson KE, Hilton J, Park A, Habeck C, Flynn J, Tycko B, Stern Y. Apoe-dependent pet patterns of brain activation in alzheimer disease. *Neurology*. 2004;63:913-915

[60] Mosconi L, Nacmias B, Sorbi S, De Cristofaro MT, Fayazz M, Tedde A, Bracco L, Herholz K, Pupi A. Brain metabolic decreases related to the dose of the apoe e4 allele in alzheimer's disease. *J Neurol Neurosurg Psychiatry*. 2004;75:370-376

[61] Grimmer T, Tholen S, Yousefi BH, Alexopoulos P, Forschler A, Forstl H, Henriksen G, Klunk WE, Mathis CA, Perneczky R, Sorg C, Kurz A, Drzezga A. Progression of cerebral amyloid load is associated with the apolipoprotein e epsilon4 genotype in alzheimer's disease. *Biological psychiatry*. 2010;68:879-884

[62] Reiman EM, Chen K, Liu X, Bandy D, Yu M, Lee W, Ayutyanont N, Keppler J, Reeder SA, Langbaum JB, Alexander GE, Klunk WE, Mathis CA, Price JC, Aizenstein HJ, DeKosky ST, Caselli RJ. Fibrillar amyloid-beta burden in cognitively normal people at 3 levels of genetic risk for alzheimer's disease. *Proceedings of the National Academy of Sciences of the United States of America*. 2009;106:6820-6825

[63] Drzezga A, Grimmer T, Henriksen G, Muhlau M, Perneczky R, Miederer I, Praus C, Sorg C, Wohlschlager A, Riemenschneider M, Wester HJ, Foerstl H, Schwaiger M, Kurz A. Effect of apoe genotype on amyloid plaque load and gray matter volume in alzheimer disease. *Neurology*. 2009;72:1487-1494

[64] Potkin SG, Guffanti G, Lakatos A, Turner JA, Kruggel F, Fallon JH, Saykin AJ, Orro A, Lupoli S, Salvi E, Weiner M, Macciardi F. Hippocampal atrophy as a quantitative trait in a genome-wide association study identifying novel susceptibility genes for alzheimer's disease. *PLoS One*. 2009;4:e6501

[65] Saykin AJ, Shen L, Foroud TM, Potkin SG, Swaminathan S, Kim S, Risacher SL, Nho K, Huentelman MJ, Craig DW, Thompson PM, Stein JL, Moore JH, Farrer LA, Green RC, Bertram L, Jack CR, Jr., Weiner MW. Alzheimer's disease neuroimaging initiative biomarkers as quantitative phenotypes: Genetics core aims, progress, and plans. *Alzheimers Dement*. 2010;6:265-273

[66] Shen L, Kim S, Risacher SL, Nho K, Swaminathan S, West JD, Foroud T, Pankratz N, Moore JH, Sloan CD, Huentelman MJ, Craig DW, Dechairo BM, Potkin SG, Jack CR, Jr., Weiner MW, Saykin AJ. Whole genome association study of brain-wide imaging phenotypes for identifying quantitative trait loci in mci and ad: A study of the adni cohort. *NeuroImage*. 2010;53:1051-1063

[67] Stein JL, Hua X, Morra JH, Lee S, Hibar DP, Ho AJ, Leow AD, Toga AW, Sul JH, Kang HM, Eskin E, Saykin AJ, Shen L, Foroud T, Pankratz N, Huentelman MJ, Craig DW, Gerber JD, Allen AN, Corneveaux JJ, Stephan DA, Webster J, DeChairo BM, Potkin

SG, Jack CR, Jr., Weiner MW, Thompson PM. Genome-wide analysis reveals novel genes influencing temporal lobe structure with relevance to neurodegeneration in alzheimer's disease. *NeuroImage*. 2010;51:542-554

[68] Ho AJ, Stein JL, Hua X, Lee S, Hibar DP, Leow AD, Dinov ID, Toga AW, Saykin AJ, Shen L, Foroud T, Pankratz N, Huentelman MJ, Craig DW, Gerber JD, Allen AN, Corneveaux JJ, Stephan DA, DeCarli CS, DeChairo BM, Potkin SG, Jack CR, Jr., Weiner MW, Raji CA, Lopez OL, Becker JT, Carmichael OT, Thompson PM. A commonly carried allele of the obesity-related fto gene is associated with reduced brain volume in the healthy elderly. *Proceedings of the National Academy of Sciences of the United States of America*. 2010;107:8404-8409

[69] Schuur M, van Swieten JC, Schol-Gelok S, Ikram MA, Vernooij MW, Liu F, Isaacs A, de Boer R, de Koning I, Niessen WJ, Vrooman H, Oostra BA, van der Lugt A, Breteler MM, van Duijn CM. Genetic risk factors for cerebral small-vessel disease in hypertensive patients from a genetically isolated population. *J Neurol Neurosurg Psychiatry*. 2011;82:41-44

[70] K TC, Lunetta KL, Baldwin CT, McKee AC, Guo J, Cupples LA, Green RC, St George-Hyslop PH, Chui H, DeCarli C, Farrer LA. Association of distinct variants in sorl1 with cerebrovascular and neurodegenerative changes related to alzheimer disease. *Archives of neurology*. 2008;65:1640-1648

[71] Liang WS, Chen K, Lee W, Sidhar K, Corneveaux JJ, Allen AN, Myers A, Villa S, Meechoovet B, Pruzin J, Bandy D, Fleisher AS, Langbaum JB, Huentelman MJ, Jensen K, Dunckley T, Caselli RJ, Kaib S, Reiman EM. Association between gab2 haplotype and higher glucose metabolism in alzheimer's disease-affected brain regions in cognitively normal apoeepsilon4 carriers. *NeuroImage*. 2011;54:1896-1902

[72] Wittenberg GM, Tsien JZ. An emerging molecular and cellular framework for memory processing by the hippocampus. *Trends in neurosciences*. 2002;25:501-505

[73] Jackson GD, Berkovic SF, Tress BM, Kalnins RM, Fabinyi GC, Bladin PF. Hippocampal sclerosis can be reliably detected by magnetic resonance imaging. *Neurology*. 1990;40:1869-1875

[74] Eriksson PS, Perfilieva E, Bjork-Eriksson T, Alborn AM, Nordborg C, Peterson DA, Gage FH. Neurogenesis in the adult human hippocampus. *Nature medicine*. 1998;4:1313-1317

[75] Gould E, Beylin A, Tanapat P, Reeves A, Shors TJ. Learning enhances adult neurogenesis in the hippocampal formation. *Nature neuroscience*. 1999;2:260-265

[76] Gallagher M, Landfield PW, McEwen B, Meaney MJ, Rapp PR, Sapolsky R, West MJ. Hippocampal neurodegeneration in aging. *Science (New York, N.Y.* 1996;274:484-485

[77] Harding AJ, Halliday GM, Kril JJ. Variation in hippocampal neuron number with age and brain volume. *Cereb Cortex*. 1998;8:710-718

[78] Cameron HA, McKay RD. Restoring production of hippocampal neurons in old age. *Nature neuroscience*. 1999;2:894-897

[79] Kempermann G, Kuhn HG, Gage FH. Experience-induced neurogenesis in the senescent dentate gyrus. *J Neurosci*. 1998;18:3206-3212

[80] Rampon C, Tang YP, Goodhouse J, Shimizu E, Kyin M, Tsien JZ. Enrichment induces structural changes and recovery from nonspatial memory deficits in ca1 nmdar1-knockout mice. *Nature neuroscience*. 2000;3:238-244

[81] Rampon C, Tsien JZ. Genetic analysis of learning behavior-induced structural plasticity. *Hippocampus*. 2000;10:605-609

[82] Kornack DR, Rakic P. Continuation of neurogenesis in the hippocampus of the adult macaque monkey. *Proceedings of the National Academy of Sciences of the United States of America*. 1999;96:5768-5773

[83] White T, Andreasen NC, Nopoulos P. Brain volumes and surface morphology in monozygotic twins. *Cereb Cortex*. 2002;12:486-493

[84] Scamvougeras A, Kigar DL, Jones D, Weinberger DR, Witelson SF. Size of the human corpus callosum is genetically determined: An mri study in mono and dizygotic twins. *Neuroscience letters*. 2003;338:91-94

17

Neuroimaging Findings in Dementia with Lewy Body: A Review

Francesca Baglio, Maria Giulia Preti and Elisabetta Farina
Fondazione Don Carlo Gnocchi ONLUS Milano
Politecnico di Milano
Italy

1. Introduction

1.1 Dementia with Lewy bodies: An overview

Dementia with Lewy bodies (DLB) is a progressive neurodegenerative disorder characterized by the core clinical features of fluctuating consciousness, visual hallucinations and parkinsonism.

The term DLB and the clinical criteria were first introduced and proposed by Mc Keith and colleagues in 1996 during the First International Workshop of the Consortium on Dementia with Lewy Bodies (McKeith et al., 1996) and were revised in 2005 to improve the sensitivity for diagnosis (McKeith et al., 2005). Interestingly, in these revised criteria, imaging with Single Photon Emission Computed Tomography (SPECT) or Positron Emission Tomography (PET) played an important role for the first time in the clinical diagnostic criteria of a dementia and was included as a suggestive feature supporting the diagnosis.

After Alzheimer's disease (AD), DLB is now considered the second most common type of degenerative dementia in elderly people (Aarsland et al., 2008; McKeith et al., 2004) observed in 15 to 25% of autopsy series (Heidebrink, 2002; McKeith et al., 1996; Perry et al., 1990). These percentages are consistent with the few available epidemiological population-based studies (de Silva et al., 2003; Herrera et al., 2002; Rahkonen et al., 2003; Stevens et al., 2002; Yamada et al., 2001; Yamada et al., 2002), which have reported the prevalence of DLB ranging from 0 to 30.5% of all dementia cases in individuals older than 65 years and from 0 to 5% in the general population (Zaccai et al., 2005). However, DLB is a regularly misdiagnosed clinical condition, with autopsy reports indicating a higher frequency than that detected in clinical settings (Farina et al., 2009; Mollenhauer et al., 2010).

The pathological background of DLB has been a matter of controversy and is a complex issue (see Fig. 1). The core neuropathological finding is the presence of α-synuclein aggregates which form neuronal inclusions called Lewy bodies (LBs). According to the consensus pathological guidelines, based on a semiquantitative scoring of α-synuclein pathology (LBs density and distribution) in specific brain regions, DLB is distinguished into three different phenotypes (brainstem, transitional/limbic, and diffuse neocortical). Moreover, DLB pathological features are often associated to various degrees of AD pathology (i.e. limbic and neocortical spread of LB lesions with or without concomitant AD amyloid plaque pathology).

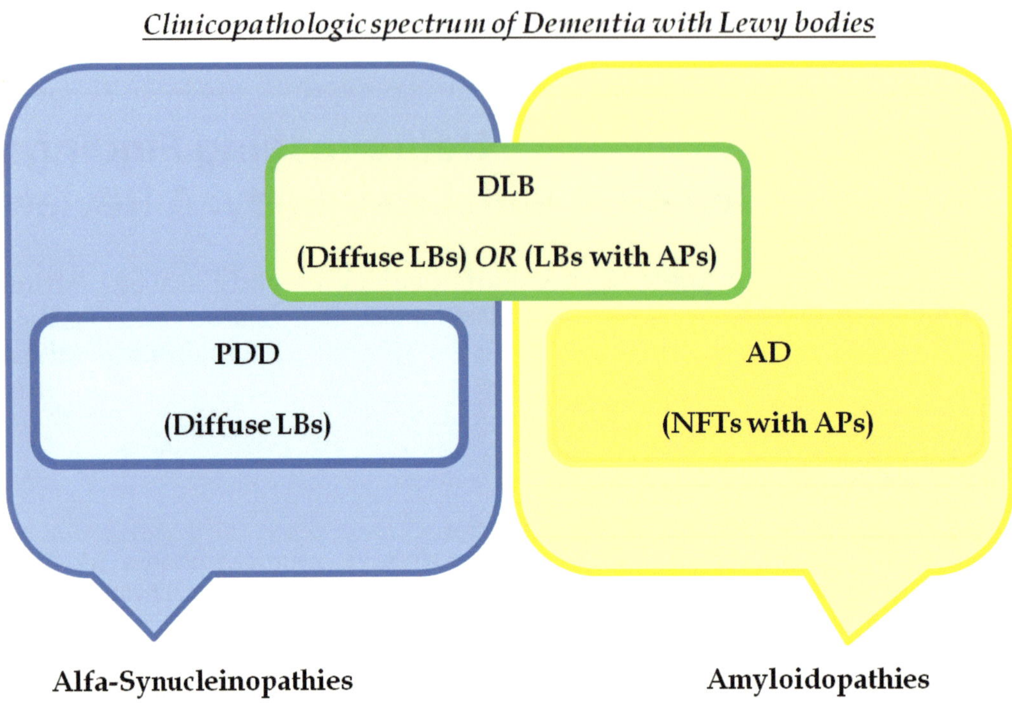

Fig. 1. Clinicopathological interaction between dementia with Lewy bodies (DLB), Parkinson's disease dementia (PDD) and Alzheimer's disease (AD). LBs: Lewy Bodies; NFTs: neurofibrillary tangles; APs: amyloid plaques.

As previously described, the clinical criteria for the diagnosis of DLB were established in 1996 (McKeith et al., 1996) and revised in 2005 (McKetih et al., 2005) to include additional suggestive clinical features (REM sleep behaviour disorder and severe neuroleptic sensitivity) as well as specific neuroradiological findings (Dopamine SPECT or PET imaging). The central feature for the diagnosis, that must be present for either probable or possible DLB, is a condition of dementia. This dementia is defined as a progressive cognitive decline of sufficient magnitude to interfere with normal social or occupational function and with prominent deficits on tests of attention, executive function, and visuospatial ability. The cognitive deficits are not necessarily associated with memory impairment at list at the early stages of the diseases. Then, "probable" DLB is characterized by the presence of this central characteristic with any two of the three core features (fluctuating cognition, recurrent visual hallucinations, or parkinsonism) or one core feature and one suggestive feature, whereas "possible" DLB is diagnosed in the absence of any core features but in the presence of one or more suggestive features. Finally, clinical criteria also includes supportive features (commonly present but not proven to have diagnostic specificity) and findings that do not support DLB (see Table 1 for a detailed description of clinical criteria).

DLB shares many common clinical (motor, cognitive, attentional, and psychiatric symptoms), neuropsychological (prominent deficits on tests of attention, executive function, and visuospatial ability) and pathological features (LBs α-synuclein aggregates) with Parkinson Disease Dementia (PDD). In the last years, in fact, DLB and PDD have been both included in the same nosological chapter of synucleinopathies, that is Lewy Body Dementias

<table>
<tr><td colspan="3">THE CLINICAL DIAGNOSTIC CRITERIA FOR DEMENTIA WITH LEWY BODIES
from the Third International report of the DLB consortium
(McKeith et al, 2005)</td></tr>
<tr><td>CENTRAL FEATURE
□ Dementia with impairment in everyday functioning.
□ Prominent or persistent memory impairment may not necessarily occur in the early stages but is usually evident with progression.
□ Deficits on tests of attention, executive function, and visuospatial ability may be especially prominent.</td><td>CORE FEATURES
□ Fluctuating cognition with pronounced variations in attention and alertness
□ Recurrent visual hallucinations
□ Parkinsonism</td><td>SUGGESTIVE features
□ REM sleep behavior disorder
□ Severe neuroleptic sensitivity
□ Reduced dopaminergic activity in basal ganglia (SPECT or PET imaging)</td></tr>
<tr><td colspan="3">For a diagnosis of "Probable" DLB:
Central feature AND two core features - OR -Central feature AND one or more core features with one or more suggestive features
For a diagnosis of "Possible" DLB:
Central feature AND one core feature - OR - Central feature AND one or more suggestive features
--
Timing cut-off
"one -year rule" between the onset of dementia and parkinsonism to distinguish DLB and PDD</td></tr>
<tr><td colspan="3">SUPPORTIVE FEATURES
these are often present but do not have diagnostic specificity
□ Repeated falls and syncope
□ Transient, unexplained loss of consciousness
□ Severe autonomic dysfunction, e.g., orthostatic hypotension, urinary incontinence
□ Hallucinations in other modalities
□ Systematized delusions
□ Depression
□ Relative preservation of medial temporal lobe structures on CT/MRI scan
□ Generalized low uptake on SPECT/PET perfusion scan with reduced occipital activity
□ Abnormal (low uptake) MIBG myocardial scintigraphy
□ Prominent slow wave activity on EEG with temporal lobe transient sharp waves</td></tr>
<tr><td colspan="3">FINDINGS THAT DO NOT SUPPORT DLB
□ Presence of cerebrovascular lesions on brain imaging (brain CT or MRI) or focal neurologic signs
□ Presence of any other physical illness or brain disorder sufficient to explain the clinical symptoms
□ Parkinsonism that occurs for the first time when dementia is severe</td></tr>
</table>

Table 1. The clinical diagnostic criteria for dementia with Lewy bodies taken from the third international report of the DLB consortium (McKeith et al., 2005). SPECT: single photon emission computed tomography; PET: positron emission tomography; CT: computed tomography; MRI: magnetic resonance imaging; MIBG: 31-iodine metaiodobenzylguanidine single photon emission computed tomography; EEG: electroencephalography.

(Lippa et al., 2007). PDD should be the suspected diagnosis in patients with Parkinson's disease (PD) who develop cognitive deficits and/or behavioural disturbances such as hallucinations during the course of their illness (Emre et al., 2007). These two diseases are so closely related that they are distinguished by an arbitrary cut-off ("one year rule") in the timing of motor compared to cognitive dimensions (PDD can be diagnosed only when cognitive deterioration supervenes after one year of the motor symptoms onset). Their response to the treatment with acetylcholinesterase inhibitors (AChEI) and the side effects associated with administration of conventional neuroleptic drugs are similar. Whether the distinction between PDD and DLB is nowadays based on an arbitrary time criterion, the distinction between DLB and other types of dementias such as Alzheimer Disease (AD) at the onset (Watson et al., 2009) is not always straightforward. Particularly, clinical differentiation between DLB and AD is sometimes difficult in the early stage because the symptoms overlap and the cognitive decline can also appear without the parkinsonism. In case of clinical uncertainty some additional investigation for differential diagnosis can be helpful: neuropsychological evaluation with formal tests, neuroimaging tools such as magnetic resonance imaging (MRI) or nuclear medical procedures (PET/SPECT), electroencephalography (EEG) and cerebrospinal fluid analysis.

2. Neuroimaging techniques contribution to DLB diagnosis

In this chapter we propose a systematic literature review concerning the principal neuroimaging techniques used for the diagnosis of DLB and their results. In contrast to PET and SPECT analysis, MRI represents a non-invasive tool to assess changes in macroscopic tissue structure (conventional MRI), microstructure (diffusion tensor imaging, DTI), metabolism (MR Spectroscopy, MRS), and cerebral activity (functional MRI, fMRI), and could bring invaluable additional information for the diagnosis of the pathology. The systematic literature search was performed using the computer database MEDLINE accessed via the Web of Knowledge. Two searches were performed including the following terms: "radionuclide imaging"[MeSH Terms] AND "lewy body disease"[MeSH Terms] for the first and "magnetic resonance imaging"[MeSH Terms] AND "lewy body disease"[MeSH Terms] for the second search. We limited the results with these criteria: Humans studies, English language, and publication date of last five years (from 2005/01/01 to 2011/03/01). The period was limited to the last five years in order to include works published after the revision of the clinical criteria for DLB (McKeith et al., 2005). This search produced a total of 165 papers, which were screened individually by title and abstract, looking for information pertaining to PET/SPECT and MR studies in DLB. Moreover, the bibliographies of relevant papers were hand searched to find additional references. In this way, 84 original research papers were identified.

2.1 Functional nuclear imaging techniques to diagnose DLB

The above mentioned techniques PET and SPECT represent well-established, reliable imaging methods to assess the functional and metabolic brain changes in DLB (McKeith et al., 2005; McKeith et al., 2007). In Box A, technical aspects of these techniques are briefly summarized. The role of these techniques is well defined in the context of DLB (McKeith et al., 2007), although these procedures are very expensive and not widely used in common radiological settings. Moreover, the need of radioactive isotope injection limits the application of these exams only to cases of uncertain or difficult diagnosis.

Box A: Functional Nuclear Imaging Techniques: PET and SPECT

Positron Emission Tomography (PET) and Single Photon Emission Computed Tomography (SPECT) are highly specialized nuclear imaging techniques which provide a means to quantitatively study the metabolic processes within the body and reliably reveal functional abnormalities in the presence of various diseases.

PET acquisitions require firstly the injection of a short-lived radioactive isotope, which combines itself with a specific biologic molecule present in the body. This procedure permits to observe the concentration of that molecule in different structures. After a determined period of time, the isotope decays with the emission of a positron which immediately annihilates with an electron, producing a pair of gamma rays in opposite directions. Particular rings of detectors containing special crystals that produce light when hit by a gamma ray are included within the PET scanner, and the scanner's electronics record these detected gamma rays during the acquisition and map an image of the area where the radiopharmaceutical is located. This process allows the observation of the metabolic activity of the biologic molecule combined with the radiopharmaceutical. For example, glucose combined with a radioisotope will show the pathway followed by glucose in the brain, in the heart, or in a growing tumour.

SPECT procedure of image acquisition is similar to PET, but simpler, as particular radiopharmaceuticals are employed, which directly emit gamma rays during their decay. Larger detectors of gamma rays rotate around the patient.

In this way, nuclear medicine techniques of neuroimaging are able to measure the physiological functioning of the brain, and can be useful to diagnose a multitude of medical conditions, e.g. heart disease, infection, the spread of cancer, thyroid disease, but also stroke, head trauma, dementia. The results of the analysis are spatial colour maps of the radioactivity distribution within tissues and with these images it could be shown that maps of activated brain regions could be produced by detecting the indirect effects of neural activity on variables such as Cerebral Blood Flux (Fox et al., 1986), Cerebral Blood Volume (Fox and Raichle, 1985) and blood oxygenation (Fox and Raichle, 1985; Frostig et al., 1990). Thanks to the double photon emission in PET, the acquisition with PET generates results faster and therefore limits radiation exposure to the patient. The amount of radiation exposure the patient receives in PET is about the same as two chest X-rays.

In respect to fMRI, PET requires multiple acquisitions and the combination of multiple individual brain images in order to obtain a reliable signal. This results in an extension of the acquisition time.

Furthermore, PET and SPECT do not provide structural information about the inspected tissues, therefore the acquisition of images using other imaging techniques such as structural MRI is needed, to precisely localize the resulting activations. Alternatively, in modern PET-CT scans the combined acquisition of a computer tomography (CT) is performed.

2.1.1 Single Photon Emission Computed Tomography (SPECT)

SPECT studies on DLB have been mainly addressed to the investigation of: 1) efficiency of dopamine transporter (DAT) in the the nigrostriatal pathway (usually referred to as DAT imaging); 2) the characteristics of perfusion within brain compartments.

DAT SPECT is useful in DLB for the investigation of dopaminergic neurons in basal ganglia (caudatum and putamen), as previous literature proved that a loss of dopaminergic neurostriatal neurons is detectable in DLB but not in AD (Piggott et al., 1999; Suzuki et al., 2002). The first ligand used in dopaminergic SPECT was [123I]-2b-carbomethoxy-3b-(4-iodophenyl) tropane (b-CIT). More recently, the ligand [123I] N-x-flouropropyl-2b-carbomethoxy-3b-(4-iodophenyl) nortropane (FP-CIT) was introduced, requiring a shorter time interval between injection and scanning (R. W. H. Walker and Z. Walker, 2009). SPECT with this ligand (FP-CIT SPECT) has been included in the last revision of the International Consensus Criteria for DLB (McKeith et al., 2005). In particular, in a phase III multicentre study among a large cohort of subjects, McKeith and co-workers (McKeith et al., 2007) determined the effectiveness of FP-CIT SPECT to distinguish DLB from other dementias (principally AD), revealing a sensitivity and specificity of respectively 78% and 90% respectively. So far, there have been published many studies that investigated DLB by dopaminergic SPECT (Colloby et al., 2005; David et al., 2008; Lim et al., 2009; O'brien et al., 2009; Roselli et al., 2009; Walker et al., 2007). All these works consistently show the diagnostic value of dopaminergic SPECT as applied to DLB, through the evaluation of the striatal dopaminergic innervations reduction, also in the distinction from other dementias (Soret et al., 2006). In particular, Lim and colleagues (Lim et al., 2009) compared b-CIT SPECT with FDG-PET in the investigation of patients with DLB and AD, concluding that SPECT shows higher accuracy than PET in improving the diagnostic confidence of DLB. Moreover, Roselli et al. (Roselli et al., 2009) found significant correlations between decreased striatal DAT levels and visual hallucinations in DLB patients. The association of behavioural disturbances and SPECT analysis was also investigated (David et al., 2008), in order to assess the relationship between apathy and DAT uptake in DLB and AD patients: a significant correlation was found between lack of initiative and bilateral putamen DAT uptake, demonstrating a relationship between apathy and DAT levels.

Perfusion SPECT studies, instead, use markers such as ^{99}mTc- hexamethylpropyleneamine oxime to identify deficits in the functional pattern of brain activity. The majority of available studies highlighted a characteristic pattern of hypoperfusion in DLB patients in parietal and occipital brain areas (Brockhuis et al., 2006; Hanyu et al., 2006a; Lobotesis et al., 2001). However, other studies also suggested the presence of hypoperfusion in the frontal, parietal, and temporal cortex and in the thalamus (Chang et al., 2008). The differentiation between AD and DLB patients was often investigated by means of this second perfusion-based SPECT approach, in order to identify characteristic features allowing to distinguish between the two most common types of dementias (Colloby et al., 2010a; Colloby et al., 2010b; Goto et al., 2010; Kasama et al., 2005; Kemp et al., 2005; Mito et al., 2005; Shimizu et al., 2005; Shimizu et al., 2008; Tateno et al., 2008a). When compared with AD, DLB patients presented a preserved perfusion in the medial temporal lobe structures and a hypoperfusion in the occipital lobes, besides an increased perfusion in the striatum and thalamus bilaterally. In a recent study by Colloby and colleagues (Colloby et al., 2010a), the utility of ^{99}mTc-exametazime SPECT in the distinction between AD and DLB was verified through a Region Of Interest (ROI) approach and the Principal Component Analysis (PCA). The ROI analysis showed decreased regional CBF in AD compared to DLB, in the medial temporal lobe, in the striatum bilaterally and in the right thalamus.

Moreover, a distinction between the two groups was possible through the analysis of the principal components (PCs). Two components, in fact, were identified as being differentially affected in AD and DLB. The former revealed concomitant decreased perfusion in the medial temporal lobes and increased perfusion in the cerebellum of AD compared to DLB patients. Conversely, the latter represented a concomitant increase of regional CBF in thalamus bilaterally ,and in the right striatum of DLB compared to AD patients.

Interestingly, SPECT imaging was also used in combination with other measures to better detect changes in DLB. Several studies (Hanyu et al., 2006b; Inui et al., 2007; Novellino et al., 2010; Tateno et al., 2008b) which combined SPECT and (1,2,3)I-metaiodobenzylguanidine myocardial (MIBG) scintigraphy reported that the accuracy power in the diagnostic process of DLB resulted increased. Furthermore, Goto and colleagues (Goto et al., 2010) proposed to combine the computation of ratios on perfusion SPECT with MRI volumetric data (hippocampal, occipital, and striatal structures) to discriminate between DLB and AD. They found that the striatal volume and the occipital SPECT ratio in the DLB group was lower than that in the AD group and concluded that the combination of SPECT and MRI might contribute to a successful differential diagnosis of DLB. Chang et al. (Chang et al., 2008), instead, demonstrated the efficacy of perfusion SPECT combined with neuropsychological evaluation to differentiate early stage DLB patients at early clinical stage from those suffering from PD. SPECT images analysed with a ROI approach resulted in a pattern of significant hypoperfusion in DLB compared with healthy controls in frontal, parietal, thalamic, and temporal areas; consistent to this imaging finding, neuropsychological tests revealed the presence of deficits in DLB patients with respect to controls including the following cognitive domains: mental manipulation, short-term memory, abstract thinking, drawing and semantic verbal fluencies. Compared with PD, DLB patients showed significantly reduced SPECT signals in temporal areas and had lower scores at neuropsychological evaluation for mental manipulation, drawing and semantic verbal fluency. Conversely, SPECT analyses (FP-CIT and DAT) were unable to discriminate DLB and PDD (Rossi et al., 2009), thus supporting the hypothesis that these two forms of dementia belong to a continuum spectrum of a unique disease.

In conclusion, the two different SPECT analyses (DAT and perfusion) have proven to be both useful, but DAT scan seems to be more robust and accurate for diagnostic purposes, as described in a recent study by Colloby and colleagues (Colloby et al., 2008). These authors directly compared the performances of the two SPECT approaches when applied to the differential diagnosis between AD and DLB, and identified dopaminergic SPECT as the technique with higher diagnostic accuracy (ROC curve area 0.83, sensitivity 78.6%, specificity 87.9% in respect to perfusion SPECT with ROC curve area 0.64, sensitivity 64.3%, specificity 63.6%).

2.1.2 Positron Emission Tomography (PET)

Together with SPECT, PET allows the functional investigation of brain activity and metabolism (see Box A) and therefore represents a powerful instrument for the early detection of dementia (Koeppe et al., 2005), since it was proven that brain function deficit in dementia occurs long before disease clinical evidences (Tartaglia et al., 2011). The use of different radioisotopes increases PET versatilities. Depending on the specific tracer used, in fact, PET imaging allows the representation of specific molecules, and therefore the analysis of different functioning systems (e.g. the neural energy metabolism with F-18 2-fluoro-2-deoxy-D-glucose; the cholinergic way with N-11C-methyl-4-piperidyl acetate; the dopaminergic with 18fluorodopa; the brain amyloid burden with Pittsburgh compound B).

The more common tracer used in PET clinical studies is the F-18 2-fluoro-2-deoxy-D-glucose (FDG), which provides information about neuronal energy metabolism, in terms of regional glucose uptake. In the context of DLB, previous FDG-PET studies revealed a pattern of hypometabolism in the medial occipital cortex (Klein et al., 2010; Perneczky et al., 2008a; Satoh et al., 2010), in agreement with the previously reported SPECT data of hypoperfusion. Furthermore, other literature data found a correlation between cerebral hypometabolism in right temporoparietal cortex, prefrontal cortex and the precuneus and patients' performance level of everyday competence (Perneczky et al., 2008b; Perneczky et al., 2009a). Moreover, a recent study by Miyazawa and co-workers (Miyazawa et al., 2010) introduced a new pattern of hypermetabolism in DLB regarding three different areas: the peri-motor area, the basal ganglia and the cerebellum. Interestingly, only patients with hypermetabolism in all these three areas experimented recurrent visual hallucinations, therefore authors concluded that this pattern may be related to the core features of this behavioural disturbance.

In recent years, these relationships between brain perfusion and symptoms domain were well investigated (Fujishiro et al., 2010; Miyazawa et al., 2010; Nagahama et al., 2008; Nagahama et al., 2010; O'Brien et al., 2005; O'Brien et al., 2008; Perneczky et al., 2010). The cognitive performances on visual spatial and attentional tasks in DLB were proved to be closely related to the frontal-subcortical network dysfunction of these patients (Nagahama et al., 2008; Perneczky et al., 2008a; Perneczky et al., 2009b; Perneczky et al., 2010). A recent FDG-PET study by Fujishiro and colleagues (Fujishiro et al., 2010) demonstrated the correlation between REM sleep behaviour disorder and the development of DLB, observing that the typical pattern of occipital hypometabolism on FDG-PET clearly manifested in patient with DLB also in prodromal stages. Furthermore, distinguishable cerebral networks were associated with different psychotic symptoms in DLB patients: dysfunctions of the parietal-occipital association cortices with visual hallucinations; dysfunctions of limbic and paralimbic structures with misidentification and relative hyperperfusion in the frontal cortex with delusions (Nagahama et al., 2010; Perneczky et al., 2008a; Perneczky et al., 2009b).

As to the comparison with PD, instead, a metabolic decrease was found in DLB in the inferior and medial frontal lobes and in the right parietal lobe (Yong et al., 2007). Moreover, a comparison with PDD revealed similar pattern of metabolism reduction for PDD and DLB, except for the anterior cingulated and these findings support the hypothesis that these types of dementias are closely related and may be included in a unique spectrum (Yong et al., 2007). These data are concordant with an innovative multitracer PET study on PDD, PD and DLB patients, which aims at highlighting the complex damage pattern at the base of these conditions (Klein et al., 2010). For the first time, a multidimensional approach was introduced to detect the complex issue of the neuropathological spectrum of Lewy Body dementias (see Fig. 1): besides FDG, 18fluorodopa (FDOPA) was used to study the dopaminergic system and N-11C-methyl-4-piperidyl acetate (MP4A) for the cholinergic one, aiming on identifying the different characteristics of these systems. The results did not succeed in the distinction between the two conditions of DLB and PDD, but allowed to identify the metabolic features of the observed neuronal systems. A dopaminergic deficit was showed in the amygdala, in the anterior cingulated and in the prefrontal cortex of patients compared to controls, whereas the analysis with MP4A highlighted a cholinergic deficit regarding the occipital cortex. As this cholinergic impairment did not regard PD patients without dementias, it seemed to be directly responsible for the development of dementia in addition to motor symptoms. In line with previous studies, FDG-PET underlined a pattern of hypometabolism in correspondence of the cholinergic deficit, in the parieto-occipital brain regions. Taken together, in agreement with Klein and co-workers, these findings strengthen the concept that PDD and DLB represent two sides of the same coin in a continuum of Lewy Body Diseases.

When facing the issue of the comparison between DLB and AD, the FDOPA PET represent an interesting way to distinguish between the two pathologies, since differently from DLB, AD is not affected by a dopaminergic dysfunction. Moreover, in this context also FDG-PET demonstrated effectiveness, revealing a decrease in the occipitotemporal metabolism of DLB, in accordance with the visual processing problems that primarily DLB patients report (Gilman et al., 2005).

The recent development of new PET ligands which can bind amyloid, such as the radiolabeled Pittsburgh compound B ([11C]PiB), opened new frontiers on the study of amyloid metabolism through PET (Tartaglia et al., 2011). This aspect appears of importance in the study of DLB, since it was proven to be associated with amyloid deposition, as it happens in Alzheimer Disease (Brooks et al., 2009). Previous literature suggested a similar pattern of amyloid high cortical deposition in AD and DLB (Backsai et al., 2007; Fodero-Tavoletti et al., 2007; Maetzler et al., 2009), whereas conflicting data are reported about the comparison between DLB and PDD. In fact, ([11C]PiB)-PET studies reported a significant increase in the amyloid load in DLB compared to PDD (Edison et al., 2008; Gomperts et al., 2008), demonstrating the efficacy of this technique in the distinction between DLB and PDD. On the contrary, Foster and colleagues (Foster et al., 2010) showed that amyloid deposition did not allow differentation between different subtypes of Lewy Body associated disorders.

In conclusion, the power of PET as well as SPECT analysis is represented by the modalities versatility, allowing the study of the different and complex neuropathological substrates of DLB which is not possible with other imaging modalities without tracers (Herholz et al., 2007; Kemp et al., 2007). Nevertheless, the limits imposed by the use of radioactive isotope injection and high costs must be taken in consideration.

2.2 MRI-based analyses techniques: Adding useful information to clinicians

The importance of introducing advanced MR imaging techniques in the DLB diagnosis beside nuclear imaging methods is due to their capability to non-invasively detect early changes which could be potential biomarkers of the pathology. These MRI-based techniques can be used in large-scale studies thanks to the wide availability of MR scanners in clinics. MRI is a complex field including different approaches which permit the investigation of several aspects of brain structure and function. The clinical utility of structural neuroimaging with MRI for diagnosis and differential diagnosis of dementias is well-established (Hentschel et al., 2005), however, conventional MRI in association with advanced methods of image processing (e.g. voxel-based morphometry) represent a powerful tool in tissue structure analysis. Moreover, the investigation of microstructural changes is permitted by DTI through the observation of water molecular displacements within tissues. Cerebral activity is also detectable by functional MRI (fMRI) techniques. In the following, we summarise the principal literature findings in the study of DLB obtained using the above mentioned MRI approaches.

2.2.1 Voxel Based Morphometry (VBM)

The analysis with the technique of voxel based morphometry (VBM) on Magnetic Resonance images is one of the most widespread MRI-based approaches aimed at quantifying regional differences across subjects in brain tissue volumes (see Box B for technical details). In the context of DLB, the use of VBM appears highly promising to investigate the pattern of gray and white matter (GM and WM) atrophy and the severity of the damage.

Several literature studies used VBM to demonstrate the differences between DLB and PDD, and converged to reveal a pattern of more pronounced gray matter atrophy in DLB compared to PDD. These results appear in concordance with the ([11C]PiB)-PET findings of greater structural cortical changes in DLB related to amyloid burden (Edison et al., 2008; Gomperts et al., 2008). However, the distribution of this GM loss appears very heterogeneous among the different studies, and regards: the temporal (Beyer et al., 2007; Tam et al., 2005), parietal and occipital lobes (Beyer et al., 2007; Lee et al., 2010a), striatal areas (Lee et al., 2010a), right premotor areas, right inferior frontal lobe and right superior frontal gyrus (Sanchez-Castaneda et al., 2009). In a recent study, Sanchez-Castaneda and colleagues (Sanchez-Castaneda et al., 2010) found a different pattern of structural and functional correlations between the two dementias, in particular: decreases in volume in associative visual areas, left precuneus and inferior frontal lobe which correlates with visual hallucinations only in DLB. A possible explanation for these different results is the heterogeneity (e.g. disease duration, stage of dementia) amongst patients with PDD (patients who developed dementia early or later in the course of their illness) who are included in these small size studies. Moreover, the same pattern of atrophy measured in GM of DLB in respect to PDD was found also in WM by Lee and co-workers (Lee et al., 2010a). In their recent study, they demonstrated a significant decrease of the WM density in DLB, specifically in the bilateral occipital and left occipito-parietal areas. Moreover, they found that the atrophy level of GM and WM was similar in DLB patients, whereas WM damage was observed to a lesser severity in respect to GM loss in PDD. Taken together, these data may reflect the different nature of neuropathological aspects or potentially the different neuropathological stages regarding PDD and DLB. Further studies including a better clinical characterisation of patients (e.g. matching for age, dementia duration, and treatments) are needed to clarify the topic and delete this potential bias.

As to the comparison between DLB and AD, the distinction in terms of cerebral atrophy between these two groups was not well defined. A few recent studies attempted to identify a pattern of cortical atrophy which could distinguish DLB patients from AD patients (Burton et al., 2009; Whitwell et al., 2007). Whitwell et al. (Whitwell et al., 2007) highlighted a more severe cortical atrophy in AD compared to DLB patients regarding the medial temporal lobe, inferior temporal regions, the hippocampus and the temporoparietal cortex. Both groups revealed a pattern of damage in the midbrain and substantia innominata, although DLB patients showed a greater loss regarding the midbrain whereas AD regarding the substantia innominata. Thus, the specific pattern of cortical atrophy able to characterize DLB from AD was identified by Whitwell as a relatively focused loss in midbrain, substantia innominata and hypothalamus, with a sparing in hippocampus and temporal cortex. Changes in substantia innominata suggesting cholinergic impairment of DLB were also detected by Hanyu and co-workers (Hanyu et al., 2005; Hanyu et al., 2007). Furthermore, other studies found that the temporal (Beyer et al., 2007; Burton et al., 2009; Takahashi et al., 2010) and frontal lobes (Beyer et al., 2007) are potentially interested by a more pronounced cortical loss in AD compared to DLB. In particular, Burton and colleagues (Burton et al., 2009) showed that medial temporal lobe atrophy on MRI had an important role by distinguishing AD and DLB in pathologically confirmed cases.

Box B: Voxel Based Morphometry

Voxel-based morphometry (VBM) of structural MRI data is a well-established technique of group analysis which allows the comparison of regionally specific differences in the local concentration of gray matter between two groups of subjects on a voxel by voxel basis. Typically T1-weighted MRI scans enter the VBM analysis and the compared groups consist in a group of subjects with a disorder and an age-matched control group of healthy subjects, in order to highlight the features characterizing pathology, in terms of brain volumes. The technique of VBM has become increasingly popular over the last few years since it is relatively easy to use. It has also been applied to assess the patterns of grey and white matter loss regarding many different pathologies (Whitwell et al., 2007). The importance of this approach is that it gives a comprehensive assessment of anatomical differences throughout the brain, without being biased to one particular structure (Ashburner and Friston, 2000), as it does not require any a priori assumptions concerning which structures to consider. This gives to the VBM a significant advantage over more traditional region of- interest (ROI) approaches, which involve the manual delineation of the structures of interest (Withwell et al., 2007), being therefore extremely operator-dependent and scarcely reproducible.

The first step of the VBM analysis involves a spatial normalization of the images of all subjects to bring them to the same stereotactic space and perform voxel-wise comparisons. This is achieved by registering every image to one previously chosen template image, with the minimization of the residual sum of squared differences between them. Then, the gray matter is extracted from the normalized images by means of a segmentation of the different brain tissues from the images. The next step is the smoothing of gray matter images, in order to compensate for normalization errors and also to render the data more normally distributed, increasing thus the validity of parametric statistical tests. The accuracy of the gray matter segmentation step is essential in order to assure that the analysis of the proper structures of interest is performed.

After that, the voxel-wise statistical analysis is performed with the aim of identifying positions in the brain where the gray matter concentration differs significantly between groups. The General Linear Model (GLM) is used for the statistical analysis, allowing many different tests to be applied, as group comparisons and identification of regions of gray matter concentration that are related to particular covariates (e.g. pathology severity, age). The output from the method is a statistical parametric map showing regions where gray matter concentration differences between the compared groups appear statistically significant.

Obviously the image pre-processing of the VBM analysis is required to be extremely accurate and rigorous to avoid errors of interpretation caused by misclassification of non-brain voxels or voxels belonging to other tissues, and to allow precise statistical analyses.

One shortcoming of the VBM approach is in fact represented by the decrease in the sensitivity for the detection of group differences, associated with the variability among individuals both due to sample heterogeneity and to inaccuracies introduced with the image pre-processing. In addition, the smoothing step involves a trade off to be considered: while high levels of smoothing increase the ability of the technique to detect group differences by reducing the variance, excess smoothing diminishes the accuracy in the localization of changes.

In conclusion, the main findings of these studies can be summarised in the following key points: 1) the rate of cerebral cortical atrophy of DLB patients appears higher than PDD but at the same time lower than AD; 2) the medial temporal lobe structures are more preserved in both DLB and PDD in respect to AD (Beyer et al., 2007; Burton et al., 2009; Tam et al., 2005; Whitwell et al., 2007); 3) DLB and PDD show greater changes in respect to AD in subcortical structures and this is due to dopaminergic system dysfunction (Hanyu et al., 2007; Summerfield et al., 2005; Whitwell et al. 2007).

2.2.2 Diffusion Tensor Imaging (DTI)

Diffusion weighted and diffusion tensor imaging (DTI) could play an important role in the study of DLB, thanks to the unique capability of these techniques to investigate white matter microstructural damages, which could help in the definition of a characteristic neurodegenerative pattern and consequently in the differentiation of DLB patients from other dementias. White matter diffusion characteristics are primarily assessed by means of the computation of Mean Diffusivity (MD) and Fractional Anisotropy (FA) (see Box C for further technical details).

Previous DTI studies on DLB were implemented initially with Regions Of Interest (ROI) based methods or voxel-based DTI and found diffusion abnormalities of the corpus callosum, pericallosal areas and the frontal, parietal, occipital and, less prominently, temporal white matter of patients compared with controls (Bozzali et al., 2005; Firbank et al., 2007a; Firbank et al., 2007b; Lee et al., 2010b). These findings in regions with a high prevalence of long connecting fibre tracts might suggest the presence of neurodegeneration involving associative cortices. Moreover, the selective involvement of parietal, frontal and occipital lobes might explain some of the clinical and neuropsychological features of DLB, providing a possible distinctive marker for this disease. The modest involvement of the temporal lobe, according to previously described VBM studies (Beyer et al., 2007; Burton et al., 2009; Tam et al., 2005; Takahashi et al., 2009; Whitwell et al., 2007), is consistent with the relative preservation of global neuropsychological measures and memory tasks in the early stage of DLB. More recently, Kantarci and colleagues (Kantarci et al., 2010) found increased MD in the amygdala and decreased FA in the inferior longitudinal fasciculus in DLB with respect to controls. Authors suggested that the former result could reflect the typical microvacuolation associated with LBs pathology in this structure, whereas the latter may be due to the presence of core symptoms of visual hallucinations. The encountered inferior longitudinal fasciculus damage in concordance with a tractography based study by Ota and colleagues (Ota et al., 2009) correlates with the pathology, as this bundle is responsible for visuospatial cognition and DLB is thought to involve an impairment of the visual association area.

In the above mentioned study by Ota et al. (Ota et al., 2009) the findings were supported by the computation of eigenvalues (λ_1, λ_2, λ_3), providing information about the magnitude of axial (λ_1) and radial (λ_2, λ_3) diffusivity. They found significantly lowered λ_2 and λ_3 in the inferior longitudinal fasciculus of DLB patients in respect to healthy controls, however no difference was found in λ_1. Furthermore, a recent study (Kiuchi et al., 2011) introduced the tractographic reconstruction of white matter fiber bundles not only for the study of DLB but also for the comparison with AD. The analysis was focused on the uncinate fasciculus, inferior fronto-occipital fasciculus and inferior longitudinal fasciculus. Although no significant differences were seen between AD and DLB, some different features in the FA evaluation were found between each patient group and controls. In particular, significantly lowered FA values were found in bilateral uncinate fasciculus for both AD and DLB, and in bilateral inferior fronto-occipital

Box C: Diffusion weighted and Diffusion Tensor Imaging

Diffusion Weighted Imaging (DWI) is an advanced MRI technique providing invaluable information concerning tissue structure at a microscopic scale, thanks to the observation of the molecular diffusion. The image contrast in DWI depends, in fact, on the entity of water molecule diffusive displacements in tissues, and consequently on tissue microstructure. The basic principles of DWI, which has been an important area of research in the past decade, were introduced in the mid-1980s and combined conventional MR imaging principles with the use of sharp bipolar magnetic field gradient pulses in order to encode molecular diffusion effects in MR signal. The physical process of molecular diffusion, first formally described by Einstein in 1905, refers to the random motion of molecules, also called Brownian motion, which results from the thermal energy carried by these molecules (Beaulieu, 2002). The erratic motion of molecules in a homogeneous solution is statistically described by a displacement distribution, which represents the probability that a particular molecule travels a given distance in a given time interval, and is governed by the diffusion coefficient D. In biological tissues, compared to solutions, the movement of molecules is hindered by macromolecules and cellular organelles and is also restricted by the confinement created by membranes. The macroscopic result is a decreased coefficient of diffusion, named apparent diffusion coefficient (ADC). In biological tissues with a highly anisotropic structure, such as white matter fibre bundles, diffusion is characterized by a specific directionality, since the peculiar structural arrangement of the medium limits molecular movement in some directions. To fully describe the diffusion process, it is thus necessary to investigate displacements of molecules not only along one direction, but along multiple dimensions. This is possible using Diffusion Tensor Imaging (DTI), which describes diffusion in the three-dimensional space using a tensor quantity D instead of a single coefficient. This provides a detailed mathematical description of diffusion and allows to compute the principal direction of diffusion in every position of the explored tissue, as the principal eigenvector of the tensor. Moreover, from the tensor eigenvalues (λ_1, λ_2, λ_3) computed in every voxel of the image, two useful scalar measures providing information about the diffusion features can be computed: the Mean Diffusivity (1)

$$MD = \frac{(\lambda_1 + \lambda_2 + \lambda_3)}{3} \qquad (1)$$

indicating the diffusion magnitude, and the Fractional Anisotropy (2)

$$FA = \sqrt{\frac{3}{2}} \frac{\sqrt{(\lambda_1 - MD)^2 + (\lambda_2 - MD)^2 + (\lambda_3 - MD)^2}}{\sqrt{(\lambda_1{}^2 + \lambda_2{}^2 + \lambda_3{}^2)}} \qquad (2)$$

providing an estimate of the degree of diffusion directionality. These metrics are commonly used to quantitatively assess diffusion features in healthy population and abnormalities in pathological tissues. Furthermore, DTI is at the base of the advanced technique of tractography (or fiber tracking), i.e. the virtual reconstruction of brain white matter tracts, starting from the assumption that the direction of major diffusion would indicate the overall orientation of the fibres in the brain. This technique represents one of the most important area of current research and, in combination with fMRI, opens a window on the important issue of brain connectivity.

Box D: BOLD signal and functional Magnetic Resonance Imaging

The functional Magnetic Resonance Imaging (fMRI) analysis provides invaluable information about the localization of neuronal activations related to a task or in a condition of rest, and for this reason is one of the most widely used method for brain mapping and measuring behaviour-related neural activity in the human brain. The development of functional techniques gives to MRI the ability to observe both the structures and also which structures participate in specific functions, gaining great power in the mapping of functional connectivity. Different fMRI techniques can be employed to measure the hemodynamic response, however fMRI based on blood-oxygen level-dependent (BOLD) contrast has gained great success due to its high sensitivity and accessibility (Logothetis, 2002). This contrast was firstly described by Ogawa and colleagues in 1990 (Ogawa et al., 1990a; Ogawa et al., 1990b), with the introduction of a high resolution gradient-echo-pulse sequence accentuating the susceptibility effects of deoxygenated Hemoglobin (dHb) in the venous blood and obtaining therefore a signal dependent on the blood oxygen level. In fact, dHb owns a paramagnetic nature which induces a local alterations of the magnetic field in correspondence of the compartments containing dHb, and a consequent modification the T2* weighted MRI signal. The increase in regional CBF caused by a neuronal activation does not correspond to an increase in the oxygen consumption rate (Fox & Raichle, 1985), thus a decreased oxygen extraction fraction is observable and this results in a lower dHb content per volume unit in activated tissues (Logothetis, 2002). For this reason, activated areas will be characterized by a higher BOLD signal in the image. However, it was demonstrated that BOLD contrast is actually a complex type of response controlled by several parameters, depending therefore not only on blood oxygenation, but also on cerebral blood flux and volume (Ogawa et al. 1993; Ogawa et al., 1998; Van Zijl et al. 1998; Weisskoff et al. 1994). Although the exact relation between the blood oxygen-level dependent (BOLD) signal and the underlying neural activity appears difficult to explicate, fMRI experiments allow to observe which brain areas activate in relation to the performance of a particular task. Patients are required to perform a specific task during the MRI acquisition, expecting the activation of specific corresponding brain areas during the task. This information is useful both in healthy subjects, to map the normal cerebral functions, and in presence of diseases, aiming on underlying possible changes of functionality in damaged brains. Moreover, fMRI opens a window on the complicated issue of neuronal connectivity, allowing the observation of functional connections between different areas in the brain, and of neuronal plasticity, i.e. the capability of the brain functions to change and adapt to external inputs, during life or in presence of pathologies. Recently, the fMRI analysis in a condition of resting (so called resting state condition) is gaining more attention in the current research, aiming on exploring the activated areas and their connections during rest. In respect to other techniques to map brain functional activity, some aspects characterizing fMRI can be listed as advantages of this technique: firstly, the signal does not require injections of radioactive isotopes as it happens for positron emission tomography (PET); the in-plane resolution of functional images could be less than 1 mm; furthermore, the total acquisition time can be very short, depending on the paradigm to perform.

fasciculus and left inferior longitudinal fasciculus for DLB with respect to controls, suggesting that DLB exhibited modifications in visual-related WM tractcs.
From all these studies, we can argue that tractographic reconstruction proved to be helpful for a better understanding of WM connectivity in DLB patients and in particular for the detection of visual related damages in this dementia.

2.2.3 Functional Magnetic Resonance Imaging (fMRI)

The most diffuse neuroimaging techniques for the evaluation of brain activity and function in DLB are undoubtedly the above mentioned PET and SPECT. Functional investigations with fMRI (details in Box D) in DLB are still developing and currently appears less widespread than nuclear imaging studies. A unique task-related fMRI study (Sauer et al., 2006) was conducted and investigated the pattern of activations in DLB and AD during visual colour, face and motor stimuli. A significantly greater activation of DLB compared to AD, independent on task performance, age or cognitive score, was found in the superior temporal sulcus during the motor task. Instead, performance-dependent differences were found in the activation patterns related to the motor and face task, in which the activity appeared higher for AD compared to DLB, and in the default mode network pattern, in which the effect was greater for AD and DLB with respect to controls. Authors concluded thus that fMRI can be reliably used for the detection of functional activity distribution patterns in these two conditions. However, the role of fMRI remains unclear in the study of those patients, as the significance of the found results are not completely understood. Further studies combining anatomical MRI, DTI, and resting state fMRI are needed, in order to verify the hypothesis that structural subcortico-cortical connections may provide integral routes for communication between cortical resting state networks, and that changes in the integrity of these connections have a role in this dementia.

3. Conclusion

In this chapter, we reviewed the literature concerning the study of DLB through imaging techniques. We have shown that the use of neuro-imaging methods could noticeably improve the differential diagnosis of DLB when several doubts exist. To solve this problem, the nuclear imaging methods (PET/SPECT) play nowadays the principal role (O'Brien et al., 2007). However, MRI techniques revealed interesting results and although they are now limited to the research field, except for the assessment of medial temporal lobe preservation with structural MRI, they seem to be a promising measure for detecting early and potentially preclinical DLB changes and for the validation of surrogate markers to be applied in longitudinal studies and pharmacological trials (von Gunten & Meuli, 2009; Watson et al., 2009). We think that the combination of different MRI methods may contribute to a better understanding of this often misdiagnosed pathology.

4. Acknowledgments

We are grateful to David T. Utriainen and Marco Bozzali for valuable advice on this chapter.

5. References

Aarsland, D.; Kurz, M.; Beyer, M.; Bronnick, K.; Piepenstock Nore, S. & Ballard, C. (2008). Early discriminatory diagnosis of dementia with Lewy bodies. The emerging role of CSF and imaging biomarkers. *Dementia and Geriatric Cognitive Disorders,* Vol.25, No.3, pp. 195-205, ISSN 1421-9824; 1420-8008

Ashburner, J. & Friston, K. J. (2000). Voxel-based morphometry--the methods. *NeuroImage,* Vol.11, No.6 Pt 1, pp. 805-821, ISSN 1053-8119; 1053-8119

Bacskai, B. J.; Frosch, M. P.; Freeman, S. H.; Raymond, S. B.; Augustinack, J. C.; Johnson, K. A.; Irizarry, M. C.; Klunk, W. E.; Mathis, C. A.; Dekosky, S. T.; Greenberg, S. M.; Hyman, B. T. & Growdon, J. H. (2007). Molecular imaging with Pittsburgh Compound B confirmed at autopsy: a case report. *Archives of Neurology,* Vol.64, No.3, pp. 431-434, ISSN 0003-9942; 0003-9942

Beaulieu, C. (2002). The basis of anisotropic water diffusion in the nervous system - a technical review. *NMR in Biomedicine,* Vol.15, No.7-8, pp. 435-455, ISSN 0952-3480; 0952-3480

Beyer, M. K.; Larsen, J. P. & Aarsland, D. (2007). Gray matter atrophy in Parkinson disease with dementia and dementia with Lewy bodies. *Neurology,* Vol.69, No.8, pp. 747-754, ISSN 1526-632X; 0028-3878

Bozzali, M.; Falini, A.; Cercignani, M.; Baglio, F.; Farina, E.; Alberoni, M.; Vezzulli, P.; Olivotto, F.; Mantovani, F.; Shallice, T.; Scotti, G.; Canal, N. & Nemni, R. (2005). Brain tissue damage in dementia with Lewy bodies: an in vivo diffusion tensor MRI study. *Brain : A Journal of Neurology,* Vol.128, No.Pt 7, pp. 1595-1604, ISSN 1460-2156; 0006-8950

Brockhuis, B.; Slawek, J.; Wieczorek, D.; Ussorowska, D.; Derejko, M.; Romanowicz, G.; Marks, W. & Dubaniewicz, M. (2006). Cerebral blood flow changes in patients with dementia with Lewy bodies (DLB). A study of 6 cases. *Nuclear Medicine Review.Central & Eastern Europe : Journal of Bulgarian, Czech, Macedonian, Polish, Romanian, Russian, Slovak, Yugoslav Societies of Nuclear Medicine and Ukrainian Society of Radiology,* Vol.9, No.2, pp. 114-118, ISSN 1506-9680; 1506-9680

Brooks, D. J. (2009). Imaging amyloid in Parkinson's disease dementia and dementia with Lewy bodies with positron emission tomography. *Movement Disorders : Official Journal of the Movement Disorder Society,* Vol.24 Suppl 2, pp. S742-7, ISSN 1531-8257; 0885-3185

Burton, E. J.; Barber, R.; Mukaetova-Ladinska, E. B.; Robson, J.; Perry, R. H.; Jaros, E.; Kalaria, R. N. & O'Brien, J. T. (2009). Medial temporal lobe atrophy on MRI differentiates Alzheimer's disease from dementia with Lewy bodies and vascular cognitive impairment: a prospective study with pathological verification of diagnosis. *Brain : A Journal of Neurology,* Vol.132, No.Pt 1, pp. 195-203, ISSN 1460-2156; 0006-8950

Chang, C. C.; Liu, J. S.; Chang, Y. Y.; Chang, W. N.; Chen, S. S. & Lee, C. H. (2008). (99m)Tc-ethyl cysteinate dimer brain SPECT findings in early stage of dementia with Lewy bodies and Parkinson's disease patients: a correlation with neuropsychological tests. *European Journal of Neurology : The Official Journal of the European Federation of Neurological Societies,* Vol.15, No.1, pp. 61-65, ISSN 1468-1331; 1351-5101

Colloby, S. J.; Williams, E. D.; Burn, D. J.; Lloyd, J. J.; McKeith, I. G. & O'Brien, J. T. (2005). Progression of dopaminergic degeneration in dementia with Lewy bodies and

Parkinson's disease with and without dementia assessed using 123I-FP-CIT SPECT. *European Journal of Nuclear Medicine and Molecular Imaging,* Vol.32, No.10, pp. 1176-1185, ISSN 1619-7070; 1619-7070

Colloby, S. J.; Firbank, M. J.; Pakrasi, S.; Lloyd, J. J.; Driver, I.; McKeith, I. G.; Williams, E. D. & O'Brien, J. T. (2008). A comparison of 99mTc-exametazime and 123I-FP-CIT SPECT imaging in the differential diagnosis of Alzheimer's disease and dementia with Lewy bodies. *International Psychogeriatrics / IPA,* Vol.20, No.6, pp. 1124-1140, ISSN 1041-6102; 1041-6102

Colloby, S. J.; Taylor, J. P.; Firbank, M. J.; McKeith, I. G.; Williams, E. D. & O'Brien, J. T. (2010a). Covariance 99mTc-exametazime SPECT patterns in Alzheimer's disease and dementia with Lewy bodies: utility in differential diagnosis. *Journal of Geriatric Psychiatry and Neurology,* Vol.23, No.1, pp. 54-62, ISSN 0891-9887; 0891-9887

Colloby, S. J.; Perry, E. K.; Pakrasi, S.; Pimlott, S. L.; Wyper, D. J.; McKeith, I. G.; Williams, E. D. & O'Brien, J. T. (2010b). Nicotinic 123I-5IA-85380 single photon emission computed tomography as a predictor of cognitive progression in Alzheimer's disease and dementia with Lewy bodies. *The American Journal of Geriatric Psychiatry : Official Journal of the American Association for Geriatric Psychiatry,* Vol.18, No.1, pp. 86-90, ISSN 1545-7214; 1064-7481

David, R.; Koulibaly, M.; Benoit, M.; Garcia, R.; Caci, H.; Darcourt, J. & Robert, P. (2008). Striatal dopamine transporter levels correlate with apathy in neurodegenerative diseases A SPECT study with partial volume effect correction. *Clinical Neurology and Neurosurgery,* Vol.110, No.1, pp. 19-24, ISSN 0303-8467; 0303-8467

de Silva, H. A.; Gunatilake, S. B. & Smith, A. D. (2003). Prevalence of dementia in a semi-urban population in Sri Lanka: report from a regional survey. *International Journal of Geriatric Psychiatry,* Vol.18, No.8, pp. 711-715, ISSN 0885-6230

Edison, P.; Rowe, C. C.; Rinne, J. O.; Ng, S.; Ahmed, I.; Kemppainen, N.; Villemagne, V. L.; O'Keefe, G.; Nagren, K.; Chaudhury, K. R.; Masters, C. L. & Brooks, D. J. (2008). Amyloid load in Parkinson's disease dementia and Lewy body dementia measured with [11C]PIB positron emission tomography. *Journal of Neurology, Neurosurgery, and Psychiatry,* Vol.79, No.12, pp. 1331-1338, ISSN 1468-330X; 0022-3050

Emre, M.; Aarsland, D.; Brown, R.; Burn, D. J.; Duyckaerts, C.; Mizuno, Y.; Broe, G. A.; Cummings, J.; Dickson, D. W.; Gauthier, S.; Goldman, J.; Goetz, C.; Korczyn, A.; Lees, A.; Levy, R.; Litvan, I.; McKeith, I.; Olanow, W.; Poewe, W.; Quinn, N.; Sampaio, C.; Tolosa, E. & Dubois, B. (2007). Clinical diagnostic criteria for dementia associated with Parkinson's disease. *Movement Disorders : Official Journal of the Movement Disorder Society,* Vol.22, No.12, pp. 1689-707; quiz 1837, ISSN 0885-3185

Farina, E.; Baglio, F.; Caffarra, P.; Magnani, G.; Scarpini, E.; Appollonio, I.; Bascelli, C.; Cheldi, A.; Nemni, R.; Franceschi, M.; Italian Group for Lewy Body Dementia and Dementias Associated to Parkinsonism; Messa, G.; Mantovani, F.; Bellotti, M.; Olivotto, F.; Alberoni, M.; Isella, V.; Regazzoni, R.; Schiatti, E.; Vismara, C.; Falautano, M.; Barbieri, A.; Restelli, I.; Fetoni, V.; Donato, M.; Zuffi, M. & Castiglioni, S. (2009). Frequency and clinical features of Lewy body dementia in Italian memory clinics. *Acta Bio-Medica : Atenei Parmensis,* Vol.80, No.1, pp. 57-64, ISSN 0392-4203; 0392-4203

Firbank, M. J.; Blamire, A. M.; Krishnan, M. S.; Teodorczuk, A.; English, P.; Gholkar, A.; Harrison, R. & O'Brien, J. T. (2007a). Atrophy is associated with posterior cingulate white matter disruption in dementia with Lewy bodies and Alzheimer's disease. *NeuroImage,* Vol.36, No.1, pp. 1-7, ISSN 1053-8119; 1053-8119

Firbank, M. J.; Blamire, A. M.; Krishnan, M. S.; Teodorczuk, A.; English, P.; Gholkar, A.; Harrison, R. M. & O'Brien, J. T. (2007b). Diffusion tensor imaging in dementia with Lewy bodies and Alzheimer's disease. *Psychiatry Research,* Vol.155, No.2, pp. 135-145, ISSN 0165-1781; 0165-1781

Fodero-Tavoletti, M. T.; Smith, D. P.; McLean, C. A.; Adlard, P. A.; Barnham, K. J.; Foster, L. E.; Leone, L.; Perez, K.; Cortes, M.; Culvenor, J. G.; Li, Q. X.; Laughton, K. M.; Rowe, C. C.; Masters, C. L.; Cappai, R. & Villemagne, V. L. (2007). In vitro characterization of Pittsburgh compound-B binding to Lewy bodies. *The Journal of Neuroscience : The Official Journal of the Society for Neuroscience,* Vol.27, No.39, pp. 10365-10371, ISSN 1529-2401; 0270-6474

Foster, E. R.; Campbell, M. C.; Burack, M. A.; Hartlein, J.; Flores, H. P.; Cairns, N. J.; Hershey, T. & Perlmutter, J. S. (2010). Amyloid imaging of Lewy body-associated disorders. *Movement Disorders : Official Journal of the Movement Disorder Society,* Vol.25, No.15, pp. 2516-2523, ISSN 1531-8257; 0885-3185

Fox, P. T. & Raichle, M. E. (1985). Stimulus rate determines regional brain blood flow in striate cortex. *Annals of Neurology,* Vol.17, No.3, pp. 303-305, ISSN 0364-5134; 0364-5134

Fox, P. T.; Mintun, M. A.; Raichle, M. E.; Miezin, F. M.; Allman, J. M. & Van Essen, D. C. (1986). Mapping human visual cortex with positron emission tomography. *Nature,* Vol.323, No.6091, pp. 806-809, ISSN 0028-0836; 0028-0836

Frostig, R. D.; Lieke, E. E.; Ts'o, D. Y. & Grinvald, A. (1990). Cortical functional architecture and local coupling between neuronal activity and the microcirculation revealed by in vivo high-resolution optical imaging of intrinsic signals. *Proceedings of the National Academy of Sciences of the United States of America,* Vol.87, No.16, pp. 6082-6086, ISSN 0027-8424; 0027-8424

Fujishiro, H.; Iseki, E.; Murayama, N.; Yamamoto, R.; Higashi, S.; Kasanuki, K.; Suzuki, M.; Arai, H. & Sato, K. (2010). Diffuse occipital hypometabolism on [18 F]-FDG PET scans in patients with idiopathic REM sleep behavior disorder: prodromal dementia with Lewy bodies? *Psychogeriatrics : The Official Journal of the Japanese Psychogeriatric Society,* Vol.10, No.3, pp. 144-152, ISSN 1479-8301; 1346-3500

Gilman, S.; Koeppe, R. A.; Little, R.; An, H.; Junck, L.; Giordani, B.; Persad, C.; Heumann, M. & Wernette, K. (2005). Differentiation of Alzheimer's disease from dementia with Lewy bodies utilizing positron emission tomography with [18F]fluorodeoxyglucose and neuropsychological testing. *Experimental Neurology,* Vol.191 Suppl 1, pp. S95-S103, ISSN 0014-4886; 0014-4886

Gomperts, S. N.; Rentz, D. M.; Moran, E.; Becker, J. A.; Locascio, J. J.; Klunk, W. E.; Mathis, C. A.; Elmaleh, D. R.; Shoup, T.; Fischman, A. J.; Hyman, B. T.; Growdon, J. H. & Johnson, K. A. (2008). Imaging amyloid deposition in Lewy body diseases. *Neurology,* Vol.71, No.12, pp. 903-910, ISSN 1526-632X; 0028-3878

Goto, H.; Ishii, K.; Uemura, T.; Miyamoto, N.; Yoshikawa, T.; Shimada, K. & Ohkawa, S. (2010). Differential diagnosis of dementia with Lewy Bodies and Alzheimer Disease using combined MR imaging and brain perfusion single-photon emission tomography. *AJNR.American Journal of Neuroradiology,* Vol.31, No.4, pp. 720-725, ISSN 1936-959X; 0195-6108

Hanyu, H.; Tanaka, Y.; Shimizu, S.; Sakurai, H.; Iwamoto, T. & Abe, K. (2005). Differences in MR features of the substantia innominata between dementia with Lewy bodies and Alzheimer's disease. *Journal of Neurology,* Vol.252, No.4, pp. 482-484, ISSN 0340-5354

Hanyu, H.; Shimizu, S.; Hirao, K.; Kanetaka, H.; Sakurai, H.; Iwamoto, T.; Koizumi, K. & Abe, K. (2006a). Differentiation of dementia with Lewy bodies from Alzheimer's disease using Mini-Mental State Examination and brain perfusion SPECT. *Journal of the Neurological Sciences,* Vol.250, No.1-2, pp. 97-102, ISSN 0022-510X; 0022-510X

Hanyu, H.; Shimizu, S.; Hirao, K.; Kanetaka, H.; Iwamoto, T.; Chikamori, T.; Usui, Y.; Yamashina, A.; Koizumi, K. & Abe, K. (2006b). Comparative value of brain perfusion SPECT and [(123)I]MIBG myocardial scintigraphy in distinguishing between dementia with Lewy bodies and Alzheimer's disease. *European Journal of Nuclear Medicine and Molecular Imaging,* Vol.33, No.3, pp. 248-253, ISSN 1619-7070; 1619-7070

Hanyu, H.; Shimizu, S.; Tanaka, Y.; Hirao, K.; Iwamoto, T. & Abe, K. (2007). MR features of the substantia innominata and therapeutic implications in dementias. *Neurobiology of Aging,* Vol.28, No.4, pp. 548-554, ISSN 1558-1497; 0197-4580

Heidebrink, J. L. (2002). Is dementia with Lewy bodies the second most common cause of dementia? *Journal of Geriatric Psychiatry and Neurology,* Vol.15, No.4, pp. 182-187, ISSN 0891-9887; 0891-9887

Hentschel, F.; Kreis, M.; Damian, M.; Krumm, B. & Frolich, L. (2005). The clinical utility of structural neuroimaging with MRI for diagnosis and differential diagnosis of dementia: a memory clinic study. *International Journal of Geriatric Psychiatry,* Vol.20, No.7, pp. 645-650, ISSN 0885-6230

Herholz, K.; Carter, S. F. & Jones, M. (2007). Positron emission tomography imaging in dementia. *The British Journal of Radiology,* Vol.80 Spec No 2, pp. S160-7, ISSN 1748-880X; 0007-1285

Herrera, E.,Jr; Caramelli, P.; Silveira, A. S. & Nitrini, R. (2002). Epidemiologic survey of dementia in a community-dwelling Brazilian population. *Alzheimer Disease and Associated Disorders,* Vol.16, No.2, pp. 103-108, ISSN 0893-0341

Inui, Y.; Toyama, H.; Manabe, Y.; Sato, T.; Sarai, M.; Kosaka, K.; Iwata, N. & Katada, K. (2007). Evaluation of probable or possible dementia with lewy bodies using 123I-IMP brain perfusion SPECT, 123I-MIBG, and 99mTc-MIBI myocardial SPECT. *Journal of Nuclear Medicine : Official Publication, Society of Nuclear Medicine,* Vol.48, No.10, pp. 1641-1650, ISSN 0161-5505

Kantarci, K.; Avula, R.; Senjem, M. L.; Samikoglu, A. R.; Zhang, B.; Weigand, S. D.; Przybelski, S. A.; Edmonson, H. A.; Vemuri, P.; Knopman, D. S.; Ferman, T. J.; Boeve, B. F.; Petersen, R. C. & Jack, C. R.,Jr. (2010). Dementia with Lewy bodies and Alzheimer disease: neurodegenerative patterns characterized by DTI. *Neurology,* Vol.74, No.22, pp. 1814-1821, ISSN 1526-632X; 0028-3878

Kasama, S.; Tachibana, H.; Kawabata, K. & Yoshikawa, H. (2005). Cerebral blood flow in Parkinson's disease, dementia with Lewy bodies, and Alzheimer's disease according to three-dimensional stereotactic surface projection imaging. *Dementia and Geriatric Cognitive Disorders,* Vol.19, No.5-6, pp. 266-275, ISSN 1420-8008; 1420-8008

Kemp, P. M.; Hoffmann, S. A.; Holmes, C.; Bolt, L.; Ward, T.; Holmes, R. B. & Fleming, J. S. (2005). The contribution of statistical parametric mapping in the assessment of precuneal and medial temporal lobe perfusion by 99mTc-HMPAO SPECT in mild Alzheimer's and Lewy body dementia. *Nuclear Medicine Communications,* Vol.26, No.12, pp. 1099-1106, ISSN 0143-3636

Kemp, P. M. & Holmes, C. (2007). Imaging in dementia with Lewy bodies: a review. *Nuclear Medicine Communications,* Vol.28, No.7, pp. 511-519, ISSN 0143-3636

Kiuchi, K.; Morikawa, M.; Taoka, T.; Kitamura, S.; Nagashima, T.; Makinodan, M.; Nakagawa, K.; Fukusumi, M.; Ikeshita, K.; Inoue, M.; Kichikawa, K. & Kishimoto, T. (2011). White matter changes in dementia with Lewy bodies and Alzheimer's disease: A tractography-based study. *Journal of Psychiatric Research,* ISSN 1879-1379; 0022-3956

Klein, J. C.; Eggers, C.; Kalbe, E.; Weisenbach, S.; Hohmann, C.; Vollmar, S.; Baudrexel, S.; Diederich, N. J.; Heiss, W. D. & Hilker, R. (2010). Neurotransmitter changes in dementia with Lewy bodies and Parkinson disease dementia in vivo. *Neurology,* Vol.74, No.11, pp. 885-892, ISSN 1526-632X; 0028-3878

Koeppe, R. A.; Gilman, S.; Joshi, A.; Liu, S.; Little, R.; Junck, L.; Heumann, M.; Frey, K. A. & Albin, R. L. (2005). 11C-DTBZ and 18F-FDG PET measures in differentiating dementias. *Journal of Nuclear Medicine : Official Publication, Society of Nuclear Medicine,* Vol.46, No.6, pp. 936-944, ISSN 0161-5505

Lee, J. E.; Park, B.; Song, S. K.; Sohn, Y. H.; Park, H. J. & Lee, P. H. (2010a). A comparison of gray and white matter density in patients with Parkinson's disease dementia and dementia with Lewy bodies using voxel-based morphometry. *Movement Disorders : Official Journal of the Movement Disorder Society,* Vol.25, No.1, pp. 28-34, ISSN 1531-8257; 0885-3185

Lee, J. E.; Park, H. J.; Park, B.; Song, S. K.; Sohn, Y. H.; Lee, J. D. & Lee, P. H. (2010b). A comparative analysis of cognitive profiles and white-matter alterations using voxel-based diffusion tensor imaging between patients with Parkinson's disease dementia and dementia with Lewy bodies. *Journal of Neurology, Neurosurgery, and Psychiatry,* Vol.81, No.3, pp. 320-326, ISSN 1468-330X; 0022-3050

Lim, S. M.; Katsifis, A.; Villemagne, V. L.; Best, R.; Jones, G.; Saling, M.; Bradshaw, J.; Merory, J.; Woodward, M.; Hopwood, M. & Rowe, C. C. (2009). The 18F-FDG PET cingulate island sign and comparison to 123I-beta-CIT SPECT for diagnosis of dementia with Lewy bodies. *Journal of Nuclear Medicine : Official Publication, Society of Nuclear Medicine,* Vol.50, No.10, pp. 1638-1645, ISSN 1535-5667; 0161-5505

Lippa, C. F.; Duda, J. E.; Grossman, M.; Hurtig, H. I.; Aarsland, D.; Boeve, B. F.; Brooks, D. J.; Dickson, D. W.; Dubois, B.; Emre, M.; Fahn, S.; Farmer, J. M.; Galasko, D.; Galvin, J. E.; Goetz, C. G.; Growdon, J. H.; Gwinn-Hardy, K. A.; Hardy, J.; Heutink, P.; Iwatsubo, T.; Kosaka, K.; Lee, V. M.; Leverenz, J. B.; Masliah, E.; McKeith, I. G.; Nussbaum, R. L.; Olanow, C. W.; Ravina, B. M.; Singleton, A. B.; Tanner, C. M.; Trojanowski, J. Q.; Wszolek, Z. K. & DLB/PDD Working Group. (2007). DLB and PDD boundary issues: diagnosis, treatment, molecular pathology, and biomarkers. Neurology, Vol.68, No.11, pp. 812-819, ISSN 1526-632X; 0028-3878

Lobotesis, K.; Fenwick, J. D.; Phipps, A.; Ryman, A.; Swann, A.; Ballard, C.; McKeith, I. G. & O'Brien, J. T. (2001). Occipital hypoperfusion on SPECT in dementia with Lewy bodies but not AD. *Neurology,* Vol.56, No.5, pp. 643-649, ISSN 0028-3878; 0028-3878

Logothetis, N. K. (2002). The neural basis of the blood-oxygen-level-dependent functional magnetic resonance imaging signal. *Philosophical Transactions of the Royal Society of*

London.Series B, Biological Sciences, Vol.357, No.1424, pp. 1003-1037, ISSN 0962-8436; 0962-8436

Maetzler, W.; Liepelt, I.; Reimold, M.; Reischl, G.; Solbach, C.; Becker, C.; Schulte, C.; Leyhe, T.; Keller, S.; Melms, A.; Gasser, T. & Berg, D. (2009). Cortical PIB binding in Lewy body disease is associated with Alzheimer-like characteristics. *Neurobiology of Disease,* Vol.34, No.1, pp. 107-112, ISSN 1095-953X; 0969-9961

McKeith, I.; O'Brien, J.; Walker, Z.; Tatsch, K.; Booij, J.; Darcourt, J.; Padovani, A.; Giubbini, R.; Bonuccelli, U.; Volterrani, D.; Holmes, C.; Kemp, P.; Tabet, N.; Meyer, I.; Reininger, C. & DLB Study Group. (2007). Sensitivity and specificity of dopamine transporter imaging with 123I-FP-CIT SPECT in dementia with Lewy bodies: a phase III, multicentre study. *Lancet Neurology,* Vol.6, No.4, pp. 305-313, ISSN 1474-4422; 1474-4422

McKeith, I. (2004). Dementia with Lewy bodies and other difficult diagnoses. *International Psychogeriatrics / IPA,* Vol.16, No.2, pp. 123-127, ISSN 1041-6102; 1041-6102

McKeith, I. G.; Dickson, D. W.; Lowe, J.; Emre, M.; O'Brien, J. T.; Feldman, H.; Cummings, J.; Duda, J. E.; Lippa, C.; Perry, E. K.; Aarsland, D.; Arai, H.; Ballard, C. G.; Boeve, B.; Burn, D. J.; Costa, D.; Del Ser, T.; Dubois, B.; Galasko, D.; Gauthier, S.; Goetz, C. G.; Gomez-Tortosa, E.; Halliday, G.; Hansen, L. A.; Hardy, J.; Iwatsubo, T.; Kalaria, R. N.; Kaufer, D.; Kenny, R. A.; Korczyn, A.; Kosaka, K.; Lee, V. M.; Lees, A.; Litvan, I.; Londos, E.; Lopez, O. L.; Minoshima, S.; Mizuno, Y.; Molina, J. A.; Mukaetova-Ladinska, E. B.; Pasquier, F.; Perry, R. H.; Schulz, J. B.; Trojanowski, J. Q.; Yamada, M. & Consortium on DLB. (2005). Diagnosis and management of dementia with Lewy bodies: third report of the DLB Consortium. *Neurology,* Vol.65, No.12, pp. 1863-1872, ISSN 1526-632X; 0028-3878

McKeith, I. G.; Galasko, D.; Kosaka, K.; Perry, E. K.; Dickson, D. W.; Hansen, L. A.; Salmon, D. P.; Lowe, J.; Mirra, S. S.; Byrne, E. J.; Lennox, G.; Quinn, N. P.; Edwardson, J. A.; Ince, P. G.; Bergeron, C.; Burns, A.; Miller, B. L.; Lovestone, S.; Collerton, D.; Jansen, E. N.; Ballard, C.; de Vos, R. A.; Wilcock, G. K.; Jellinger, K. A. & Perry, R. H. (1996). Consensus guidelines for the clinical and pathologic diagnosis of dementia with Lewy bodies (DLB): report of the consortium on DLB international workshop. *Neurology,* Vol.47, No.5, pp. 1113-1124, ISSN 0028-3878; 0028-3878

Mito, Y.; Yoshida, K.; Yabe, I.; Makino, K.; Hirotani, M.; Tashiro, K.; Kikuchi, S. & Sasaki, H. (2005). Brain 3D-SSP SPECT analysis in dementia with Lewy bodies, Parkinson's disease with and without dementia, and Alzheimer's disease. *Clinical Neurology and Neurosurgery,* Vol.107, No.5, pp. 396-403, ISSN 0303-8467

Miyazawa, N.; Shinohara, T.; Nagasaka, T. & Hayashi, M. (2010). Hypermetabolism in patients with dementia with Lewy bodies. *Clinical Nuclear Medicine,* Vol.35, No.7, pp. 490-493, ISSN 1536-0229; 0363-9762

Mollenhauer, B.; Forstl, H.; Deuschl, G.; Storch, A.; Oertel, W. & Trenkwalder, C. (2010). Lewy body and parkinsonian dementia: common, but often misdiagnosed conditions. *Deutsches Arzteblatt International,* Vol.107, No.39, pp. 684-691, ISSN 1866-0452; 1866-0452

Nagahama, Y.; Okina, T.; Suzuki, N. & Matsuda, M. (2010). Neural correlates of psychotic symptoms in dementia with Lewy bodies. *Brain : A Journal of Neurology,* Vol.133, No.Pt 2, pp. 557-567, ISSN 1460-2156; 0006-8950

Nagahama, Y.; Okina, T.; Suzuki, N. & Matsuda, M. (2008). Cerebral substrates related to impaired performance in the clock-drawing test in dementia with Lewy bodies. *Dementia and Geriatric Cognitive Disorders,* Vol.25, No.6, pp. 524-530, ISSN 1421-9824; 1420-8008

Novellino, F.; Bagnato, A.; Salsone, M.; Cascini, G. L.; Nicoletti, G.; Arabia, G.; Pugliese, P.; Morelli, M.; Paglionico, S.; Cipullo, S.; Manna, I.; De Marco, E. V.; Condino, F.; Chiriaco, C.; Morgante, L.; Zappia, M. & Quattrone, A. (2010). Myocardial (123)I-MIBG scintigraphy for differentiation of Lewy bodies disease from FTD. Neurobiology of Aging, Vol.31, No.11, pp. 1903-1911, ISSN 1558-1497; 0197-4580

O'Brien, J. T.; McKeith, I. G.; Walker, Z.; Tatsch, K.; Booij, J.; Darcourt, J.; Marquardt, M.; Reininger, C. & DLB Study Group. (2009). Diagnostic accuracy of 123I-FP-CIT SPECT in possible dementia with Lewy bodies. *The British Journal of Psychiatry : The Journal of Mental Science,* Vol.194, No.1, pp. 34-39, ISSN 1472-1465; 0007-1250

O'Brien, J. T.; Colloby, S. J.; Pakrasi, S.; Perry, E. K.; Pimlott, S. L.; Wyper, D. J.; McKeith, I. G. & Williams, E. D. (2008). Nicotinic alpha4beta2 receptor binding in dementia with Lewy bodies using 123I-5IA-85380 SPECT demonstrates a link between occipital changes and visual hallucinations. *NeuroImage,* Vol.40, No.3, pp. 1056-1063, ISSN 1053-8119; 1053-8119

O'Brien, J. T. (2007). Role of imaging techniques in the diagnosis of dementia. *The British Journal of Radiology,* Vol.80 Spec No 2, pp. S71-7, ISSN 1748-880X; 0007-1285

O'Brien, J. T.; Firbank, M. J.; Mosimann, U. P.; Burn, D. J. & McKeith, I. G. (2005). Change in perfusion, hallucinations and fluctuations in consciousness in dementia with Lewy bodies. *Psychiatry Research,* Vol.139, No.2, pp. 79-88, ISSN 0165-1781; 0165-1781

Ogawa, S.; Lee, T. M.; Kay, A. R. & Tank, D. W. (1990a). Brain magnetic resonance imaging with contrast dependent on blood oxygenation. *Proceedings of the National Academy of Sciences of the United States of America,* Vol.87, No.24, pp. 9868-9872, ISSN 0027-8424; 0027-8424

Ogawa, S.; Lee, T. M.; Nayak, A. S. & Glynn, P. (1990b). Oxygenation-sensitive contrast in magnetic resonance image of rodent brain at high magnetic fields. *Magnetic Resonance in Medicine : Official Journal of the Society of Magnetic Resonance in Medicine / Society of Magnetic Resonance in Medicine,* Vol.14, No.1, pp. 68-78, ISSN 0740-3194; 0740-3194

Ogawa, S.; Menon, R. S.; Tank, D. W.; Kim, S. G.; Merkle, H.; Ellermann, J. M. & Ugurbil, K. (1993). Functional brain mapping by blood oxygenation level-dependent contrast magnetic resonance imaging. A comparison of signal characteristics with a biophysical model. *Biophysical Journal,* Vol.64, No.3, pp. 803-812, ISSN 0006-3495; 0006-3495

Ogawa, S.; Menon, R. S.; Kim, S. G. & Ugurbil, K. (1998). On the characteristics of functional magnetic resonance imaging of the brain. *Annual Review of Biophysics and Biomolecular Structure,* Vol.27, pp. 447-474, ISSN 1056-8700; 1056-8700

Ota, M.; Sato, N.; Ogawa, M.; Murata, M.; Kuno, S.; Kida, J. & Asada, T. (2009). Degeneration of dementia with Lewy bodies measured by diffusion tensor imaging. *NMR in Biomedicine,* Vol.22, No.3, pp. 280-284, ISSN 0952-3480; 0952-3480

Perneczky, R.; Drzezga, A.; Boecker, H.; Forstl, H.; Kurz, A. & Haussermann, P. (2008a). Cerebral metabolic dysfunction in patients with dementia with Lewy bodies and visual hallucinations. *Dementia and Geriatric Cognitive Disorders,* Vol.25, No.6, pp. 531-538, ISSN 1421-9824; 1420-8008

Perneczky, R.; Drzezga, A.; Boecker, H.; Ceballos-Baumann, A. O.; Granert, O.; Forstl, H.; Kurz, A. & Haussermann, P. (2008b). Activities of daily living, cerebral glucose metabolism, and cognitive reserve in Lewy body and Parkinson's disease. *Dementia and Geriatric Cognitive Disorders,* Vol.26, No.5, pp. 475-481, ISSN 1421-9824; 1420-8008

Perneczky, R.; Haussermann, P.; Drzezga, A.; Boecker, H.; Granert, O.; Feurer, R.; Forstl, H. & Kurz, A. (2009a). Fluoro-deoxy-glucose positron emission tomography correlates of impaired activities of daily living in dementia with Lewy bodies: implications for cognitive reserve. *The American Journal of Geriatric Psychiatry : Official Journal of the American Association for Geriatric Psychiatry,* Vol.17, No.3, pp. 188-195, ISSN 1545-7214; 1064-7481

Perneczky, R.; Drzezga, A.; Boecker, H.; Wagenpfeil, S.; Forstl, H.; Kurz, A. & Haussermann, P. (2009b). Right prefrontal hypometabolism predicts delusions in dementia with Lewy bodies. *Neurobiology of Aging,* Vol.30, No.9, pp. 1420-1429, ISSN 1558-1497; 0197-4580

Perneczky, R.; Drzezga, A.; Boecker, H.; Ceballos-Baumann, A. O.; Valet, M.; Feurer, R.; Forstl, H.; Kurz, A. & Haussermann, P. (2010). Metabolic alterations associated with impaired clock drawing in Lewy body dementia. *Psychiatry Research,* Vol.181, No.2, pp. 85-89, ISSN 0165-1781; 0165-1781

Perry, R. H.; Irving, D. & Tomlinson, B. E. (1990). Lewy body prevalence in the aging brain: relationship to neuropsychiatric disorders, Alzheimer-type pathology and catecholaminergic nuclei. *Journal of the Neurological Sciences,* Vol.100, No.1-2, pp. 223-233, ISSN 0022-510X; 0022-510X

Piggott, M. A.; Marshall, E. F.; Thomas, N.; Lloyd, S.; Court, J. A.; Jaros, E.; Burn, D.; Johnson, M.; Perry, R. H.; McKeith, I. G.; Ballard, C. & Perry, E. K. (1999). Striatal dopaminergic markers in dementia with Lewy bodies, Alzheimer's and Parkinson's diseases: rostrocaudal distribution. *Brain : A Journal of Neurology,* Vol.122 (Pt 8), No.Pt 8, pp. 1449-1468, ISSN 0006-8950; 0006-8950

Rahkonen, T.; Eloniemi-Sulkava, U.; Rissanen, S.; Vatanen, A.; Viramo, P. & Sulkava, R. (2003). Dementia with Lewy bodies according to the consensus criteria in a general population aged 75 years or older. *Journal of Neurology, Neurosurgery, and Psychiatry,* Vol.74, No.6, pp. 720-724, ISSN 0022-3050; 0022-3050

Roselli, F.; Pisciotta, N. M.; Perneczky, R.; Pennelli, M.; Aniello, M. S.; De Caro, M. F.; Ferrannini, E.; Tartaglione, B.; Defazio, G.; Rubini, G. & Livrea, P. (2009). Severity of neuropsychiatric symptoms and dopamine transporter levels in dementia with Lewy bodies: a 123I-FP-CIT SPECT study. *Movement Disorders : Official Journal of the Movement Disorder Society,* Vol.24, No.14, pp. 2097-2103, ISSN 1531-8257; 0885-3185

Rossi, C.; Volterrani, D.; Nicoletti, V.; Manca, G.; Frosini, D.; Kiferle, L.; Unti, E.; De Feo, P.; Bonuccelli, U. & Ceravolo, R. (2009). "Parkinson-dementia" diseases: a comparison by double tracer SPECT studies. *Parkinsonism & Related Disorders,* Vol.15, No.10, pp. 762-766, ISSN 1873-5126; 1353-8020

Sanchez-Castaneda, C.; Rene, R.; Ramirez-Ruiz, B.; Campdelacreu, J.; Gascon, J.; Falcon, C.; Calopa, M.; Jauma, S.; Juncadella, M. & Junque, C. (2009). Correlations between gray matter reductions and cognitive deficits in dementia with Lewy Bodies and

Parkinson's disease with dementia. *Movement Disorders : Official Journal of the Movement Disorder Society,* Vol.24, No.12, pp. 1740-1746, ISSN 1531-8257; 0885-3185

Sanchez-Castaneda, C.; Rene, R.; Ramirez-Ruiz, B.; Campdelacreu, J.; Gascon, J.; Falcon, C.; Calopa, M.; Jauma, S.; Juncadella, M. & Junque, C. (2010). Frontal and associative visual areas related to visual hallucinations in dementia with Lewy bodies and Parkinson's disease with dementia. *Movement Disorders : Official Journal of the Movement Disorder Society,* Vol.25, No.5, pp. 615-622, ISSN 1531-8257; 0885-3185

Satoh, M.; Ishikawa, H.; Meguro, K.; Kasuya, M.; Ishii, H. & Yamaguchi, S. (2010). Improved visual hallucination by donepezil and occipital glucose metabolism in dementia with Lewy bodies: the Osaki-Tajiri project. *European Neurology,* Vol.64, No.6, pp. 337-344, ISSN 1421-9913; 0014-3022

Sauer, J.; ffytche, D. H.; Ballard, C.; Brown, R. G. & Howard, R. (2006). Differences between Alzheimer's disease and dementia with Lewy bodies: an fMRI study of task-related brain activity. *Brain : A Journal of Neurology,* Vol.129, No.Pt 7, pp. 1780-1788, ISSN 1460-2156; 0006-8950

Shimizu, S.; Hanyu, H.; Kanetaka, H.; Iwamoto, T.; Koizumi, K. & Abe, K. (2005). Differentiation of dementia with Lewy bodies from Alzheimer's disease using brain SPECT. *Dementia and Geriatric Cognitive Disorders,* Vol.20, No.1, pp. 25-30, ISSN 1420-8008; 1420-8008

Shimizu, S.; Hanyu, H.; Hirao, K.; Sato, T.; Iwamoto, T. & Koizumi, K. (2008). Value of analyzing deep gray matter and occipital lobe perfusion to differentiate dementia with Lewy bodies from Alzheimer's disease. *Annals of Nuclear Medicine,* Vol.22, No.10, pp. 911-916, ISSN 0914-7187; 0914-7187

Soret, M.; Koulibaly, P. M.; Darcourt, J. & Buvat, I. (2006). Partial volume effect correction in SPECT for striatal uptake measurements in patients with neurodegenerative diseases: impact upon patient classification. *European Journal of Nuclear Medicine and Molecular Imaging,* Vol.33, No.9, pp. 1062-1072, ISSN 1619-7070; 1619-7070

Stevens, T.; Livingston, G.; Kitchen, G.; Manela, M.; Walker, Z. & Katona, C. (2002). Islington study of dementia subtypes in the community. *The British Journal of Psychiatry : The Journal of Mental Science,* Vol.180, pp. 270-276, ISSN 0007-1250; 0007-1250

Summerfield, C.; Junque, C.; Tolosa, E.; Salgado-Pineda, P.; Gomez-Anson, B.; Marti, M. J.; Pastor, P.; Ramirez-Ruiz, B. & Mercader, J. (2005). Structural brain changes in Parkinson disease with dementia: a voxel-based morphometry study. Archives of Neurology, Vol.62, No.2, pp. 281-285, ISSN 0003-9942; 0003-9942

Suzuki, M.; Desmond, T. J.; Albin, R. L. & Frey, K. A. (2002). Striatal monoaminergic terminals in Lewy body and Alzheimer's dementias. *Annals of Neurology,* Vol.51, No.6, pp. 767-771, ISSN 0364-5134; 0364-5134

Takahashi, R.; Ishii, K.; Miyamoto, N.; Yoshikawa, T.; Shimada, K.; Ohkawa, S.; Kakigi, T. & Yokoyama, K. (2010). Measurement of gray and white matter atrophy in dementia with Lewy bodies using diffeomorphic anatomic registration through exponentiated lie algebra: A comparison with conventional voxel-based morphometry. *AJNR.American Journal of Neuroradiology,* Vol.31, No.10, pp. 1873-1878, ISSN 1936-959X; 0195-6108

Takahashi, R.; Ishii, K.; Shimada, K.; Ohkawa, S. & Nishimura, Y. (2010). Hypoperfusion of the motor cortex associated with parkinsonism in dementia with Lewy bodies.

Journal of the Neurological Sciences, Vol.288, No.1-2, pp. 88-91, ISSN 1878-5883; 0022-510X

Tam, C. W.; Burton, E. J.; McKeith, I. G.; Burn, D. J. & O'Brien, J. T. (2005). Temporal lobe atrophy on MRI in Parkinson disease with dementia: a comparison with Alzheimer disease and dementia with Lewy bodies. *Neurology,* Vol.64, No.5, pp. 861-865, ISSN 1526-632X; 0028-3878

Tartaglia, M. C.; Rosen, H. J. & Miller, B. L. (2011). Neuroimaging in dementia. *Neurotherapeutics : The Journal of the American Society for Experimental NeuroTherapeutics,* Vol.8, No.1, pp. 82-92, ISSN 1878-7479; 1878-7479

Tateno, M.; Utsumi, K.; Kobayashi, S.; Takahashi, A.; Saitoh, M.; Morii, H.; Fujii, K. & Teraoka, M. (2008a). Usefulness of a blood flow analyzing program 3DSRT to detect occipital hypoperfusion in dementia with Lewy bodies. *Progress in Neuro-Psychopharmacology & Biological Psychiatry,* Vol.32, No.5, pp. 1206-1209, ISSN 0278-5846; 0278-5846

Tateno, M.; Kobayashi, S.; Shirasaka, T.; Furukawa, Y.; Fujii, K.; Morii, H.; Yasumura, S.; Utsumi, K. & Saito, T. (2008b). Comparison of the usefulness of brain perfusion SPECT and MIBG myocardial scintigraphy for the diagnosis of dementia with Lewy bodies. *Dementia and Geriatric Cognitive Disorders,* Vol.26, No.5, pp. 453-457, ISSN 1421-9824; 1420-8008

van Zijl, P. C.; Eleff, S. M.; Ulatowski, J. A.; Oja, J. M.; Ulug, A. M.; Traystman, R. J. & Kauppinen, R. A. (1998). Quantitative assessment of blood flow, blood volume and blood oxygenation effects in functional magnetic resonance imaging. *Nature Medicine,* Vol.4, No.2, pp. 159-167, ISSN 1078-8956; 1078-8956

von Gunten, A. & Meuli, R. (2009). Delineating dementia with lewy bodies: can magnetic resonance imaging help? *Frontiers of Neurology and Neuroscience,* Vol.24, pp. 126-134, ISSN 1660-4431; 0300-5186

Walker, Z.; Jaros, E.; Walker, R. W.; Lee, L.; Costa, D. C.; Livingston, G.; Ince, P. G.; Perry, R.; McKeith, I. & Katona, C. L. (2007). Dementia with Lewy bodies: a comparison of clinical diagnosis, FP-CIT single photon emission computed tomography imaging and autopsy. *Journal of Neurology, Neurosurgery, and Psychiatry,* Vol.78, No.11, pp. 1176-1181, ISSN 1468-330X; 0022-3050

Walker, R. W. & Walker, Z. (2009). Dopamine transporter single photon emission computerized tomography in the diagnosis of dementia with Lewy bodies. *Movement Disorders : Official Journal of the Movement Disorder Society,* Vol.24 Suppl 2, pp. S754-9, ISSN 1531-8257; 0885-3185

Watson, R.; Blamire, A. M. & O'Brien, J. T. (2009). Magnetic resonance imaging in lewy body dementias. *Dementia and Geriatric Cognitive Disorders,* Vol.28, No.6, pp. 493-506, ISSN 1421-9824; 1420-8008

Weisskoff, R. M.; Zuo, C. S.; Boxerman, J. L. & Rosen, B. R. (1994). Microscopic susceptibility variation and transverse relaxation: theory and experiment. *Magnetic Resonance in Medicine : Official Journal of the Society of Magnetic Resonance in Medicine / Society of Magnetic Resonance in Medicine,* Vol.31, No.6, pp. 601-610, ISSN 0740-3194; 0740-3194

Whitwell, J. L.; Weigand, S. D.; Shiung, M. M.; Boeve, B. F.; Ferman, T. J.; Smith, G. E.; Knopman, D. S.; Petersen, R. C.; Benarroch, E. E.; Josephs, K. A. & Jack, C. R.,Jr. (2007). Focal atrophy in dementia with Lewy bodies on MRI: a distinct pattern from

Alzheimer's disease. *Brain : A Journal of Neurology,* Vol.130, No.Pt 3, pp. 708-719, ISSN 1460-2156; 0006-8950

Yamada, T.; Hattori, H.; Miura, A.; Tanabe, M. & Yamori, Y. (2001). Prevalence of Alzheimer's disease, vascular dementia and dementia with Lewy bodies in a Japanese population. *Psychiatry and Clinical Neurosciences,* Vol.55, No.1, pp. 21-25, ISSN 1323-1316; 1323-1316

Yamada, T.; Kadekaru, H.; Matsumoto, S.; Inada, H.; Tanabe, M.; Moriguchi, E. H.; Moriguchi, Y.; Ishikawa, P.; Ishikawa, A. G.; Taira, K. & Yamori, Y. (2002). Prevalence of dementia in the older Japanese-Brazilian population. *Psychiatry and Clinical Neurosciences,* Vol.56, No.1, pp. 71-75, ISSN 1323-1316; 1323-1316

Yong, S. W.; Yoon, J. K.; An, Y. S. & Lee, P. H. (2007). A comparison of cerebral glucose metabolism in Parkinson's disease, Parkinson's disease dementia and dementia with Lewy bodies. *European Journal of Neurology : The Official Journal of the European Federation of Neurological Societies,* Vol.14, No.12, pp. 1357-1362, ISSN 1468-1331; 1351-5101

Zaccai, J.; McCracken, C. & Brayne, C. (2005). A systematic review of prevalence and incidence studies of dementia with Lewy bodies. *Age and Ageing,* Vol.34, No.6, pp. 561-566, ISSN 0002-0729; 0002-0729

18

Endoscopic Intracranial Imaging

Oscar H. Jimenez-Vazquez
"Dr. Miguel Silva" Hospital General Morelia, Michoacan, Mexico

1. Introduction

The fundamental aim of the chapter is to create awareness in the general medical community about the benefits of neuroendoscopy imaging for prompt and effective diagnosis and treatment of lesions within or adjacent to fluid-filled intracranial cavities.
Neuroendoscopy is a surgical diagnostic and therapeutic modality that has suffered an oscillating course in history, regarding its indications and applications. At present, it enjoys another thrust of popularity, which may be evident by the increasing number of publications and academic events world-wide related to this discipline. It has been evolving continuously, allowing for new indications, applications, and results.
Neuroendoscopy is not a novel technique. According to a large number of articles and books, the application of lenses to observe internal parts of the body without a wide exposure, was initiated in the 19th century, and such technology was soon applied to the intracranial space. Very primitive equipment was used to explore the ventricular system and to excise the choroid plexus. Since the beginning of this new technology, it has suffered continuous modifications that have improved optical quality and surgical capability, resulting in better surgical outcome (1).
As a typical example of a minimally invasive neurosurgical technique, neuroendoscopy has led to improvement in diagnosis, therapy, and prognosis in many intracranial lesions. Practically all intracranial compartments may be reached with an endoscope, whether it is rigid or flexible, and indications have increased dramatically. It is now possible to diagnose and treat through direct observation intraventricular, as well as subarchnoid and parenchymal lesions.
Hoping to avoid a shunt placement and its complications, third-ventriculostomies were initially adopted as promising procedures for most cases of hydrocephalus. Although it has not been associated with the postoperative results that were hoped for, it has today very clear indications. Hypertensive and obstructive hydrocephalus due to different pathologies in the cerebral aqueduct, the posterior part of the third ventricle, or the fourth ventricle, may be some of the ideal cases for a third-ventriculostomy. Although some factors may vary when performing a third ventriculostomy, such as early age, a final word has not been said in this regard, since the controversy continues. Shunt systems, nevertheless, continue to be an important part of the instruments needed in the treatment of hydrocephalus.
Congenital cysts in or adjacent to the ventricular system acting as space occupying lesions and hydrocephalus may be another clear indication for endoscopic exploration and cavity communication, sometimes requiring a shunt system. Although not as frequent as the

previous case, septum cavum pellucidum cysts have been other clear indications for endoscopic fenestrations, either with mechanical means (like the endoscope itself) or with laser beams. In such cases raised intracranial pressure is normalized and symptomatology slowly resides.

Catheter placements and revisions may represent frequent indications for endoscopic shunt revisions, given the large number of shunt operations that take place daily throughout the world, so dysfunction of these systems are to be expected. The causes for shunt dysfunction are many, but may not be evident with image studies (CT or MRI scans), therefore intraventricular endoscopy offers a direct diagnostic method which may yield clear images in real time. It also allows the opportunity to apply therapeutic measures during the same operation.

Haematoma drainage, membrane fenestrations, tumour biopsies and resections, and open neurosurgical assistance, may be other common procedures that may be assisted with the endoscope. Although indications may vary according to the local neuropathological illnesses and diagnostic capabilities, it is largely dependent on the neurosurgeons experience.

As published elsewhere (2), there is a need to stress that precise diagnosis is a key factor for a correct planning of a successful neuroendoscopic procedures, since conventional image studies may be deficient in resolution. This is certainly the case in modest medical facilities, where computed tomography (CT) and magnetic resonance imaging (MRI) scanners may not be available or updated. This fact may represent a high proportion of primary medical care systems world-wide, and it is certainly true for hospitals of our community. To demonstrate this fact, the results obtained in our series of endoscopy cases, preoperative image studies (CT and MRI) have yielded unparallel results compared with those obtained with endoscopy in roughly half of the cases. This is especially true in the beginning of the case recollection, because image studies were more primitive than the images obtained from more modern machines, and the images were more modest in resolution.

Neuroendoscopy may yield high quality images which may confirm or discard diagnostic possibilities during the surgical procedure, making often times in-situ modifications necessary. Derived from the previous statement, and because the original preoperative diagnosis was different from the intraoperative endoscopical image, the surgical treatment that was finally performed was different from the one originally planned in about a third of the cases. In this context, other surgical procedures, including open procedures, were avoided, and therefore additional risks and costs to the patient were reduced.

Neuroendoscopy in our hospitals has been performed by the same neurosurgeon in 102 procedures. With its limitations, it has demonstrated benefits, as well as drawbacks. Among the former, accuracy in diagnosis of lesions that were subject to several differential diagnosis, especially when they were based on low definition image studies. Full details of our cases can be observed in table 1.

Endoscopy equipment, in our experience, has changed through different times. Initially, a pediatric cystoscope was used and procedures were limited to observations and few cystic perforations. Septostomies also were commonly performed. Most of these procedures were not recorded in image documents. The same was true for a second generation of instruments, which included a semi-rigid, 2mm diameter fibroscope, a new light source, but no camera or video-recorder. Our present endoscope is a 4mm rigid Richard Wolf, with three working channels, a video system and a high definition screen.

Case	Age	Sex	Clinical Diagnosis	Image Diagnosis	Endoscopic Diagnosis	Ct/Endo Correl	Tx Modif
1	30	M	RICP, SD.	Global Hydrocephalus. No visible cause.	Adherence of the catheter to choroid plexus.	NO	NO
2	19	M	RICP.	Supratentorial hydrocephalus. Cysticercal ependymitis. 3rd ventricle calcifications.	Ventriculomegaly with NO ependymitis or calcification.	NO	YES
3	17	M	RICP.	Supratentorial hydrocephalus. Ependymitis. Intra-ventricular septi and/or 3rd ventricle cysticerci.	Ventriculomegaly with NO ependymitis, cysticerci or septi.	NO	YES
4	43	M	RICP; Dementia.	Parenchymal calcifications. Global hydrocephalus.	Ventriculomegaly.	YES	NO
5	26	F	RICP, SD*.	Hydrocephalus. Thalamic tumour with 3rd. ventricle infiltration and shunt involvement.	Ventricular compression with NO tumour infiltration. Catheter in inter-ventricular septum*.	NO/ NO	YES/ YES
6	26	F	RICP.	Supratentorial hydrocephalus. 3rd ventricle tumour invasion.	3rd ventricle tumour invasion with ventriculomegaly.	NO	NO
7	39	M	RICP.	Global hydrocephalus. Cysticercal basal arachnoiditis.	Multiple ependymal calcifications. Ventriculomegaly.	YES	NO
8	30	M	RICP.	Left ventricular cyst.	Septum in ventricle without cystic lesion.	NO	YES
9	42	F	CSF fistula, SD.	Pneumocephalus with hydrocephalus.	Ventriculomegaly with pneumocephalus.	YES	NO
10	34	M	RICP.	Supratentorial hydrocephalus. Cerebellar tumour with 3rd ventricle invasion.	Ventriculomegaly with NO 3rd ventricle invasion.	NO	YES
11	57	M	RICP, Dementia.	Supratentorial hydrocephalus.	Ventriculomegaly.	YES	NO
12	18	F	Epilepsy.	Mild global cortical atrophy.	Determination of callosotomy extent.	YES	NO

Case	Age	Sex	Clinical Diagnosis	Image Diagnosis	Endoscopic Diagnosis	Ct/Endo Correl	Tx Modif
13	28	M	RICP, SD.	Global hydrocephalus.	Ventriculomegaly. Multiple intraventricular adherences*.	NO/ NO	NO/ NO
14	31	F	RICP.	Global hydrocephalus.	3rd ventricle septum. Ventriculomegaly.	NO	YES
15	29	M	RICP, Dementia.	Supratentorial hydrocephalus. Porencephalic cyst NOT communicated with ventricles.	Partial communication of cyst to dilated ventricles.	NO	YES
16	32	F	Seizures.	Right parietal lobe cystic tumour with septi.	Parietal tumour with independent cysts.	YES	NO
17	17	M	RICP, SD.	Supratentorial hydrocephalus. Two ventricular catheters.	Fibrosis of 3rd ventricle floor with one catheter. Adherence of second catheter to choroid plexus.	NO	YES
18	21	M	RICP.	Hydrocephalus. Thalamic tumour.	Ventriculomegaly. Callosotomy assistence*.	YES/ YES	NO/ NO
19	54	F	RICP; Dementia.	Occipital tumour with ventricular deformation. Hydrocephalus.	Extrinsic 3rd ventricle dysplacement. Ventriculomegaly.	YES	NO
20	60	M	RICP, Hemipare sis.	Subacute subdural hematoma with septi.	NO septi in hematoma.	NO	YES
21	52	M	RICP, SD, Infection.	3rd and left lateral ventricle hydrocephalus. Purulent ependymitis.	Ventriculomegaly and abundant adherences* No purulent ependymitis.	NO	YES
22	43	M	RICP.	Global hydrocephalus. Septum in right lateral ventricle. Pineal calcification within the 3rd ventricle.	NO septum. Pineal calcification not visible.	NO	YES
23	46	M	RICP.	Hydrocephalus. Cortical cyst.	Ventriculomegaly.	YES	NO
24	46	M	Stroke with dysartria and hemiparesis	Hydrocephalus. 3rd ventricle displacement by arachnoid cyst.	Discrete 3rd ventricle with adherences in the lateral ventricle. Ventriculomegaly.	NO	NO

Case	Age	Sex	Clinical Diagnosis	Image Diagnosis	Endoscopic Diagnosis	Ct/Endo Correl	Tx Modif
25	77	F	Headache, seizures.	Hydrocephalus. Multiple parenchymal calcifications and cysts.	Ventriculomegaly with adhesive ependymitis. NO cysts.	NO	NO
26	77	M	RICP, coma.	Supratentorial hydrocephalus.	Ventriculomegaly with a small viable cysticercus in choroid plexus.	NO	YES
27	18	F	RICP.	Compressive septum pellucidum cyst.	Dilated, isolated and hypertensive septum pellucidum cyst.	YES	NO
28	29	F	Epilepsy.	Dilated left temporal ventricle.	Dilated left temporal lateral ventricle.	YES	NO
29	65	M	RICP, coma.	Parenchymal haemorrhage in frontal lobe.	Parenchymal haemorrhage in frontal lobe.	YES	NO
30	19	M	RICP, SD, infection.	Supratentorial hydrocephalus.	Severe adhesive 3rd ventricle ependymitis.	NO	NO
31	32	F	Epilepsy.	Loss of white-gray matter interface in left temporal lobe. Normal ventricles.	Narrow left temporal ventricle.	YES	NO
32	37	F	RICP.	Supratentorial hydrocephalus. Right supra- infratentorial arachnoid cyst.	Ventriculomegally. Right supra-infratentorial arachnoid cyst.	YES	NO
33	27	M	Dementia.	Hydrocephalus. Porencephalic cyst.	Cyst independent from dilated ventricles.	YES	NO
34	30	M	RICP, SD. Left hemiparesis	Supratentorial hydrocephalus. 4th ventricle cyst.	Ventriculomegaly with extensive intraventricular fibrosis.	NO	NO
35	50	M	RICP, social neglect.	Supratentorial hydrocephalus.	Ventriculomegaly.	YES	NO
36	35	M	RICP, signs and symptoms of infection.	Supratentorial hydrocephalus with ependymitis.	Ventriculomegaly with NO ependymitis. Abundant fibrosis in 3rd (with small compartments) and lateral ventricles*.	NO/ NO	YES/ YES

Case	Age	Sex	Clinical Diagnosis	Image Diagnosis	Endoscopic Diagnosis	Ct/Endo Correl	Tx Modif
37	**46**	**M**	Epilepsy.	Left temporal lobe atrophy.	Intraventricular electrode placement control. Ventriculomegaly.	YES	NO
38	**21**	**M**	Epilepsy.	Left temporal lobe epileptogenic focus.	Narrow ventricle. Failed endoscopy.	--	--
39	**41**	**F**	Arnold Chiari and RICP.	Ventriculomegaly.	Ventriculomegaly.	YES	NO
40	**46**	**M**	Brain injury sequels.	Ventriculomegaly.	Turbid CSF poor visualization.	--	--
41	**19**	**M**	RICP.	Supratentorial hydrocephalus.	Ventriculomegaly. Granular ependymitis.	NO	NO
42	**23**	**M**	RICP.	Universal hydrocephalus.	Fibrous bands and ependymitis with Monroe obstruction.	NO	YES
43	**45**	**M**	Chiasmal syndrome.	Hypophyseal macroadenoma.	Bloody tumour bed.	--	--
44	**35**	**F**	Acromegaly	Supratentorial tumour.	Bloody tumour bed.	--	--
45	**42**	**M**	Vague neurological symptoms.	Universal hydrocephalus. HIV +.	Hypertrophic ependymitis with fibrous deposits in the III ventricle floor. Generalized tissue paleness.	NO	YES
46	**27**	**M**	Postra-umatic hydro-cephalus.	Dilated independent supratentorial ventricles.	Normal pressure ventriculomegaly due to Munro foramen obstruction.	NO	YES
47	**23**	**M**	Postra-umatic hydro-cephalus.	Supratentorial ventriculomegaly.	Three ventricle dilatation with thin 3rd ventricle floor.	YES	NO
48	**26**	**F**	Amenor-rhoea, galactor-rhoea, and mild headache.	Hydrocephalus, Lateral ventriculomegally with sellar arachnoidocele.	Ventriculomegaly, Munro foramen obstruction due to arachnoid membranes.	NO	YES
49	**47**	**M**	Epilepsy, dementia.	Hydrocephalus, Multiple cerebral cysticerci.	Viable cysticerci with scolex contained in turbid fluid* (both endoscopies).	YES/ YES	NO/ NO

Case	Age	Sex	Clinical Diagnosis	Image Diagnosis	Endoscopic Diagnosis	Ct/Endo Correl	Tx Modif
50	56	M	RICP.	Hypodense images in 3rd ventricle and basal cisterns.	Viable cysticerci in 3rd ventricle contained in turbid fluid, obstructing visualization of the floor.	YES	NO
51	42	F	RICP.	Supratentorial hydrocephalus with widened infundibular recess.	Ventriculomegaly with widened infundibular recess.	YES	NO
52	54	M	RICP, mood changes, episodic fever.	Global hydrocephalus.	Ventriculomegaly.	YES	NO
53	34	F	RICP, Right frontal cystic tumour	Cystic hypodense tumour.	Cerebral surface cyst wall	YES	NO
54	15	M	RICP, SD, Arnold-Chiari.	Three ventricle hydrocephalus, corpus callosum agenesis, cephalic catheter in brain tissue.	Ventriculomegaly, ventricular septum agenesis, cephalic catheter in brain tissue.	YES	NO
55	21	M	RICP, SD, Arnold-Chiari.	Three ventricle hydrocephalus, corpus callosum and septum agenesis, cephalic catheter in ventricle.	Ventriculomegaly, ventricular septum agenesis, granular ependymitis, cephalic catheter in ventricle.	NO	NO
56	32	M	RICP.	Left and 3rd ventricle hydrocephalus.	Isolated right ventricle	YES	NO
57	25	M	RICP, dizziness, confusion, dementia, meningeal signs. HIV +	3-ventricle hypertensive hydrocephalus	Turbid dense liquid, pale tissue covering ependymal walls, with adhesive clots and membranes	NO	YES

Case	Age	Sex	Clinical Diagnosis	Image Diagnosis	Endoscopic Diagnosis	Ct/Endo Correl	Tx Modif
58	**57**	**M**	RICP. Incoherent language, Dizzyness	Hydrocephalus, granular ependymitis.	Ventriculomegaly, granular ependymitis with café au lait spots and verrucae, 3rd ventricle floor stiffness.	NO	NO
59	**39**	**F**	RICP, diplopia.	Triventricular hydrocephalus.	Ventriculomegaly with severe septum lacerations.	YES	NO
60	**33**	**M**	RICP.	Hydrocephalus	Ventriculomegaly, severe septum lacerations, granular ependymitis and verrucae.	NO	NO
61	**44**	**M**	Headache, seizures.	Viable cysticerci in brain parenchyma and cisterns.	Viable parenchymal and cisternal cysticerci.	YES	NO
62	**44**	**M**	RICP, cysticercos is.	Hydrocephalus, 3rd ventricle and cisternal cysticerci.	Ventriculomegaly, 3rd ventricle and cisternal cysticerci.	YES	NO
63	**44**	**M**	Shunt dysfunctio n	Hydrocephalus.	Ventriculomegaly, cysticercus in shunt tip.	NO	NO
64	**58**	**M**	RICP, ataxia, Parinaud, diplopia.	Hydrocephalus, pineal tumour with possible 3rd ventricle involvement.	Ventriculomegaly, pineal tumour with 3rd ventricle involvement.	YES	NO
65	**44**	**M**	RICP.	Shunt dysfunction.	Cysticercus in shunt tip.	NO	NO
66	**28**	**F**	RICP, left hemi-paresis.	Right frontotemporoparietal cyst.	Cystic breast cancer metastasis.	YES	NO
67	**40**	**F**	RICP. macroceph alus	Severe hydrocephalus.	Ventriculomegaly, fibrous ependymal and cisternal bands, atrophic choroid plexus.	NO	NO
68	**16**	**F**	Headache, dizziness	Hydrocephalus, rare images in 3rd ventricle floor.	Ventriculomegaly.	NO	NO

Case	Age	Sex	Clinical Diagnosis	Image Diagnosis	Endoscopic Diagnosis	Ct/Endo Correl	Tx Modif
69	33	M	Headache, dizziness, ataxia.	Hydrocephalus, right hemisphere cerebellar tumour.	Ventriculomegaly.	YES	NO
70	39	M	RICP, dizziness.	Three-ventricle hydrocephalus, occluded aqueduct.	Ventriculomegaly, prepontine and premesencephalic adherences.	NO	NO
71	73	F	Sudden dysphasia and headache.	Hydrocephalus and a 4th ventricle hemorrhage	Ventriculomegaly and an active 3rd ventricle hemorrhage.	NO	YES
72	61	F	Hakim-Adams triad, progressive headache	Three-ventricle hydrocephalus, occluded aqueduct.	Ventriculomegaly	YES	NO
73	40	M	RICP, headache, confusion, fever, meningeal signs, ataxia. HIV +	Hydrocephalus, thalamic tumour with 3rd ventricle involvement.	Ventriculomegaly, pale granular ependyma, no tumour in 3rd ventricle.	NO	YES
74	41	F	RICP, previous posterior fossa operation	Three-ventricle hydrocephalus.	Ventriculomegaly, adhesive arachnoiditis in premesencephalic and prepontine cistern.	NO	YES
75	31	M	RICP	Three-ventricule hydrocephalus	Ventriculomegaly, cisternal cysticercosis	NO	NO
76	67	M	Headache, tremor, confusion, incoherent language	Hydrocephalus, ventricular cysticerci	Ventriculomegal, aracnoid cyst	NO	YES
77	65	M	Headache, aggressive behavior, somnolence	Cystic lesions in Sylvian sulcus	Epidermoid in Sylvian sulcus.	NO	YES
78	72	M	Hakim-Adams triad, progressive headache	Three-ventricle asymmetric hydrocephalus, occluded aqueduct.	Ventriculomegaly, ependymitis with opaque epithelia.	NO	YES

Case	Age	Sex	Clinical Diagnosis	Image Diagnosis	Endoscopic Diagnosis	Ct/Endo Correl	Tx Modif
79	81	M	Right hemi-paresis, memory dysfun-ction, visual and auditive halluci-nations.	Hydrocephalus, diencephalic lesion affecting 3rd ventricle.	Ventriculomegaly, thinning and protruding cyst in 3rd ventricle wall.	NO	YES
80	40	F	Seizures, RICP.	Three-ventricle hydrocephalus, increased prepontine cistern, brain calcifications.	Ventriculomegaly, cysticerci in prepontine and premesencephalic cistern.	YES	NO
81	27	M	RICP, ataxia, dystonia.	Brain stem tumour with 3rd and 4rd ventricle involvement.	Ventriculomegaly, tumour invading 3rd ventricle.	YES	NO
82	54	M	RICP.	Three-ventricle hydrocephalus, cisternal cysticerci. Post ETV and cysticercal removal. Hydrocephalus.	Ventriculomegaly, cisternal cysticercosis.	YES	NO
83	54	M	RICP	Post ETV and cysticercal removal. Hydrocephalus.	Ventriculomegaly, severe ventriculitis-arachnoiditis. Ventriculomegaly, severe ventriculitis-arachnoiditis	NO/ YES	NO/ NO
84	39	F	RICP	Hydrocephalus, 3rd ventricle tumour.	Ventriculomegaly, tumour in 3rd ventricle.	YES	NO
85	62	F	Headache, memory loss.	Three-ventricle hydrocephalus.	Ventriculomegaly.	YES	NO
86	33	M	RICP, myalgia.	Hydrocephalus, ependymitis.	Ventriculomegaly, granular ventriculitis and arachnoiditis	YES	YES
87	59	M	RICP.	Three-ventricle hydrocephalus.	Ventriculomegaly, cisternal cysticercosis	YES	NO

Case	Age	Sex	Clinical Diagnosis	Image Diagnosis	Endoscopic Diagnosis	Ct/Endo Correl	Tx Modif
88	64	M	Dysartria, ataxia, dementia, headache	Three-ventricle hydrocephalus, cisternal cysticercosis	Ventriculomegaly, cisternal cysticercosis	YES	NO
89	69	F	Headache, seizures, aphasia, weakness	Three-ventricle hydrocephalus.	Ventriculomegaly, mild arachnoiditis	NO	NO
90	32	F	RICP	Hydrocephalus	Ventriculomegaly	YES	NO
91	37	F	RICP, ataxia, vertigo	Three-ventricle hydrocephalus, cystic cerebellar tumour	Endoscopy-assisted resection of haemangioblastoma	YES	NO
92	26	M	RICP, ophtalmo-plegia, somnolence	Three-ventricle hydrocephalus, thalamic tumour.	Ventriculomegaly, 3rd ventricle compression, sponge-like tumour.	YES	NO
93	37	M	RICP	Isolated cyst from shunted ventricles.	Ventriculomegaly, intracystic cysticerci, isolated from shunt tip	NO	YES
94	42	F	RICP, seizures	Communicating hydrocephalus	Ventriculomegaly, cisternal fibrosis unable to pass the endoscope	NO	YES
95	48	M	RICP	Three-ventricle hydrocephalus	Ventriculomegaly	YES	NO
96	40	F	RICP, colloid cyst in the 3rd ventricle	Three-ventricle hydrocephalus, colloid cyst in 3rd ventricle roof	Ventriculomegally, colloid cyst. Partial resection in second endoscopy	YES/ YES	NO/ NO
97	33	M	RICP	Hydrocephalus	Ventriculomegaly	YES	NO
98	37	F	RICP	Three-ventricle hydrocephalus, colloid cyst in 3rd ventricle	Ventriculomegaly, colloid cyst. Total resection through vellum interpositum	YES	NO
99	16	F	Epilepsy	Arachnoid cyst in left sylvian fissure	Thick and stiff onion-skin cystic walls. Cystic communication to basal cisterns	YES	NO
100	53	M	RICP, dementia	Three-ventricle hydrocephalus, third ventricle tumour	Ventriculomegaly, third ventricle craniopharyngioma	YES/ YES	NO/ YES

Case	Age	Sex	Clinical Diagnosis	Image Diagnosis	Endoscopic Diagnosis	Ct/Endo Correl	Tx Modif
101	**70**	**M**	RICP, dementia	Communicating hydrocephalus	Ventriculomegaly	YES	NO
102	**82**	**M**	RICP, dementia	Three ventricle hydrocephalus	Ventriculomegally. Cysticercal resection in basal cistern. Widespread ependymitis on a second operation.	NO/ NO	YES/ NO
103	**24**	**F**	RICP	Right lateral ventricle hydrocephalus	Right lateral ventriculomegally due to Monroe foramen blocking by ependymal lining	NO	YES
104	**46**	**F**	CSF fistula	Right frontal floor defect with encephalocele	The same	YES	NO
105	**28**	**M**	RICP	Universal hydrocephalus due to intraventricular firm tumour	Soft bloody intraventricular tumour	YES	YES

*Diagnosis and findings of second endoscopy.
RICP: Raised Intracranial Pressure. **SD**: Shunt dysfunction. **CSF**: Cerebrospinal Fluid. **M**: Male. **F**: Female.

Table 1. Endoscopy Cases Characteristics.

Among our cases, 72% have been admitted with raised intracranial pressure. Most of these consisted of hypertensive hydrocephalus, although some were diagnosed as intracranial haematomas, cystic tumours with no hydrocephalus, arachnoid and cysticercal cysts, and other diagnosis. All of them but a few were resolved with endoscopic procedures, including drainage, resection and fenestration.

Focal neurological dysfunction was the second syndromic diagnosis which was associated with brain infarcts, visual or other cranial nerve impairment. Some of these cases shared other syndromes such as raised intracranial pressure, meningismus, etc., since these diagnoses were not exclusive.

Dementia was associated with 14% of the cases explored with endoscopy. Not attributed to raised intracranial pressure, necessarily, although shared by this syndrome was a constant feature. Many of these patients were diagnosed as Hakim syndromes and had some improvement of the dementia component after endoscopic exploration and subsequent shunting.

Seizures as an epileptic entity or an isolated event was present in 13% of the cases studied. In some patients epileptic fits were an integral part of the disease, especially in those which were operated on for seizure control under endoscopical supervision. Such cases have been subject to other publications (2) nevertheless it is worth stressing that endoscope-assisted procedures in open neurosurgeries for patients with pharmacological deficient control, have made substantial contributions to the success in the treatment of those patients.

Central nervous system infection (4%), cerebrospinal-fluid fistula (2%), chiasmal compression syndrome (2%), and endocrine syndrome (2%) were other pathological entities encountered in the series.

Neurocysticercosis is a parasitic disease that has been diagnosed not only in some developing countries, where it is considered endemic, but also in developed countries, where it is experiencing a continuous increase. The cause of this increase is an ever growing migrant population towards many countries of Northamerica, Europe, etc. Many series of cases of neurocysticercosis highlight the role for endoscopy in order to achieve two main purposes: to diagnose with precision in cases of intracranial and intraspinal cysts where no scolex has been observed with image studies, and to establish a treatment protocol for different pathological entities related to the parasite, such as hidrocephalus, associated with different degrees of ventricular/cisternal inflammatory lesions, as well as its appropriate timing. According to our observations, individual therapeutic measures may be indicated for different time spans in regard to cysticercal disease. The removal of the cyst may be only a limited part of the treatment when dealing with a complex case, in which other anti-cystciercal measures have failed. In such cases, different treatment modalities may be included simultaneously, given the extensive clinico-pathological polymorphism of this disease.

Cysticercosis cases have presented in our hospitals with many clinical manifestations, such as raised intracranial pressure due to mass effect and/or hypertensive hydrocephalus, meningitis, stroke, dementia, epilepsy, etc. It is not uncommon to include in the treatment protocol several drugs, such as one or more antiepileptics, analgesics, immune depressors, gastric protectors, antibiotics, anticysticercals, etc. Moreover, the treatment modalities include one or more surgical operations which may commonly include endoscopic procedures that the neurosurgeon must be ready to perform.

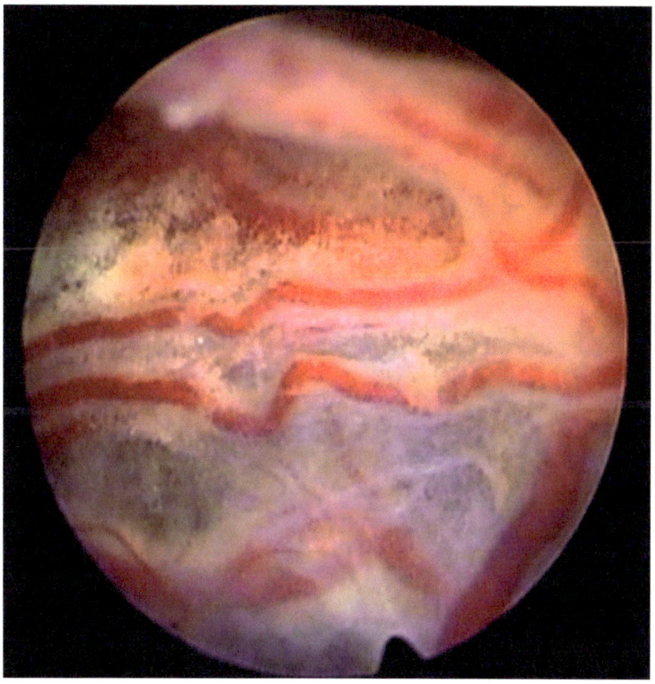

Fig. 1. Vascularised capsule from cyst containing live cysticerci.

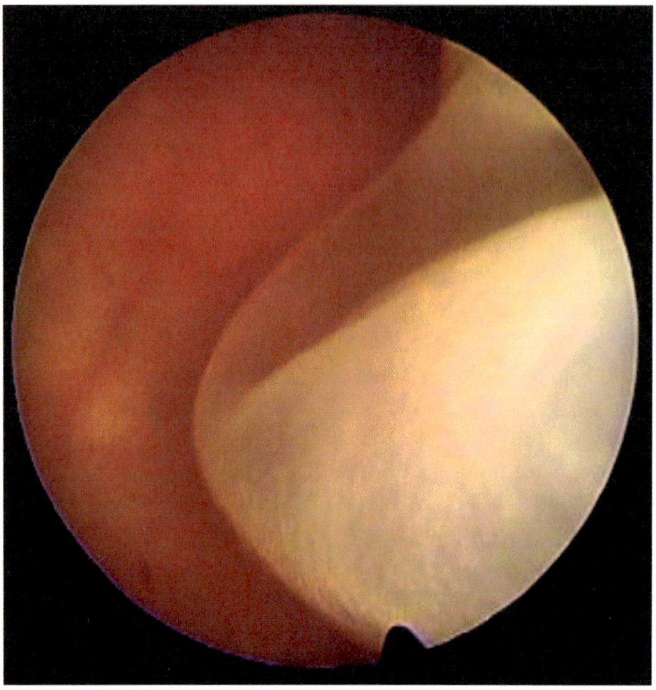

Fig. 2. Intracapsular view of the viable cysticerci and the characteristics of the highy vascularised capsule wall.

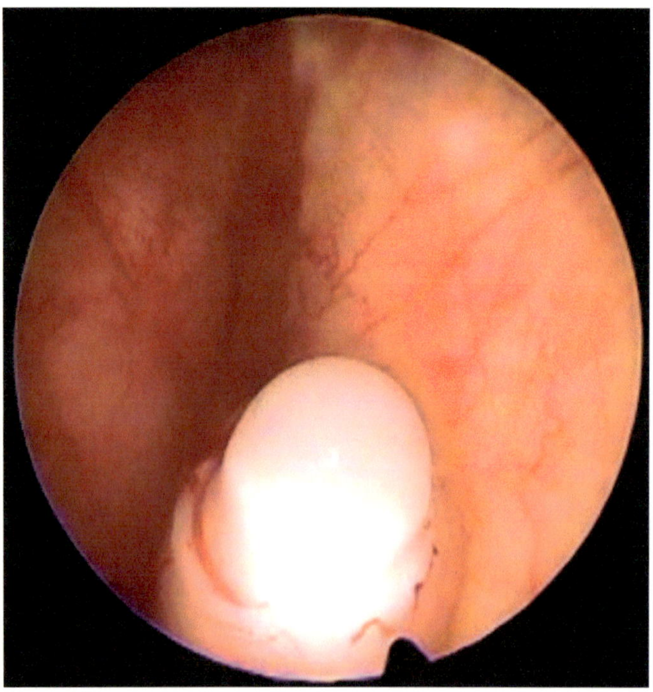

Fig. 3. Intracapsular communication with the ventricular catheter from the shunt system.

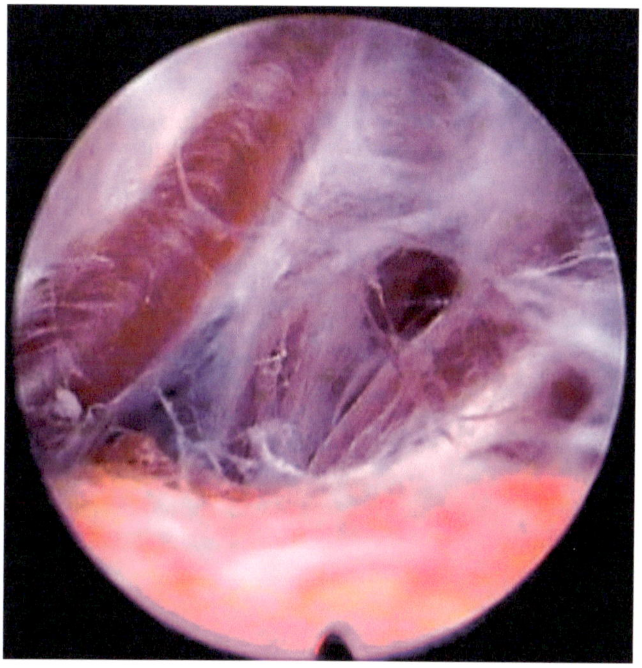

Fig. 4. Firmly adhered capsule to pericystic blood vessels in a case of an arachnoid cyst in the left Sylvian fissure.

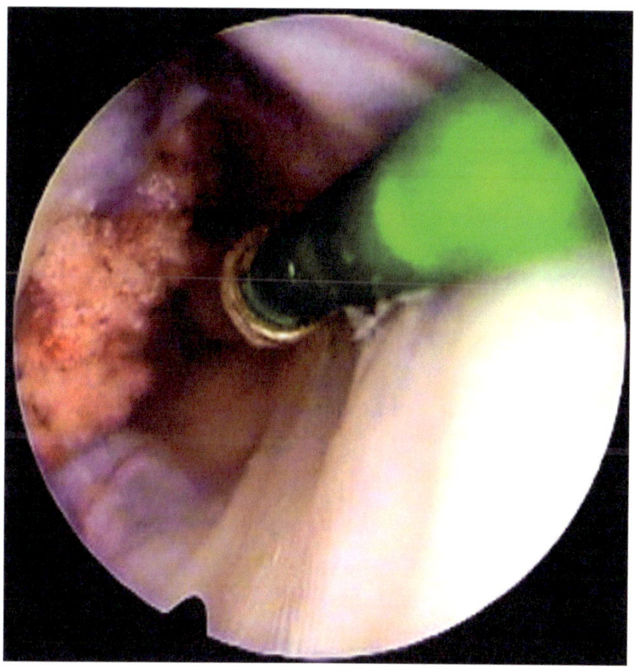

Fig. 5. Colloid cyst capsule involvement of the choroid plexus and foramen of Monroe. Wall characteristics resemble closely those of an aracnoid cyst in vascularity, firm consistency and piercing resistance.

As opposed with some centers in which complicated patients are sent home to meet their fate, all the patients in our hospitals receive some kind of treatment, regardless of their condition. Cases of so called malignant cysticercosis are treated with all the therapeutic resources at hand, with an aggressive treatment that matches the malignancy of the disease.

Some unusual cases of neurocysticercosis have been described previously (7). Although some cases may be considered as coincidences, others may be pathological enigmas. One of these latter cases is a patient who was initially diagnosed as having an interhemispheric arachnoid cyst. During endoscopic exploration, a cyst with a highly vascularised hard capsule was encountered. After several perforations were made, a transparent yellow fluid escaped from the interior of the cyst and several viable cysticerci were also found. The parasites and several blood clots adhered to de walls of the cyst were then removed and finally the cyst was communicated with the ventricluar system where a functional shunt system was previously installed (figures 1-3). After a thorough search in the literature, cyst formations in the subarachnoid space that surrounded live cysticerci have not been previously described. The capsule was similar in resistance, vascularity, and rigidity to those found in other cystic lesions, like arachnoid and colloid cysts (figures 4-5). This could mean that cystcerci may also colonize arachnoid cysts or, on the other hand, they may form a capsule quite similar to that of a congenital condition.

Although few endoscopically accessible tumours can be resected completely, biopsies of larger and more vascularised lesions can be taken with precision from selected areas, considering the amount vascular proliferation, its location and associated phenomena. Because of blurring of the entire field, which may be time-consuming to clear and sometimes difficult to achieve, a bloody fluid-filled space is a major drawback during the tumour resection. Among the tumour type that have been reported to complete or almost complete resection, colloid cysts, some astrocytomas, subependymomas, third ventricle craniopharingiomas, etc, may be mentioned. Hydrocephalus, if present, can be treated during the same exploratory procedure.

Our experience with endoscopy in tumour cases has included 19 cases. Biopsies have been performed in 11 cases while resections have been accomplished in 8. Some of the tumour types include meningiomas and craniopharingiomas within the third ventricle, exophytic gliomas, cystic astrocytomas and carcinomas. Although some intracranial lesions don't have a neoplastic nature strictly speaking, colloid, porencephalic, and arachnoid cysts may also be included in this section because of its commonly associated mass effect.

Endoscopic views from the tumour capsule and surface may have a characteristic appearance when its fluid is clear or has been washed with physiologic solution. There is usually a vascular mesh composed of layers of nets imposed one on top of the other, as onion skins. The vascular proliferation as observed with endoscopy vary according to the tumour type, and it is most abundant as more malignant the tumour is (figs 6-7).

Endoscopic assistance in open cranial neurosurgery has been described for several years, according to the articles written by Perneczky and coworkers, among others (4). Indications of endoscopy related to this modality have also increased, and ongoing publications of new indications are constantly appearing in the words neurosurgical literature. It is frequently used to reach spaces that are normally difficult to observe with the microscope, making the surgical procedure safer. Aneurysm clipping, cranial nerve dissection, are some among many the operations that may normally be assisted with endoscopes.

New indications for endoscopy imaging have been appearing continuously, not only to obtain a precise diagnosis, but also to assist in open surgical procedures. It is now possible to measure the extent of callosal section with endoscopy assistance, as well as ventricular exploration before electrode implantation during epilepsy surgery (3). Among our cases, an endoscopical exploration of the temporal horn of the lateral ventricle was explored previous to electrode placement for resective epilepsy surgery in three patients. In another 2 patients, the endoscope was used to assess the extent of the callosal section. There were no complications derived from these procedures which take only several additional minutes in the operating period. Other authors have inserted electrodes within the ventricles for the same purpose, and their conclusions are similar to ours (5).

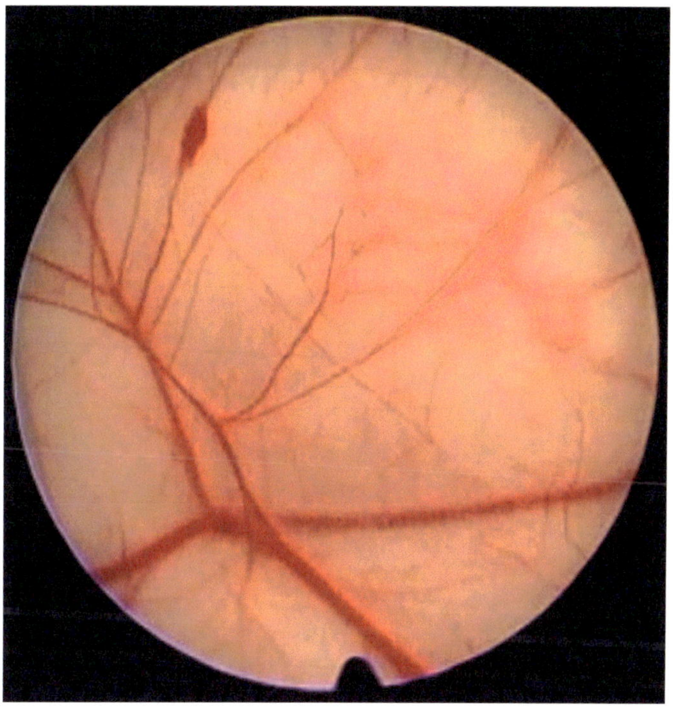

Fig. 6. Visceral cyst wall in a case of cystic astrocytoma. Large vessels organized in several leyers with different depths, occasionally with varicous formations.

HIV-associated hydrocephalus has been explored endoscopically in three patients. Clinically, they have been diagnosed following a continuously deteriorating and waisting condition that suddenly involved the central nervous system. Other common clinical data, like diarrhea, weight loss, cutaneous lesions, etc. were present at the time of hydrocephalus diagnosis. CT scans demonstrated obstructive hydrocephalus with a variable degree of inflammatory ependymal reaction which was confirmed with endoscopical observations. Grayish-white exudates in the ependymal lining, pseudo-membrane formation, inflammatory bands, etc. and other lesions that blocked the cerebro-spinal fluid drainage systems, like the foramen of Monroe and the cerebral aqueduct, were constant findings. Similar to the tuberculous leptomeningitis, the clinical course in these patients was a progressive deterioration regardless of the pharmacological and surgical treatments.

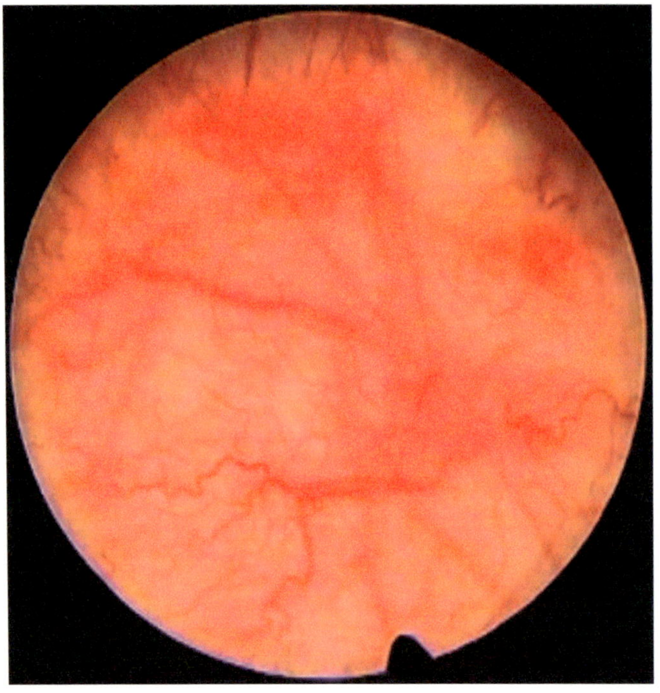

Fig. 7. Dense proliferation resembling a multi-leyer vascular mesh in a case of cystic carcinoma. Opaque yellow fluid has been removed and substituted with saline solution.

Postoperative complications after the use of endoscopical equipments are very rare, owing to the minimally-invasive nature of the procedure and the relative ease which the equipment may be handled. Some of these complications reported in the literature have been cases of infections, haemorrhages, or additional cerebral lesions caused by the surgeon; raised intracranial pressure during the procedure caused by defective fluid drainage-related at the time of endoscopy, which may account for neurological deterioration and death, has become a recent concern that was largely ignored in the past.

Among our cases, the complications that have been observed were accidental punctures to the ventricle walls and lacerations to the borders of the foramen of Monroe. These lesions have apparently been clinically silent. Unsuccessful endoscopical procedures may sometimes be considered as surgical complications, considering the cerebral laceration that is necessary to have access to the ventricles. Taking into account those cases, we would have a higher rate of complications, especially in early procedures when the endoscopic equipments were more modest.

Although not described by other authors, and even denied by some (6), the endoscopic findings encountered during a second procedure in patients with persistent hydrocephalus following cyticercal resection, have consisted of different types of inflammatory lesions. Because the release of the cyst content has been the probable cause for such inflammatory lesions, these findings that appear in the postoperative period, may be considered by some as complications. Four patients diagnosed as persistent cysticercal hydrocephalus, in which we have performed a second endoscopical observation, could then have increased our complication rate.

Technological progress has included endoscopy as well as other similar procedures that may be yield similar images, like virtual endoscopy. Until now the special lenses-based Hopkins system images may be superior compared to those obtained through a pixel-based computer reconstruction, although digital technology may be superior to optic technology at some point.

2. References

[1] Chrastina J, Novak Z, Riha I. (2080) Neuroendoscopy. Brastisl Lek Listy. 109 (5): 198-201.

[2] Jimenez-Vazquez OH, Nagore N. (2008) The impact of neuroendoscopy in the emergency setting-a retrospective study of imaging, intraoperative findings, and surgical outcome in 55 patients. Clin Neurol Neurosurg 110: 539-543.

[3] Jimenez O, Leal R, Nagore N. (2002) Minimally invasive electrodiagnostic monitoring in epilepsy surgery. Brit J Neurosurg 16 (5): 498-500.

[4] Perneczky A, Fries G. Endoscope-assited brain surgery: part 1. Evolution, basic concepts, and current technique. (1998) Neurosurg 42: 219-224.

[5] Song JK, Abou-Khalil B, Konrad PE. Intraventricular monitoring for temporal lobe epilepsy: report on technique and initial results in eight patients. (2003) J Nneurol Neurosurg Psychiatry. 74: 561-5.

[6] Cappabianca P. Application of neuroendoscopy to intraventricular lesions. (2008) Neurosurgery 62[shc suppl 2]:shc575–shc598.

[7] Jimenez O, Nagore N. (2000) Cystic lesions associated with meningiomas. Report of three cases. Br J Neurosurg 14(6): 595-596.